# Musculoskeletal Disorders

# Musculoskeletal Disorders

## Healing Methods From

## Chinese Medicine, Orthopaedic Medicine

## and Osteopathy

by

Alon Marcus, DOM, LAc, DAAPM

North Atlantic Books
Berkeley, California

Musculoskeletal Disorders

Published by
North Atlantic Books
P.O. Box 12327
Berkeley, CA 94712

Cover Art: Keri Maxfield, American Association of Oriental Medicine
Cover design: Nancy Koerner

Printed in the United States of America

*Musculoskeletal Disorders: Healing Methods from Chinese Medicine, Orthopaedic Medicine and Osteopathy* is sponsored by the Society for the Study of Native Arts and Sciences, a nonprofit educational corporation whose goals are to develop an educational and crosscultural perspective linking various scientific, social, and artistic fields; to nurture a holistic view of the arts, sciences, humanities, and healing; and to publish and distribute literature on the relationship of mind, body, and nature.

**Library of Congress Cataloging-in-Publication Data**

Marcus, Alon.
  Musculoskeletal Disorders : healing methods from Chinese Medicine,
  orthopaedic medicine, and osteopathy / Alon Marcus.
      P.   cm.
  Includes bibliographical references and index.
  ISBN 1-55643-282-8 (hardcover)
  1. Musculoskeletal system--Diseases. 2. Medicine, Chinese.
3. Orthopedics.   4. Osteopathic medicine.   I. Title.
  [DNLM: 1. Musculoskeletal Diseases--rehabilitation. 2. Medicine,
Chinese Traditional.   3. Manipulation, Orthopedic--methods.
4. Osteopathic Medicine--Methods.   WE  140  M322m  1999]
RC925.5.M36 1999
616.7--DC21
DNLM/DLC
for Library of Congress                                      98-34889
                                                                 CIP

To my patients and family, Ruti, Sivan and Noam

## Chapter 11: The Lower Extremities 547

# List of Tables

# Foreword

The healing arts professions and the public they serve are confronted by many dilemmas as we approach the next millennium. The Twentieth Century has seen the development of extraordinary advances in medical science. Surgical techniques and medical therapeutic substances have revolutionized health care. With those advances have come major concerns about health care cost and access. Most recently there has been an increasing interest by the public in alternative forms of health care and a willingness to pay for these alternatives out of pocket when not covered by health insurance. We have seen the rise of terms like "alternative," complementary," and "integrative," both in the medical community and the public, seeking to broaden options available for care. This has not been easy as much alternative health care brings with it different belief systems and paradigms than orthodox medical practice.

One of the major interests in alternative care is Oriental Medicine and the use of Acupuncture. Recently a NIH Consensus Panel found needle acupuncture to have efficacy in a number of conditions, and to be helpful as adjunctive care in many others. The panel did not review other aspects of Oriental Medicine. To date there have been few attempts by medical writers to bridge the Eastern and Western medical traditions to assist the practitioner in integrating these different approaches.

Alon Marcus has met that challenge with this work *Musculoskeletal Disorders: Healing Methods from Chinese Medicine, Orthopaedic Medicine and Osteopathy*. He has given us a concise, easily readable text dealing with musculoskeletal problems that represent a large portion of presentations to the health care system. He has blended Oriental Medicine and Traditional Medicine approaches with excellent use of the literature in both fields as background. It provides information for the practitioner that is useful both for understanding multiple approaches, and as "how to" book for performing many of the recommended procedures. It serves as a reference text as well as a user-friendly manual to guide the practitioner in assisting the patient. It is not a book that will languish on the shelf but will be well worn by continued use.

It is refreshing to see the orthodox medical community beginning to look at alternative forms of healing. The challenge to the alternative practitioner will be to demonstrate the efficacy and mechanisms of action on these approaches through the scientific method. Dr. Marcus had helped by providing one of the first road maps for integrating Oriental Medicine into traditional practice. Bring on the next millennium. We are ready for it.

Philip E. Greenman, DO, FAAO
Professor, College of Osteopathic Medicine at Michigan State University
Past President, North American Association of Musculoskeletal Medicine
President, American Back Society

# *Foreword*

I have known Alon Marcus for many years. I cannot actually remember how we met, but soon after that fateful occurrence, Alon was visiting my orthopedic medicine office at least weekly, an event that went on for months and then years. From the first, the teaching went both ways. He made a broad study of orthopedic medicine and was a regular at orthopedic medical meetings, where he was one of the very few non-Western medical physicians. It did not take long for Dr. Marcus to reach expert status in his orthopedic knowledge and practice. Alon and I have taught classes together with both Western medical and Asian physicians in attendance, attempting to merge Traditional Chinese Medicine with the logic of the thoroughly allopathic orthopedic medicine. We have had excellent success from both points of view.

From the beginning of our relationship, Alon's goal has always been to educate his Asian medicine colleagues, trying to expand their ability to accurately diagnose and treat musculoskeletal problems, while maintaining and using the strengths and methods of their Chinese medical heritage. He has published studies in both the orthopedic medical and acupuncture literature, showing that acupuncture applied at both the precise site of the lesion (diagnosed by specific orthopedic medical examination), used as a local irritant, and also applied along the meridians through its classical methods, can be used to treat various ligamentous and tendonous lesions in the spine and peripheral joints.

Over the years, we found that many of our patients needed more than just treatment of their orthopedic lesions. They had nutritional, biochemical, and spiritual problems that would not allow their bodies to heal, no matter how they were needled, injected, manipulated or medicated. We also discovered that some of what we had been taught was wrong. These revelations led to whole new realms of study that both complicated our lives and forced us to change our methods. Eventually, a new " holistic" paradigm emerged. We merged the diagnostic strength of Cyriax' Orthopaedic Medicine, the energy of Chinese Medicine, the ligament diagnostics of Hackett, Ongley and Dorman, the biochemistry of nutrition, and the spinal diagnostics and philosophy of osteopathy. Eventually, a new "holistic" paradigm emerged. Dr. Marcus has chronicled it in *Musculoskeletal Disorders: Healing Methods form Chinese Medicine, Orthopaedic Medicine and Osteopathy*.

Dr. Marcus has been working assiduously on this text for a long time. I have seen new drafts, modifications, and even completely re-written chapters necessitated by new knowledge and new theory. There are contributions by the most knowledgeable and published authors in their particular fields. What has finally emerged is a massive, work that encompasses and coalesces the many and seemingly disparate fields that any sophisticated practitioner must use to understand and treat his or her patients. I am not aware of any previous work that brings together this type of cross-disciplinary knowledge. This is a text for any practitioner who wants to learn about musculoskeletal medicine. It is useful as a text and reference for the beginner and to the expert. Bravo and well done!

Richard I. Gracer, MD, DABFP, DAAPM
Asst. Clinical Professor, UC San Francisco School of Medicine
Co-chair In-house Education, Health Medicine Forum

# Foreword

Musculoskeletal pain is an all too common and extraordinarily neglected subject in medicine. Many patients endure chronic pain unnecessarily. There is a great need for practitioners skilled in systems and modalities of treatment that until recently were considered "alternative". Scientific inquiry into the healing methods of acupuncture, manipulative therapy, and Chinese medicine has demonstrated considerable efficacy in the treatment of pain and the promotion of healing. Further evaluation will reveal greater insights yet.

*Musculoskeletal Disorders: Healing Methods from Chinese Medicine, Orthopaedic Medicine and Osteopathy* is a comprehensive book in scope and is an important contribution to practitioners interested in these areas. Dr. Marcus has been ambitious in his desire to be as inclusive as possible and should be commended for his success in bringing together a vast amount of information. This is a laudable and a difficult task considering the multiple paradigms and complexities of between near polar opposites. To this add the technical aspects of Chinese medicine, acupuncture needling techniques, advanced imaging, manipulative medicine, as well as the theoretical background of Oriental and Occidental orthopedic medicines, and you have a book whose scope is as broad as the disparate culture's approach to the treatment and evaluation of the puzzle of pain.

Even if the reader does not intend to use all the treatments described in the text, this book still serves a valuable reference and will enhance practitioners' understanding of musculoskeletal care. I predict it will facilitate a greater understanding and integration of this approach with improved outcome among those practitioners applying these insights. In short, the publication of this book will do much to "mainstream" these methods and alleviate the unnecessary suffering of many.

Rick Marinelli ND, MAAcOM, LAc, DAAPM

Past President, Naturopathic Physician's Acupuncture Academy
Clinical Professor at National College of Naturopathic Medicine

# Foreword

Thousands of people consult Oriental medicine practitioners for musculoskeletal pains every year, and they often get good clinical results. However, based on my years of teaching experience all over America, when it comes to systematically evaluating and treating musculoskeletal disorders, I must state, that many acupuncturists are still very much in the dark.

*Musculoskeletal Disorders: Healing Methods from Chinese Medicine, Orthopaedic Medicine and Osteopathy* by Alon Marcus DOM, LAc, DAAPM is a marvelous piece of work in terms of its content and timing of publication. As suggested by the title, it deals not only with traditional Oriental approaches of acupuncture, herbs and manipulative massage but also Western orthopedic and Osteopathic strategies in musculoskeletal disorders. Just when the profession of Oriental medicine needed a book like this for upgrading of our educational standards, it appears in front of our eyes. Throughout the book, the author systematically discusses, in a very practical manner, all relevant clinical aspects of orthopedic problems that acupuncturists confront in daily practice. And, in each problem, be it neck pain or lower back pain, he gives an extremely useful overview of methodologies of examination and treatment. His traditional Oriental interpretations of orthopedic problems are precious caveats of clinical knowledge that only an experienced practitioner can give through years of practice.

I met Alon years ago when he was just starting up his private practice and I always found him extremely bright and observant. It has been a great joy for me to watch him mature as a clinician and instructor. Now, after spending eight years in teaching and writing, he has done excellent work bridging the two different medical systems of orthopedic medicine from the East and the West. I must state that he has acquired an amazing degree of understanding of both systems and their integration. Without which, this book would never have been possible.

Our profession has needed this book in order to facilitate communication between Western health care providers and practitioners of traditional Oriental medicine. As a matter of fact we need a book like this for all the fields of medicine. Since I began my practice and teaching in 1979, I have been an adamant advocate for integrating traditional Oriental medicine into the main stream of medical practice in America.

Now is the time for all of us in the health care field to become "complementary" rather than "alternative" to each other. This book is a very good place to start.

Miki Shima, OMD, LAc
President Japanese-American Acupuncture Foundation
Past President The California Acupuncture Association
Past Member California Acupuncture Examining Committee

# Preface

All over the world, health professionals are discovering successful healing techniques different from the methods on which they usually rely. Some of the procedures are new; others come from healing systems many thousands of years old. Musculoskeletal complaints are very common and often are challenging to medical practitioners. Now health care practitioners can learn an integration of "alien" techniques and traditional methods that can be more effective than exclusive use of any one method.

*Musculoskeletal Disorders: Healing Methods from Oriental Medicine, Orthopaedic Medicine and Osteopathy* is a basic clinical text for medical practitioners interested in complementary approaches to medicine. The text describes an approach to musculoskeletal medicine that combines the benefits of Western science with principles and techniques developed throughout the world. It introduces integrated methods that have been of significant benefit to patients, some of whom have not responded to other traditional approaches. The text summarizes allopathic and nonallopathic approaches. It aims to open a new understanding, and to help the practitioner develop a set of integrated techniques that can be fine-tuned for each patient. It incorporates expertise from systems such as updated Cyriax's approach to Orthopaedic Medicine (specific soft tissue diagnosis and treatment); Osteopathic medicine (evaluation and treatment of tissue motion restrictions) and Oriental medicine (OM) (understanding of systemic prodromal relationships and a different approach to the classification of symptoms and signs and specific treatment methods). This text presents a practical approach to the diagnosis and treatment of musculoskeletal conditions through methods which include manual therapy, acupuncture, injection therapy, medicinal therapy and exercise therapy.

Oriental medicine, especially acupuncture, is gaining great popularity in the western world and is now entering a creative (updating) stage. The lexicon developed to describe Oriental medicine is very old and reflects the philosophy of it's time. These seemingly "primitive" descriptions do however make clinical sense and can be updated to reflect more recent scientific knowledge (and can be shown to have many similarities with modern biomedical theory). A few ideas in this text are original but the majority of them are derived from my teachers and available literature.

The reader is introduced first to basic concepts of Oriental medicine and their application in musculoskeletal medicine. OM theory is related to the modern biomedical model. Then the reader is introduced to basic biomedical concepts as applied to musculoskeletal medicine. A review of musculoskeletal disorders follows. Next basic examination and diagnostic principles are covered, followed by a review of treatment principles and methods used in this text. Further sections cover regional disorders. An appendix summarizing nutritional influences on musculoskeletal disorders follows.

I hope the reader will be stimulated to pursue additional development of such methods and find them clinically helpful.

Alon Marcus

# Acknowledgements

The preparation of a text such as this cannot be accomplished without direct and indirect input from many people. I would like first to thank Richard Gracer, M.D., for introducing me to Orthopaedic Medicine and graciously allowing me to precept in his office for several years. I would also like to extend my gratitude to the following friends: Thomas A. Dorman, M.D., for his contribution to the text, teaching and input at various stages of the manuscript; Thomas H. Ravin, M.D., provided all the materials on imaging as well as strong encouragement; Stephen M. Levin, M.D., for contributing to the text and for his greatly appreciated reviews of early stages of the manuscript; Lennord S. Horwitz, D.P.M., provided materials for the foot and ankle section as well as valuable teaching and support; Fred L. Mitchell, Jr., D.O., for helpful discussions and for generously providing figures; Bob Starr, P-AC., for his friendship, support and useful reviews; my wife, Ruth P. Goldenberg, M.D., for her support and valuable input; my father, Joseph Marcus, M.D., for his encouragement, help in creating many of the figures, and helpful input; Michael Brown, D.C., P-AC., for his suggestions, tremendous knowledge and enlightened views; David Molony, LAc., for his friendship, support and encouragement; Keri Maxfield for creating acupuncture figures and for her artistic input; and Fang Yao-hui, M.B., LAc, R.N., for his friendship and for translating Chinese texts.

Finally I would especially like to thank Judith O'Dell for the countless hours she put in preparing this text and her unremitting support and encouragement, enabling this project to go forward.

# Contributors

**Thomas Dorman MB ChB MRCP (UK) FRCP (UK).**

Dr. Dorman is an internist in private practice in Washington, USA. He had a mixed up-bringing, before turning to medicine, which included service in the Israeli paratroopers in the 1956 Sinai campaign. He graduated from Edinburgh University Scotland and then followed an eclectic career in several branches of medicine. This was followed by a residency equivalent in internal medicine and cardiology which led to the Membership in the Royal College of Physicians of the United Kingdom. During a sojourn in Canada, he was a Fellow of the Royal College of Physicians of Canada and became board certified in internal medicine in the United States. Academically, pursuing the problems of chest pain of non-cardiac origin, progressed to an interest in orthopedic medicine in which his main contributions to medicine ensued.

Dr. Dorman has practiced and studied the use of prolotherapy extensively and has contributed substantially to research in this area. Most ligament failure affects the low back and the neck. Studying this area led Dr. Dorman into developing a new understanding of the role of the human pelvis in locomotion in which ligaments play a sentinel role. Dr. Dorman is one physician who describes himself as a ligament doctor. His research and writing have led him to prominence in select national and international forms. He has also been a popular speaker in "alternative" circles. He published an important text on orthopedic medicine and numerous research papers on the subject. He has produced a newsletter monthly since April 1979 which covers a broad range of subjects in medicine, science and philosophy. The newsletter can be described as revisionist, which is reflected in its title FACT FICTION AND FRAUD in Modern Medicine. Many of his articles are available on his web site http://www.dormanpub.com

**Lennord Horwitz DPM.**

Dr. Lenny Horwitz graduated from Podiatry school in 1963. He then did a one year internship followed by a residency in foot surgery. After fifteen years of limiting his practice exclusively to foot surgery, he had an opportunity to be at a chiropractic meeting. There he discovered that joints, muscles and pain have a relationship. He gave up doing surgery and naturally progressed to proliferative therapy, acupuncture and homeopathy for the alleviation of foot pain and dysfunction. He is board certified by the American Academy of Pain Management. He lectures, writes and teaches throughout the year at different professional schools, seminars and medical conventions. He and his wife Phyllis chose to live in the heart of Appalachia. He practices his specialty in Bluefield, Virginia, USA.

**Stephen M Levin MD FACS FACOS.**

Dr. Levin is a board certified orthopedic surgeon and is the Director of the Potomac Back Center, Vienna, Virginia, USA. He began his orthopedic practice as a general orthopedic surgeon in Alexandria, VA and was Chief Orthopedic Surgeon at Alexandria Hospital. In the past 10 years, he has limited his practice to the diagnosis and treatment of back pain, initially including both surgical and nonsurgical methods; the practice is now solely nonsurgical.

Dr. Levin is Past President of the North American Academy of Musculoskeletal Medicine and a member of the North American Spine Society, The American Back Society, the American Society of Biomechanics, and several other professional and research organizations. Academic appointments include being a former Associate Clinical Professor of Orthopedic Surgery, Michigan State University; Assistant Clinical Professor of Orthopedic Surgery, Howard University; Distinguished Visiting Professor Orthopedic Surgery, Louisiana State University, USA.

## Thomas H Ravin MD.

Dr. Ravin practices full time as a musculoskeletal physician in Denver, Colorado, USA. At one time, he was a diagnostic radiologist and a nuclear medicine physician, but his interest in hands-on patient care led him into a medical practice that includes manipulation and injection therapies as well as some radiography. His background in radiology has been translated into an interest in imaging of the musculoskeletal system, particularly of the spine, ankles, and wrists.

Dr. Ravin's special interests are in teaching ligamentous injection techniques and how to use imaging to aid in diagnosis of ligamentous laxity. He has written numerous articles and taught seminars on these subjects for the American Association of Orthopaedic Medicine (AAOM) and the American Academy of Osteopathy. He is the immediate Past President of the AAOM.

# Introduction

This book's integrated (and complementary) paradigm includes three approaches; Medical; Functional; and Energetic for evaluating and treating musculoskeletal disorders (Table 1 on page xxxiv). Although the text describes these approaches as separate sections, it is the author's contention that integration (often within the same session) of these techniques is a better approach than using any one alone. The text proposes some **theoretical** parallels between the biomedical and oriental medical (OM) approaches. These theoretical analogies however must be viewed with caution, as the biomedical model and OM have completely different origins in their understanding and descriptions of health and disease. For example, a patient with joint arthrosis (a biomedical classification) most often presents with a syndrome which is classified as deficiency of Defensive and True Qi (types of bodily energies), weakness of Kidneys and accumulation of Dampness and Wind in OM. On the other hand a patient with septic arthritis (a biomedical classification) will present usually with acute (branch) symptoms that are most often classified as Damp Heat and Toxin in the OM model. Treatment can, to some extent, be designed on the basis of the biomedical classification. A fine tuning, based on OM diagnosis can then be added to the particular patient's OM diagnosis.

Different systems have advantages and weaknesses. This text for example, combines the strength of Orthopaedic Medicine diagnosis, which yields a much more lesion specific diagnosis than possible with OM methods by themselves, with the channel theory of OM. Acupuncture channels and points are then chosen based on Orthopaedic diagnosis. Herbs are also prescribed based on common presentation associated with each orthopedic disorder and their OM counterpart.

When using manual therapy emphasis is put on Orthopaedic and Western osteopathic techniques because in the opinion of the author they are more useful and usually more gentle than Tui-Na (OM) techniques.[1] It must however, be emphasized that Tui-Na and western techniques are often identical, except in theoretical description; Tui-Na "treats" "channels," "energies" as well as localized tissues, while the western models rely on orthopedic diagnosis and biomechanical models. Cross fiber massage, which is used often in the text, is a very common technique used by both Tui-Na (on local areas) and by Orthopaedic Medicine. Both, western models and Tui-Na, utilize high velocity techniques and soft tissue mobilization in their treatment armamentarium. Many of Tui-Nas' other techniques are used to treat the affected channels (the author prefers acupuncture to treat the channels).

The herbal formulas utilized in this text come from a category known as experience formulas in OM. These types of formulas have been clinically tested, and usually on biomedically defined disorders.

---

1. There are many manual therapy techniques in OM. such as; Tui-Na, Shiatsu, Amma, acupressur, Jin-shin-jutsu, Ampuku, Do-in, Te-ate and others (CAAOM Scope of Practice for Licensed Acupuncturists).

The formulas in this text originate from the Tui-Na department, and practitioners, in Guangzhou Municipal Hospital China, where the author served a clinical internship. Other formulas are taken from literature such as, Simple and proved recipe, and Chinese medicine secret recipe. This approach to herbal therapy is best suited for this text.

Next I would like to present two cases which illustrate the integrated and complementary approach used in the text.

## FIRST CASE

Lori is a 59 year old female, referred by her family practitioner, for treatment of severe neck pain. Lori is an administrator at a university and spends many hours in front of her computer. Lori stated that she had been suffering from neck stiffness, and after spending many hours in front of the computer, mild pain as well. She related that about 4 months prior she had to leave the country, rather unexpectedly, for the funeral of her brother. Following the trip she awoke one morning with severe neck pain and limited movements. She related that her family accused her of being "too American" because she did not show much emotion during the funeral and subsequent visit.

At her first office visit Lori described having severe pain, which she rated at 8-9 on the VAS scale. She stated that the pain involved her neck, head, right shoulder, arm and forearm. She also suffered from constant "pins and needles" in her right arm, which followed the distribution of C6 dermatome, or Large and Small Intestine acupuncture channels. She described moderate difficulties with lifting of even light objects, and running. She also described mild limitations in bending, standing, walking, sitting, climbing stairs and resting in bed.

Her systems review enumerated aversion to cold and damp weather (although she "cannot stand" hot and muggy weather as well). She fatigues easily and feels weakness in her legs and knees. She has difficulty sleeping due to pain, mostly between 12-3am. Lori lost her olfactory sense following a respiratory infection several years ago. No other pertinent information was revealed.

Lori's past treatments included 25 visits with a physical therapist and one "cortisone" injection neither of which gave her any relief at all.

Her sensory and motor examination were within normal limits. Her neck movements were quite limited with extension, right sidebending and rotation being the most limited and difficult. When attempting to look forward Lori has to hyperextend her lumbar and thoracic spine. When asked to rotate her neck she compensates by rotating her trunk instead. Palpation revealed extreme muscle tightness in her scalenes, SCM, trapezius, and levator scapula. I, and apparently her medical doctor, have never seen a patient with such tight musculature. An attempt to assess cervical joint play and function was impossible, both in the supine and seated positions. She had palpatory tenderness which followed much of the Small Intestines channel. Her tongue was slightly pale and otherwise unremarkable. Lori's pulses were thready with a slight slippery quality in her right deep bar position. Lu-1 and right subcostal area were tender to palpation. Her lower abdomen lacked resiliency and light pressure resulted in deep penetration of the pressing hand. The rectus abdominus muscles were tight bilaterally.

Her X-ray report stated that Lori's cervical spine is degenerated globally, with somewhat more degeneration at her C-4-C5 joint and disc space.

An OM analysis of Lori's symptoms suggests weakness of the Lung system, weakness in the Kidney system, Emptiness of Liver Blood, contraction of the Lung and Stomach Sinews channels, and retention of pathogenic factors. Her Lung and Defensive Qi weakness both contributed to her severe respiratory infection and loss of olfactory sense, and allowed for external pathogenic factors to penetrate. Her lower abdomen, weakness of legs and knees suggests deficiency in the Kidney system. Her severely tight muscles, pale tongue and subcostal sensitivity suggest weakness in Liver Blood. Inability to extend the spine with bilaterally tight rectus muscles suggested that the Stomach Sinews channel is affected (probably a result of chronic Liver dysfunction). No clear orthopedic diagnosis was possible because of the inability to perform many of the necessary evaluations. However, due to the severity of her symptoms, and to limited extension, an internal disc derangement or spinal stenosis were most probable.

I decided to address Lori's Kidney weakness and Liver Blood emptiness first. Stimulation of K-3 followed by GB-25 (Kidney Alarm point) and UB-23 (Kidney back Shu point) was used to strengthen her Kidneys. Moxa was added to UB-23 point to warm her energy. The needles were removed after 10 minutes and Sp-4 and P-6 were added to activate the Penetrating (Chong) and Yin Linking (Wei) channels. K-9 was used to further activate the Yin Linking (Wei) channel. These two channels activate the Blood system and address Lori's abdominal presentations. Hot cervical ear points (by impedance measurement) were needled at the same time. Shen Men/Spirit Gate, Sympathetic, Thalamus/ Pain Control and Stress Control/Adrenal were added to reinforce the relaxing effects of the treatment. After 20 minuets these needles were removed and reevaluation of Lori's ROM showed no change. However, it was now possible to perform mechanical evaluations of the cervical joints, with Lori in the supine position. Her cervical joints revealed restrictions in extension and right sidebending and rotation, FRS (lt) from C-3 to C-6. Muscle energy technique was used to address the joint dysfunction and this resulted in some improvement in joint play.

I then asked Lori to sit up and evaluate the treatment by rotating her head from side to side (which showed about 10% improvement) for about five minutes. When I returned, Lori was in tears, stating that this was the first time in months that she had any relief from her pain. The "pins and needles" in her arm dissipated. Although rotation movements improved, no change was noted in her ability to extend the neck. A biweekly treatment plan was initiated.

Lori was seen again in two days and stated that she was "much better" and was no longer suffering from "pins and needles" down her arm. Examination however, revealed no improvement in extension. Rotations were increased by about 10-15%. Mechanical examination was possible and revealed some increased joint play, reduced guarding, and joint restrictions similar to those found in her first visit. Lori's treatment was repeated and herbal medication (formula for cervical spondylopathy, see neck section) was added to her treatment program.

This treatment protocol was continued for three weeks, with some additions to address her Lung system which was further damaged by her unexpressed grief (the emotion of the Lung system). On every other treatment session local myofascial needling techniques were used (see treating myofascial tissues). And the Stomach and Lung Sinews channels were activated. Deep needling was extremely difficult as her cervical intrinsic muscles were extremely tight and this often resulted in bent needles. At the end of the three weeks Lori's attitude was much improved, and she felt more hopeful that her condition can improve. Her pain was reduced to around 5 on the VAS scale (still a fairly severe rating). Extension was still limited.

Because no significant change was gained in extension flexibility and her pain only improving about 40%, it was decided that an MRI evaluation was needed. The MRI showed spondylytic changes with disc, or osteophyte, seen at C3-4, C4-5, and C6-7. These changes resulted in mild cord compression at C3-4 on the right, and at C4-5 on the left. At C5-6 stenosis was present, without cord compression. In addition, neural foraminal narrowing was present at multiple levels.

Lori's case illustrates the advantage of combining several treatment approaches which allowed for better utilization of manual therapy techniques and improved clinical outcome, despite her severely pathologic cervical spine. Acupuncture alone did not improve her ROM and only resulted in less guarding when Lori was in a supine position.

Also "her pins and needles" disappeared following manual therapy but did not respond to acupuncture. On the other hand, it was the acupuncture treatment which allowed for treatment with manual therapy. Some relief was obtained even though injection and physical therapy were unsuccessful in giving any relief at all.

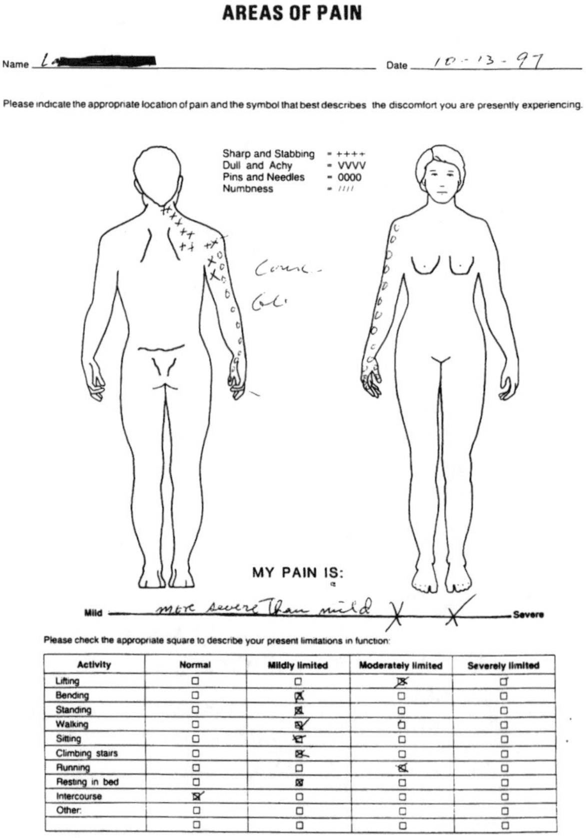

**AREAS OF PAIN**

Name _____ Date _10-13-97_

Please indicate the appropriate location of pain and the symbol that best describes the discomfort you are presently experiencing.

| | |
|---|---|
| Sharp and Stabbing | = ++++ |
| Dull and Achy | = VVVV |
| Pins and Needles | = 0000 |
| Numbness | = //// |

**MY PAIN IS:**

Mild ——— more severe than mild X ——— X ——— Severe

Please check the appropriate square to describe your present limitations in function:

| Activity | Normal | Mildly limited | Moderately limited | Severely limited |
|---|---|---|---|---|
| Lifting | □ | □ | ☒ | □ |
| Bending | □ | ☒ | □ | □ |
| Standing | □ | ☒ | □ | □ |
| Walking | □ | ☒ | □ | □ |
| Sitting | □ | ☒ | □ | □ |
| Climbing stairs | □ | ☒ | □ | □ |
| Running | □ | □ | ☒ | □ |
| Resting in bed | □ | ☒ | □ | □ |
| Intercourse | ☒ | □ | □ | □ |
| Other: | □ | □ | □ | □ |
| | □ | □ | □ | □ |

*Figure1- 1:*Lori's intake drawing and VAS scale.

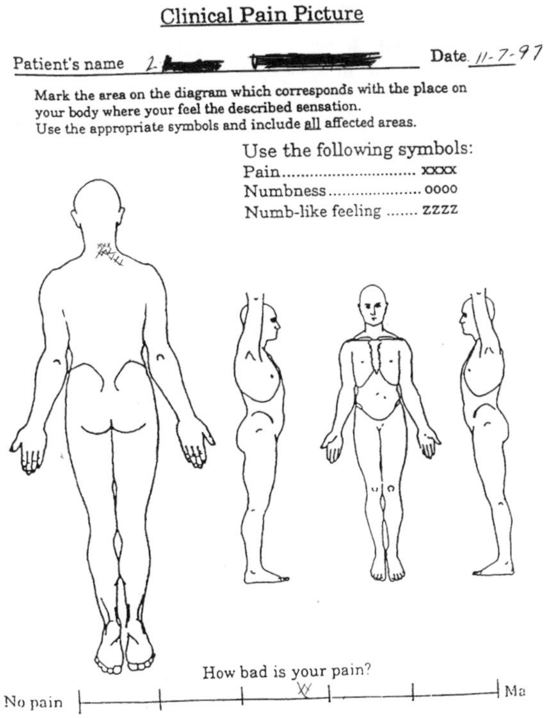

## Clinical Pain Picture

Patient's name  2.~~[redacted]~~   Date _11-7-97_

Mark the area on the diagram which corresponds with the place on
your body where your feel the described sensation.
Use the appropriate symbols and include **all** affected areas.

Use the following symbols:
Pain............................ xxxx
Numbness..................... oooo
Numb-like feeling ....... zzzz

How bad is your pain?

No pain |——————|——————|——————X——————|——————| Ma

*Figure1- 2:*Lori's drawing and VAS scale at discharge.

The second case, that of Moris, is presented to illustrate an approach which actually integrates information and utilizes it in the management of shoulder pain.

## SECOND CASE

Moris is a 59 year old university professor. He has an extremely intellectual personality and spends little time on other activities, including exercise. Moris is a regular patient and receives general health supporting treatments. On one of his visits he complained of increasingly worsening shoulder pain of four week duration, pointing at his deltoid muscle. He could not identify any injury; however, on questioning he realized that he had been working on an article and was reaching up to pull books quite frequently. As Moris is 59

years old I suspected that he suffered from Cyriax's traumatic capsulitis. Examination however, showed full external rotation and glenohumeral abduction. Resisted muscle testing was painful on external rotation only. No painful arc was noted, and the distal end of the infraspinatus tendon insertion was quite sensitive to pressure. Cervical examination revealed no significant medical involvement. Joint dysfunction, FRS (rt) was found at the C4-C5 joint. On palpation many tender points were found which would have not illuminated the source of his symptoms.

As Mori's general health was addressed at regular intervals, treatment focused on his shoulder pain alone. The Sinews channel most similar to the infraspinatus muscle, in location and function, is the Small Intestine. I began the treatment with 5 minutes of cross fiber massage at the inferior aspect of the tendon insertion. Then the Small Intestine Sinews channel was activated by needling SI-1 and GB-13. Triggers at the muscle belly as well as SI-11, 10, and TW-14 were then added. An electrical stimulator was connected with the (-) pole at SI-11 and (+) electrode at TW-14. At the end of the session the cervical dysfunctions were addressed with muscle energy techniques.

Moris was told to avoid lifting objects above shoulder level. He was also educated on how to minimize usage of the infraspinatus muscle. The exact treatment protocol was repeated 2 more times, within the same week, at which point his symptoms disappeared and resisted external rotation was non-symptomatic. Moris remained symptom free for two years when the same symptoms and history reoccurred. This time it was a little more difficult to treat and Moris received eight treatments to his shoulder before he was symptom free.

All of Moris's treatment decisions were made based on Orthopaedic Medicine diagnosis. The information was then used to design a treatment plan that mainly utilized acupuncture with the addition of some manual therapy. The channels, points, and use of electrical stimulation were based on clinical findings that pointed to the infraspinatus muscle (a biomedical orthopedic diagnosis).

*Table 1.* **APPROACHES TO MUSCULOSKELETAL DISORDERS**

| **MEDICAL** | Description | Used to understand the reductionist effect of a "lesion." Attempts to isolate a particular site and prescribe specific, appropriate treatments |
| | Strength | Often the most effective method of providing quick relief from symptoms |
| | Weakness | Treatments often result in side effects<br>Rarely considers underlying factors and recurrence of symptoms are frequent<br>If clinical presentation not within current pathological models (or if "objective data" is difficult to obtain by acceptable methods), "blame" often shifted to patient; genuine complaints often ignored |
| **FUNCTIONAL** | Description | Used to evaluate, in a somatic system, clinically-observable dysfunctions that may be more difficult to quantify by reductionist methods<br>Several biomechanical standards and approaches |
| | Strengths | Often allows for identification of underlying mechanical perpetuating factors or underlying pain generators |
| | Weaknesses | Some studies show poor inter-rater reliability of physical signs |
| **ENERGETIC** | Description | Used to identify symptoms and signs complexes that are very different from the "scientific paradigm" (such as the influence emotional states have on particular systems and tissues)<br>These may often present in a prodromal stage of dysfunction and/or pathology<br>These complexes may be at the root of patients' constitution and symptoms |
| | Strength | Can be helpful for addressing weak and sensitive patients, who otherwise do not respond to more direct treatment methods |
| | Weakness | Subjectivity of symptoms and signs used in assessment<br>Treatment less regimented |

# Chapter 1: *Oriental Medicine*

This chapter covers essential principles of Oriental Medicine (OM) and is not intended to replace a basic text on the subject. OM principals are related to musculoskeletal disorders and to biomedical orthopedics.

Among OM methods, Traditional Chinese Medicine (TCM) may be the best-documented. Created following China's Communist Revolution to unify segments of existing methods, TCM is derived from the entire history of Chinese Medicine.[1] TCM attempts to unify these segments by creating a common theoretical framework

that can be used to categorize medical conditions in organized *patterns*. Table 1-1 lists some of the most important OM literature.

The TCM approach has both strengths and weaknesses, among them. Diagnosis and treatment are relatively simple; however, the clinical relevance for many conditions has not been proven. Many TCM *pattern discriminations* (syndromes, zheng) are theoretical and probably oversimplified. Nevertheless, TCM methodologies have been established as useful for many maladies and disorders, including musculoskeletal conditions, that affect humans and other animals, as well.

1. For an OM reading list, see "Works Consulted" in references.

*Table 1-1.* CHINESE MEDICINE: TREATISES AND MEDICAL THEORIES

| TREATISE/MEDICAL BOOK | DATE | | |
|---|---|---|---|
| Book of Changes | About | 7th | Century B.C. |
| Yellow Emperor | About | 3rd | Century B.C. |
| Pulse Classic | About | 3rd | Century B.C. |
| Book of Difficulties | About | 1st | Century B.C. |
| Herbal Classic of Shen Nong (Divine Plowman) | About | 1st | Century B.C. |
| Theses on Exogenous Febrile Diseases | About | A.D. | 220 |
| Nong's Newly Revised Materia Medica | About | A.D. | 659 |
| Cooling School | | A.D. | 1120-1200 |
| Purgative School | | A.D. | 1156-1228 |
| Gastrosplenic Supplementation School | | A.D. | 1180-1251 |
| Great Compendium of Acupuncture | | A.D. | 1368-1644 |
| Compendium of Materia Medica | | A.D. | 1518-1593 |
| Yang Supplementation School | | A.D. | 1522-1640 |
| Pestilence School | | A.D. | 1582-1652 |
| Thermic Heat Disease School | | A.D. | 1667-1746 |
| Traditional Chinese Medicine (TCM) (Post-Communist Revolution) | Modern China | | |

In this text the term TCM is used to refer to modern mainland Chinese style medicine and OM to the diverse systems of medicine in the orient.

# Basic Oriental Medicine Concepts

Western medicine and OM differ greatly in their approaches to, and understanding of, the human body. Western medicine is a reductionist, causal-analytic system that looks for the microscopic etiology of disease. Health is defined on a "statistical norm" scale. Oriental medicine takes a qualitative approach, giving more credence to empirical experience and subjective complaints than to quantitative objective data. In OM, emphasis is on the host's reaction to the disease rather than on the disease state; on human potential rather than the "norm." This method allows for greater individual variation.

Oriental medical science views all life forms as being similar in energetic essence, as sharing the vital forces of the universe.[1] Accordingly, all matter is affected similarly by natural forces such as wind, cold and damp. Oriental science uses this type of relationship to explain everything in the universe, including human physiology and pathology.

OM is a holistic method that evolved from the way body systems affect one another. As in Western medicine, OM recognizes that some bodily functions have both local and general/systemic effects.

Many similarities can be demonstrated between western medicine and OM, even though each is constructed from a distinct perspective and uses an altogether different language. Many of the systems that OM describes are surprisingly similar to the current biomedical model.

---

1. A view which is certainly supported to some extent by DNA research.

**NOTE:** Clinical parallels must be viewed with caution.

## Principles of OM

Within its own parameters, OM is comprehensive, logical and consistent.

OM sees the human body as a combination of vital *energies* and material substances that must stay in balance for health to be preserved. The bulk of OM theory and practice is the description and manipulation of the functional relationships, *patterns of correspondences*, and quality of the body network of *channels*, *Organs*, fluids and *energies*. This approach allows for a great amount of flexibility.[2]

## OM Terminology

Through the ages, the oriental sciences have developed many theories to describe and treat the human body. Some of the language used to describe these theories might seem to belong to poetry rather than to medical science; however, terms such as Five Elements, Yin-Yang and Eight Principles (Parameters/Entities) denote specific, identifiable, ordered and classified hypotheses. In *modern* times (post-Communist Revolution) these theories have been integrated into TCM.

### OM & Anatomical Terminology

The OM anatomical model, which has been explained by observable phenomena (including some dissection),[3] describes:

---

2. It can also result in intertherapist disagreements and inconsistencies.

3. In the past Chinese physicians rarely used dissection to study human anatomy and physiology. A dead body, which lacks Qi energy, was considered of limited value for studying health. Instead, physicians explored the human body using self-awareness, meditation and trial and error. The resulting model had little relationship to biomedical anatomy.

- A system of channels responsible for circulation.
- Organs that, when compared to the biomedical model, are somewhat different in shape, location and number.

To comprehend OM, the western trained practitioner must first let go of the western understanding of human organs. For example, the Liver:

- Houses the Blood.
- Controls smooth flow of Qi (vital energy).
- Controls smoothness of the flow of substances in the body.
- The state of the Liver is reflected by the health of the sinews.

*OM & Physiological Terminology*

Chinese sciences use language from the observable environment to explain human physiology and pathology. A study of oriental medical vocabulary reveals an ordered system that describes complexes of symptoms and signs (syndromes) through terminology such as Generating, Controlling, Excess/Fullness, Deficiency/Emptiness, Wind, Wet, Heat, Qi, Blood, Phlegm, and Stagnation.

## Diagnosis

OM uses a differential diagnosis method that involves groups of symptoms and signs called pattern discriminations. This text covers the orthopedic aspect of the pattern discriminations known as:

- Eight Principles.
- Five Phases.
- Organ/Bowel.
- Channel and Connecting Channel.
- Qi and Blood.
- Disease Cause.
- Body Fluids.
- Six Stages.

The other principal pattern discriminations, Four Stages and Triple Warmer, are not within the scope of this text.

Once a practitioner has come to an understanding of the OM view of human organs, a closer look reveals many similarities between the OM and western systems. This section introduces the relationship among OM principals, orthopedics and modern biomedicine.

## Qi

Qi (pronounced "chee") is the life force within all living matter. The concept of a "universal energy" is central to OM and is used to describe both function and dysfunction. The Chinese character that makes up the word Qi is composed of two characters that represent steam/gas and rice. When combined, the two characters signify the dynamic fluid quality of Qi: Qi can manifest differently and transform, performing different functions in different situations, and even manifesting as either form or energy.

The movement of steam (and Qi), which has a spiraling quality, has been compared to the double helix of DNA, and is thought to be the shape of the energy that binds the universe, living and non-living things.[4]

In medicine the term Qi usually refers to the dynamic movement and functional aspects of physiology. Table 1-1 on page 6 describes several types of Qi that exist in the body. The Qi disorders are deficiency (emptiness, vacuity) and stagnation (fullness, repletion). Each of these disorders consists of a group of conditions that can occur due to:

---

4. The shape of hexagrams, from the *Book of Changes,* that are composed of various combinations of broken and unbroken lines and are supposed to symbolize all phenomena, together with the spiraling movement of Qi, have provocative similarities to DNA.

**1.** Qi deficiency, characterized by general physical weakness.

   If severe, this can lead to sinking of Qi causing prolapse of Organs.

**2.** Qi stagnation, loss of the dynamic character of Qi, with pain described as a feeling of distention or throbbing.

   If severe, this can lead to rebellious Qi (reverse flow of Qi), with symptoms such as nausea, vomiting or cough.

## Pain & Qi

Pain can result from deficiency of Qi and stagnation of Qi.

### Qi Deficiency

Pain due to Qi deficiency is intermittent, chronic, dull, deep and achy. Associated with weakness, it becomes worse in the afternoon or, at times, at night.[5] This type of pain responds to palpation and massage. If associated with excess Cold (Yin), the pain is aggravated by cold or wet weather and can respond poorly to deep palpation and massage. Qi deficiency pain is commonly seen in patients who have chronic myofascial pain and fibromyalgia.

### Qi Stagnation

Pain due to Qi stagnation usually is felt as distending, throbbing or pulsating (especially if associated with Heat) and is poorly localized. This type of pain can change in location and character. It can become aggravated by lack of movement and can be alleviated with subsequent movement (this is typical of ligamentous pain).[6]

Qi stagnation pain can be susceptible to emotional aggravation. Often it is associ-

ated with numb-like sensation (usually from associated Wind and/or Blood deficiency).

Qi stagnation pain is commonly a component of sclerotomal pain of ligamentous origin (see chapter 3). Although Qi stagnation usually is classified as an *excessive* condition, pain that is caused by Qi stagnation often responds, at least initially, to heat and deep, invigorating massage.

**NOTE:** This type of treatment may result in increased pain one or two days later.

## Defensive Qi

Defensive Qi plays a particularly important role in musculoskeletal medicine. The classic *Simple Questions* states that Defensive Qi is slippery and rough in nature and cannot enter the channels. It circulates under the skin and between the muscles, vaporizes (giving it a material aspect) between membranes, and disseminates over the chest and abdomen. *Spiritual Axis* says that Defensive Qi warms the muscles. The least refined of the Qi's, Defensive Qi, is rooted in Ming-Man (Kidney Yang). The production of Defensive Qi depends greatly on Kidney and Ming-Man function, (and True Qi) assisted by the Lung, Liver, Spleen, Large and Small Intestine.[7]

### Defensive Qi & Biomedical Analogies

Defensive Qi is responsible for elimination of Exogenous factors and for reaction to the environment. Reflexive, inherent and instinctual (automatic), it performs these functions automatically. Defensive Qi is similar in many ways to the autonomic and immune system in biomedicine.

**TEMPERATURE REGULATION.** Among the areas

---

5.  Night pain is more often due to Blood stagnation.

6.  The hallmark of ligamentous pain in Orthopaedic Medicine is posain, pain aggravated by lack of movement. Ligaments are also a common source of a numb-like sensation called nulliness.

7.  The Transporting/Shu points for these organs can be used to treat weakness of Defensive Qi manifesting as susceptibility to external influences and in patients that are weak and fatigued.

of influence of Defensive Qi is temperature regulation—opening the skin pores to release heat or closing the pores in reaction to cold *(biomedicine: an autonomic nervous system function)*. The "battle" between Defensive Qi and pathological influences is responsible for the development of fever and inflammation *(biomedicine: immune system, which is closely related to autonomic system reaction)*. The Defensive Qi function of warming the muscles is also related closely to the biomedical autonomic nervous system function that regulates circulation of blood to the muscles and skin.

**DEFENSIVE QI: SKIN & FASCIA.** Defensive Qi protects the Organs and appears to have some functions relating to skin and fascia that are similar to functions in the biomedical model.

Skin and fascia are made of collagen and elastic fibers, ground substance and cellular elements that protect muscles and organs and provide storage of elastic energy. Defensive Qi supplies energy to the Sinews *(tendinomuscular)* channels and therefore provides potential energy, as well.

Skin and fascia also are continuous throughout the body. Fascia sometimes is described as uniting in the abdomen (as is Defensive Qi) and can provide support and warmth to muscles, joints, vessels, nerves and organs.

Fascia is covered by slippery fluid, allowing movements between tissues. Defensive Qi moves through the Cou Li *(the space between the skin and muscles)*, where fluids also circulate.

Skin and fascia contain small-caliber nerve fibers that play a role in the immune system (Ochoa and Mair 1969). In OM, Defensive Qi is the main immune energy that circulates in skin and fascia.

Patients suffering from fibromyalgia (chronic generalized muscular aches) often suffer from disturbed sleep. Defensive Qi circulates at the Exterior (muscles and skin) during the day and in the Interior (Organs) during the night. When sleep is disturbed, the formation/supplementation of Defensive Qi from True Qi is disturbed, and the moistening and warming of muscles are affected. Treatment directed at defensive Qi is used often for fibromyalgia patients.

Defensive Qi can become disharmonious with Nourishing Qi, resulting in excessive sweating and heat *(biomedicine: activation of the sympathetic nervous system)*. When this kind of disharmony affects the joints, they can become inflamed and swollen as seen in Heat Bi *(biomedicine: inflammatory arthritis)*. Disharmonious Defensive and Nutritive Qi is a common finding in patients who have chronic fatigue syndrome, myofascial pain syndromes and fibromyalgia.[8]

## Ancestral (Chest) Qi

Ancestral (Chest) Qi provides another example of similarities between OM theory and biomedicine. Centered at the chest region, this Qi is derived from the interaction of Food-Qi and air: Food-Qi is transported to the Lungs, where it combines with air and becomes Ancestral (Chest) Qi.

Blood is closely related to Ancestral (Chest) Qi, postnatal Qi and prenatal Qi. The functions of Ancestral (Chest) Qi are to control respiration, generation and nourishment of Blood *(biomedicine: oxygenation of blood)*; and to circulate Qi and Blood throughout the body. The condition of Ancestral (Chest Qi) can be assessed by looking at the respiratory and circulatory systems. Ancestral (Chest) Qi clearly represents many of the biomedical functions of the respiration, blood formation, oxygenation, and cardiovascular systems in general.

---

8. These conditions are commonly treated by harmonizing the Nourishing and Defensive Qi, using variations of Cinnamon Twig Decoction (Gui Zhi Tang +/-).

*Table 1-1.* **TYPES OF QI**

| | |
|---|---|
| **TRUE** | • Formed by Ancestral and Original Qi<br>• Assumes two forms; Defensive Qi and Nourishing Qi |
| **ORGAN** | • The physiological activity of the organ |
| **CHANNEL** | • Transmitted and conveyed through a conduit system that is part of the body |
| **DEFENSE** | • Flows outside of vessels<br>• Coarse and slippery in nature<br>• Cannot enter the channels; however, enters the organs at night<br>• Warms and moistens the muscles and skin<br>• Controls the skin pores, regulating sweat<br>• Main function: defense against exogenous, pathological Qi |
| **NOURISHING** | • Moves with the Blood<br>• Helps the Blood in nourishing functions |
| **ORIGINAL** | • Inherited vitality and constitution; closely related to Essence<br>• Precursor to all other Qi<br>• Not renewable[a]<br>• Resides in the Kidney and nourishes Kidneys<br>• Has a historical aspect<br>(memory of old trauma can be stored in Original Qi) |
| **ANCESTRAL/ CHEST** | • Formulated from the interaction of Food Qi and air<br>• The force and strength of respiration that circulates Qi and Blood by regulating the heart function<br>• The force that nourishes the Heart and Lungs<br>• Limb circulation and movement depends largely on Ancestral Qi |

a. Treating source points CV-4 through 7 and GV-4 and the use of many herbs can support Original Qi.

# 陰陽 Yin & Yang

Yin and Yang is one of the earliest concepts described in Chinese sciences. First described around 700 B.C., Yin and Yang are relative, interdependent forces that both oppose and complement each other.[9]

The Chinese character for Yin describes the shady side of a mountain while the character for Yang the sunny side. One cannot exist without the other, and each transforms into the other. This concept is exemplified by the effects of morning and evening sun that result in opposite sides of the same mountain being more Yin or Yang at different times. A basic tenet of Yin Yang principles is that all subsystems (including the musculoskeletal system) are united, are part of a metasystem that are independent and interdependent at the same time. Although there may be local and specific variations the underlying principles cannot be violated—disease begins when harmony is disturbed.

According to Yin-Yang theory, the seasonal cycle is the outcome of the mutually regulating, mutually generating and mutually consuming activities of Yin and Yang. Either side of the two opposites always regulates and acts on the other. This process of mutual regulation and interaction is at the heart of Yin and Yang theory, without which change would not occur. Therefore, the two opposites of Yin and Yang do not exist as an entity in a still or inactive state. They constantly interact with each other and allow for alteration and development of objects and phenomenon.

The most basic tenets of the Yin-Yang concept are:

- Everything in the universe contains both Yin and Yang.

*Spiritual Axis* states, Yin and Yang could amount to ten in number, be extended to one hundred, to one thousand, to ten

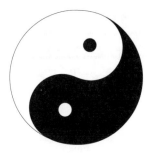

*Figure 1-1:* Yin and Yang Symbol.

thousand and even to the infinite....Man has physical shape which is inseparable from Yin and Yang.

- The entire universe consists of dynamic interdependent interactions between pairs of opposites (Yin and Yang).

*Spiritual Axis* states, Yin is installed in the interior as the material foundation for Yang, while Yang remains on the exterior as the manifestation of the Yin function.

- Yin and Yang can transform into each other.

*Spiritual Axis* states, Extreme Cold will bring about Heat, and extreme Heat will induce Cold... [furthermore], Excessive Yin may cause Yang syndromes or tend to transform into Yang and vice versa.

- Disease begins when balance is disturbed.

*Spiritual Axis* states, When Yin keeps balance with Yang and both maintain a normal condition of Qi, then health will be high-spirited. A separation of Yin and Yang will lead to the exhaustion of essential Qi.

Compared to Yin, Yang is more active, warmer, faster and lighter (less dense). Yin pertains to dense material substances. Yang pertains to function. Entities such as the *Exterior* (skin, skeletal muscles, head, limbs and trunk), upper, outer or dorsal aspects of the body are considered Yang, as compared to the *Interior* (the viscera and the deep channels), lower and anterior aspects of the body (Table 1-2).

9. Although the emperor Sheng Nung, about 2800 B.C., is believed to be the source of the duality principles of the Yin Yang.

*Table 1-2.* **BASIC YIN AND YANG ASPECTS**

| YIN ASPECTS | YANG ASPECTS |
|---|---|
| Interior | Exterior |
| Lower | Upper |
| Anterior | Outer or Dorsal |
| Less active | More active |
| Cooler | Warmer |
| Slower | Faster |
| Substance | Function |

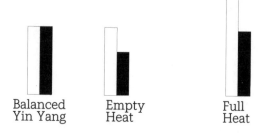

*Figure 1-2:* Yin Yang balance.

Interior, deficiency, and Cold syndromes are considered Yin, while Exterior, excess, and Heat syndromes are considered Yang. A boisterous voice indicates Yang, a low voice is Yin. Bright color is Yang, dim color is Yin. Feeble and weak respiration is Yin, coarse breathing is Yang. Superficial, rapid, and forceful pulses are Yang, slow, deep feeble, and weak pulses are Yin.

A few examples of Yin-Yang pairs are Qi and Blood, Exterior and Interior, Cold and Hot, Emptiness and Fullness.

**QI - BLOOD.** Qi, the vital force responsible for all life and all physiological activity, is more Yang than Blood.

Blood, which is denser, is more Yin. Blood is similar to biomedical blood but has different origins (to some extent) and additional physiological and pathological attributes.

**EXTERIOR - INTERIOR.** Exterior (Yang, functional, muscular, hollow organ) conditions are considered to be less serious than interior (Yin, substance, bone, solid organ) conditions.

**COLD - HOT.** Cold can be caused either by exogenous pathogens or by insufficiency of the body's Yang. When compared to Heat, it is considered to be Yin.

Heat is considered Yang in function or pathology. It can be caused by exuberant Yang energy (full Heat) or by relative weakness of Yin (empty Heat). Heat also can be caused by exogenous influences (Figure 1-2).

**EMPTINESS - FULLNESS.** Emptiness, which is also called deficiency or vacuity, refers to a condition of insufficiency of any body substance or energy (Yin, Yang, Qi, Blood, Essence, Fluids). It is Yin in nature.

Fullness (also called repletion or excess), which refers to any condition associated with exuberant pathogenic Qi or overaccumulation/stagnation, is Yang in nature.

## Biomedicine & Yin-Yang

Biomedical physiology describes balanced, interrelated and interdependent systems, as well. Many neural and endocrine functions are interdependent and interrelated, are opposing in some situations and cumulative in others. Some are inhibitory; some are complementary. Goldenberg N. (1973) for example, compared the functions and relationships of cyclic adenosine monophosphate (cAMP) and cyclic guanosine monophosphate (cGMP) to Yin and Yang OM principals.[10] The density of cAMP and cGMP in cells are interrelated, at times oppose each other, and perform different functions in different cells.

---

10. cAMP and cGMP mediate (second messenger) action of catecholamines, cholinergic receptors in parasympathetic nerve, vasopressin, adrenocorticotropic hormone, and other hormone functions.

## Yin Yang & Musculoskeletal Medicine

In orthopedics, Yin and Yang can be expressed in various ways. For example, muscles that produce motion, acceleration or concentric action can be considered Yang in nature. Muscles that stop motion, decelerate, and are eccentric in action may be considered more Yin in nature. Contractile aspects of muscles, myosin and actin (see chapter 2), may be considered Yang. Tendons, which are noncontractile and denser, more Yin.

To maintain normal gait and joint control, concentric Yang (*agonist*) muscles must interact constantly and sustain a working balance with eccentric Yin (*antagonist*) muscles. This interdependence between agonist and antagonist muscles is a good example of Yin-Yang principles and interdependence.

## Yin Yang & Muscles

The biomedical model categorizes white muscles as having phasic functions and red muscles as having postural functions.

Phasic muscles are more Yang in nature. They tend to be located more superficially, can produce more force and are fast acting.

Postural muscles may be classified as Yin: they tend to be more deep in the body, more vascular (increased density) and more resistant to fatigue than phasic muscles.

Postural Yin (red) muscles tend to develop Yang dysfunctions such as tightness. Phasic Yang (white) muscles tend to develop Yin dysfunction such as weakness (see chapter 2).

# Disease Etiology

OM etiology classifies causes of disease (*factors*) as exogenous, endogenous, independent and miscellaneous.

## Exogenous Pathogenic Factors

The *exogenous factors*—environmental influences that can cause disease—are Wind, Cold, Fire, Damp, Dryness and Summer-Heat (Table 1-3 on page 10). These environmental factors, which are associated with climatic influences, often manifest as acute disorders.[11]

In OM, all pain is caused by obstruction of either Qi energy or Blood flow. Exogenous factors can result in obstruction and therefore pain.

The exogenous factors often invade the Exterior and obstruct the flow of Qi and Blood. These pathological influences also can cause obstruction by invading the Interior. Reiter's Syndrome, an acute asymmetric arthritis that is accompanied by urethritis, conjunctivitis, and/or cervicitis, is one example of a condition in which pathogenic factors affect both the Exterior and the Interior.

INFLAMMATION. Inflammation is a reaction of the body Defensive Qi to insult.[12] Because inflammation usually is associated with tissue warmth and swelling, it is often classified as Wet Heat. Inflammation rids the body of foreign matter (exogenous or endogenous pathological factors), disposes of damaged cells, and initiates wound healing.

When inflammation affects a joint (Heat Bi) such as in rheumatoid arthritis, the cartilage can be damaged by Heat which injures fluids and joint nutrition (*biomedicine: by neutrophils and lysosomal enzymes that enter that area*).

The body reacts to injury and infection similarly, since both activate Defensive Qi. In biomedicine, injury or infection also can result in similar reactions (see inflammation chapter 3).

---

11. Wind, Cold, Fire, Heat, Damp and Dryness also can be generated internally. In such cases these factors manifest with similar symptoms that are unrelated to climatic influences.

12. A Yang Ming reaction.

*Table 1-3.* **EXOGENOUS FACTORS**

| FACTOR | SYMPTOMS | COMMON IN |
|---|---|---|
| Wind | Suddenness and changeability | Paresthesias, neuralgia |
| | Symptoms with unfixed location | |
| | Upper body symptoms | |
| | Labile emotions | |
| Cold | Slowness and contraction | Pain |
| | Subjective feeling of cold | |
| | White appearance | |
| Heat | Restlessness (less so than with Fire) | Inflammation |
| | Thirst | |
| | Subjective sensation of heat | |
| | Objective sensation of heat | |
| | Red appearance | |
| Fire (a degree of heat) | Thirst | Muscle atrophy and neuritis |
| | Subjective sensation of heat | |
| | Objective sensation of heat | |
| | Red appearance | |
| | Restlessness, rage | |
| Damp | Subjective sensation of heaviness and stickiness (symptoms of fixed location), persistent, difficult to cure | Swelling, arthrosis, edema, myalgia |
| | Feeling of sluggishness or apathy | |
| Dryness | Dryness, such as of skin, lips | Spasms, contracture, paresthesias |
| | Constipation | |
| Summer Heat | High fever and profuse sweating | Not related to orthopedic disorders |
| | Seasonal in nature | |

**LATENT PATHOGENIC FACTORS.** The concept of an incubation period was described early in the classic *Canon of Internal Medicine* Book of *Simple Questions*, which says that the injuries caused by the:

| | |
|---|---|
| cold of the winter | cause a recurrence of the illness in spring |
| wind of spring | make people unable to retain food in the summer |
| heat of summer | cause intermittent fever in fall |
| humidity of fall | cause a cough in winter |

The etiology of painful disorders is often said to be related to external pathogenic factors; however, patients rarely relate this kind of history. Latent pathogenic factors may be one explanation.

## Endogenous Factors

In OM, the body and mind affect each other directly in an integrated system in which the internal Organs play a direct role. Emotional effects are not seen as secondary influences that stress the human system, but rather as factors directly responsible for disease (Table 1-4).[13]

OM considers the mind to be part of the five solid Organ systems, especially the Heart. The classic text *Spiritual Axis* states:

> The organ that is responsible for performance of mental activities is the heart....The heart is the monarch of the five solid and six hollow organs... Therefore, grief and sorrow also disturb the heart, and a disturbance of the heart affect the five solid and six hollow organs.

Because the Heart controls the Blood vessels, and therefore the Blood, Blood is said to be the foundation of mental activity. If there is plenty of Heart Blood, the mind is clear, thinking is brisk, and one is full of spirit and vigor.

The endogenous factors—influences that originate from within—consist of the *seven affects*: Joy, Anger, Sorrow, Anxiety, Preoccupation, Fear and Fright/Shock (Table 1-4 on page 12). Imbalance in one or more of these emotions can disturb the homeostasis leading to endogenous damage and disharmonies of the Organs. These disharmonies can progress to Heat, Fire, Cold, Wind, Damp, Qi or Blood stagnation, channel obstruction, and tissue damage.

Unbalanced emotions often affect the Liver and Heart, resulting in decreased Blood circulation, Blood deficiency and

generation of Internal Wind. Decreased Blood circulation and Blood deficiency can lead to musculotendinous tension, and rigidity. Internal Wind can result in symptoms such as numbness, paresthesias, neck pains and headaches.

Anxiety and preoccupation can weaken the Spleen/pancreas and cause accumulation of Dampness. Weakness of the Spleen/pancreas also affects muscle strength, especially of the four extremities. Dampness often penetrates the muscles and joints which become heavy and achy.

The classic text *Simple Questions* summarizes the relationship of the mind, emotions and spirit and implies a psychosomatic relationship between pain and pain perception:

> When the Heart is peaceful,
> any pain is negligible.

**BIOMEDICINE & EMOTIONAL EFFECTS.** The human brain has as many as 400,000 synaptic terminals in a single axon, and it contains one hundred billion neurons. These connections constantly form new connections, some of which can become permanent. Emotions may result in neuropsychological changes that can become "*hard wired*" in the brain, resulting in permanent, new synaptic connections. Biomedical sciences have shown physiological effects from emotions via the limbic, reticular and autonomic systems (see chapter 2). These neural changes may explain some of the endogenous factor effects that OM describes.

Although emotional effects may be viewed in a cultural framework, as they may be expressed and experienced differently in different cultures, they do seem to have physiologic effects that are more universal. For example, in OM anger (both expressed and non-expressed) is considered a primary factor in the etiology of high blood pressure.[14]

---

13. Emotions can also arise as a direct result of Organic dysfunction.

14. In the Framingham study anger was not an independent predictor of hypertension in western patients, however, anxiety was a predictor in middle-aged western men.

*Table 1-4.* **ENDOGENOUS FACTORS**

| FACTOR | CAN AFFECT AND BE AFFECTED BY | EFFECT |
|---|---|---|
| Over Joy | Heart | Disperses Qi and makes it circulate slowly |
| | | Symptoms that result from excessive lifestyle (burning the candle at both ends) |
| | | Disordered thinking |
| Expressed Anger | Liver | Causes Qi to rise |
| | | Often head and neck symptoms |
| Repressed Anger | Liver | Knots Qi Mental depression, subcostal distension and distension pain |
| Over Sorrow | Lung | Constricts and depletes Qi |
| | | Fatigue, breathlessness, difficulty "letting go" |
| Anxiety/ Preoccupation | Spleen/pancreas | Causes Qi to slow and knot (stagnate) |
| | | Drains/disorganizes Qi |
| | | Digestive system symptoms; fatigue, weakness, Wetness/Phlegm |
| Fear | Kidney | Causes Qi to descend |
| | | Kidney symptoms (increased urination, day/night urination w/fear, etc.) |
| | | Bone and spine disorders (spinelessness, lack of will) |
| Fright/Shock | Kidney | Qi drops, scatters and flows disorderly |
| | | Heart and Kidney symptoms |
| | | Insomnia, palpitations, pronounced fear |

Biomedical studies have shown a relationship between expressed anger and blood pressure (Laude, Girard, Consoli, Mounier-Vehier, and Elghozi 1997; Shapiro, Goldstein and Jamner 1996). The outward expression of anger has been linked to higher cardiovascular reactivity and risk of heart attacks (Siegman and Snow 1997; Verrier and Mittleman 1996). In a recent study a correlation between anger and platelet aggregation has been shown (Wenneberg et al. 1997). Shapiro et al. (1997) have shown that healthy college students with high anger and sadness scores had significantly higher diastolic blood pressure at night, taken with automatic periodic recordings, than those with high happiness and pleasantness scores.

In OM anger affects mostly the Liver and is said to engender Fire, both of which affect blood circulation (Fire can thicken the Blood or possibly cause platelet aggregation). The effects of Liver Fullness (from acute anger) on the Heart can be explained by the Five Phases theory—Wood insulting Fire (see Five Phases chapter 1).

**INCREASED RISK OF DISEASE FROM DEPRESSION.** More recently, biomedicine has shown that certain emotional states result in increased risk for various diseases. For example, depression is a risk factor in the development of osteoporosis (Schweiger, Deuschle, Korner, Lammers, Schmider, Gotthardt, Holsboer and Heuser 1994).[15] Researchers speculate that changes in appetite, decreased activity and increased cortisol levels are responsible for this kind of effect.

In OM, depression is related to the Liver and Kidneys, with repressed anger (often Liver related) and loss of will (often Kidney related) at the root. Stagnation of Liver Qi results in poor Blood circulation, formation of Heat and, through Five Phases theory, in draining of Kidneys. Poor circulation and Heat can result in disturbed sleep. Liver stagnation can also affect the Spleen/pancreas (Five Phases theory), influencing appetite. Kidney weakness, which has been shown to correlate to changes of steroid levels, also affects the libido. The Kidney controls the marrow and the strength of the bones.

EMOTIONS AND PAIN. Studies have shown a link between symptom-specific physiological reactivity and pain severity in reaction to stressful events, especially in depressed patients (Burns et al. 1997). Anxiety sensitivity or the fear of anxiety-related bodily sensations, arising from beliefs that the sensations have harmful consequences is associated with pain behavior and disability (Asmundson and Taylor 1996). Pain is often made worse by fear, by anger, or by a sense of isolation. The pain may be diminished if the patient understands the cause and loses his fear. Patients who keep busy find that sensory and other distractions relieve pain (Brand 1997) (see chapter 2).

Biomedical risk factors for development of pain chronicity are (CSAG 1994):

- Personal problems such as marital and financial.

- Psychologic distress and depression.

- Adversarial medicolegal problems.

- Low job satisfaction.

- Disproportionate illness behavior.

---

15. Depression is associated with insomnia, changes in appetite, inactivity or agitation, and loss of libido.

In cases of pain chronicity, Endogenous factors must be addressed medically and through education, meditation, self awareness and exercises for internal cultivation (breathing exercises). This is important, because dysfunctional behavior is a common factor in patients suffering from chronic pain and may affect tissue and organ function.

## Independent Factors

Independent factors (Table 1-5) are related to lifestyle. Diet, sexual activity, excessive consumption of physical resources, trauma, parasitic infection and poisons can all damage the Interior or Exterior and can lead to obstruction and tissue damage. OM stresses moderation as a way of maintaining health and longevity. Lack of moderation in any of these lifestyle factors can result in disease. The exploration to pathogenesis chapter in the classic *Simple Question* states that excessive:

| | |
|---|---|
| use of the eyes | injures the Blood |
| lying down | injures the Qi |
| sitting | injures the muscles |
| standing | injures the bones |
| exercise | injures the sinews |

By and large, dietary imbalance weakens the Spleen/pancreas; Spleen/pancreas weakness results in insufficiency of Nutritive Qi, Blood and Dampness; Dampness obstructs the channels; and lack of Nutritive Qi and Blood results in insufficiency of raw materials needed for normal tissue renewal.

*Simple Questions* also states that excess of:

| | |
|---|---|
| salty flavor | hardens the pulse |
| bitter flavor | withers the skin |

| pungent flavor | knots the muscles and injures the skin and hair |
| sour flavor | toughens the flesh |
| sweet flavor | causes aches in the bones |

The treatise cites the importance of appropriate balanced flavors in keeping the Organs and tissues healthy, adding that:

| sour flavor | strengthens the Liver |
| the Liver | nourishes the muscles |
| the muscles | strengthen the Heart |

Excessive sexual activity depletes the Essence,[16] Original Qi and Kidney energy, all of which can lead to joint and bone disorders, particularly of the lower spine and knees.

Consumption of an individual's resources taxes the ability to self-heal (diminishes homeostasis).

**EFFECTS OF SMOKING.** Smoking, which is not traditionally included as an independent factor,[17] is a risk factor for many diseases. Smoke is a hot toxin that injures Yin substance, resulting in Yin deficiency, Empty Heat and reduced nutritional supply to tissues.

In biomedicine, smoking has been shown to decrease fibrinolytic activity and nutritional supply to tissues, including intervertebral discs. Decreased nutritional supply can lead to increased risk of poor healing and can cause disc pathologies, surgical and fracture nonunion. Smoking lowers the interdiscal pH (Humbly and Moony 1992) and has been shown to increase the rate of disc degeneration (Battié et al. 1991; Holm et al. 1981). This may

---

16. Essence; sperm, egg and genetic strength.

17. As early as 1800, an OM treatise described smoking as having hot, drying and toxic effects.

*Table 1-5.* **INDEPENDENT (LIFESTYLE) FACTORS**

| FACTOR | AFFECTS (MOSTLY) |
|---|---|
| Diet | Spleen/pancreas |
| Sexual Activity | Kidney |
| Excessive Consumption | Kidney, Spleen, Lung |
| Trauma | Exterior (skin, muscles, etc.) |
| Parasitic Infection and Poisons (smoking) | Spleen, Liver, Intestine (Lungs, Kidneys, Yin, Yang, Soft tissues) |

explain why patients who smoke often develop chronicity (Holm and Nachemson, 1988).

## Miscellaneous Factors

The miscellaneous factors—secondary pathogenic factors that can lead to disease—are Phlegm and Static Blood (Table 1-6). These factors arise due to dysfunctions in other systems.

Disorders of the Spleen, Lung and Kidney can result in Dampness and Phlegm production. Disorders of the Liver, Lung and Heart can result in Blood stagnation.

Excessive Heat or Cold can result in Blood stagnation and Phlegm production. Both Phlegm and Static Blood can cause channel obstruction, leading to painful symptoms.

**PHLEGM FACTOR.** Phlegm is a factor when swelling takes shape and is localized. By comparison, Dampness usually pertains to a more generalized edema or symptoms of heaviness (with the appropriate signs). Swelling due to Phlegm feels harder than swelling that is due to Dampness. Phlegm is associated with arthritic and muscular disorders.

**STATIC BLOOD FACTOR.** Blood stagnation is a common pathology seen in musculoskeletal disorders (especially when trauma is involved) and in the elderly. Blood stagnation often is a consequence of many

*Table 1-6.* MISCELLANEOUS FACTORS

| FACTOR | SYMPTOMS |
|---|---|
| Phlegm | (depending on where it lodges)<br>• Cough<br>• Dizziness<br>• Nausea<br>• Many other symptoms, including elusive ones |
| Static Blood | • Stabbing, fixed pain and/or lumps, night pain<br>• Blue-green appearance |

chronic dysfunctions. When Phlegm, Dampness and Blood stagnation combine (seen commonly in severe arthritis), swelling and/or lumps develop that are severely tender and difficult to treat.

# Eight Principles

Eight Principles is a system that classifies disease according to Yin-Yang, Hot-Cold, Internal-External and Deficiency-Excess. The classic treatise *Difficult Issues* states:

Frequent movement in the vessels indicates an illness in the palaces.

Slow movement in the vessels indicates an illness in the depots.

Frequency indicates Heat.
Slowness indicates Cold.

Yang symptoms are caused by Heat.
Yin symptoms are caused by Cold.
These principles can be employed to distinguish illnesses in the depots and palaces.

The Eight Principles comprise a method by which disease can be localized, its major characteristics can be categorized, and the progression of symptoms can be understood. Pain from muscle strain provides a good example.

## Pain from Muscle Strain

Pain from muscle strain is a common occurrence. Accompanied by swelling and warmth, it is acute, sharp, burning, intense, and relatively superficial. The condition is classified as Yang, Hot, External and Excessive because:

| | |
|---|---|
| Yang | The condition is acute and the pain is sharp and intense. |
| Hot | The tissue feels warm and responds to icing, and the pain can have a burning quality. |
| External | The lesion is located in the muscle. |
| Excessive | The area is sensitive to touch. |

TREATMENT PRINCIPLES. In designing treatment principles for this condition, the practitioner considers that, because the condition is:

| | |
|---|---|
| Yang and Excessive | Strong techniques that have a Yin effect are appropriate. |
| External and Hot | Superficial and cooling techniques (such as bleeding acupuncture points) on the Yang channels are appropriate. |

## Chronic Muscular Pain (Fibromyalgia)

An example of a condition that is often classified as Yin, Cold, Internal and Deficient is chronic muscular pain or fibromyalgia. The patient may have pain that, for the most part, is constant, chronic, dull, deep, achy (moderate intensity), and aggravated when the patient is tired, in the afternoon and possibly at night. The patient may feel cold and may find relief from heat and pressure (massage).

The practitioner uses treatments that are Yang in nature because the condition is Yin and Deficient. Energy from Yang channels is directed deeply to Yin channels (by selection of points and deep needling). Warming and tonifying techniques are used.

The Eight Principles is one of the major systems used currently when prescribing herbal medicines.

# Five Phases

The Five Phases theory, one of the oldest in OM, suggests that all phenomena in the universe are made of five energetic phases (qualities) that are subject to positive and negative feedback mechanisms.

The Phases—five elemental configurations that can be found in all material and natural order—are Wood, Fire, Earth, Metal and Water. Physiologically, the Five Phases theory explains the unity of the mutual relationships between the Organs and body tissues, as well as between the human body and nature. In medicine, the Five Phases are patterns of associative relationships between different physiological and natural phenomenon. For example, each of the seasons (late summer being a separate season) is related to one of the Phases and their associated Organ. (Although the concept of a seasonal organ functional relationship seems obscure, a recent study of the effects of academic stress on the hypophyseal-pituitary-adrenal axis hormones has shown seasonal relationships [Malarky et al. 1995].)

The physiological activities of the Organs can be classified according to the different characteristics of the Five Phases:

• Wood (Liver) is associated with germination, extension, softness, and harmony.

Therefore, anything that has these characteristics can be categorized as having Wood Phase qualities.

• Fire (Heart) is associated with Heat and flaring up of emotions.

• Earth (Spleen/pancreas) is associated with growing, nourishment, and change.

• Metal (Lung) is associated with separation, death, strength, and firmness.

• Water (Kidney) is associated with cold, moisture, and downward flowing.

The positive feedback component of the Five Phases theory is called the generation cycle; the negative feedback component is called the control cycle.

The generation cycle is an activating, generating and nourishing sequence of elemental relationships.

Wood→Fire→Earth→Metal→Water

The control cycle is a sequence of elemental relationships that restrict and inhibit

Wood→Earth→Water→Fire→Metal

The *Classic of Categories* states:

If there is no generation, then there is no growth and development. If there is no restriction, then endless growth and development will become harmful. [18]

Therefore, the movement and change of all things exists through their mutual generating and controlling relationships. These relationships are the basis of the never ending cycle of natural elements.

The *Simple Questions* states:

When the Qi of one of the Five Phases is excessive, it will overwhelm its subjugated [controlled] Phase [such as Wood overwhelming Earth] and counter-control its own subjugating Phase [such as Wood counter-regulating Metal].....The East generates wind, wind generates Wood, Wood generates sour, sour generates Liver, Liver generates Sinews.... The Five Phases theory is applied to the physiology and pathology of the human body by using the relationships of generation and control to guide clinical practice.

---

18. Interestingly this is the current thinking about cancer.

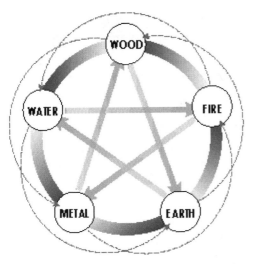

*Figure 1-3:* Generation cycle, inner thick circle; control cycle, thick inner arrows; over-regulation (insult) dysfunction outer thin circle.

Table 1-7 lists the associations between elements and Organs in the Five Phases theory

*Table 1-7.* **FIVE PHASES: ELEMENT-ORGAN ASSOCIATIONS**

| ELEMENT | ORGANS |
| --- | --- |
| Wood | Liver and Gall-Bladder |
| Fire | Heart and Small Intestines |
| Earth | Spleen and Stomach |
| Metal | Lung and Large Intestines |
| Water | Kidney-Bladder |

## Five Phases Disorders

Five Phases theory is used also to demonstrate transformation of pathological influences. The Classic of *Internal Medicine* states:

> When the Liver is diseased, the Liver will transmit {the disease} to the Spleen, and so one should replenish the Qi of the Spleen.

Diseases of the Liver and Spleen/pancreas often interact with each other. For example, Liver disease may affect the Spleen/pancreas because Wood can over-control Earth, while Spleen/pancreas illness may affect the Liver because Earth can counter-control (insult) Wood. Liver disease may also influence the Heart by "mother affecting son" illness. If Liver disease is transmitted to the Lung it can be categorized as Wood counter-controlling (insulting) Metal. If it is transmitted to the Kidney, then it is considered a "son affecting mother" illness. The other Organs follow the same principles.

The controlling relationships among Organs can be expressed as follows:

- The Lung's (Metal) function of clearing and descending can restrict the hyperactivity of Liver (Wood) Yang.

- The Liver's function of regulating the smooth flow of Qi is capable of reducing stagnation at the Spleen/pancreas (Earth).

- The Spleen's transportation and transformation function is able to subdue the overflowing of Kidney Water.

- The Kidney's nourishing and moistening function can prevent flaring up of Heart Fire.

- The Heart's Yang can prevent hyperactivity of the Lung's (Metal) clearing and descending functions.

Therefore, the application of the Five Phases theory in explaining the complicated interaction between the solid Organs can be summed up by these four relationships: over-regulation, counter-regulation, mother affecting son, and son affecting mother (Figure 1-3).

Some acupuncture systems rely almost entirely on the Five Phases theory for diagnosis and treatment. It is most useful for treatment of mental disorders; it is less effective for musculoskeletal disorders except when used as part of a larger treatment plan. Table 1-8 on page 18 summarizes the Five Phases characteristics.

*Table 1-8.* **CATEGORIZATION OF OBJECTS AND PHENOMENA ACCORDING TO THE FIVE ELEMENTS**

| PHASE CHARACTERISTICS | WOOD | FIRE | EARTH | METAL | WATER |
|---|---|---|---|---|---|
| TONE | Jiao | Zheng | Gong | Shang | Yu |
| FLAVOR | Sour | Bitter | Sweet | Pungent | Salty |
| COLOR | Green/Cyan | Red | Yellow | White | Black |
| CHANGE | Germination | Growth | Transformation | Harvest | Storage |
| CLIMATE | Windiness | Warmness | Dampness | Dryness | Coldness |
| DIRECTION | East | South | Center | West | North |
| SEASON | Spring | Summer | Late Summer | Autumn | Winter |
| ORGAN | Liver/ Gall Bladder | Heart/ Small Intestine | Spleen/ Stomach | Lung/ Large Intestine | Kidney/ Urinary Bladder |
| SENSE | Eye | Tongue | Mouth | Nose | Ear |
| TISSUE | Sinew | Vessel | Muscle | Skin & Hair | Bone |
| EMOTION | Anger | Joy | Rumination/ Excessive thinking | Melancholy/ Mourning | Fear |
| SOUND | Shouting | Laughing | Singing | Crying | Moaning |

# Blood

In OM, the term Blood pertains to the same red fluid described in the biomedical model.[19]

Blood is formed and maintained by interaction of the Spleen/pancreas, Liver, Lungs, Heart and Kidneys. It is derived from interaction of Food-Qi, Lung-Qi, and Heart Qi, all of which take root from Original Qi and Essence. A relationship between the Spleen/pancreas (Food-Qi), Lungs (Air), Heart and Essence (Kidney / bone marrow), and the creation and function of Blood was recognized in the Qing dynasty (Maciocia 1989).[20]

## Function

The main function of Blood is nourishing and moistening of the entire body. As Blood flows throughout the channels and Organs, it has multiple functions and can develop various dysfunctions. Table 1-9 on page 19 lists disorders of the Blood with their principal characteristics, symptoms and signs.

Blood plays an important role in the nourishment and moistening of sinews as was emphasized in the *Spiritual Axis*:

> When the Blood is harmonized...the sinews are strong and the joints are supple.

### Blood Disorders (Musculoskeletal Effects)

Lack of nourishment due to Blood deficiency, or stagnation, can result in stiff-

---

19. OM attributes other functions to this fluid.

20. Many of these systems are associated with biomedical blood, as well.

ness and fragility of the tendons, ligaments and other sinews. Blood deficiency often results in generation of internal Wind with symptoms such as paresthesia (pins and needles), numbness, unfixed or radiating pain, and upper body symptoms. Deficient Blood, a Yin substance, can also result in empty Heat with burning pain *(biomedicine: neuropathies)* and bleeding.

**RELATIONSHIP OF BLOOD WITH LIVER AND KIDNEY.** The relation of the Blood to the Liver and Kidney is especially important in musculoskeletal medicine. Athletic activity demands increased blood circulation to muscles. Blood circulation is dependent on normal function of the Liver, because Liver stores and regulates (releases) Blood.

Stagnation of the Liver can result in decreased Blood flow during physical activity, leading to a lack of nourishment of muscles and sinews. Patients who experience increased symptoms during or after physical activity often suffer from Liver Blood and Kidney disorders *(biomedicine: often adrenal disorders)*. Increased physical activity must be balanced with rest, because Blood regenerates itself in the Liver when the person is lying down.

Blood and Essence are interdependent. The Kidneys are the root of Essence (which is made by refinement of Blood) and whole body Yin and Yang. Kidneys control the bone marrow and therefore generation of Blood *(Biomedical: marrow as well)*.

**RELATIONSHIP OF BLOOD WITH LUNGS AND SPLEEN/PANCREAS.** The Lungs and Spleen/pancreas (the root of postnatal Qi) are important because Qi holds the Blood in the blood vessels. When Qi cannot hold the blood, microbleeding can result in fixed, sharp pain of unknown origin. However, from a clinical standpoint bleeding is more often caused by Blood Heat. Weakness of the Lung can result in pooling of blood in the lower extremities and formation of varicose veins (Lung function is important in venous circulation).

*Table 1-9.* **DISORDERS OF THE BLOOD**

| DEFICIENCY | CHARACTERISTICS |
|---|---|
| Blood deficiency | • Lusterless appearance<br>• Dizziness when standing |
| Blood Stasis | • Impairment of flow or local accumulation of blood for various reasons<br>• Characteristically gives rise to lumps and/or pain in fixed location |
| Blood Heat | • Results from heat toxin or empty heat entering the Blood<br>• Usually characterized by bleeding |

**RELATIONSHIP OF BLOOD WITH HEART.** When Heart Blood is weak, the patient is restless, and sleep quality is affected. Chronic poor sleep is a common factor in patients who suffer from myalgias and other chronic pain syndromes.

# Essence

Essence, which is part of the Kidney system, is the material basis of life. Essence has two aspects:

• Inherited Essence (prenatal), which cannot be altered.

• Acquired Essence (postnatal), which can be supplemented and can reinforce inherited Essence.

A fluid-like substance, Essence relates to the sperm and the egg. It forms the basis of growth, sexuality, reproduction and aging.

Abnormal bone and mental growth is associated with lack of Essence. Since Essence determines each person's constitution, it is associated with many conditions that manifest by weakness, such as a weak immune system, life-long lack of endurance and general weakness, reproductive disorders, and brain disorders. The patient often relates frequent childhood diseases.

Excessive sexual activity depletes Essence. Weak Essence is a common factor in early degenerative joint disease, early degenerative disc disease and other degenerative spinal and bone disorders. According to *Simple Questions*:

> Essence is the root of the body, if it is protected and stored, latent pathogenic heat will not appear in spring time.

In many ways, acquired Essence resembles genetic material and the inborn, constitutional condition of the individual.

# Fluids

Fluids such as urine, sweat, tears and saliva moisten and nourish the skin, flesh, muscles, sensory organs and excretory organs.

Fluids that are clear, light and thin circulate with Defensive Qi, moistening the muscles and skin are called *Jin*. Controlled by the Lungs, they fill bursas that can be treated through the Sinews channels and Lungs.

A thicker, denser Fluid called *Ye* (liquid) circulates more deeply and is related to Nutritive Qi. Ye is related to the Spleen/pancreas and Kidney. Its function is to moisten and nourish the joints, brain, cerebral spinal fluid and bone marrow.

**BIOMEDICINE & YE**. Ye may be closely correlative to biomedical synovial fluid. The Synovium (see chapter 2) is a colorless, viscid fluid that lubricates and nourishes the joint, including the avascular articular cartilage. The Synovium plays a significant role in infection control (*OM: Spleen, Kidney, Essence and marrow function*) and in production of hyaluronate, which gives synovial fluid its viscosity.

# The Channels (Meridians)

The body consists of matter and energies that circulate through a network of channels and Organs. The channels, also called meridians, connect all types of tissues.

OM uses the concept of *channels* to describe various systems: the circulatory, lymphatic, and nervous systems among them. Throughout OM history, as the need to explain medical phenomena and prevailing philosophies have changed, channel theories have evolved and their sophistication has increased.

## The Channels & Acupuncture

The channels are at the root of acupuncture theory: the belief is that acupuncture produces a physiological affect via the channels. Researchers have attempted to verify the existence of acupuncture channels; however, no linear relationship has been demonstrated between a singular channel and any known anatomical or physiological entity or system. Attempts to document the existence of acupuncture channels resulted in varied conclusion. De Vernejoul et al. (1985) injected radioactive technetium to a number of acupuncture and nonacupuncture points and showed a scintigraphic evidence of specific radioactive paths which could be interpreted as acupuncture channels. Lazorthes et al. (1990) attempted to reproduce this study but failed to show any such distribution.

Many similarities can be demonstrated using a less rigid approach. For example, many back Shu (Transport) points and Alarm (Mu) points are on appropriate dermatomal segments for the organ they affect. Myofascial and sclerotomal triggers *(biomedicine: referred pain patterns)* often have distributions that are similar to that of the Sinews channels.[21]

---

21. For a review of the modern research on the channels and points, see *The Vital Meridian* (Bensoussan 1991).

Table 1-10. PHYSIOLOGIC ACTIVITY OF THE CHANNELS

| CHANNELS (MERIDIANS) | PHYSIOLOGIC ACTIVITY |
|---|---|
| Sinews | • Location of Defense Qi circulation<br>• Connection between Main channels and connective tissue and skin<br>• With the muscles, provide a protective layer<br>• Important in acute disorders such as sprain/strain and in disorders of bursae<br>• Important in musculoskeletal disorders |
| Connecting | • Link Main channels with surrounding tissues<br>• Part of the blood vessel system<br>• Provide a functional connection between the ventral-dorsal and Yin-Yang aspects<br>• Store energy and blood and release them to the Main channels when needed<br>• Important in prevention of chronicity, emotional disorders, excess conditions |
| Main | • Connect Organs to rest of system<br>• The main channel system |
| Divergent | • Reinforce Main channels<br>• Provide functional connection between Yin-Yang Channels and Organs<br>• Balance between the right and left<br>• Important in Yin (substance) anatomical/pathological disorders |
| Extra | • Store extra Qi and Blood<br>• Release Qi and Blood when Main channels are vacuous<br>• Balance between the left-right, superior-inferior, and diagonal aspects<br>• Important in chronic disorders |

## Channel Distribution

Distributed from Exterior to Interior, the channels are arranged such that they cover the body in all directions and dimensions (Table 1-11 on page 22).

Each channel corresponds to a functional and dysfunctional *level* within the body.

## The Channels & Patterns of Discrimination

Use of pattern discriminations by channel systems (for diagnosis) is the oldest type of pattern discrimination in OM. Responsible for communication between tissues in a closed/opened feedback system, each channel has its own physiologic activity and pathologic manifestations. The OM attribution of many conditions to distal Organs can be traced to the existence of the channels.

All channels, regardless of their location, are more superficial energetically than the Organ system. Often Painful Obstruction (*Bi*) syndromes (*biomedicine: musculoskeletal disorders*) are obstructive channel disorders. When a patient has musculoskeletal pain without any Organ symptoms, the condition can be considered purely of channel origin. Because the channels and Organs are interrelated, and because channel energy enters into the deeper Organ system at the Sea points, Organic symptoms can be a part of the pattern discriminations of the internal course of the channel.

### Importance in Musculoskeletal Medicine

Channel discrimination is especially important in musculoskeletal medicine. The channels can be invaded by exogenous pathogens, or they can develop dysfunctions due to endogenous disharmonies. Exogenous pathogenic factors, by and large, penetrate the body from the more superficial channels and travel through the channel system into deeper energetic or anatomic levels.

The musculoskeletal system, including several aspects of the joints, is part of the Exterior energy system and of the external pathways of the Main channels. Other aspects of the musculoskeletal system that relate to structure and biochemistry relate more to the deeper channel systems.

Table 1-10 on page 21 describes the physiologic activities of the channels.

## The Sinews Channels

The most superficial of the channels, the Sinews (tendinomuscular) channels are the locus for circulation of Defense Qi. With the muscles, the Sinews channels:

- Provide the protective layer of the body.

- Govern movement.

- Serve as the connection between the Main and Divergent channels to the muscles, connective tissues and skin.

Defensive Qi circulates through the Sinews channels. Patients who have myofascial pain syndromes and fibromyalgia often develop stagnation of Defensive Qi (especially the fluid quality). Fluid stagnation transforms to Phlegm that becomes nodules (*biomedicine: fibrositic nodules*) called myofascial trigger points in biomedicine and Ashi points in OM. Treatment of local Ashi (trigger) points mobilizes the Sinews channels and disperses stagnation.

The Sinews channels support and maintain skeletal integrity by connecting the "hundred bones," thereby playing an important role in locomotion, the immune system, and the individual's sense of physical and emotional boundaries.

Although early Chinese writing does not describe the exact anatomical and functional delineations of single muscles, the classic descriptions of general muscular functions and distribution through the

*Table 1-11.* **CHANNEL DISTRIBUTION**

| CHANNELS | DISTRIBUTION |
|---|---|
| Main | Longitudinal |
| Connecting | Join the Main Yang channel to its paired Main Yin channel anteroposteriorly |
| Divergent | Cover the sagittal and axial plains |
| Extra | Add a diagonal axis |

Sinews channels are accurate and reflect both function and dysfunction (*biomedicine: pain distributions*) of muscles. As previously stated the Sinews channels do not resemble any single muscle or group of muscles; however, their distribution often reflects functional muscle unit action on joint structures. Also, their distribution is similar to myofascial and sclerotomal referred pain patterns, which suggests that the Sinews channels were partly surmised following the distribution of needle sensation when muscles were stimulated.

### Sinews Channels & the Brain

The Sinews channels and the Main channels follow approximately the same external path. The Sinews channels are wider than the Main channels, and their energies always flow proximately and terminate in the head region ("brain" in Taoist tradition).[22] This functional connection between the Sinews channels (*biomedical: motor units*) and the brain (*biomedical: upper motor neuron*) provides another example of the sophistication of the channel theory. It is through the Sinews channels that OM assesses motor activity and movement.

**RELATIONSHIP TO POINTS.** The Sinews channels do not have acupuncture points; however, their source and activating points are the Well points (most distal point) of

22. Some sources describe the Yin leg channels as terminating at CV-3.

related Main channels. Sinews channel energy is said to accumulate around the joints as it rises toward the Termination point on the trunk or head. Ashi (trigger, sensitive) points often manifest in the Sinews channels system.

As the fairway of Defensive Qi—the least refined and most reflexive Qi—the Sinews channels can amplify and externalize more endogenous and/or deeper dysfunctions. Since muscle tension can serve as a diagnostic lens into the interior of the body, (visceral disorders often result in muscle tension and pain that can be used in diagnosis), interruption of muscle tension must be performed carefully.

## Symptoms & Signs

The Sinews channels provide an approach to the locomotive unit (*biomedicine: muscles, joints, ligaments, tendons, bursae and fasciae*). They are important in the treatment of acute conditions such as musculoskeletal sprains and strains, trauma, edema, and skin diseases including burns. They are often used in the initial stage of external pathogenic invasion. Acupuncture (by and large) functions through tapping the Defensive Qi and directing it to tissues, and deeper channels. The Sinews channels play an important role in this action.

### Fullness in the Sinews Channels

Acute injuries, or invasion of pathogenic factors, often results in fullness of the Sinews channel and relative emptiness of the related Main channel. This occurs as a result of release of Defensive Qi from the Main Channel to the Sinews channel (in order to help fight the pathogenic factors). Therefore, when the Sinews channel is full its corresponding Main channel is empty. Symptoms and signs of fullness in the Sinews channels are related mainly to strong sensitivity to light pressure (hyperesthesia), severe pain, muscular spasms and contractions, edema and signs of inflammation.

### Emptiness in the Sinews Channels

Chronic disorders can deplete the Sinews channels and result in further movement of pathogenic factors to the Main channels which may result in a relative fullness of the Main channels. Therefore, when a Sinews channel is empty, its corresponding Main channel is full. Symptoms and signs of emptiness in the Sinews channels are related principally to dull and often deep ache, pain on deep pressure, lack of skin tone, hypoesthesia, muscular atonia and atrophy, numbness, coldness and pruritus.

## Sinews Channel Functions: Yin Yang Pairs, Six Energetic Zones

OM classifies Sinews channel functions in Yin Yang pairs and within the Six Energy Zones (stages).[23]

The Six Energy Zones are layers of functional/pathological categories that describe the transformation of pathological influences from the External (Yang/energetic) to the Internal (Yin/substance) levels. They are:

- Tai (great) Yang.
- Yang Ming (bright).[24]
- Shao (lesser) Yang.
- Tai Yin.
- Shao Yin.
- Jue (terminal) Yin.

The Six Energetic Levels were described first in the classic *Yellow Emperor's Cannon of Internal Medicine* and *Classic of Difficult Issues* and were expanded on in the *Theses on Exogenous Febrile Diseases*. The latter book related these levels mainly to the staging and development of infectious diseases.

---

23. A Yin channel and its paired Yang channel.

24. In *Theses on Exogenous Febrile Diseases*, Shao Yang precedes Yang Ming (Yang Ming Organ is the first stage of Internal invasion). However, when considering common clinical presentations, especially in musculoskeletal disorders, Shao Yang can be considered as the level between the External and the Internal.

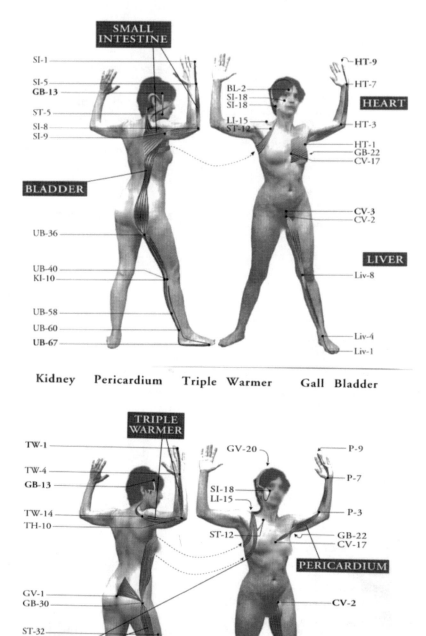

*Figure 1-4:*    Sinews channels

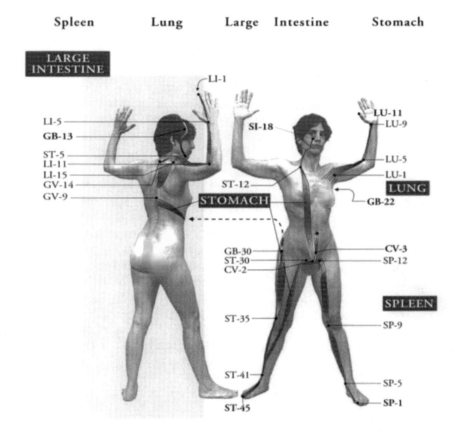

*Figure 1-5:* Sinews channels.

### Tai Yang Level (Urinary Bladder, Small Intestine)

The most superficial layer of the channels, and anatomically the broadest of channels, the Tai Yang level (Urinary Bladder and Small Intestine channels) is the first layer of defense against climatic and worldly influences. Said to open to the Exterior, the Tai Yang channels are strongly related to upright posture and movements that involve extension.

Tai Yang disorders can also result in disorders of joint depression, rotation, adduction and flexion. When the Tai Yang external channels are affected, symptoms mostly are functional and have little or no affect on structure.

### Yang Ming Level (Stomach, Large Intestines)

The Yang Ming level (Stomach and Large Intestines channels) is the location where:

- The immune system is activated (by infection or injury).

- Inflammation (fever/heat, struggle between Defensive and pathologic Qi) is induced.

The Yang Ming level is said to close on the Exterior. When soft tissue or joint inflammation is apparent, the Yang Ming level must be attended.

Yang Ming channel disorders commonly result in problems of joint elevation and depression and may also result in flexion, extension, and abduction disorders.[1]

*Shao Yang*
*(Gall Bladder & Triple Warmer)*

The Shao Yang level (the Gall Bladder and Triple Warmer channels) is an intermediate level between the External and the Internal.[2] Relating mostly to rotational movements, the Shao Yang is said to pivot.

Shao Yang disorders also may result in symptoms related to rotation, sidebending, extension, abduction and adduction. When affected, symptoms may have both functional and mild structural/cellular/inflammatory components: the immune system (acute/chronic inflammation) is still activated, but symptoms of weakness and possibly muscle atrophy are emerging. Both Cold and Heat are present and often alternate.

*Yin Levels*

When pathological influences enter the Interior, they begin to take form, and structural damage can be demonstrated. Soft tissue weakness is more pronounced. Flexion dysfunctions are more apparent and often involve the most superficial Tai Yin channels—the Spleen/pancreas and Lung channels. Once pathology enters the *Jue* (terminal) Yin channels (Liver and Pericardium), significant anatomical damage has occurred and paralysis/atrophy (Wei syndrome) may set in.[3]

---

1.  Inflammation, the normal reaction to injury, should not be inhibited too quickly following the injury, as this may interfere with proper healing, and chronicity may develop. For many inflammatory musculoskeletal disorders, especially for those that occur from injuries, only mildly cooling medications (herbs) should be used, with emphasis on vitalizing of Blood (see chapter 6). Modern anti-inflammatory agents may lead to chronicity, as well.

2.  The typical alternating hot and cold symptoms of Shao Yang are considered as having both Tai Yang and Yang Ming (External/Internal) symptoms.

3.  Wei syndromes are conditions that involve wasting of muscular function such as myasthenia gravis.

*Disorders of Six Energetic Zones*

One example of the effects of the Six Energetic levels on muscles can be seen in the patient who has abnormal forward head posture. Along with Defensive Qi, the Tai Yang energetic level functions to maintain the defenses and psychological boundaries. Poor self esteem, especially during the teen years, often results in bad attitude and in slouched and forward head posture.

This posture stresses the Tai Yang level and affects the Urinary Bladder and Small Intestines Sinews channels. Such posture can result in fatigue of the suboccipital muscles, levator scapulae, and upper fibers of the trapezius, all of which can shorten as they work harder to maintain the head upright. The upper flexor muscles (Yang Ming/Tai Yin) can become inhibited, stretched and weak, a Yin Yang reaction. If this posture (and psychological state) remains, the upper flexor muscles, the sternocleidomastoid and scalene muscles (Yang Ming, Tai Yin) become rigid and inflamed. Hyperactivity of Yang Ming and Tai Yin muscles can result in headaches and can, by a Yin Yang reaction, stretch and facilitate the suboccipital neck extensors and the levator scapulae, which often develops trigger (Ashi) points at their attachments to the scapula. Long-term dysfunction results in the involvement of the deeper Yin channels, and structural changes occur. When the deeper Yin channels are affected, it may be difficult to influence the patient's posture.

## Connecting Channels

The Connecting channels (Luo vessels) (Figure 1-6, Figure 1-7), which run deeper then the Sinews channels, provide a defense system secondary to that of the Sinews channels. According to *Canon of Internal Medicine* book: *Spiritual Axis*, the Connecting channels (vessels) float to the surface of the body, where they are visible; therefore they are related to superficial vasculature.

## Yin and Yang Channels of the Arm

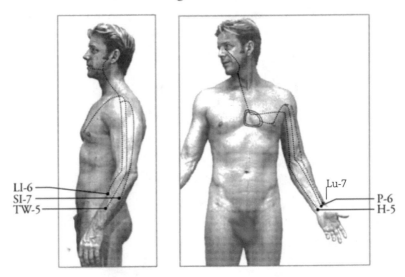

## Yin and Yang Connecting Channels of the Leg

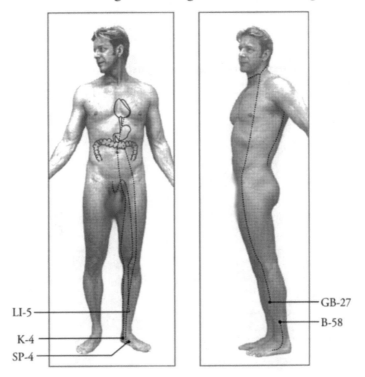

*Figure 1-6:* Connecting channels.

## Great Connecting Channels of the Spleen and Stomach

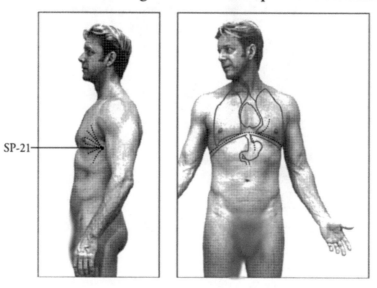

## Conception and Governing Channels

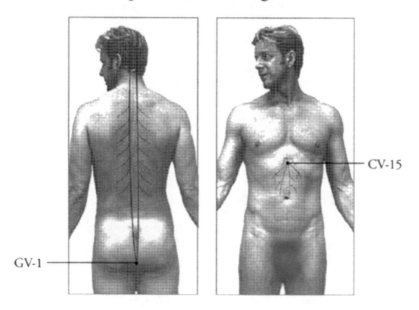

*Figure 1-7:* Connecting Channels.

The Connecting channels divide into three smaller channels—Minute, Superficial and Blood vessels—that branch throughout the body. Described earlier than the Main channels, the Connecting channels were used when primitive needles were used for bleeding (Pirog 1996).

The Connecting channels link the 12 Main, Governing and Conception channels with each other and with the surrounding tissues. In addition to these 14 Connecting channels, A Great Connecting channel of the Spleen/pancreas links all of the Connecting channels. "Whole" body pain is often said to involve the Great Connecting channel of the Spleen/pancreas.[4]

Each Connecting channel separates from the Main channel at the connecting (Luo) point and connects with its paired channel at the source point. These channels, along with blood vessels, strengthen the Yin-Yang relationship between associated pairs of Main channels, and they connect the Main channel to its associated Organ. Connecting channels reinforce physiologically the ventral and dorsal somatic relationship of the Yin and Yang aspects. Surplus energy can be stored in the Connecting channels and released to the Main channel when needed.

The Connecting channels relate mainly to movement of Nourishing Qi and related Blood; however, the Connecting channels also can be affected by exogenous pathogenic factors before they penetrate to the deeper Main channels. According to the *Spiritual Axis*:

The Connecting channels are unable to flow through the great joints. They must move by various routes to tissues and enter. Then they collect together on the skin, where their meeting points can be seen on the surface. Therefore, when needling the connecting channels, one must needle the places where they collect together on the surface, where there may be an accumulation of blood. Even if there is no [local] concentration [of pathogens], one must needle quickly to disperse the pathogen and let out its blood. If allowed to remain, it will cause a painful obstruction [*Bi* syndrome].

Symptoms of the Connecting channels are related to those of the Main channel and vascular systems. The condition of the Connecting channels can be assessed by looking at superficial vasculature and possibly the lymph system. The Connecting channels are often affected by strains, sprains and contusions. They are used mainly in disorders of circulation, especially involving superficial blood vessels, and when visible swelling occurs. Pain of both the Yin and Yang aspect of a limb or joint may be due to pathology in the Connecting channels. When the Connecting channels are involved, pain usually is local, although it may begin to expand as pathogenic influences move through the blood vessels and enter the Main channels.

The Connecting channels can be used to disperse external pathogens and to prevent formation of painful obstruction (*Bi* syndrome). They can be used to treat emotional disturbances, as well.

## The Twelve Main Channels

The Twelve Main channels which perform the most significant of the channel functions, lie both in the deepest and the outer external layers of the body.[5] All other channels reinforce the Main channels, which connect the Organs to the rest of the system.

Each Main channel reflects three aspects in its name:

1. External course (important in musculoskeletal medicine).

2. Location on the body, with Yin or Yang somatic aspects.

3. Associated Organ and internal course.

Each Main channel is associated with an Organ and has both internal and external pathways. The external aspects of the Main channels relate to somatic components they influence. The internal aspects

---

4.  Sp 21 is used often for "whole" body pain.

5.  However, the Divergent and Extra channels often are more important for treating chronic and deep disorders.

relate to the viscera. The accessory channels (Divergent, Connecting, and Extra) supplement, and share points with, the Main channels.

Of the Main channels, six are Yin and six are Yang, three each on the upper and lower extremities. Each Yin channel has a paired Yang counterpart, and vice versa. The balance of the Main channels determines health. Table 1-12 on page 35 and Table 1-13 on page 36 describes the principal symptoms and signs that indicate dysfunction of the Main channels (Figure 1-8 through Figure 1-12 on page 34).

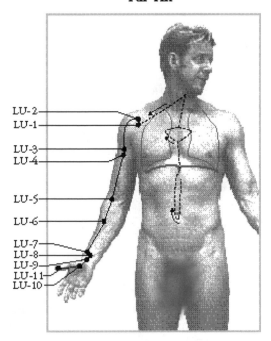 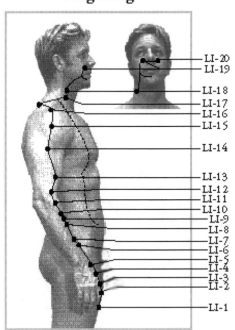

*Figure 1-8:*    Lung and Large Intestine Main channels.

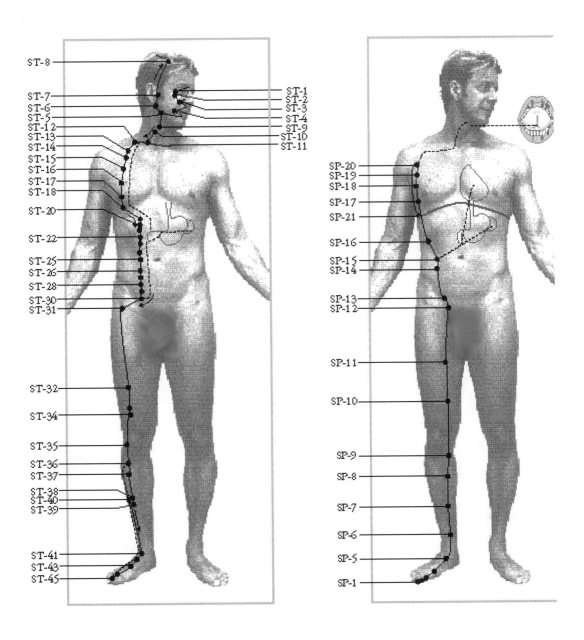

*Figure 1-9:* Stomach and Spleen Main channels.

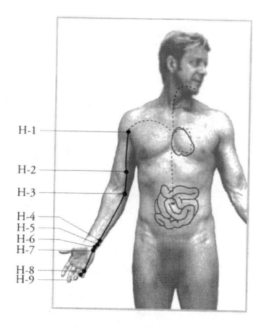
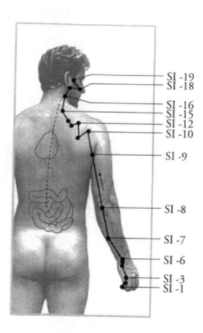

*Figure 1-10:*    Heart and Small Intestine Main channels.

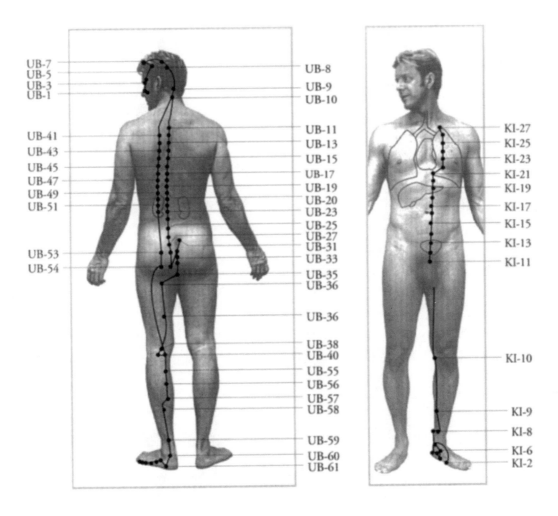

*Figure 1-11:* Kidney and Urinary Bladder Main channels.

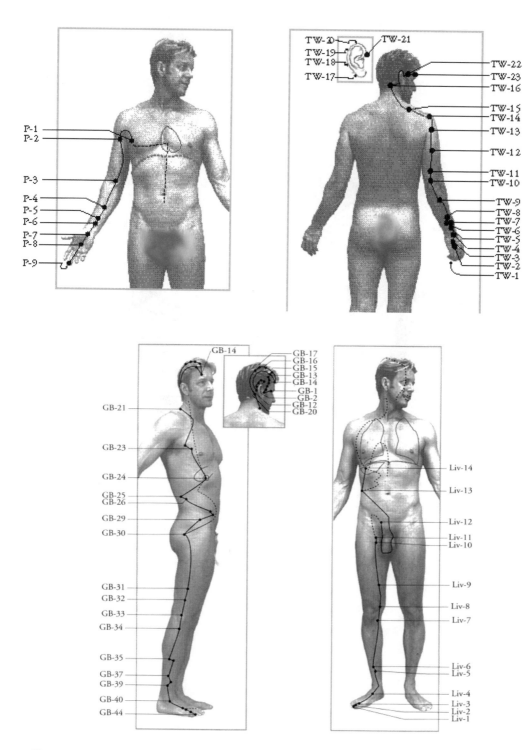

*Figure 1-12:*    Pericardium, Triple Warmer and Liver Gall Bladder Main channels.

Table 1-12. THE MAIN CHANNELS

| MAIN CHANNEL/ ASSOCIATED ORGAN | PRINCIPAL SYMPTOMS AND SIGNS |
|---|---|
| HAND TAI YIN<br>Lung | **External.** Pain at the arm, supraclavicular fossa, shoulder, neck and upper back along the channel, usually associated with fever and/or chills; shoulder, elbow, wrist flexion disorders<br><br>**Internal.** Organic symptoms such as cough, dyspnea, sore throat |
| HAND YANG MING<br>Large Intestine | **External.** Swelling of the neck; locomotor dysfunction or pain of the fingers, wrist extensors, shoulder or upper arm elevators, SCM muscle; fever; dry mouth; sore throat; toothache<br><br>**Internal.** Lower abdominal pain; stool disorders |
| FOOT YANG MING<br>Stomach | **External.** Swelling of the lower limbs and/or neck; pain along its path; SCM muscle, knee extensors, foot dorsiflexion and trunk stabilizer disorders; dry mouth; sore throat; fever<br><br>**Internal.** Abdominal distention and pain; fever; thirst; loose stools; mania |
| FOOT TAI YIN<br>Spleen/pancreas | **External.** Fatigue, weakness, atonia and flexion disorders of muscles of the limbs; lower limb adduction disorders; pain in the posterior mandibular area and lower cheek; cold along the inside of the thigh and knee; swelling of the leg and feet<br><br>**Internal.** Diarrhea; reduced food intake; abdominal pain |
| HAND SHAO YIN<br>Heart | **External.** Pain in the scapular region and/or medial aspect of the forearm; shoulder flexion disorders; coldness of extremities; general feverishness<br><br>**Internal.** Chest pain; essence-spirit disorders |
| HAND TAI YANG<br>Small Intestine | **External.** Stiffness of the neck; pain along the lateral aspect of the shoulder and upper arm; levator scapula disorders, numbness of tongue; pain in the cheek<br><br>**Internal.** Pain in the lower abdomen radiating to the lower back or genitals; dry stools |

*Table 1-13.* THE MAIN CHANNELS

| MAIN CHANNEL/ ASSOCIATED ORGAN | PRINCIPAL SYMPTOMS AND SIGNS |
|---|---|
| FOOT TAI YANG<br>Bladder | **External.** Stiff neck; headache; pain along channel, or intrinsic spine muscle disorders, of the cervical; thoracic or lumbar spine; pain in the posterior aspect of the thigh, leg and foot; eye disease; alternating chills and fevers |
| | **Internal.** Various urinary disorders and mental disorders |
| FOOT SHAO YIN<br>Kidney | **External.** Back pain; quadratus lumborum dysfunction; pain in the lateral gluteal region and in the posterior aspect of the thigh; pain in the soles of the feet; weakness of the legs and knees; dryness of the mouth |
| | **Internal.** Shortness of breath; urinary disorders; impotence; vertigo; blurred vision |
| FOOT JUE YIN<br>Pericardium | **External.** Stiffness of the neck; spasm of the limbs; subaxillary swelling; hypertonicity of the elbow and arm |
| | **Internal.** Delirious speech; palpitations; restlessness; mental disorders |
| HAND SHAO YANG<br>Triple Burner | **External.** Pain behind the ears, cheeks and jaw, or at the posterior aspect of the shoulder and the upper arm; disorders of shoulder and elbow extensors, suboccipital and intrinsic cervical muscles; rotation disorders and atonia |
| | **Internal.** May include abdominal distention and water metabolism disorders |
| FOOT SHAO YANG<br>Gall Bladder | **External.** Pain under the chin, in the lateral aspect of the buttocks, thigh, knee, and leg; rotation disorders; fever alternating with chills |
| | **Internal.** Vomiting; bitter taste in the mouth; chest pain |
| FOOT JUE YIN<br>Liver | **External.** Spasms of the limbs; upper motor (spastic) paralysis; headache; vertigo; tinnitus |
| | **Internal.** *(*May include) lower abdominal pain, oppressive feeling in chest |

## Divergent Channels

The Divergent channels depart from the Main channels at origin points near articulations (hands, shoulders, pelvis, hips and knees) and are branches of the Main channels. The Divergent channels reinforce the Main channels and are the functional/ structural connection between the Yin-Yang channels and the Organs. Therefore, they may be considered as having a deeper function than that of the Main channels. They function to substantiate (internalize/ materialize) functional (Yang), autonomic, instinctual experiences from Defensive Qi (which is one type of their Qi) into Original Qi (transform into Yin substance).[6]

### Yang Divergent Channels

From their points of origin on the limbs, the Yang Divergent channels enter the Organs that are in the abdominal and chest cavities. Moving through these cavities, they enter the other Organs and then resurface at the neck, where they rejoin the Main channels at the return points.[7]

### Yin Divergent Channels

The Yin Divergent channels converge with the Yang Divergent channels (with which they are associated in a Yin-Yang relationship) and then join the Main Yang channel. A Yin Divergent channel does not return to its own Yin Main channel (Figure 1-13).

---

6.  Where postnatal Qi influences prenatal Qi

7.  The origins of the Divergent channels near major articulations and resurfacing at the neck, and the relation between Defensive Qi (immune system) and Original Qi (substance), have been compared to the lymphatic system.

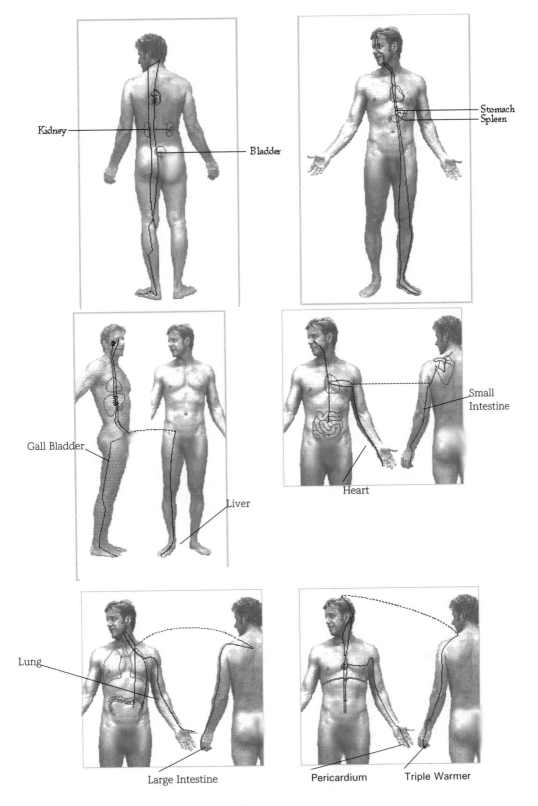

*Figure 1-13:* Divergent Channels

*Use of Divergent Channels*

The Divergent channels are important for treating Interior-Exterior coupled disorders and pathologic (beyond functional) disease processes. Long-term dysfunctions, including gait and posture disorders, can be addressed via the Divergent channels, which reinforce left (Yang) and right (Yin) channel relationships, as well.

The Divergent channels are important in treatment of fibromyalgia and chronic fatigue syndrome. Defensive Qi circulates outside the channels during the day and via the Divergent channels to the Organs at night. Any sleep disturbance (common in pain patients and with fibromyalgia) interrupts this process and may result in Organic dysfunction and chronicity. Disruption of Defensive Qi day/night circulation may result in intermittence of symptoms (also common in fibromyalgia patients).

## Eight Extra Channels (Curious Channels, Extra Vessels)

The eight Extra channels (Figure 1-14 through Figure 1-16), (also called the Eight Curious channels or Eight Extra vessels), which also lie deep, are an important part of the channel system. The theory of eight Extra channels originated in the Classic *Difficult Issues,* which says the eight Extra channels are separated from the circulation of the Main channels, even though the majority of these channels branch from the Main channels and share the Main channel function of circulating Qi (especially Original/Yuan Qi). The eight Extra channels also store extra Qi and Blood, releasing them when the Main channels are empty, and they provide additional connections among the twelve Main channels. The association with Original Qi, and their ability to release Qi and Blood explains their use in constitutional illnesses and general weakness.

The Extra channels also absorb excess pathogenic factors that were not expelled by the Sinews, Connecting and Main channels, a circumstance that may explain the use of TW-5 in disorders of external origin (Pirog *ibid*). Since the eight Extra channels are said to have little circulation, pathogenic factors can accumulate in them and therefore, conditions that involve swelling and heat (especially chronic) are associated with the Extra channels. Tenderness will be found in large regions and scattered throughout the territories of several channels. With time disorders of the bones, including hypertrophy (spurs) can develop.

Later in OM history, several Master points were created and use of the Extra channels was expanded (Pirog *ibid*).[8] Use of these channels has been expanded greatly in modern times, especially in Japan.

*Extra Channel Use*

The Extra channels are especially effective for treating chronic, deep seated or constitutional conditions. They are also effective for treating other conditions that involve several channels (wide spread pain), and that involve left right or diagonal energetic dysfunctions.

---

8.   Said to control and activate the Extra channels.

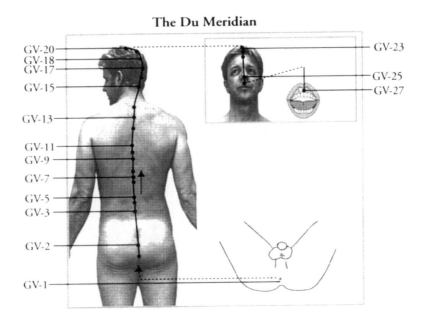

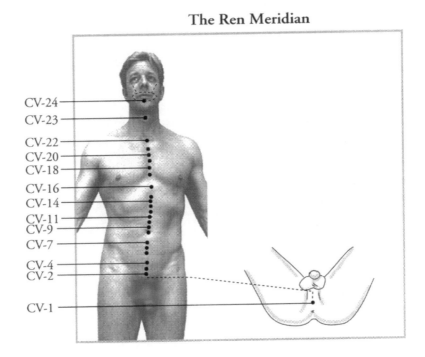

*Figure 1-14:*   Extra channels.

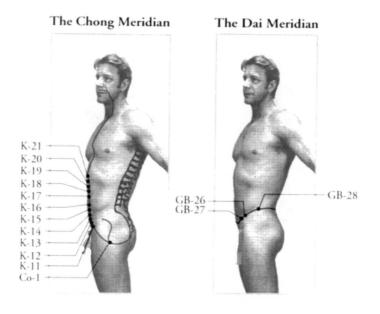

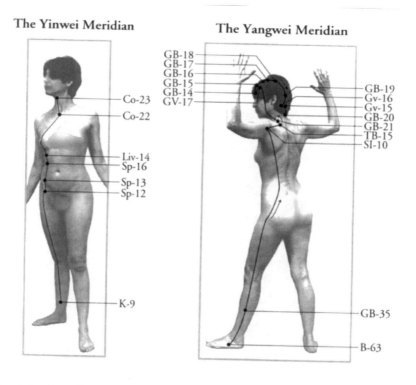

*Figure 1-15:* Extra channels.

## The Yangqiao Meridian                    The Yinqiao Meridian

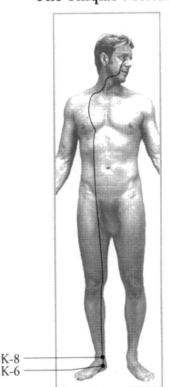

B-1
S-1
S-3
S-4
LI-15

GB-20
LI-16
SI-10

GB-29

B-59
B-61
B-62

K-8
K-6

*Figure 1-16:* Extra channels.

Each Extra channel is associated with specific pathological signs. Usually pain that involves the Extra channels is seen over large regions and may occur in several sites.

Of particular importance for musculoskeletal disorders are:

• The Governing (Du) channel is used often in disorders of the head, neck and back, especially midline pain. A sense as though one cannot hold the head up is often associated with the Governing (Du) channel.

• Girdle (Dai) and Yang Linking (Wei) channels support and keep the muscles and Sinews strong and tight. The Girdle (Dai) channel influences the low back and pelvis while the Yang Linking (Wei)

has more generalized effects. Both of these channels are associated with pain elicited by rotation. They both treat weakness and instability.

• Yin and Yang Motility (Qiao) channels are often associated with imbalances between the medial and lateral legs and postero-lateral and antero-medial areas with difficulties in walking or standing. Symptoms that are worse in the day or night are associated, as well. Fullness in the Yin Motility (Qiao) is associated with limpness of the postero-lateral aspects of the leg and back and symptoms increasing during the day. Fullness in the Yang Motility (Qiao) is associated with limpness of the antero-medial aspects of the leg and back and symptoms increasing during the night.

• The Penetrating (Chong) channel, which controls the Blood, is associated with an inability to express a source for symptoms (vague symptoms), often due to internal Wind arising from deficient Blood.

Tables Table 1-15 through Table 1-21 on page 49 summarize the Extra channels, the principal symptoms and signs associated with them, and their Master (Meeting), Activating and Departure points. The tables integrate various ideas and sources both modern and classic.

*Table 1-14.* **GOVERNING (DU) CHANNEL**

| FUNCTION | Controls/governs Yang channel function; absorbs Yang surplus (both healthy and pathologic)<br>Home to Brain and Kidney (marrow)<br>Affects mental and reproductive functions, spine, nerves, and cerebrospinal fluid<br>Influences musculoskeletal and sensory activity; expels pathogens |
|---|---|
| GENERAL SYMPTOMS | Lowered immunity, weakness of many Yang functions<br>Symptoms of upper body<br>Spinal pain (especially midline) and stiffness<br>Heavy sensation in head<br>Vertigo<br>Urinary retention<br>Hemorrhoids and mental/neurological disorders<br>Anterior-posterior Qi disharmony |
| DEFICIENCY/EMPTINESS SYMPTOMS | Lack of strength<br>Stiffness of spine<br>Heavy head<br>Sterility<br>Impotence<br>Hemorrhoids<br>Phlegm epilepsy<br>Weak character |
| PHYSICAL FINDINGS | Pulse floating and uninterrupted in all three positions (proximal [chi], middle [bar] and distal [inch]), wiry and long<br>Tenderness along mid-back, top of head, GV-20, and SI channel, especially SI-3 |
| MASTER/MEETING POINT | SI-3 |
| COUPLED POINT | UB-62 |
| ACTIVATING POINT | GV-1 |

*Table 1-15.* CONCEPTION (REN) CHANNEL

| | |
|---|---|
| **FUNCTION** | Called the Sea of Yin |
| | Controls lower abdomen and anterior chest and abdomen |
| | Regulates menstruation |
| | Nurtures the fetus |
| | Nourishes the uterus |
| | Controls body fluids, especially in the abdomen |
| **GENERAL SYMPTOMS** | Urogenital disorders |
| | Lower abdominal symptoms |
| | Pains in the genitalia or the umbilicus with radiation to the chest and tense |
| | Abdomen |
| | Reproductive disorders |
| | Anterior/posterior Qi disharmony |
| | Phlegm anywhere in the body[a] |
| | Cough |
| | Bronchitis |
| | Asthma |
| | Emphysema |
| **EXCESS/FULLNESS SYMPTOMS** | Menstrual problems |
| | Vaginal discharge |
| | Male genitourinary disorders |
| | Head and neck pain |
| | Mouth sores |
| | Hernia |
| | Abdominal distention |
| **DEFICIENCY/EMPTINESS SYMPTOMS** | Miscarriage |
| | Uterine hemorrhaging |
| | Sterility |
| | Enuresis |
| | Menstrual problems |
| | Skin disorders |
| **PHYSICAL FINDINGS** | Pulse tight at the distal (inch) position; thin, full and long from distal to middle (bar) positions |
| | Abdominal tenderness and tightness along channel |
| | Tenderness along Lu channel, especially Lu-1 and Lu-7 |
| **MASTER/MEETING POINT** | Lu-7 |
| **COUPLED POINT** | Ki-6 |
| **ACTIVATING POINT** | Ki-1 |

a.  Lu-7 is the commend point which may explain this function

*Table 1-16.* PENETRATING (CHONG) CHANNEL

| | |
|---|---|
| **FUNCTION** | The Central reservoir (Sea) of Blood and Essence<br>Called the Sea of the Twelve Channels<br>Source of Qi for channels<br>Governs sexual characteristics<br>Regulates menstruation<br>Connects prenatal/postnatal Qi<br>Governs reproduction<br>Affects gastrointestinal system and heart |
| **GENERAL SYMPTOMS** | Urogenital disorders<br>Sexual symptoms, both sexes<br>External/internal Qi disharmony |
| **EXCESS/FULLNESS SYMPTOMS** | Sensation as though body increasing in size<br>Inability to express a source for symptoms (vague symptoms)<br>Deficient lactation<br>Impotence<br>Menstrual irregularities |
| **DEFICIENCY/EMPTINESS SYMPTOMS** | Inability to express a source for symptoms (vague symptoms)<br>Contracture<br>Pain<br>Prostatitis<br>Urethritis<br>Orchitis<br>Seminal emission<br>Menorrhagia<br>Hematemesis |
| **PHYSICAL FINDINGS** | Pulse firm and uninterrupted in all three (proximal [chi], middle [bar] and distal [inch]) positions; wiry and full<br>Tenderness around the umbilicus SP channel, in particular SP-6, 4 and suprapubic |
| **MASTER/MEETING POINT** | SP-4 |
| **COUPLED POINT** | PC-6 |
| **ACTIVATING POINT** | K-3 |

*Table 1-17.* **Girdle (Dai) Channel**

| | |
|---|---|
| **Function** | Connects all channels at the trunk<br>Regulates balance of Qi between upper and lower body<br>Supports the abdomen and low back |
| **General Symptoms** | Limpness of the lumbar region (instability)<br>Menstrual disorders<br>Lumbar/hip dysfunction<br>Lumbar pain radiating to abdomen, pelvis, genitals or medial thigh<br>External/internal Qi disharmony<br>Paralysis<br>Deficiency in lower body<br>Excess in upper body<br>Laxity of ligaments |
| **Excess/Fullness Symptoms** | Excess of the Yang channels<br>Weakness of upper extremities<br>Lumbar or loin pain<br>Unilateral weakness in eye, breast or ovary |
| **Deficiency/Emptiness Symptoms** | Weak loins or lumbar ("feels like sitting in water")<br>Hypermobility (laxity of ligaments)<br>Pain in opposite shoulder, eye, breast or ovary<br>Abdomen distention |
| **Physical Findings** | Pulse tight at proximal (cubit) position and beats that vibrate left and right<br>Tenderness around umbilicus, along the channel, and at GB-41 and UB-23 |
| **Master/Meeting Point** | GB-41 |
| **Coupled Point** | TW-5 |
| **Activating Point** | GB-26 |

*Table 1-18.* **YANG MOTILITY (QIAO) CHANNEL**

| | |
|---|---|
| **FUNCTION** | Rules the left side of the body (Yang)<br>Regulates the movement of Yang Qi and fluids<br>Regulates muscular activity<br>Nourishes the muscles and joints of lower extremities<br>Controls opening and closing of eyes<br>Fullness condition of this channel implies an Emptiness condition of the Yin Qiao Mai, and vice versa |
| **GENERAL SYMPTOMS** | Pain in lumbar region and/or spasm along lateral lower extremity, with corresponding weakness along the medial aspects<br>acute headaches and wind problems (CVA, etc.)<br>Muscular problems of a Yang nature (tightness, spasm) on dorsal unilateral aspect of body<br>Symptoms often bilateral, however worse one side or show an opposite reaction on opposite side |
| **EXCESS/FULLNESS SYMPTOMS** | Deficiency/Emptiness of Yin organs and Excess/Fullness of Yang organs<br>Upper body Excess<br>Symptoms worse at night<br>Restlessness<br>Anger<br>Epilepsy during the day<br>Eye diseases<br>Open eyes (will not close)<br>Excess tearing<br>Throat pain<br>Male genitourinary conditions<br>Shoulder pain<br>Pain of the lateral leg |
| **DEFICIENCY/EMPTINESS SYMPTOMS** | Deficiency/Emptiness of Yang with Excess/Fullness of the Yin organs<br>Upper body Empty<br>Complaints worse during day<br>Night epilepsy<br>Inability to keep eyes open<br>Hypersomnia<br>Migraines<br>Throat pain<br>Difficulty breathing<br>Lower Warmer Excess/Fullness<br>Gynecological problems<br>Waist pain<br>Tightness of medial leg<br>*Bi* syndromes of joints |
| **PHYSICAL FINDINGS** | Pulse tight at distal (inch) position, beats vibrate to the right and left<br>Tenderness around ASIS, on or around the GV channel, especially upper back superpubic; and posterior axilla |
| **MASTER/MEETING POINT** | UB-62 |
| **COUPLED POINT** | SI-3 |
| **ACTIVATING POINT** | UB-59 |

*Table 1-19.* YIN MOTILITY (QIAO) CHANNEL

| | |
|---|---|
| **FUNCTION** | Rules the right side of the body (Yin)<br>Regulates Yin aspect of movement of Qi and fluids (quality and flexibility, essence and free movement); opening and closing of eyes; muscular activity<br>Excess/Fullness condition of this channel implies Deficiency/Emptiness condition of *Yang Qiao Mai*, and vice versa |
| **GENERAL SYMPTOMS** | Tightness and spasms along medial lower limb with flaccidity along lateral aspect of limb<br>Unilateral headache near eye<br>Tightness of back muscles with weakness of rectus abdominus<br>Eye, circulatory, gynecological disorders |
| **EXCESS/FULLNESS SYMPTOMS** | Deficiency/Emptiness of Yang organs with Excess/Fullness of Yin organs (worse during day)<br>Night epilepsy<br>Inability to keep eyes open<br>Hypersomnia<br>Difficulty breathing<br>Feeling cold<br>Migraine<br>Throat pain<br>Lower Warmer Excess/Fullness (gynecological problems, waist pain, tightness of the medial leg, *Bi* syndromes of joints) |
| **DEFICIENCY/EMPTINESS SYMPTOMS** | Excess/Fullness of Yang channels (fever; headache with heat)<br>Symptoms worse during weather changes |
| **PHYSICAL FINDINGS** | Pulse tight at proximal (cubit) position, beats vibrate to the right and left<br>Tenderness/tightness along CV channel, especially above and below umbilicus, suprapubic periumbilical mid-clavicle and SCM (ST-9) Lu-1, Lu-7; K channel along abdomen and K-8, K-6 and Ki-3 |
| **MASTER/MEETING POINT** | Ki-6 |
| **COUPLED POINT** | Lu-7 |
| **ACTIVATING POINT** | Ki-8 |

*Table 1-20.* **Yin Linking (Wei) Channel**

| | |
|---|---|
| **Function** | Carries Ancestral Qi and functions on deepest level of Yin, ruling Interior<br>Links the Yin of the body |
| **General Symptoms** | General weakness<br>Lumbar or genital pain<br>Vague thoracic heaviness (chest oppression) and pain dyspnea<br>Circulatory problems<br>Distension in subcostal region<br>Ache in waist<br>Insomnia<br>Nightmares<br>Restlessness, anxiety, fear; timidity, depression<br>Easily angered<br>Palpitations<br>Delirium<br>Weakness of homolateral upper extremity and contralateral lower extremity |
| **Excess/Fullness Symptoms** | Delirium<br>Nightmares<br>Weakness of homolateral upper extremity and contralateral lower extremity<br>Dyspnea<br>Chest oppression |
| **Deficiency/Emptiness Symptoms** | Pain in homolateral upper extremity and contralateral lower extremity<br>Hypotension<br>Hypothyroidism<br>Impotence<br>Rectal prolapse<br>Depression<br>Timidity<br>Fear<br>Nervous laughter |
| **Physical Findings** | Pulse at the proximal (cubit) position seem to roll toward the little finger or up, beats are sinking; big and full<br>With excess deep pulses stronger than superficial ones<br>With deficiency, deep pulses weaker than superficial ones<br>Subcostal tenderness or tightness, especially on right<br>Tenderness of medial clavicle, suprapubic, periumbilical and SP-6 |
| **Master/Meeting Point** | PC-6 |
| **Coupled Point** | Sp-4 |
| **Activating Point** | Ki-9 |

*Table 1-21.* **YANG LINKING (WEI) CHANNEL**

| | |
|---|---|
| **FUNCTION** | Unites and regulates Yang channel activity<br>Impacts Wei Qi (rules exterior; superficial and acute pathologies; pathologies having to do with rotations and extension) |
| **GENERAL SYMPTOMS** | Unilateral symptoms<br>Neck-shoulder pain, especially with headache radiating from base of head to forehead or ipsilateral eye<br>Pain in lateral aspect of body<br>Headaches, especially unilateral<br>Muscular fatigue and/or stiffness<br>Arthritis with sensitivity to weather changes<br>Vertigo<br>Fevers<br>Chills |
| **EXCESS/FULLNESS SYMPTOMS** | Excess of Yang channels<br>Fever<br>Headache with heat<br>Symptoms worse during weather changes<br>Mumps |
| **DEFICIENCY/EMPTINESS SYMPTOMS** | Deficiency of Yang channels<br>Lack of body heat<br>Loss of strength, especially during rainy or cold weather |
| **PHYSICAL FINDINGS** | Pulse at proximal (cubit) position seem to roll toward little finger or up, beats are floating; big and full<br>Tenderness/ tightness around ASIS, especially left side<br>TW-5 along GB channel — GB-21 to GB-29 and GB-35, GB-34 |
| **MASTER/MEETING POINT** | TW-5 |
| **COUPLED POINT** | GB-41 |
| **ACTIVATING POINT** | UB 63 |

# Organs

The anatomy, physiology and pathology of OM Organs are quite different from those of the scientific medical model. OM emphasis is on the relationships of the Organs to related systems. The *Spiritual Axis* states:

> The five solid Organs store up essential Qi and regulate its outflow. The six Hollow organs transform and transport substances without storing them and for this reason they may be over-filled but cannot be filled to capacity.

The Organs influence distal tissues through the systems' channels. The Liver, for example, controls nourishment to the eyes. The Kidney influences hearing. These types of physiologic attributions, their relationships, and their balance are at the root of OM Organ pattern discrimination.[1] Nonetheless, many similarities between biomedicine and OM Organs can be demonstrated. One example is the OM Kidney system, which controls growth, the bones, fluids, reproduction and hearing. It houses the prenatal Qi, store Essence and Original Qi, thereby governing the body's energy reserves and ability to cope with stress. Kidneys are the root of Qi and respiration. The taste related to the Kidneys is saltiness. Most chronic disease processes eventually affect the Kidneys.

---

1. OM is a system in flux and ideas have changed with time. For example, most mental and cognitive functions are attributed to the Heart and Kidneys. In the Yuan and Ming dynasty however, some physicians have attributed these functions to the brain. Also, the sea of marrow (brain) has always been thought to be under the influence of the Kidneys, showing some understanding of the role of the brain in early writing, as well. The *Spiritual Axis* says the spirit Qi comes from the brain.

## Gate of Fire.

The Yang of the Kidney, also called the Gate of fire (*Ming Man*), is located between the Kidneys (the right K in some texts). This separate location may reflect the biomedical adrenal system, as adrenal insufficiency has been shown to correlate closely with Kidney (mostly Yang) deficiency.

### *Suprarenal (Adrenal) Glands*

The adrenal glands, which are located at the upper end of each kidney, are important in the regulation of many bodily functions, including the nervous system. Each adrenal gland has an external layer of cortex and an internal layer of myelonic material. The adrenal cortex and myelonic material secrete hormones that have direct effects in the regulation of various nutritional and defense activities. Their action is also important in the process of acupuncture analgesia and anesthesia.

SUPRARENAL MYELONIC MATERIAL. Suprarenal myelonic material is controlled by fibers of the anterior lowest splanchnic nerve that contains the sympathetic fibers for the renal plexus. It secretes adrenaline and demethyladrenaline (noradrenaline, norepinephrine), and in action is similar to sympathetic nerves.

SUPRARENAL CORTEX. The suprarenal cortex secretes many adrenocortical hormones—corticosteroids and sex hormones—that are necessary for maintaining many of the basic activities of life. Adrenocortical hormones can strengthen the body's capacity to resist harmful factors such as injuries, diseases, infections, and painful stimulation. Excessive hormonal secretion, as seen in high stress states, may be deleterious to soft tissues (*OM: all of which are related to Kidney function in OM*).

Table 1-22 on page 51 highlights some similarities of biomedical renal and adrenal disease and OM Kidneys. Also a recent study has demonstrated that in woman 65-

85 year old hearing loss and bone mass are related (Clark 1995), a relationship clearly defined by OM since the Kidneys control both hearing and bone.

Table 1- 22. BIOMEDICAL AND OM KIDNEY SYSTEMS

| CONDITION | BIOMEDICAL RENAL AND ADRENAL | OM KIDNEYS AND GATE OF FIRE |
|---|---|---|
| MULTIPLE CAUSES | Causes of renal failure and disease are numerous and multisystemic Acute adrenal insufficiency can result from many severely stressful circumstances | Causes of K disorders are numerous as most disorders eventually affect K energy |
| PREGNANCY | Disorders often related to pregnancy | Ks control reproduction and are affected by pregnancy |
| GROWTH FAILURE | Preadolescence adrenal insufficiency is related to growth failure and delayed puberty | K essence deficiency is related to growth failure and delayed puberty as well |
| IMPOTENCE AND AMENORRHEA | Disorders are associated with development of impotence and amenorrhea | Ks regulate reproduction and are associated with impotence and amenorrhea |
| GYN ANOMALIES | GYN congenital anomalies are highly associated with renal system anomalies | Ks house the prenatal Qi and GYN disorders and anomalies are related to the Ks |
| PULMONARY CONGESTION AND CONGESTIVE HEART FAILURE | Disorders of renal and adrenal system are associated with pulmonary congestion and congestive heart failure, both of which result in shortness of breath and edema | Disorders of Ks are related to pulmonary congestion and shortness of breath as the Ks are the root of breath and control fluid |
| BONES | Chronic renal disease can result in osteodystrophy Cushing's (adrenal excess) is related to osteoporosis | K disorders are related to osteoporosis and osteodystrophy as the Ks control the growth and strength of bones |
| PROTEINURIA | Proteinuria seen in renal disease, (protein in urine) can result in cloudy urine | Loss of Essence can manifest as cloudy urine as well |
| MENTAL SYMPTOMS | Encephalopathy can be seen with renal disease | Symptoms of cognition and brain function often are related to K disorders as the Ks control the Essence and sea of Marrow (brain) |
| SKIN PIGMENTATION | Hyperpigmentation is a common sign of renal or adrenal disease | Darkening of skin is associated with K disorders as well |
| DIGESTIVE SYMPTOMS | Anorexia, nausea, vomiting, and diarrhea are associated with renal failure | K and Sp interrelation (dysfunctions through Five Phases theory) are associated with same symptoms |
| SALT | Salt overload can result from renal disease | Saltiness is the taste associated with the Ks |
| STRESS TOLERANCE AND WEAKNESS | Adrenal cortex glucocorticoid hormone insufficiency results in weakness, dizziness and reduced stress tolerance | Dizziness is a symptom associated with K and Essence deficiency. The Body's ability to cope with stress (energy reserves) is controlled by the Ks |
| TEMPERATURE | Heat and cold intolerance is seen with renal and adrenal disorders | Heat and cold intolerance are commonly related to K disorders as all of the body's Yin Yang is rooted in the Ks |
| FATIGABILITY | Fatigability, especially in afternoon, is commonly seen in renal and adrenal disorders | Afternoon fatigue is a K associated symptom as the Ks circadian time is in afternoon |
| HAIR LOSS | Hair loss seen with adrenal disorders | Hair loss is a symptom of K disorders |
| APATHY | Apathy commonly seen with both renal and adrenal disorders | Apathy is a common manifestation of K disorders as the emotion associated with the K's is the will |
| LIBIDO | Loss of libido can be seen with adrenal and renal disorders | Libido is a cardinal function of K |

Other examples of similarities between OM and Biomedical organ functions are bleeding, Liver disorders and Spleen/pancreas disorders.

**BLEEDING.** Bleeding and thrombotic disorders are related to the Liver and Spleen in both OM and biomedicine. Liver disease results in deficiencies of all clotting factors except factor VIII. The OM Liver controls the storage of Blood. In OM the Spleen/pancreas holds the blood in the vessels and is dependent on proper digestive function. Vitamin K deficiency impairs production of clotting factors II, VII, IX and X. The major source of vitamin K is dietary and therefore is dependent on good digestive function. Infections are related to bleeding in both models.

**LIVER DISORDERS.** In biomedicine, liver disease often results in anorexia, nausea, vomiting, diarrhea, fatigue, weakness, fever, jaundice, amenorrhea, impotence and infertility. Signs such as spider telangiectasis, palmar erythema, nail changes, Dupuytren's contracture, testicular atrophy and gastrointestinal bleeding are recognized.

In OM, via the Five Phases theory, Liver disorders affect the Spleen/Stomach and also lead to anorexia, nausea, vomiting, diarrhea, fatigue and weakness. Heat and Damp in the Liver or Gall Bladder results in fever and jaundice. Interruption of the Liver's function of regulating the Blood can result in amenorrhea, infertility and bleeding disorders. The Liver channel passes through the penis and testicles; hence disorders of the Liver channel and Organ are associated with impotence and testicular atrophy. The Liver controls the sinews; the nails reflect its condition. When Liver Blood fails to nourish the sinews, soft tissue contracture (including Dupuytren's) results. Nail changes, including Muehrcke lines, Terry's nails and finger clubbing are manifestations of Liver disorders.

**SPLEEN DISORDERS.** As in biomedicine, in OM the Spleen is associated with the immune system (Defensive and Lung Qi production). Dysfunction of the OM Spleen can result in Phlegm production and lymph node enlargement (seen also with biomedical spleen disorders).

The biomedical spleen is part of the extramedullary hematopoiesis system and therefore is associated with blood formation in both OM and biomedicine.

The Spleen in OM is associated with digestive functions, more appropriately attributed to the pancreas in biomedicine. This apparent difference may be in name only. One section in the classic *Difficult Issues* includes the pancreas as part of the Spleen:

> The Spleen weighs 2 pounds and 3 ounces. It is 3 inches wide, 5 inches long and has ½ pound of fatty tissue surrounding it.

The "fatty tissue" probably represents the pancreas (Maciocia 1989).

Many of these examples are related to severe, and often end-stage, biomedical diseases. The question arises as to whether OM symptom–sign differentiation might represent early, pre-disease (or dis'ease) functional stages of similar biomedical advanced diseased states. If this were to prove true, OM might provide a way of preventing the development of such diseases. (This would be difficult to assess or prove).

## Extraordinary Organs

There is another category of Organs called the extraordinary hollow Organs which include the brain, marrow, bone, vessels, gall bladder, and uterus. They are named hollow but their functions are considered as similar to that of the five solid Organs.

**YIN ORGANS.** Table 1-23 on page 53 through Table 1-27 on page 57 are brief descriptions of the Yin Organ functions and patterns.

**YANG ORGANS.** The Yang organs, which also have patterns of symptoms and signs, are located more superficially and therefore are considered by many to be less important.

Table 1-28 on page 58 through Table 1-33 on page 61 summarize the general characteristics of the Yang organs.

*Table 1- 23.* **YIN ORGANS: KIDNEY/WATER (K)**

| | |
|---|---|
| FUNCTION | Growth; reproduction; regeneration; stores Essence (fullest at birth, depreciates throughout life); metabolizes fluid |
| GOVERNS | The bones, fluids, Yin and Yang of the entire body |
| OPENS | Into the ears |
| HOUSES | The will |
| EXPRESSES | Ambition, creativity, vigor, focus |
| HEALTHY EXPRESSIONS | Gentleness, endurance and groundedness |
| UNHEALTHY PSYCHOLOGICAL EXPRESSIONS | Fear, indecisiveness, apathy, discouragement, negativity, lack of will, impatience |
| PERSONIFIES | Philosopher |
| PAIR EXTERNAL ORGAN | The Bladder |
| DISEASE PATTERNS | Kidney disease patterns and their characteristic symptoms include: |
| KIDNEY YANG DEFICIENCY (KYAD) | Painful or limp knees and lumbar regions, fatigue, tinnitus, coldness<br>Pulse: deep or floating at the proximal (*cubit*) position, slow and weak; may be slippery<br>Tongue: pale, flabby, moist, and possibly thick, white fur |
| SPLEEN AND KYAD | Symptoms seen in KYaD, persistent diarrhea |
| K FAILURE TO HOLD THE QI | Symptoms seen in KYaD, asthma, rapid and short breath |
| HEART AND KYAD | Symptoms seen in KYaD, palpitation, dyspnea, edema |
| INSUFFICIENCY OF K ESSENCE | Soft bones, intellectual deficiency, slow growth, hair loss, low energy reserves |
| INSECURITY OF K QI | Polyuria or incontinence, low back pain |
| K YIN DEFICIENCY (KYID) | Dry throat and lips, dizziness, tinnitus, back pain<br>Pulse: deep at proximal (*cubit*) or floating at distal (*inch*) position, Quick and Weak<br>Tongue: Red, thin, dry, fissures, little or no fur |
| HEART AND KYID | Symptoms seen in KYiD; palpitation; insomnia |
| LIVER AND KYID | Symptoms seen in KYiD; headache; flowery vision (floaters); severe dizziness |
| LUNG AND KYID | Symptoms seen in KYiD; dry cough; night sweats |

*Table 1- 24.* **Yin Organs: Liver/Wood (LIV)**

| | |
|---|---|
| **Function** | Free flowing of Qi |
| **Governs** | Storage and movement of Blood, and nourishment of sinews (seen in nails), muscle tone and strength |
| **Opens** | At the eyes |
| **Houses** | The ethereal soul |
| **Expresses** | Decisiveness, control of emotions, principle of emergence (spring and the power of action) |
| **Healthy Expressions** | Kindness, spontaneity and ease of movement |
| **Unhealthy Psychological Expressions** | Anger, erratic behavior, tension, depression (repressed anger), frustration and resentments, feeling stuck, and dysthymia (blahs), lack of direction in life |
| **Personifies** | Pioneer |
| **Pair External Organ** | Gallbladder |
| **Disease Patterns** | Liver disease patterns and their characteristic symptoms include: |
| **Liv Blood deficiency** | Dizziness, insomnia, flowery vision and/or restriction of movement, tightness of sinew-muscular components and/or tingling and numbness of the limbs, headache (especially on left side) and pale complexion<br>Pulse: thready, wiry, choppy, possibly quick<br>Tongue: pale |
| **Upflaming of Liv fire (UfLivf)** | Short temper, headache, dizziness, red eyes, sudden tinnitus, red complexion<br>Pulse: wiry, quick, weak or strong<br>Tongue: red, thin or flabby, yellow fur |
| **Hyperactive Liv Yang** | Symptoms seen in UfLivf, pain of lower back<br>Pulse: wiry, quick and weak<br>Tongue: red, thin, fissures, no or little fur |
| **Liv Wind** | Rigidity of the neck, tremors or jerking, headache, convulsions<br>Pulse: wiry, quick or slow, tight, floating<br>Tongue: red, thin or flabby, often yellow fur |
| **Stagnation of Liv Qi (SLivQ)** | Mental depression, painful distention of the subcostal regions<br>Pulse: wiry<br>Tongue: normal |
| **Invasion of Stomach by Liv** | Symptoms seen in SLivQ; nausea; vomiting; acid reflux |
| **Liv and Spleen Disharmony** | Symptoms seen in SLivQ; abdominal pain and diarrhea, both of which are exacerbated by emotional factors |

*Table 1- 25.* **YIN ORGANS: SPLEEN/PANCREAS/EARTH (SP)**

| | |
|---|---|
| **FUNCTION** | Governs digestion, helps in production of Blood, contains the Blood in the vessels |
| **GOVERNS** | Flesh (muscle bulk, mass) |
| **OPENS** | Into the mouth |
| **HOUSES** | Thought |
| **EXPRESSES** | Centeredness, persistence, care |
| **HEALTHY EXPRESSIONS** | Fairness, openness, deep thinking, recollection |
| **UNHEALTHY PSYCHOLOGICAL EXPRESSIONS** | Excessive use of the mind (obsessiveness), melancholia, agitated sleep and nightmares, stubbornness and rigidity, excessive ruminating on the past |
| **PERSONIFIES** | Care giver, farmer |
| **PAIR EXTERNAL ORGAN** | Stomach |
| **DISEASE PATTERNS** | Spleen disease patterns and their characteristic symptoms include: |
| **SPLEEN (SP) QI DEFICIENCY (SPQD)** | Fatigue, thin or loose stools, abdominal discomfort<br>Pulse: weak, soft, deep, especially in middle (*bar*) position; slow or fast<br>Tongue: flabby, moist, thin or thick white fur |
| **SPLEEN YANG DEFICIENCY** | Symptoms seen in SPQD; abdominal pain relieved by warmth and pressure; drained, white complexion, sensitivity to cold |
| **CENTRAL QI SAGGING** | Spleen and Stomach, frequently referred to as Central QI Symptoms seen in SPQD, bloating after meals, sagging distention of abdomen, prolapse of viscera |
| **SPLEEN FAILURE TO MANAGE THE BLOOD** | Hemorrhage (mainly menorrhagia hemafecia occurring with Spleen deficiency symptoms) |
| **CENTRAL QI DEFICIENCY COLD** | Abdominal pain relieved by pressure, warmth and food |

*Table 1- 26.* **YIN ORGANS: LUNG/METAL (LU)**

| | |
|---|---|
| **FUNCTION** | Governs respiration Qi and regulates the flow of waterways |
| **GOVERNS** | Surface and skin |
| **OPENS** | At the nose |
| **HOUSES** | Corporeal soul |
| **EXPRESSES** | Expression, clarity of speech |
| **HEALTHY EXPRESSIONS** | Appropriate sadness and cheerfulness |
| **UNHEALTHY PSYCHOLOGICAL EXPRESSIONS** | Grief, worry, sadness, difficulty letting go |
| **PERSONIFIES** | Sensitive type |
| **PAIR EXTERNAL ORGAN** | Large intestine |
| **DISEASE PATTERNS** | Lung disease patterns and their characteristic symptoms include: |
| **LU QI DEFICIENCY** | Cough, shortness of breath, low voice, weak enunciation<br>Pulse: weak, floating or deep, slow or fast<br>Tongue: normal or flabby |
| **LU YIN DEFICIENCY** | Dry cough, night sweating, flushed cheeks, afternoon fevers<br>Pulse: weak, floating or deep, especially in distal (inch) position; quick<br>Tongue: red, thin, fissures, little or no fur |
| **NONDIFFUSION OF LU QI** | Paroxysmal cough and/or dyspnea |
| **IMPAIRED DEPURATIVE DOWNBEARING OF LU QI** | Persistent cough and/or water metabolism disorders |

*Table 1- 27.* **YIN ORGANS: HEART/FIRE (H)(PERICARDIUM/FIRE {P}**

| | |
|---|---|
| **FUNCTION** | Supplies Blood to the entire body |
| **GOVERNS** | Said to govern the vessels |
| **OPENS** | Into the tongue |
| **HOUSES** | The spirit |
| **EXPRESSES** | Clarity of thought |
| **HEALTHY EXPRESSIONS** | Rosy complexion, clarity, ordered thinking and expression |
| **UNHEALTHY PSYCHOLOGICAL EXPRESSIONS** | Disturbances of mental function, irrational behavior, hysteria, delirium, bipolar mood disorders, coma |
| **PERSONIFIES** | Intellectual |
| **PAIR EXTERNAL ORGAN** | Small Intestine |
| **PERICARDIUM** | Closely related to Heart function<br>Protects the Heart<br>Associated with sympathetic nervous system |
| **DISEASE PATTERNS** | Heart disease patterns and their characteristic symptoms include: |
| **H QI DEFICIENCY (HQD)** | Dizziness, palpitations, shortness of breath, tendency to perspire, fatigue<br>Pulse: weak, especially at distal (*inch*) position<br>Tongue: normal or; flabby, pale |
| **H YANG DEFICIENCY** | HQD symptoms, cold limbs, cold sweat, edema, dull white complexion<br>Pulse: weak, deep, slow may be slippery<br>Tongue: flabby, pale, thin or thick white fur |
| **H BLOOD DEFICIENCY (HBD)** | Dizziness, palpitation, lusterless complexion, shortness of breath, insomnia, poor memory<br>Pulse: weak, thready, quick, choppy<br>Tongue: pale |
| **H YIN DEFICIENCY (HYID)** | HBD symptoms with night sweating, restlessness and flushing red complexion<br>Pulse: weak, floating, quick, especially at distal (inch) position<br>Tongue: thin, red, dry, no or little fur |
| **UPFLAMING OF H FIRE** | Restlessness, insomnia, red complexion<br>Pulse: quick, weak or strong, deep or floating<br>Tongue: red tip |
| **HEART OBSTRUCTION** | Angina, purple complexion<br>Pulse: weak or strong, choppy<br>Tongue: purple |

*Table 1- 28.* **YANG ORGANS: URINARY BLADDER/WATER**

| FUNCTION | Receives the "impure/dirty'" part of fluids after the Small Intestine separates the fluid from the "pure/clean" fluids |
|---|---|
| | • In charge of Qi transformation (transforming and excreting fluids by the power of Qi—fluid disorders due to Qi dysfunction) |
| | • Controls storing of fluid |
| HEALTHY INDICATIONS | Balanced mental state |
| EMPTINESS/DEFICIENCY | • Fright affects the Bladder adversely (loss of urine) |
| | • Paranoia/suspicion and jealousy |
| | • Back and neck pain |
| | • Neurological disorders |
| | • Lack of confidence |
| | • Lethargy |
| | • Low sexual energy; frequent, excessive or cloudy urination; incontinence |
| | • Epistaxis |
| | • Fear |
| EXCESS/FULLNESS | • Agitation |
| | — Excessive erections |
| | — Headaches |
| | — Olfactory problems |
| | • Pain along spine or waist |
| MENTAL SYMPTOMS | • Changeable moods |
| | • Over-enthusiasm |
| | • Suspicion, jealousy |
| | • Lack of confidence |
| PRINCIPAL SYMPTOMS | • Stiff neck |
| | • Pain along cervical, thoracic or lumbar spine |
| | — Headache |
| | — Pain in posterior aspect of thigh, leg and foot |
| | — Eye disease |
| | — Alternating chills and fevers |

*Table 1- 29.* **Yang Organs: Small Intestine/Fire**

| FUNCTION | • Separates the "pure" from the "impure"<br>• Controls fluid reabsorption<br>• Responsible for quality of Blood<br>• Proclaims Qi<br>• Protects spirit by filtering out negative input |
|---|---|
| **HEALTHY INDICATIONS** | • Confidence<br>• Appropriateness and sharp mindedness |
| **MENTAL SIGNS** | Poor mental assimilation<br>• Feeling of mental deficiency due to inability to assimilate Ideas<br>• Insecurity |
| **EXCESS/FULLNESS** | • Small intestine organ disorders<br>• Pain, discomfort or abnormal sensations in lower abdomen<br>• Tenderness in hypogastric area<br>• Pain at temples and sides of neck<br>• Flaccidity of arm muscles and joints, especially elbows<br>• Cystitis, urethritis<br>• Over-confidence, delusions |
| **EMPTINESS/ DEFICIENCY** | • Swelling and nodules<br>• Hemicrania/Migraine<br>• Tinnitus; pain around ear<br>• Cystitis, urethritis<br>• Mental deficiency |
| **PRINCIPAL SYMPTOMS** | • Neck stiffness<br>• Tongue numbness<br>• Urethritis, cystitis and small intestine organs disorders |

*Table 1-30.* **YANG ORGANS: TRIPLE WARMER/FIRE**

| | |
|---|---|
| **FUNCTION** | • Regulates metabolism (water)<br>• Regulates basal temperature<br>• Helps communication among lower, middle and upper parts of body<br>  — Upper Warmer<br>  — mist/fog (water vapor)<br>  — Middle Warmer<br>  — foam (gruel)<br>  — Lower Warmer<br>     swamp/dregs (waste water)<br>• Associated with the parasympathetic nervous system |
| **HEALTHY INDICATIONS** | Balanced mental state |
| **MENTAL SIGNS** | • Poor elimination of harmful thoughts<br>• Emotional upsets caused by breaking of friendships or family relations<br>• Suspicion<br>• Anxiety |
| **PRINCIPAL SYMPTOMS** | • Abdominal distension; hardness and fullness lower abdomen<br>• Urinary difficulty or frequency<br>• Edema<br>• Pain behind ears, cheeks, neck and jaw or at posterior aspect of shoulder and upper arm |

*Table 1-31.* **YANG ORGANS: LARGE INTESTINE/METAL**

| | |
|---|---|
| **FUNCTION** | • Elimination<br>• Absorbs water<br>• Drains turbid, retains clear |
| **HEALTHY INDICATIONS** | • Appropriate sadness<br>• Cheerfulness |
| **MENTAL SIGNS WEAKNESS, DYSFUNCTION, ILLNESS** | • Sadness<br>• Grief<br>• Worry |
| **EXCESS/FULLNESS** | Heat and swelling along channel<br>• Dryness, thirst, dark urine<br>• Abdominal distention, dizziness, constipation |
| **EMPTINESS/DEFICIENCY** | • Coldness<br>• Borborygmus<br>• Diarrhea |
| **PRINCIPAL SYMPTOMS** | Stagnation of Qi in the Large Intestine produces:<br>• Spastic abdominal pain<br>• Constipation<br>• Alternating small stools and diarrhea |

*Table 1- 32.* **YANG ORGANS: GALL BLADDER/WOOD**

| FUNCTION | • Stores and secretes bile<br>• Provides expression through the sinews (ligaments, tendons and other soft tissues)<br>• Serves as the source of courage and initiative<br>• Responsible for proper judgment, clarity of vision, decision-making<br>• Controls circulation of the nourishing and protecting energies |
|---|---|
| HEALTHY INDICATIONS | Good judgment and confidence |
| MENTAL SIGNS WEAKNESS, DYSFUNCTION, ILLNESS | • Impulsive behavior<br>• Rashness of judgment<br>• Indecisiveness |
| FULLNESS/EXCESS | • Abdominal, head, shoulder discomfort or pain, lateral headache (especially right side)<br>• Muscular spasms<br>• Tinnitus<br>• Agitation, impulsiveness |
| EMPTINESS/ DEFICIENCY | • Wandering pains; pains and dysfunctions in sides of body, neck or head<br>• Weakness in muscles and tendons of legs<br>• Difficulty standing<br>• Chest pain<br>• Vertigo chills<br>• Insomnia<br>• Timidity, indecisiveness, excessive sighing |

*Table 1- 33.* **YANG ORGANS: STOMACH/EARTH**

| FUNCTION | • Receives and ripens food<br>• Serves the sense of taste<br>• Moves food and Qi downwards<br>• Regulates body flesh |
|---|---|
| HEALTHY INDICATIONS | • Balanced mental state |
| MENTAL SIGNS WEAKNESS, DYSFUNCTION, ILLNESS | • Bipolar mood disorder<br>• Erratic behavior<br>• Delusions |
| FULLNESS/EXCESS | • Painful, burning sensation in stomach<br>• Hunger, halitosis, mouth ulcers and bleeding of gums<br>• Vomiting and constipation<br>• Pains and cramps in legs<br>• Laud psychotic behavior; manic phase of bipolar mood disorder |
| EMPTINESS/DEFICIENCY | • Nausea<br>• Hiccough<br>• Loss of appetite<br>• Leg weakness<br>• Worry, obsessiveness; depressive phase of bipolar mood disorder |

# Diagnosis

OM diagnosis is accomplished through the Four Examinations: visual, audio-olfactory, inquiry and palpation.

## Visual Examination

Table 1-34 on page 64 and Table 1-35 on page 65 describe the visual examination. One of the most useful visual signs in OM diagnosis is the tongue. Each area of the tongue represents various Organs and/or regions of the body. Figure 1-17 depicts the areas of correspondence on the tongue.

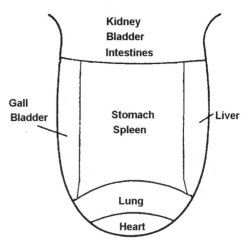

*Figure 1-17:* Areas of correspondence on the tongue.

## Audio-Olfactory Examination

Auscultation (listening) is part of the basic examination. The practitioner observes quality of voice and enunciation, verbal expression, respiration, cough, and breath.

- Loud, pressured speech often indicates Heat and/or Liver and Heart disorders.
- Unclear thinking may indicate Heart and Pericardium disorders, especially with phlegm.
- Weak enunciation and a dislike to talk may indicate deficiency, especially Lung Qi.
- Muttering to oneself often indicates Heart Qi deficiency.
- Stuttering suggests upward disturbance of Wind and Phlegm.
- A fast respiratory rate can indicate Heat or deficiency.
- A dry cough may indicate Dryness and deficiency of Yin.
- A rattling cough may indicate Phlegm and Dampness.
- Foul breath suggests pathogenic Heat in stomach, indigestion, tooth decay or unclean mouth.
- Foul offensive secretion or excretion usually indicates Heat syndrome.

- A stinking smell may indicate a Cold syndrome.

## Examination by Inquiry

The practitioner poses questions to the patient about his chief complaint and about temperature, perspiration, the head, the body, stools and micturation, diet, chest, hearing, thirst, and history of present and past illnesses. Table 1-36 on page 66 summarizes examination by inquiry.

## Examination by Palpation

During palpation the practitioner examines the radial pulse, skin, limbs, chest, abdomen, channels, Back Shu, Alarm (Mu) and Command points.

### Palpation: Radial Pulse

Palpation of the radial pulse is one of the most difficult and important aspects of OM diagnosis. Each of six positions has three depths and at least 28 qualities that

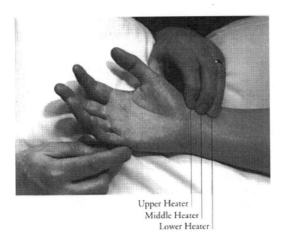

Upper Heater
Middle Heater
Lower Heater

*Figure 1-18:* OM radial pulse taking.

reflect different Organs or pathologies. Different areas around the radial pulse represent different regions and Organs in the body (Figure 1-18).

THE MOST IMPORTANT QUALITIES ARE PULSE RATE, DEPTH AND STRENGTH.

- A pulse that is quick, superficial and strong indicates a Yang condition.
- A pulse that is slow, deep and weak indicates a Yin condition.

IN MUSCULOSKELETAL PRACTICE THE MOST FRE-QUENTLY ENCOUNTERED PULSES ARE:

- *Tight* or *bowstring* in patient in pain from, Cold or Liver disorders.
- *Slippery* in patients with Dampness and Phlegm disorders.
- *Difficult/choppy* in patients with Blood stagnation and/or emptiness of Qi and Blood.
- *Floating* in patients with Wind and/or emptiness of Yin or Yang.

In the Classic of *Difficult Issues* different depths within the radial artery were said to represent various tissues and organs. The fifth difficult issue states:

The [movement in the] vessels may be light or heavy. What does that mean? It is like this. First one touches the vessel [at the inch-opening[2] by exerting a pressure] as heavy as three beans and one will reach the lung section on the [level of the] skin [and its] hair. If [one exerts a pressure] as heavy as six beans, one will reach the heart section on the [level of the] blood vessels. If [one exerts a pressure] as heavy as nine beans, one will reach the spleen section on the level of the flesh. If [one exerts a pressure] as heavy as twelve beans, one will reach the liver section on the level of the muscles. If one presses down to the bones and then lifts the fingers until a swift [movement of influences] arrives, [the level reached] is the kidneys [section]. Hence, one speaks of "light" and heavy".

The general qualities of the pulse can be assessed at the carotid artery as well. (For more information on pulse diagnosis, see the Meridian Therapy chapter 5.)

## Diagnostic Priorities

Since in OM diagnosis is established by the history and physical alone (with no lab work),[3] the practitioner must rely upon data collected through the five senses. Often patients present with conflicting information that must be prioritized.

THE FOLLOWING ARE GENERAL RULES THAT CAN AID IN THE DIAGNOSTIC PROCESS:

- Physical signs take prescience over symptoms.

- Information concerning the entire body takes precedence over data concerning any one part of the body.
  For example, patients with low tolerance to physical activity (become fatigued easily) are usually of a weak constitution type, even though they may look strong and muscular.

---

2. A location on the radial artery see meridian therapy for detail.

3. In modern times laboratory work is being incorporated increasingly into the OM paradigm.

• The condition of uppermost areas (head, upper back) take precedence over the condition of the lower parts.
For example, a patient with red complexion, and a feeling of warmth in the head, tight subcostals, with cold feet (a possible Cold sign), usually has a primary Heat or stagnation (Excess) disorder.

• The patient's general constitution is more important than any information concerning excretions and secretion.
For example, treatment of a weak patient (see abdominal diagnosis chapter 5) that also has yellow phlegm, and constipation, (a possible sign of Excess), is mostly by strengthening. Herbs that deal with Excess Heat may be added.

• Almost all chronic disorders are Internal conditions.

• Almost all acute disorders are External conditions.
However, acute abdominal disorders for example, usually are Internal or mixed conditions.

• In the presence of both Dampness and Dryness, Dampness usually is treated first.

*Table 1-34.* VISUAL EXAMINATION GENERAL

| | |
|---|---|
| **OBSERVATION OF SPIRIT** | Brightness of eyes, facial expression, clarity of speech, coordination, alertness. A patient who has spirit is fundamentally healthy; the prognosis is good |
| **OBSERVATION OF BODY** | **Complexion, Skin Color** <br> • Red— Heat <br>   — Malar flush with bright red color—empty Heat <br> • White—Cold and/or deficiency <br>   — Lusterless, pale with swelling—Qi deficiency <br>   — Emaciated face—Blood deficiency <br> • Cyan/Bluish <br>   — Stagnation <br>   — Cold <br>   — pain <br>   — convulsion <br> • Yellow—Dampness, Spleen deficiency <br>   — Flabby—Damp accumulation due to Spleen failure of transportation transformation <br>   — Jaundice, orange yellow or bright—Damp Heat <br>   — Jaundice, dark—Cold Damp <br> • Black, Gray—Kidney deficiency, Essence depletion, Blood Stasis, Phlegm accumulation <br>   — Deep in color and withered—serious disease with damage to Qi and Essence <br>   — Dark gray around eyes—Phlegm due to Kidney deficiency <br> **Weight** <br> • Excessive weight results in dampness. <br> • Excessive leanness is often due to Yin Emptiness or Spleen and Stomach weakness <br> **General condition** <br> • Muscular indicates a strong (Yang) constitution. <br> • Weak muscles indicate a weak (Yin) constitution |

*Table 1-35.* **VISUAL EXAMINATION TONGUE**

| | |
|---|---|
| **TONGUE** | Reflects the state of Qi and Blood, progression and location of disease, degree of Cold and Heat, depth of penetration of exogenous pathogens, condition of organs |
| **TONGUE FORM (BODY)** | **Enlargement.** A swollen, enlarged Tongue indicates Qi deficiency/emptiness or Water-Damp condition. Seen in edema, digestive disorders, chronic nephritis and other chronic illness. Swollen, enlarged Tongue is due to hyperplasia of connective tissue, tissue edema, or blood and lymphatic drainage disturbances |
| | **Shrinkage.** A thin, shrunken tongue indicates Yin Liquid deficiency/emptiness |
| | **Speckles and Prickles (elevated papillae, or flakes of fur on papillae).** Indicate excess Heat. Occurs in patients suffering from constipation, insomnia and lung and other infections |
| | **Fissures.** May indicate fluid depletion and conditions that affect the Spleen and Stomach; however, this condition also may be normal |
| | **Mirror (Shiny Tongue).** Seen in Yin/Humor/Fluid Depletion |
| **TONGUE MOVEMENT** | **Trembling.** Often seen in diseases such as Wind, Hyperactivity of Liver Yang, excess Heat, Qi deficiency/emptiness |
| | **Stiffness (Wry).** Seen in serious diseases such as Wind-Strike (stroke), Heat in the Pericardium, diseases of the sea of marrow (brain) |
| **TONGUE COLOR** | Pale                deficiency/emptiness, hypofunction, cold<br>Red                 Heat<br>Purple           Stagnation |
| **TONGUE FUR** | **General indications**<br>Slimy                Damp, Phlegm and digestate accumulation<br>Peeling, patchy   Yin Insufficiency or emptiness of Stomach Qi<br>White               Cold<br>Yellow            Heat<br>Black             abundant pathogen |

*Table 1- 36.* **EXAMINATION BY INQUIRY**

| TOPIC | INDICATION |
|---|---|
| Aversion to cold with fever | **At beginning of disease indicates Exterior syndrome**<br>• If with thirst and perspiration due to Heat |
| High fever without chills | May be due to exogenous pathogenic chill penetrating the Interior<br>Or Interior Heat |
| Tidal fever | **Yin deficiency**<br>• Usually in afternoon or night<br>**Yang Ming Heat**<br>• Usually start at dusk with constipation and abdominal distension |
| Alternating chills and fever | May indicates pathogenic factors are between Internal and External |
| Perspiration | • Exterior syndrome without sweat indicate Cold, with sweat indicate Heat<br>• Night sweat usually indicate Yin deficiency<br>• Spontaneous sweating usually indicate Qi or Yang deficiency<br>• Profuse sweating with night fever usually indicate internal Heat<br>• Dripping with severe weakness can be from total collapse of Yang<br>• In head may be from Heat in upper Warmer or Wet Heat in middle Warmer |
| Appetite | • No appetite usually indicate Spleen dysfunction<br>• No appetite with chest fullness usually indicate Phlegm<br>• Repulsion to food usually indicate food stagnation<br>• Excessive appetite usually indicate Stomach Heat<br>• Hunger, but unable to eat, usually indicate Stomach Yin deficiency<br>• Craving for dirt usually indicate pestilence disease |
| Thirst | **Generally indicate the condition of the body fluid**<br>**Excessive thirst may indicate:**<br>• Consumption of Yin or stagnation of the body fluids which fail to rise to the upper warmer<br>• Heat syndromes<br>• Extreme thirst with preference for hot drinks can indicate a Phlegm obstruction<br>• High fever, thirst, but patient can not drink, can indicate pathogenic factors in the Nourishing Qi and Blood |
| Taste | • Bitter taste in mouth usually indicate Heat, especially in Liver and Gall Bladder<br>• Sweet taste in mouth usually indicate Damp Heat in the Spleen and Stomach<br>• Sour taste in mouth usually indicate accumulation of Heat in Liver and Stomach<br>• Tastelessness in the mouth usually indicates dysfunction in Spleen |
| Hearing | **In general related to Kidney health**<br>• Acute tinnitus often due to Heat in Gall Bladder or Triple Warmer<br>• Chronic tinnitus often related to Kidney |

*Table 1- 36.* **EXAMINATION BY INQUIRY (CONTINUED)**

| TOPIC | INDICATION |
|---|---|
| Stool | • Dry stool shaped like sheep-dung usually indicate stagnation of Heat or fluid exhaustion<br>• Loose bowels following a dry stool usually indicate dysfunction of the Spleen and Stomach with imbalance of Dryness and Dampness<br>• Alternating dry and loose stools usually indicate Liver Qi stagnation and Spleen weakness<br>• Watery stools with undigested food usually indicate Yang deficiency of Kidney and Spleen<br>• Diarrhea with yellow burning anus usually indicate Damp Heat<br>• Formed stool with undigested food and foul smell usually indicate food stagnation<br>• Tarry (black) stool usually indicate hemorrhaging in the Spleen and Stomach (Intestines)<br>• Mild prolapse of anus during bowel movements may be due to chronic diarrhea and Spleen Qi deficiency<br>• Tenesmus usually is a sign of Qi stagnation or Damp Heat<br>• Irregular habit often is caused by Liver failing to regulate the Spleen and Stomach<br>• Diarrhea soon after abdominal distension and pain, which than relieves the pain, usually indicate food stagnation<br>• Abdominal pain not relieved by bowel movements can be due to Spleen deficiency and Liver over-controlling Spleen (Wood attack Earth) |
| Urine | • Deep yellow urine usually indicate Heat<br>• Clear and profuse urine usually indicate Cold<br>• Turbid or a mixture of urine and sperm may indicate Damp Heat<br>• Brownish urine may indicate Heat damage to Blood vessels<br>• Increased urine volume usually indicate Kidney Qi deficiency<br>• Decreased urine volume is caused by consumption of body fluid or by dysfunction of Qi<br>• Dribbling or retention of urine can indicate exhaustion of Kidney Qi or Damp Heat<br>• Stabbing pain accompanied by urgency and burning indicates Damp Heat<br>• Pain after urination usually indicate Kidney weakness<br>• Nocturnal urination is usually caused by Kidney Qi deficiency |

*Table 1- 36.* **EXAMINATION BY INQUIRY (CONTINUED)**

| TOPIC | INDICATION |
|---|---|
| Pain | **Wandering pain**<br>• Mostly from Wind<br>**Pain with Heaviness**<br>• Mostly from Dampness<br>**Severe pain**<br>• Often from Cold<br>**Pain with redness and swelling**<br>• Mostly from Damp Heat<br>**Pain and distension**<br>• Mostly Qi stagnation<br>**Pain aggravated by pressure**<br>• Mostly excess condition<br>**Pain alleviated by pressure**<br>• Mostly deficiency condition<br>Vague pain<br>• Mostly Blood deficiency and Chong channel disorder<br>**Headache**<br>• Occipital referring to the nape and upper back—Tai Yang channel<br>• Frontal referring to supraorbital ridge—Yang Ming channel<br>• Temporal—Shao Yang channel<br>• Vertex—Jue Yin channel<br>• With teeth pain—Shao Yin channel invaded by Cold<br>**Chest**<br>• Mostly obstruction of Phlegm and Blood with Qi stagnation<br>**Hypochondriac**<br>• Mostly by obstruction or dysfunction of the Liver and Gall Bladder<br>**Epigastric**<br>• Mostly by disorders of the Stomach<br>**Abdominal**<br>• Lower lateral pain mostly by Liver Qi stagnation, intestinal obsess (appendicitis) or hernia<br>• Umbilical pain mostly by parasites, food stagnation, constipation, and Spleen or Large intestine disorders<br>• Lower abdominal pain and distension mostly by Urinary disorders. If without urinary symptoms mostly by food stagnation<br>**Low back**<br>• Mostly by Kidney deficiency, Cold Damp painful Obstruction, or Blood stagnation<br>**Limbs**<br>• Mostly by painful Obstruction syndromes (Bi) |
| Sleep | **Insomnia**<br>• With palpitations, dreams and nervousness mostly by Heart Blood deficiency<br>• With restlessness of mind, and difficulty falling asleep mostly by Yin deficiency<br>• With bitter taste, vomiting, irritability and difficulty falling asleep mostly by Phlegm Fire<br>• Restless mind during sleep often due to Stomach dysfunction<br>**Hypersomnia**<br>• Mostly Qi deficiency caused by chronic disease, or failure of Spleen Yang to rise<br>• Exogenous pathogenic factors |

*Table 1- 36.* **EXAMINATION BY INQUIRY (CONTINUED)**

| TOPIC | INDICATION |
|---|---|
| Menstruation and Leukorrhea | • Early menses with red colored blood may indicate Heat |
| | • Early menses with light-colored blood may indicate Qi and Blood deficiency |
| | • Late menses with dark purple blood and pain mostly indicate Cold |
| | • Late menses with scanty light-colored blood mostly indicate Blood deficiency |
| | • Irregular menses mostly indicate Liver Qi stagnation |
| | • Amenorrhea may be caused by pregnancy, Blood stasis, Blood exhaustion, consumptive diseases and Liver Qi stagnation |
| | • Heavy flow is mostly due to Heat, if with dark purple blood, clots and pain may indicate deficiency of Penetrating (Chong) and Conception (Ren) channels or sinking of Central Qi (Spleen Qi) |

# Chapter 2: *Pain*

The complementary approach to musculoskeletal medicine combines the benefits of western science with principles and techniques developed throughout the world. Complementary methods have significant benefit to patients, some of whom have not responded to traditional approaches. This section summarizes some biomedical principals that are important for the application of this approach. The chapter presents a brief review of basic concepts and builds on information gradually, so that practitioners with limited western science training, and scientifically trained practitioners, can follow and benefit.

## Pain: The Most Common Complaint

Pain—a sensation in which a person experiences discomfort, distress, or suffering—is the most common complaint with which patients present to the doctor. For the family physician, the incidence of patients who request treatment for back pain is second only to that of patients whose complaint is a common cold. Some 40% of the American population (and of the populations of other industrialized countries) is afflicted with acute or chronic pain that requires medical management. Inadequate management and out-and-out mismanagement of these patients is common (Bonica 1990).

Musculoskeletal pain may occur due to:

• Injury.

• Unsound posture and uncoordinated movements.

• Mechanical stresses to soft tissue from dislocation of bony structures or other restrictions of tissue motions.

• Muscular imbalances.

• Inflammatory processes from acute trauma, immune dysfunctions, metabolic and repetitive injuries such as tendinitis and degenerative conditions.

• Abnormal neurological self-regulation (facilitated segment, neuropathy, psychological and neuropsychological).

• (Possibly) environmental factors such as Wind-Wet.

These disorders are usually accompanied by some degree of mechanical dysfunction, degenerative conditions such as ligament and tendon insufficiency, fibrosis, and myotendinosis in muscles or other tissues. Injury can cause sensory, motor, and/or autonomic dysfunctions in the corresponding dermatome, myotome and sclerotomes. Neoplastic and other medical diseases must be kept in mind, since they can result in pain that seems to have musculoskeletal origin.

# Neural Mechanisms of Pain

A complex experience in which psychological factors play a critical role, pain can even influence the sensory transmission processes, i.e., it can change the circuitry in the nervous system.

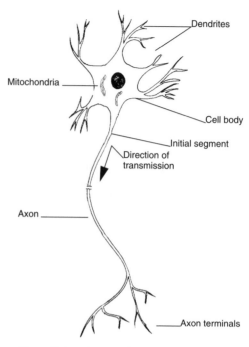

Figure 2-1:    Axon and processes.

## Basic Elements of the Nervous System

In order to consider the neural mechanisms of pain, the practitioner must have a fundamental understanding of the nervous system. The basic functional and structural component is the *neuron*, which receives information, processes it, and sends it to other neurons. A neuron is composed of a cell body (like all normal cells) and its processes, a single *axon*, and one or more—often several more—*dendrites* (Figure 2-1).

An axon is the process of a neuron by which impulses travel away from the cell body. A dendrite is a tree-like, branched process of a neuron. Dendrites conduct impulses to the cell body from the axons of other neurons. Dendrites are believed to produce graded electrical responses, in contrast to the all-or-nothing responses produced by the axon and cell body. At the other end of the axon (away from the cell body) are terminals called *synaptic bulbs*. These are buttons or knobs that form a functional connection to other nerve cells (to the cell body or to the dendrites of the next neuron) through *synaptic transmission*. Information travels down an axon by a *nerve impulse* (also called *action potential*), an all-or-nothing response. A nerve impulse is created by depolarization of the axon, which is caused by the inflow of sodium ions across the cell membrane from the outside to the inside, giving the inside of the membrane a positive charge. When triggered at the origin of the axon, the information travels all of the way down the axon. The amount of stimulation needed to initiate a nerve impulse reaction in the axon is called the *threshold*

Many characteristics give a neuron its identity or phenotype. These include its shape, location, the type(s) of transmitters and neuropeptides it produces and uses to communicate with other neurons, the cell with which it forms connections (both presynaptic and postsynaptic), and the types of receptors it bears on its cell surface to "hear" what other neurons have to say (Koslow et al. 1995).

Abnormalities in, or loss of, communication between neurons result in neurological disorders such as Alzheimer's disease, Parkinson's disease, amyotropic lateral sclerosis (ALS), and congenital epilepsy.

### The Synapses

*Synapses* are functional connections between nerve cells. They are located between the synaptic bulbs and the adjacent target nerve fibers, often a dendrite

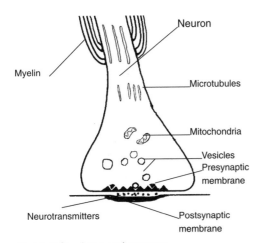

*Figure 2-2:* Axon and synapse

of the next cell. The bulb of the source nerve is covered by a membrane called the *presynaptic membrane*. The membrane of the adjacent neuron at the synapse, called the *postsynaptic membrane*, contains receptor sites for chemicals released from vesicles in the bulb (Figure 2-2). Synapses are among the most abundant structures in the brain, estimates suggest that a mammalian brain may contain $10^{15}$ (Koslow et al. 1995).

Synaptic transmission occurs across the thin synaptic space between the two neurons via the release of these chemicals, called *neurotransmitters*. The neurotransmitter diffuses within the synapse and binds to its receptor, a large protein embedded in the membrane of the receiving neuron. Some examples of neurotransmitters are epinephrine, norepinephrine, serotonin, acetylcholine, histamine, dopamine, and even some amino acids such as Gamma-aminobutyric acid (BABA) and glycine. This chemical release is initiated by the nerve impulse (action potential) travelling down the axon to the bulb.

Neurotransmitter substances may be inhibitory or excitatory, and therefore may either promote or inhibit nerve impulses. When enough synaptic excitation occurs to reach the threshold, the *sodium gate* opens. (A sodium gate is a gate in the membrane of the nerve that keeps

the sodium outside until the threshold is reached). The opening of this gate causes the interior of the membrane to be charged more positively than the outside of the membrane, and it initiates a nerve impulse in the axon. However, if synaptic inhibition occurs, the cell membrane becomes more negatively charged, often by opening some chloride channels in the cell membrane. This prevents the membrane from reaching the threshold (Waxman and deGroot 1985). Recently neurotransmitters have been shown capable of triggering gene expression providing a means by which neuronal activity can produce long-term changes in the activity at a synapse (Koslow et al. 1995).

Other modes of chemical-mediated communication between cells include dendrite release of chemical transmitters and the recently discovered systems involving small, soluble gases such as nitric oxide whose mode of action is still unclear (Koslow et al. 1995).

The synapses are probably the most important part of the system that regulates transmission across neurons. Their regulatory effect is achieved by (Ornstein and Thompson 1984):

• Directing the direction of transmission.

• Allowing for facilitation and inhibition.

• Creating summation by allowing weak and repetitive stimuli (subthreshold) to produce an accumulation of chemical transmitters, which eventually leads to a level equal to the threshold.

• Creating a synaptic delay due to the time it takes to release neurotransmitters.

• Causing fatigue due to neurotransmitter depletion.

• Allowing for the action of drugs [or acupuncture], on the secretion, removal and blocking of neurotransmitters.

Recent information has shown that neuronal and synaptic transmission do not follow linear models. It is not unusual for a neuron to receive thousands of synaptic inputs arising from diverse sources in the central nervous system. These effects will not be the same from moment to moment. Such non-linearity gives neurons integrative and computational capabilities previously unimagined. Retrograde[1] transmission as been documented as well (Koslow et al. 1995).

**PRESYNAPTIC INHIBITION.** Binding of neurotransmitters to axo-axonic synapses (the receptors that mediate presynaptic inhibition) leads to a reduction in the amount of neurotransmitter liberated by the postsynaptic axon. Presynaptic inhibition provides a mechanism by which the "gain" at a particular synaptic input to a neuron can be lowered without reducing the efficacy of other synapses that might impinge on that neuron (Waxman, deGroot 1995).

## Types of Nerve Fibers

Nerve fibers can be *myelinated* (laminated) or *unmyelinated* (unlaminated). Myelinated nerve fibers are surrounded by *Schwann cells* (a type of fatty glial cell), which wrap the nerve tightly in a multilayered structure, called a myelin sheath, that serves as an electrical insulator. Unmyelinated nerves do not have this sheath. Myelinated nerves—one of the nerve types in the peripheral nervous system—are fast conductors of information.

Nerve fibers are divided by their fiber diameters, conduction velocities and physiologic characteristics. The three categories of nerve fibers (A, B and C fibers) each have several subtypes.

Nociceptors (pain receptors) belong to A-*delta* and C afferents that are equipped in the periphery with receptors that are sensitive to noxious or potentially-noxious mechanical and chemical stimuli. Pain receptors are divided into three categories, each of which is activated by different mechanisms and is made of different fiber types (Table 2-1).

1. Transmission going in the other direction.

*Table 2-1.* **TYPES OF NOCICEPTORS**

| | |
|---|---|
| MECHANICAL | Mechanoreceptors, activated by mechanical stimulation. |
| THERMAL | Activated by injuries induced by thermal input of approximately $45^0$ Celsius and higher. |
| POLYMODAL | C fiber nociceptors, a catch-all for all other nociceptive signals. Also can respond to mechanical and thermal stimulation. |

### A-Fibers

A-fibers which are large, somatic and myelinated, are fast conductors. They:

- Act as proprioceptors (respond to stimulation within the body itself and function as sensors of posture and equilibrium).
- Provide motor supply to muscle spindles (see muscle spindle in this chapter).
- Receive pain, temperature, touch and pressure sensations.

### A-Delta Fibers

A-Delta fibers also called *high-threshold mechanoreceptors*, are medium-diameter (1-5 $\mu$m in diameter) fibers that connect A-fiber nociceptors (pain sensors) to the dorsal horns of the spinal cord. In muscles, A-delta fibers are called *type III receptors*. Pain from A-delta fibers is felt as a local sharp, and relatively brief pain. Found mostly just under the skin, these fibers transmit messages principally from the skin and mucous membrane. They are important for superficial acupuncture stimulation.

### A-Alpha Fibers

A-Alpha fibers are large (12-20 $\mu$m in diameter) and conduct at a rate of 70-120 meters per second. They function as proprioceptors, and they innervate the muscle spindles, annulospiral endings and golgi tendon organs (see muscles this chapter).

In muscles these fibers are known as *type I receptors*.

### A-Beta Fibers

A-Beta fibers are low-threshold mechanoreceptors found in skin, muscle, tendons and joints. These fibers are connected to the dorsal horns of the spinal cord via large-diameter, A-beta, myelinated fibers 5-15 μm in diameter. Relatively fast conductors, they conduct at a velocity of 30-120 meters per second. In muscles they are known *type II receptors*.

### B-Fibers

B-fibers are smaller, autonomic, myelinated fibers—are fast conductors that are slower than A-fibers and that function as preganglionic sympathetic fibers (see sympathetic system this chapter).

### C-Fibers

C-fibers also known as C-polymodal nociceptors, are found everywhere in the body except the brain. They carry pain signals from peripheral cells, transmitting messages from deep tissues and from the skin and mucous membrane, as well. These unmyelinated fibers measure 0.25-1.5 μm in diameter, the smallest of the nerve fibers. C fibers are the slowest conductors, with conduction velocity rates of 0.5-2 meters per second. (Some C fibers are thought to be very slow, taking up to five seconds to conduct from the foot to the cord). They:

- Function as pain fibers.

- Function in reflex responses.

- Are also postganglionic sympathetic fibers.

- Are known in muscles as *type IV fibers*.

- Are activated by mechanical, thermal or chemical stimuli.

When stimulated electrically, C fibers can produce pain. Pain in deep tissues felt as a deep-seated, ill-defined and widespread ache (such as seen in sclerotomal and myotomal pain), is produced by stimulation of C fibers. Gunn (1977) has demonstrated that painful stimuli from muscles have implicated muscle fiber types III and IV.

Researchers have shown that cutaneous nerves have more than four times the number of small-diameter, A-delta and C fibers than larger, myelinated A-beta fibers (Ochoa and Mair 1969). Kruger, McMahon and Kolzenbug posit that this occurs because, apart from their function of pain transmission, nociceptors serve several other regulatory and trophic functions, such as regulating:

- Blood flow and vascular permeability in both visceral and somatic tissues.

- Trophic functions such as maintenance and repair of skin integrity.

- Immunological processes, such as emigration of leukocytes at sites of tissue injury (OM: *Defensive Qi circulates largely in the skin*).

- Activity of autonomic ganglia and visceral smooth muscle.

The very slow-conducting C fibers may explain in part the "Ta Qi Phenomenon" (needling sensation) of acupuncture, which is also slow conducting.

## Brain

The brain (Figure 2-3) is composed of neurons and glia[2] and their specific interactions with one another. It can be categorized as having a brain stem, cerebellum, limbic system, and cerebrum. Unlike other organs which are composed of a relatively homogenous population of cells, the brain is diverse.

---

2. Glia is the non-nervous or supporting tissue of the brain and spinal cord.

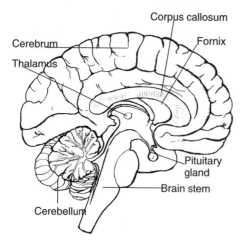

Cerebrum

Thalamus

Corpus callosum

Fornix

Pituitary gland

Brain stem

Cerebellum

*Figure 2-3:* Brain.

the spinal cord and to the central nuclei related to cranial nerves (Waxman and deGroot 1995).

CLINICAL DEFICIT. Lesions in the brainstem result primarily in sensory loss (proprioception, discriminative touch and vibratory sense) from the body and face; loss of motor control (spastic paralysis, also called ataxia) in the limbs; loss of pain and temperature sensations from the body and face; loss of hearing or balance; loss of speech (dysphagia) and swallowing (dysarthria); paralysis of the tongue; heart arrhythmias; dyspnea; and/or coma and death (Willard 1993).

## Brain Stem

The brain stem, thought to be the oldest part of the brain ontogenically (500 million years), resembles the entire brain of a reptile. Giving rise to 10 of the 12 pairs of cranial nerves, it determines the general level of alertness and warns the organism of important incoming information; directs attention to specific events; and handles basic bodily functions such as respiratory and heart rates (Ornstein and Thompson 1984). Often involved in post-traumatic injuries, the brain stem is also implicated in chronic pain syndromes that involve the cranial nerves, which in part innervate shoulder and neck muscles. Osteopathic functional techniques may be effective in treating such injuries (Ward 1995).

RETICULAR SYSTEM. The reticular system is a diffusely-organized neural apparatus that extends through the central region of the brainstem into the subthalamus and the intralaminar nuclei of the thalamus.[3] A complex system that occupies a large portion of the brainstem, the reticular structure has major ascending sensory tracts to the cerebrum and cerebellum, and descending (reticulospinal) motor tracts to

## Cerebellum

The cerebellum, which is attached to the rear of the brain stem, is mainly involved with the motor system and with maintaining posture, balance and skeletal muscle function. It maintains, adjusts and directs the coordination of muscular movement, and it stores memories for simple, learned responses (Ornstein and Thompson *ibid*).

CLINICAL DEFICIT. Lesions in the cerebellum can result in coma and death; loss of primary sensory modalities (vibratory sense, discriminative touch, and proprioception) and loss of pain and temperature sensations from the body and face; abnormal motor control (ataxia and paralysis); eye movement dysfunction; and decerebrate posturing, with the upper and lower limbs going into extreme, extensor-dominated positions (Willard 1985).

3. The thalamus is a pair of oval shaped organs forming most of the lateral walls of the third ventricle of the brain and part of the diencephalon. The diencephalon is the division of the brain between the cerebrum and mesencephalon. Consisting of the hypothalamus, thalamus, metathalamus and epithalamus.

## Cerebrum

The cerebrum, the largest part of the human brain, is divided into hemispheres that each control a side of the body. The two hemispheres are connected by the corpus callosum, a band of some three hundred million nerve cell fibers.

The cerebral cortex, which is thought to have evolved some 200 million years ago, has several lobes: frontal, temporal, parietal and occipital. The cortex allows humans to organize, remember, communicate, understand, appreciate and create (Ornstein and Thompson *ibid*).

**LONG TERM POTENTIATION (LTP).** LPT is a mechanism by which short-term memory is converted to long-term memory, as a result of frequent stimulation. It was observed first at synapses in the hippocampus,[4] which may play a role in associative learning. In early stages of development and in primitive mammals, the hippocampus is located anteriorly and constitutes part of the outer mantle of the brain. The hippocampus is involved in converting short-term memory of up to 60 minutes to long-term memory of several days or more. The anatomic substrates for long-term memory probably include the temporal lobes as well (Waxman and deGroot 1985). Studies on LPT suggest that postsynaptic neuron may release one or more diffusible substances, so-called retrograde transmitters, that affect the presynaptic neuron. In other words, LTP is initiated by events that occur in the postsynaptic neuron. The presynaptic neuron then undergoes some change that perpetuates the phenomenon. Opioid peptides may serve as retrograde inhibitory transmitters. LTP currently is the most compelling model in the mammalian brain for a neural mechanism related to

---

4. The hippocampus is an elevation of the floor of the lateral ventricle of the brain. It is an important component of the limbic system and its efferent projections form the fornix of the cerebrum. The fornix is nerve fibers that lie beneath the corpus callosum (band of fibers that connect the two cerebrum hemispheres).

learning and memory (Koslow et al. 1995).

A speculative possibility as to why acupuncture reports from China are more positive than reports from the west is that in China treatment is given daily and therefore may provoke *LTP like* mechanisms.

**CLINICAL DEFICIT.** Clinical deficit ranges from specific sensory and motor losses to alterations of cognitive functions such as language, speech, writing, reading; and to changes in awareness, social mores, memory, or consciousness. Damage to the subcortical structures can result in memory loss, aberrant emotional behavior, personality changes; and movement disorders such as hyperkinesia or hypokinesia (Willard 1985).

## Limbic System

The limbic system, a group of cellular structures rather than a single brain region, is located between the brain stem and the cortex. It interconnects structures within the cerebrum, frontal lobe, temporal lobe, thalamus, hypothalamus, and circuitous neuron pathways that connect all parts. The limbic system, which contains the hypothalamus and the pituitary gland, is involved in many of the body's self-regulating systems and is strongly involved in the emotional reactions that have to do with survival (Ornstein and Thompson *ibid*).

## The Brain & Pain

Although researchers have identified several spinal-supraspinal tracts that are involved in transmission of pain, current data suggests that nociception is not related solely to a unique or exclusive system of pathways. Several neurons within a number of reticular, cortical and diencephalic structures are responsive to noxious stimulation and are not associated with these tracts (Wall *ibid*). Axons from the thalamic nuclei, which ascend to the cerebral cortex, have been defined as three

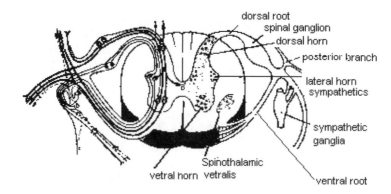

dorsal root
spinal ganglion
dorsal horn
posterior branch
lateral horn
sympathetics
sympathetic
ganglia
ventral root
Spinothalamic
vetral horn  vetralis

*Figure 2-4:*  Spinal cord and nerve roots.

thalamocortical projections, each of which relates to a different aspect of pain (Table 2-2). (Melzack, Casey *ibid*; Hand, Morrison 1970; Desijaru, Purpura 1970; Newcombe 1972).

## Spinal Cord

The spinal cord (Figure 2-4) is an intricate core with complex circuitry and biochemistry that receives sensation and routs motor signals and reflexes. This system is important in pain perception and modulation, and in integration of sensory, motor, central and sympathetic signals. The spinal cord has two horns, with laminae that have specialized functions.

### Spinal Cord Core

Each segment of the spinal cord has an inner column of gray matter that contains nerve cell bodies, and an outer sheath of white matter. A cross-section of the spinal cord reveals a central, H-shaped area. Table 2-3 and Figure 2-4 on page 79 lists sections of the H-shaped area, and the areas and/or functions they affect.

*Table 2-2.*  **THALAMOCORTICAL PROJECTIONS AND RELATED ASPECTS OF PAIN**

| PROJECTION | TERMINATION | ASPECT OF PAIN |
|---|---|---|
| 1 | Superior paracentral of cortex | Perception (localization) |
| 2 | Frontal lobe | Emotion |
| 3 | Ipsilateral temporal lobe | Recent and long-term memory |

*Table 2-3.*  **SPINAL CORD CORE**

| Section | Location | Affected System |
|---|---|---|
| Dorsal Horn | Posterior | Processing of sensory information from <br>• somata <br>• viscera (internal organs) |
| Ventral Horn | Anterior | Motor system |
| Intermediary Region | Between the dorsal and ventral horns | Formed by interneurons linking the <br>• sensory system (from dorsal horn) <br>• suprasegmental system (brain) <br>• motor system |

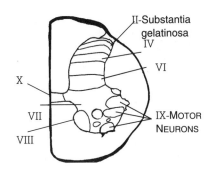

*Figure 2-5:* Spinal cord laminae (After Willard).

THE CORE SPINAL LAMINAE. Bror Rexed discusses the core spinal segments in terms of laminae of the neural tube. This tube gives rise to neurons that compose the sensory nuclei of the spinal cord and the brainstem. Each lamina organizes connections. Some neurons, such as at laminae I and V (which contribute significantly to perception of pain), cross to the contralateral side and ascend to the brain. At lamina V, somatic and visceral input converge with fibers that descend from the brain. Other laminae— II to III —integrate multiple segments without exiting the spine. Since incoming information converges, cells in these laminae contribute to referred pain (Willard *ibid*), (Figure 2-5).

Table 2-5 on page 80 summarizes functions of the laminae

*A-delta* nociceptive fibers terminate in laminae I and V. *C nociceptive* fibers terminate mainly in laminae I and II, and also in lamina III, where their axon terminals secrete substance P (Thompson 1988). Nociceptor sensory *C* fibers enter the spinal cord, where they divide into short, descending and ascending branches. Some of the sensory nociceptor fibers cross the cord to the contralateral side and form the anterolateral spinal tract. This anterolateral tract, called the *spinothalamic tract*, connects the basal spinal nucleus with the thalamic nuclei (Willard *ibid*).

SPINAL INNERVATION. The spinal cord receives approximately 31 pairs of spinal nerves. Each pair of nerves has a ventral and a dorsal root, made up of 1-8 rootlets. A spinal segment is defined by the level at which an associated nerve enters the cord. One segmental level can innervate more than one type of tissue. For example, dermatome, myotome and sclerotome receive their innervation from the same segmental level, the nerve root. However, conscious perceptions of sensation from these tissues do not overlap and may be separated by considerable distance see Figure 2-6 on page 81 and Figure 2-7 on page 81 (Willard *ibid*).

*Table 2-4.* CORE BRAIN SEGMENTS AND NEURAL TUBE LAMINAE

| CORE SEGMENT | LAMINA(E) | ARRANGEMENT |
|---|---|---|
| Dorsal Horn | I to VI | Posterior to anterior |
| Ventral Horn | VIII to IX | Posterior to anterior |
| Intermediary | VII | Between ventral and dorsal |
| Auxiliary Column of Cells | X | Concentrated around central canal |

*Table 2-5.* **SPINAL CORD LAMINA** (WAXMAN AND DEGROOT 1995)

| | |
|---|---|
| **LAMINA I** | A thin marginal layer<br>• Contains neurons that respond to noxious stimuli |
| **LAMINA II** | Also called *substantia gelatinosa*<br>• Made up of small neurons, some of which respond to noxious stimuli |
| **LAMINAE III-IV** | Known together as *nucleus proprius*<br>• Main input from fibers that convey position and light-touch senses |
| **LAMINA V** | Contains cells that respond to noxious and visceral afferent stimuli |
| **LAMINA VI** | Deepest layer of dorsal horn<br>• Contains neurons that respond to mechanical signals from joints and skin |
| **LAMINA VII** | Large zone that contains<br>• cells of dorsal nucleus medially<br>• large portion of the ventral gray column<br>• intermediolateral nucleus in thoracic and upper lumbar regions<br>• preganglionic sympathetic fibers that project to sympathetic ganglia<br>Dorsal nucleus contains cells that give rise to posterior spinocerebellar tract |
| **LAMINAE VIII AND IX** | Motor neuron groups in medial and lateral portions of ventral gray column<br>• Medial portion contains lower motor neurons that innervate axial musculature<br>• Lateral motor neuron column contains lower motor neurons that innervate distal muscles of arm and leg<br>Flexor muscles are innervated by motor neurons located centrally in the ventral horn, close to the central canal<br>Extensor muscles are innervated by motor neurons located more peripherally |
| **LAMINA X** | Represents small neurons around central canal or its remnants |

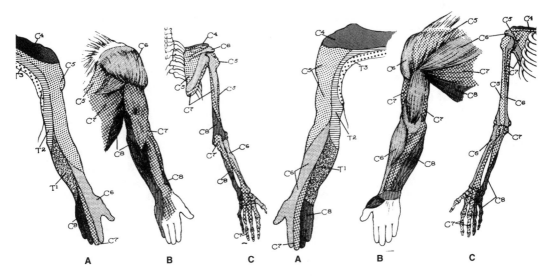

*Figure 2-6:* Segmental innervation: A—Dermatome, B—Myotome, C—Sclerotome (Reproduced with permission, Inman VT. Referred pain from skeletal structures J Nerv Ment Dis 99:660, 1944).

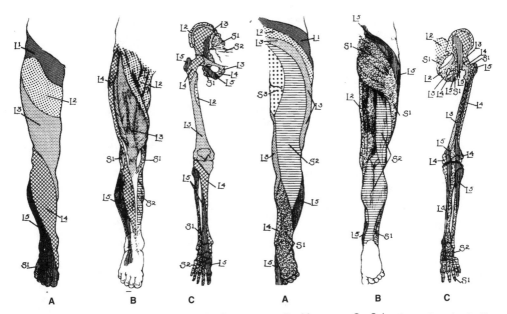

*Figure 2-7:* Segmental innervation: A—Dermatome, B—Myotome, C—Sclerotome (Reproduced with permission, Inman VT. Referred pain from skeletal structures J Nerv Ment Dis 99:660, 1944).

## Innervation: Dorsal Horn

The dorsal roots (except C1) contain afferent (sensory) fibers from the nerve cells in their ganglia. The roots also contain a variety of fibers from cutaneous and deep structures. Most of the axons in the dorsal nerve roots are small C-unmyelinated fibers and A-delta myelinated fibers that carry information about noxious and thermal stimuli. The dorsal roots also contain large A-alpha fibers that come from muscle spindles, and medium-size A-bata fibers that come from mechanoreceptors in skin and joints (Waxman and deGroot 1985).

Once thought to be a simple relay station, the dorsal horn is a complex, medullary core. The intricate circuitry of the dorsal horn includes diverse types of neurons and synaptic connections that have prolific biochemistry. These aspects of the dorsal horn make possible, not only reception and transmission of nociceptive (pain) input, but also sensory processing, such as integration of several signals, selection of signals from numerous signals, abstraction (removal) of particular signals, and appropriate dispersion of sensory impulses. This complex local processing is activated by:

- Central convergence. The coming together of several sensory receptors on one or few motor neurons.

- Central summation. Cumulative action of stimuli.

- Excitatory and inhibitory influences that come from the periphery, local interneurons and the brain (Bonica 1990).

The functional state of the dorsal horn varies according to the circumstances of somatosensory involvement. The dorsal horn can function in a:

- Normal control state.

- Suppressed state.
  A higher threshold of pain is achieved by descending inhibition (commonly seen acute in athletic injuries).

- Sensitized state.
  A low threshold to pain.

Sensitization of the dorsal horn can occur following peripheral tissue injury or inflammation, and as a result of damage to the peripheral and central nervous systems. In some instances, a pathological response can form a reorganized state in which abnormal synaptic circuitry is established. This reorganization, which can be irreversible, is thought to be secondary to degeneration of various elements of the system and to the formation of new inputs. Following injury, such reactions have been documented in both the PNS and the CNS (Woolf 1979).

Table 2-1 on page 621 (appendix B) summarizes the segments of the Central Nervous System (as this book addresses them).

## Innervation: Ventral Horn

The ventral horn roots carry the axons of large-diameter *alpha* motor neuron axons to extrafusal skeletal muscle fibers (contractile muscle fibers); smaller axons of *gamma* motor neuron to intrafusal (spindles) muscle fibers, preganglionic autonomic fibers, and a few afferent, small-diameter axons that arise from cells in the dorsal root ganglia and convey sensory information from the thoracic and abdominal viscera (Waxman and de Groot *ibid*).

## The Peripheral Nervous System

The peripheral nervous system (PNS) is composed of 43 pairs of nerves (Table 2-6 on page 83),

- The cranial nerves (12 pairs) connect with the brain.

- The spinal nerves (31 pairs) connect with the spinal cord.

- Estimated to extend 93,000 miles within the body.

Each peripheral nerve is comprised of smaller functional units—nerve fibers (an axon and its sheath). A nerve trunk is

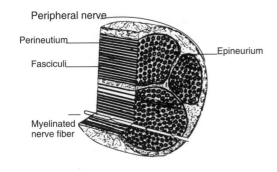

*Figure 2-8:* Peripheral nerve.

composed of different fasciculi (bands of fibers), bound together by epineurium. The epineurium consists of longitudinal collagen and fibers, fat cells, fibroblasts, blood and lymph vessels (Figure 2-8).

*Afferent & Efferent Nerves*

The PNS (Table 2-6) has both *afferent* (sensory) and *efferent* (motor) nerves.

• Afferent nerves (sensory nerves) convey information from receptors in the periphery to the CNS. The cell bodies of afferent neurons are located in structures called ganglia, which are close to the spinal cord and brain.

*Table 2-6.* **THE PERIPHERAL NERVOUS SYSTEM**

Composed of nerves
  — 43 pairs
  — 12 connected to brain
  — 31 connected to spinal cord
  — Afferent (sensory) nerves
  — cell bodies of sensory nerves located in
    ganglia, close to spinal cord and brain
• Efferent (motor) nerves
  — comprised of somatic nervous system
  — innervates the musculoskeletal system

Includes autonomic nervous system
• Innervates smooth muscles, cardiac muscles,
  blood vessels, glands
• Recent investigation demonstrated autonomic
  innervation of skeletal muscle, as well
• Associated sympathetic and parasympathetic
  nervous systems

• The efferent system (motor system) projects from the CNS to the periphery. It has an autonomic nervous system and a somatic nervous system.
— The autonomic nervous system innervates smooth muscles, cardiac muscles, glands and skeletal muscles. The somatic nervous system innervates the musculoskeletal system.

The peripheral somatic neurons are made up of large-diameter, myelinated axons, often called *motor neurons.*

## The Autonomic Nervous System

The autonomic nervous system (ANS), (Figure 2-9), involving elements of both the CNS and PNS, is controlled by the hypothalamus gland, and pertains to the automatic regulation of all body processes, such as breathing, digestion and heart rate. The autonomic nervous system is highly integrated, in both structure and functionality, with the rest of the nervous system and with the body structures. Although the autonomic nervous system has been thought to perform almost entirely involuntarily, this system responds to conscious stimulation, as well. For example it is well documented that by vasodilation, blood pressure can be lowered with meditation or biofeedback training.

*The Sympathetic & Parasympathetic Nervous Systems*

According to Korr (1970), usually the sympathetic and parasympathetic systems have been thought of as two, antagonistic, regulatory systems (negative feedback systems); however, they have different origins and functional organization, and their distributions work on different areas. This separation is easy to see by looking at the somatic structures that receive only sympathetic innervation.

Recent information shows that the sympathetic segments of the autonomic

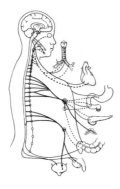

*Figure 2-9:* The autonomic nervous system.

*Table 2-7.* **GANGLIA AND GANGLIONIC FIBERS**

| | |
|---|---|
| Sympathetic Ganglia (Sympathetic Trunks) | Many close to the cord All others between the spinal cord and the organs they innervate |
| Parasympathetic Ganglia | Within the walls of the effector organs |
| Preganglionic Fibers | Between the CNS and the sympathetic and parasympathetic ganglia |
| Postganglionic Fibers | Between the ganglia and the effector organs |

nervous system play an important role in sensory processing. Investigations have also demonstrated autonomic innervation of skeletal muscle (Baker and Banks 1986). Axons that stain positive for tyrosine hydroxylase and neuropeptide Y (which suggests sympathetic efferent function) also have been found in the posterior longitudinal ligament, the ventral dura, the periosteum of the vertebral body, the intervertebral disc, and the vertebral body that reaches into the marrow cavities (Ahmed et al. 1993).

Sympathetic fibers exit the spinal cord from the thoracic and lumbar regions (thoracolumbar division). The parasympathetic fibers originate from the brain and the sacral portion of the spinal cord (craniosacral division).

After exiting, the CNS autonomic fibers synapse in cell clusters called *sympathetic ganglia* and *parasympathetic ganglia* (Table 2-7).

**ERGOTROPIC FUNCTION.** When postural and musculoskeletal demands change, changes also occur in physiologic demands of circulatory *(OM: Liver)*, metabolic and visceral activity. Hess (1954) labeled this regulatory sympathetic nervous system (SNS) task an *ergotropic function*. For the SNS to perform this task, it must receive sensory input from the musculoskeletal system, directly through segmental afferent pathways and indirectly through the higher centers, (Korr 1987).

Segmental (vertebral) dysfunction can disturb this activity and therefore can have systemic affects (see facilitated segment).

**SYMPATHETIC INNERVATION.** Most structures of the body receive their sympathetic innervation from the thoracic nerves, from where the preganglionic sympathetic cell bodies emanate. The exceptions are structures that are innervated by sympathetic cell bodies that originate at L1 and L2 (Table 2-2 on page 622 in appendix B summarizes the innervation levels).

# Pain Mechanisms

Control of nociception (pain) requires a multi-level mechanism that involves not only the brain, but peripheral and spinal controls, as well. Among the many hypotheses proposed to explain the origin, mechanisms and regulation of pain are central biasing, hypersensitivity, loss of inhibitory function leading to recruitment of other relay stations, ectopic (extra) impulses, the Gate Control Theory, and several chemical theories (Bonica 1990).

## Gate Control Theory

Melzack and Wall's Gate Control Theory (gate theory) (Melzack and Wall 1965) is the most comprehensive hypothesis on the nature of pain, encompassing even emotional and cognitive facets (Bonica *ibid*). Melzack and Wall have modified their theory several times as information has become available, and many components have been proven with newer evidence. Several elements of the gate theory are applicable broadly (Baldry *ibid*). Wall uses it mostly to explain what he refers to as the "immediate" phase of acute pain.

Normally, noxious and non-noxious stimuli transmit from small-diameter (nociceptive pain) nerve fibers to second-order neurons in the spinal cord (Willard *ibid*). According to Melzack and Wall (*ibid*), before transmission continues up to the brain, a sensory input "gate"—speculated to be located in the dorsal horn of the spinal cord (substantia gelatinosa on lamina II)—is opened by activity of small-diameter nociceptive nerve fibers, and it is closed by activity in large-diameter afferent nerve fibers, inhibiting painful stimuli transmission temporarily. They suggest that this gate regulates transmission by integrating information that is coming from the periphery, from the brain, and from within the dorsal horn itself.

The "opening" part of the gate theory has been challenged and still has not been substantiated. However, the conceptual closed gate that inhibits transmission has been verified satisfactorily (Schmidt 1971). The information that Melzack and Wall have incorporated recently includes:

- The existence of both excitatory and inhibitory interneurons in the substantia gelatinosa.

- The existence of postsynaptic inhibition in addition to the originally-posited presynaptic inhibition.

Although Wall and Melzack believed at first that large fibers always inhibit small fibers, they now confirm that, at times, large and small fibers may summate (an additive action) (Baldry *ibid*). Also stimulation of A-alpha and beta (large) fibers of the tibial nerve resulted in only slight inhibition of the C-fiber evoked cell activities of the spinothalamic tract. However, when the stimulus intensity which activates A-delta (smaller) fibers was increased, a more powerful inhibition was observed (Chung, Lee, Hori, Endo, and Willis 1984).

Signals from peripheral sensory C-nociceptor fibers (pain fibers) travel at a relatively slow rate of 0.5 to 2 meters per second. Faster A-delta (pain fibers) fiber signals travel at 5-15 meters per second. The A-delta fibers transmit signals from the skin and mucous membrane. C-fibers transmit both from deep tissues and from skin. Nonpainful impulses for pressure and temperature transmit via A-beta mechanoreceptors at a faster rate of 30-70 meters per second, and by A-gamma fibers that transmit touch and pressure at velocity rates of 15-40 meters/sec. All these various signals are routed together with painful signals toward the spinal cord. Painful signals and nonpainful signals converge in the dorsal horn and terminate primarily in the upper two lamina (Waxman and deGroot 1985; Willard *ibid*).

The gate control theory suggests that increased activity of large-diameter mechanoreceptive fibers, and other afferent (sensory) fibers that are in competition with or inhibit the slower painful messages, may "close or crowd the gate" to pain signals. Since information travels faster via large-diameter fibers, their stimulation causes them to arrive faster at the spinal cord, thereby inhibiting the pain messages from small-diameter fibers.

Also, stimulation of low-threshold mechanoreceptive fibers located in the skin, tendons and joints may be able to activate an opioid peptide-mediated serotinergic inhibitory descending system and inhibit pain transmission to the brain (a brain component of the theory). A-beta fibers from mechanoreceptors travel up the cord to the medulla oblongata's gracile and cuneate nuclei.[5] Axons from these nuclei, and those from the medial lemniscus after it dessicates[6]in the medulla, terminate principally in the ventrobasal thalamus. The medial lemniscus is connected to the periaqueductal grey area in the midbrain, at the upper end of the opioid-peptide mediated serotinergic descending inhibitory system (Baldry 1993), (Figure 2-10).

It is known now that many of the gate theory mechanisms are regulated chemically. For example, stimulation of certain neurons by acupuncture needles can lead to action potentials of the neuron, which then releases its neurotransmitter and neuropeptide substances. In turn, the neuropeptide substances are thought to be responsible for pain inhibition, or, in Wall and Melzack's terminology, the closing of a gate. To stop pain, the practitioner can stimulate these fast-conducting nerves by using shallow subcutaneous acupuncture to stimulate the local A-delta and larger fibers. The gate theory is used to explain the action of treatments such as counterirritation therapies (TENS; topical application of tingling, cooling or warming ointments; manual therapy; and acupuncture).

## Chemical Theories

The discovery of endogenous opiates such as endorphins and enkephalins (Snyder 1977) contribute significantly to the understanding of pain perception.

*Opioid Peptides* are any of the opioid like endogenous opiates that are composed of many amino acids (peptides) that are secreted by the pituitary gland and that act on the central and peripheral nervous systems. Generally, opioid peptides are divided into three distinct peptide families: enkephalins, endorphins, and dynorphins.[7] These peptides are known to have

a direct effect on pain awareness and on emotional behavior (Thompson 1984).

Endorphins function as synaptic neurotransmitters, possibly modifying the movement of sodium and potassium across nerve membranes and affecting action potentials. Researchers have isolated several endorphins, such as *alpha*, *beta* and *gamma* endorphins (Wall *ibid*).

*Enkephalins* are two closely related polypeptides found in the brain called *met*-enkephalin and *leu*-enkephalin. Frequently enkephalinergic interneurons are localized in the same areas as opiate receptors that produce pharmacological effects similar to morphine. The amino acid sequence of met-enkephalin has been found in alpha-endorphin and beta-endorphin. The amino acid sequence of beta-endorphin has been found in *beta-lipotropin*, a polypeptide secreted by the anterior pituitary gland (Snyder 1977). Plasma met-enkephalin levels have no relation to other endorphins during circadian studies and corticosteroid suppression tests. Unlike other endorphins, which are produced in the pituitary, met-enkephalins seem to be produced in the adrenal gland, gut, sympathetic ganglia and peripheral autonomic neurons (Baldry *ibid*).

The inhibition of pain that occurs in the substantia gelatinosa (lamina II) of the spinal cord—as proposed in the gate theory—is achieved in part by chemical mechanisms through the production of enkephalins that interrupt nociceptive transmissions.

*Substance P*, one of the first polypeptides to be discovered,[8] is a neurotransmitter messenger formed by 11 amino acids found in the hypothalamus, substantia nigra, and dorsal roots of the spinal nerves. It acts to stimulate vasodilation and contraction of intestinal and other smooth muscles. Substance P also serves as

5.  The medulla oblongata is the most vital part of the brain continuing as the bulbous portion and the spinal cord.

6.  Cross in the form of an "X".

7.  Recently two novel opioid peptides were reported, Orphanin and endomorphin.

8.  Discovered by Von Eurler in 1931. It was not recognized as an endorphin.

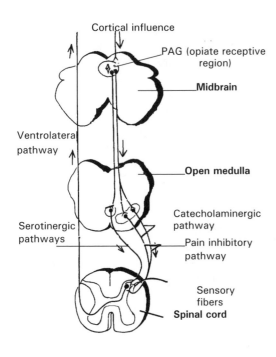

*Figure 2-10:* Schematic of pain suppression by periaqueductal gray (PAG) matter (opiate) and serotinergic systems (After Waxman and deGroot 1995).

a transmitter for signals carried by alpha and delta nerve axons traveling to and from the periphery, into the dorsal horn of the spinal cord (Marx 1979), where it can mediate long-lasting excitation. Substance P in particular, appears to transmit and mediate pain signals up the spinal cord segments (Henry 1976). In the brain it may have an analgesic effect, as well (Stewart et al. 1976). Research has suggested that the "gate" in the substantia gelatinosa is partly mediated through release of Substance P (Marx 1977).

Peripheral electrical stimulation and acupuncture have been demonstrated capable of releasing Substance P (Jin Wenquan et al. 1985) as well as other endorphins (Han *ibid*).

## Other Chemical Theories

Other important chemicals involved in pain are inflammatory mediators such as bradykinin, histamines and prostaglandins; neurotransmitters such as serotonin, norepinephrine, dopamine, gamma-aminobutyric acid (GABA), acetylcholine, glutamate and histamine; gut brain peptides such as neurotensin and Substance P; simple ions such as calcium an magnesium ions, and even adenosine triphosphate (ATP) the energy source of all cells.

**INFLAMMATORY MEDIATORS.** The nociceptors (pain receptors) belong predominantly to the small and medium size neurons in which algogens such as weak acids,[9] bradykinin[10] and serotonin produce inward currents that can generate impulse activity (Vyklicky and Knotkova-Urbancova 1996). Nociceptive receptors can be sensitized by chemicals that are secreted by injured tissues. Prostaglandins,[11] for example, make nociceptors fire more easily. As a result, the nociceptor endings become even more sensitive and reactive to chemicals such as bradykinin and histamines, which are capable of firing these pain nerves. The analgesic activity of NSAIDs such as aspirin may be the result of prostaglandins inhibition which may desensitize nociceptors (Wall *ibid*).

**NEUROTRANSMITTERS.** Serotonin, norepinephrine and GABA have been implicated in pain perception by acting as synaptic inhibitors and by influencing the release of Substance P. Medications that affect serotonin, such as anti-depressants, are used often to treat pain, and decreased level of blood serotonin has been shown in chronic pain patients (Barson and Solomon 1998). Sensitivity to norepinephrine is

9.  Pain produces.

10. Bradykinin is a peptide of nonprotein origin containing nine amino acid residues. It is a potent vasodilator.

11. Prostaglandins are eicosanoids formed by fatty acids which are part of the arachidonic acid inflammatory cascade.

seen often in sympathetic nerve fibers post-traumatically. This sensitivity is thought to be one of the causes of sympathetically-maintained pain (reflex sympathetic dystrophy), (Wall *ibid*).

- Serotonin ascending fibers have been demonstrated to run from the midline raphe nuclei in the midbrain, and ventromedial reticular formation, with axons projecting through the ventral tegmentum and medial forebrain bundle, to innervate forebrain structures. Descending serotonin fibers have been demonstrated to run from the raphe magnus nucleus, with axons projecting through the anterior and lateral funiculi, to innervate the spinal cord dorsal horn, and sympathetic lateral column cells (Kho and Robertson 1997). Increasing serotonin levels raise the pain threshold. Drugs such as clomipramine and pargyline, that raise serotonin levels, can potentiate acupuncture analgesia (Zao, Meng, Yu, Ma, Dong and Han 1987).

- Norepinephrine has complex effects, being different in the brain and spinal cord, and in different animals. In the brain, norepinephrine seems to have an antagonistic effect on analgesia produced by acupuncture and morphine, whereas, in the spinal cord, it potentates acupuncture analgesia (Han et al. *ibid*; Xie, Tong and Han 1981). Studies of norepinephrine networks in primary somatosensory cortex have shown that the net effect of norepinephrine release is to raise the signal-to-noise ratio of neural signals (Koslow 1995).

- GABA has two different effects on morphine and acupuncture analgesia, and probably pain perception. In the brain GABA seems to be antagonistic, whereas, in the spinal cord, it may have agonistic effects (Fan, Qu, Zhe and Han 1982; Pomeranz and Nguyen 1987).[12]

- Dopamine seems to have antagonistic effects in the brain, and acupuncture analgesia results in decreased concentration in the caudate nucleus in rats (Sun, Boney and Lee 1984).

- Acetylcholine reduction, by administration of hemicholine (HC-3) to the intracerebroventricular, does not alter the pain threshold but does reduce the analgesic effects of acupuncture (Ren, Tu and Han 1987).

Acupuncture and electroacupuncture have been shown to stimulate the release of all of the above neurotransmitter mediators with different electrical frequencies stimulating different neurotransmitters (see chapter 5), (Han *ibid*).

**ATP.** ATP has been shown recently to bind to P2X-3 protein. P2X-3 is a gene that encodes a protein found to exist only in sensory C-fibers. This creates a protein that floats on the surface of nociceptors and helps mediate specific biochemical properties of the pain-mediating neurons, giving the neuron its uniquely defined function. When ATP binds to this protein the nerve fires. Since ATP is found in all cells (giving cells energy), when the cells are destroyed, ATP is released into the extracellular space, where it can come in contact with this protein, on nociceptor nerves, and initiate pain sensation.

The initial pain, from tissue damage, may result from the release of cytoplasmic components that act upon nociceptors.[13] ATP was proposed to fill this role, because it elicits pain when applied intradermally and may be the active compound in cytoplasmic fractions that cause pain. Additionally, ATP opens ligand-gated ion channels (P2X receptors) in sensory neurons, and only sensory neurons express messenger RNA for the P2X3 receptor (Cook, Vulchanova, Retrieves, Elde and McCleskey 1997).[14] Administration of ATP

---

12. The drug Valium, which increases central GABA levels, has antagonistic effects on acupuncture analgesia.

13. Cytoplasm is all of the substance of a cell other than the nucleus.

results in a delayed time-course effect and suggests that it may occur concert with other mediators that are recruited by the inflammatory process, rather than reflecting a direct depolarization of sensory nerves (Sawynok and Reid 1997). Localized acidosis, associated with tissue injury, may enhance pain perception via an action on ATP-gated ion channels on mammalian sensory neurons. (Li, Peoples, Weight and Li 1996).

## Ancillary Pain Mechanisms

Researchers have posited several ancillary pain mechanisms.

### Peripheral Mechanisms

Most types of musculoskeletal pain probably occur due to peripheral (non-central nervous system) mechanisms, especially when the pain involves nerve endings (Bonica *ibid*). Most causes of musculoskeletal pain probably are secondary to direct irritation of the peripheral nervous system (Asbury and Fields. 1984). This assertion is supported by the fact that treatment of the peripheral joint often relieves pain. Involvement of the peripheral nervous system can be due to noxious stimulation such as inflammation, hypersensitivity of nerves due to nerve injury (Cannon and Rosenblueth's law of supersensitivity in denervation) and joint dysfunctions (lack of normal motion) (Iggo 1984), and various reflexes and other mechanical dysfunctions that probably stimulate one of the above conditions.

### Peripheral-Central Mechanisms

Peripheral-central mechanisms, or the interaction of peripheral and central pathways, are seen in the vicious cycle of

reflex pain. Livingston has described a vicious cycle of reflexes in which nociception increases in the primary afferent and then activates preganglionic sympathetic neurons (between the ganglia and the CNS). This leads to activation of postganglionic neurons that sensitize and activate primary afferent nociceptors, which feed back to the spinal cord, maintaining the pain cycle. This cycle can also be set up by painful input that leads to muscle spasm, which activates more motor neurons, sustaining the spasm. The spasm activates nociceptors, which feed back to the spinal cord, creating a vicious cycle. In severe manifestations of peripheral central mechanisms (such as reflex sympathetic dystrophy), the peripheral-central reflex commonly is due to a more serious lesion in the peripheral, dorsal root, and ganglion. These are often due to deafferenation (Bonica *ibid*).[15]

The *facilitated cord segment* is an important concept in osteopathic evaluation and treatment of both musculoskeletal and organ dysfunctions, by peripheral-central mechanisms. Sherington and Korr have proposed that a low threshold exists in this syndrome, and that any sensory excitation via somatovisceral (the body structure influencing the organs) or viscerosomatic (the viscera influencing the body structure) mechanism can cause a reflex and a vicious cycle of dysfunction and pain. The segment is said to be in a hypersensitive state, and it is said to produce exaggerated responses to any stimulation. (*OM: Peripheral-central reflex mechanisms fit very well with OMs internal-external channel Organ relationship and coactivation theories*).

### Nerve Sprouting

It has been shown that injury can induce sprouting of nerves in the injured area, and can lead to the creation of connections between motor (including sympathetic) and sensory (afferent) nerves.

---

14. Ligand is an organic molecule attached to a specific site on a surface or to a tracer element, like vitamin B12.

15. Interruption in the efferent nerve system.

These pathological neural circuits, along with a decrease of synaptic thresholds—probably due to neuropeptides such as substance P, inflammatory mediators and other neuromuscular and atrophic changes—lead to increased pain activation by other normal motor nerves. This may explain why mild activity aggravates pain in chronic pain sufferers (Willard 1995).

### Sympathetic Nervous System Involvement

The sympathetic nervous system is often involved in chronic pain. Lately this system has been shown to innervate muscles, ligaments, and discs (Raja *ibid*). Sympathetic ectopic foci (extra-firing of nerves) may be responsible for Travell's trigger point activity (see chapter3).

### Sensitization/Deafferenation

The exact changes and causes in peripheral nervous sensitization (pain of neuropathic origin) that occur in the presence of chronic pain and dysfunction are unknown. Perl et al. (1976) have eliminated acetylcholine, histamine, 5-HT, bradykinin, pH, potassium, and prostaglandins as being the cause of sensitization in unmyelinated afferents. Later studies show that sensitization by prostaglandins and norepinephrine is implicated with pain that is maintained sympathetically. Tasker (1991) proposed that the use of "deafferenation pain" is appropriate for all conditions that commonly are called neuropathic pain (Bonica *ibid;* Wall *ibid*).

Sensitization also can occur in the central nervous system. For example, magnetoencephalograpic and evoked potential studies in patients who have chronic back pain have demonstrated central nervous system hyper-responsiveness in the primary somatosensory cortex (Flor, Birbaumer Fust 1993; Flor, Birbaumer Fust 1993).

Many other hypotheses have been used to explain the mechanisms of pain

(and causalgia), such as central biasing, hypersensitivity, loss of inhibitory function leading to recruitment of other relay stations, and ectopic (extra) impulses (Bonica 1990). More details on some of these can be found in the "Referred Pain" section of this chapter.

# Aspects of Pain

An understanding of the three principal aspects of pain—phase, perception and localization, and source and severity—is helpful in determining an approach to treatment.

The phases of pain can be described as acute or chronic.

## Acute Pain

Bonica has defined acute pain as

> ...a complex or constellation of unpleasant sensory, perceptual, and emotional experiences and certain associated autonomic, psychologic, emotional and behavioral responses.

Acute pain results from noxious stimulation produced by injury or disease. Its function is to warn the individual that something is disordered. It may limit the patient's activity, thereby preventing further injury, or it may cause the patient to seek attention and/or to pay attention. Associated physiological responses such as increased respiration, circulation and inflammation also aid in healing.

In the case of acute trauma, a painless period (stress analgesia) following the injury is common and serves to allow the "fight or flight" (help-seeking) option. Injury elicits impulses in all types of fibers. Some are inhibitory impulses that may deter further excitation of the neuron, such as large, myelinated A-beta fibers, and some are excitatory impulses, such as unmyelinated C-fibers and myelinated A-delta fibers (Bonica *ibid*).

Wall divides acute pain into two stages that he calls *immediate* and *acute*.

### Wall's Immediate Pain Stage

Wall's *immediate* (nociceptive) pain signals tissue distress and/or damage quickly. This happens, for example, when one is slapped on the face. The quick signal occurs by way of injury-sensitive A-delta and C-fibers.

Immediate pain is associated with activation of the nervous system, not with injured tissues. However, it can change the subsequent excitability (threshold) of these nerve terminals. As a response to the initial excitation, some terminals become more sensitive, and others become less sensitive. Therefore, even brief pain is dynamic rather than static, and it can cause changes within the nervous system. A short, quick trauma may change the circuitry and the perception of pain for a longer duration. Immediate pain is not considered a significant cause of chronic pain (Wall *ibid*).

### Wall's Acute Pain Stage

The second of Wall's acute-pain stages is usually caused by tissue damage such as occurs in trauma. This kind of trauma fires nerve endings by mechanical, thermal or chemical effects. Inflammatory processes that occur in this phase are due to the production of substances such as vasoactive amines,[16] acidic lipids, lysosomal components and lymphocyte products. Some of these inflammatory mediators can activate nociceptors, as well. Various chemicals such as bradykinin, histamine, prostaglandins and potassium ions are capable of sensitizing C (type IV) and A-delta (type III) sensory nerves. These chemicals, especially bradykinin, also can

---

16. Amine is a type of organic compound that contains nitogen.

sensitize sympathetic nerve fibers (Bonica *ibid;* Wall *ibid*).

Acute pain sets in motion:

- Diminishing of inhibition.
- Change in the environment of nerve endings.
- Change in the cord reaction to some types of peripheral stimulation.

This results in an increase in all remaining sensory input, which usually consists of painful stimuli (Wall 1984). In Wall's acute phase, the pain is thought to be mostly due to C-afferent fibers, and possibly to various chemical mediators that act intraspinally.

## Chronic Pain

Chronic pain is not simply a repetition of acute pain. The patient's anxious, emotional response to acute pain is replaced by a depressed, obsessed and irritable mood. Bonica defines chronic pain as:

> ...pain that persists a month beyond the usual course of an acute disease or a reasonable time of an injury to heal, or that is associated with a chronic pathologic process that causes continuous pain, or pain that recurs at intervals for months or years.

Others define chronic pain as having more than a six-month duration. Chronic pain is different from and less understood than acute pain. Often this type of pain does not produce the obvious autonomic nervous system reactions that result from acute pain. Usually such reactions are present, but tend to be less obvious.

Chronic pain is caused by pathologic processes in the soma (non-internal organ parts of the body) and viscera (internal organs); by inflammation, by changes within the nervous system, and by psychological factors. Often acute pain is followed by functional and structural changes within the central or peripheral nervous system (Gunn *ibid*). These includes alterations of cell phenotype; changes in the expression of proteins such as receptors, transmitters and ion channels; and modifications of neural structure. (Dray, Urban, Dickenson 1994). These changes often result in sensitization of nociceptors that may acquire ongoing (spontaneous) discharge, a lowered activation threshold, and an increased response to subthreshold stimuli and stimulation from other, possibly normal, tissues (Bonica *ibid;* Wall *ibid;* Willard *ibid*).

Chronic pain can develop when pain is due to tissue damage. If the pain results from mechanical forces such as subluxation, ligament and tendon overstress and/or weakening, trigger point activation, or inflammation (repeated irritating injuries as in tendinitis), stimulation of pain receptors can be ongoing and continuous. Chronic inflammation that appears as redness, increased local temperature, and swelling (such as rheumatoid arthritis and lupus) is most often caused by abnormal immunologic responses. Chronic inflammation (Ryan and Majno 1983) also can be present without these obvious signs.

Most chronic musculoskeletal pain is probably due to mechanical dysfunctions that lead to, or are caused by, disturbances of tissue structure and function. Often these result from degenerative processes and the reactions to them (secondary factors). Subtle changes affect the mechanically-linked systems of the musculoskeletal body, causing stresses on tissues, injuring them and leading to activation of the nervous pain perception systems. The nervous mechanisms can become facilitated and cause pain on their own.

## Psychological Influences on Pain

Psychological causes of chronic pain are complex and may represent a psychiatric disorder, or a complex dynamic reorganization among converging neurons. Considering that it has been estimated that the brain has as many as 400,000 synaptic terminals in a single axon, and that it has 100 billion neurons (Melzack 1984), it is not surprising that many neuropsychological changes occur with chronic pain (Bonica *ibid*).

Secondary psychosocial (abnormal) illness behavior, including depression, inactivity, and pain avoidance, are the consequent rule in chronic pain sufferers (Naliboff et al. 1985). Studies have shown a link between symptom-specific physiological reactivity and pain severity in reaction to stressful events, especially in depressed patients (Burns et al. 1997). Anxiety, sensitivity, or the fear of anxiety-related bodily sensations, arising from beliefs that the sensations have harmful consequences is associated with pain behavior and disability (Asmundson and Taylor 1996). Pain is often made worse by fear, by anger, or by a sense of isolation. The pain may be diminished if the patient understands the cause and loses his/her fear. Patients who keep busy find that sensory and other distractions relieve pain (Brand 1997). Depression, hypochondriasis, anxiety and hysteria are related to poor outcome (Cats-Baril and Frymoyer 1991). Case histories of patients who later developed low back pain show that often the patient was under stress before experiencing pain, and that the episode of trauma that resulted in pain was minor (Kirkaldy-Willis 1990).

The patient's emotional response to pain can become the major component of his or hers suffering. In such cases, relief from the pain can become an obsession. This must be kept in mind when evaluating and treating such patients. It must be stressed however, that physicians often shift blame to the patient when the pain is poorly understood—and usually incorrectly. Slater and Glithero (1965) for example, showed that 60% of patients diagnosed by neurologists as having hysteria did not have hysteria, and that eventually they developed symptoms that related to a physical disease that could account for their symptoms. Hendler and Kolodny

(1992) have estimated that the true incidence of "psychological pain" is about one in 3000 patients. Bugdok (1997) has shown that in patients with neck pain, related to whiplash injury, successful treatment can resolve all psychological distresses that were previously considered to be of nonphysiological origin. Bugdok also states that he can identify the cause of low back pain (by anesthetic techniques) in 60-70% of patients, in spite of the literature which states that 80% of low back pain is idiopathic (unknown origin).

These behaviors, whether primary or secondary, must be addressed. Often, changing this kind of pain behavior takes some time. Treatment should focus on function, not pain reduction. Early return to activity and work may help prevent the emergence of chronic pain syndromes and reduce the costs of back care (Deyo et al. 1986). Herbal therapy and anti-depressant medications can be very useful.

DIFFERENTIATING NONORGANIC PAIN. To differentiate "nonorganic" back pain from other types of back pain,[17] Waddell devised the "Waddell signs"—seven signs elicited by the practitioner while observing patient responses (Waddell et al. 1980):

1. Superficial or nonphysiologic tenderness that is widespread to light touch.

2. Pain provoked by axial loading when light pressure is applied to the top of head.

3. Pain when rotating the trunk fully (rotating from the pelvis, to avoid twisting the spine).

4. A contradiction in sitting and supine straight-leg raising, one being painful while the other is not.

5. Nonphysiologic weakness.

6. Nonphysiologic sensory disturbance (uncoordinated motor and sensory signs).

7. Patient exaggeration response to all provocative testing.

## Gender Variations

A critical review of research examining gender variations in clinical pain experience demonstrates that women are more likely than men to experience a variety of recurrent pains. In most studies, women report more severe levels of pain, more frequent pain and pain of longer duration than do men. Women may be at greater risk for pain-related disability than men but women also respond more aggressively to pain through health related activities. Women may be more vulnerable than men to unwarranted psychogenic attributions, by health care providers to their pain (Unruh 1996).

# Pain Perception & Localization

For the patient, the most compelling aspect of pain is perception, which is subjective and should be accepted accordingly. The patient's impression of the pain is often the first clue the practitioner has for diagnosing and localizing the pain.

The patient's perception and localization take place through complex mechanisms within the nervous system. Pain signals travel mainly via A-delta and C-fibers to the limbic system in the brain, where pain is perceived first. The faster, A-delta signals travel in the anterolateral spinothalamic tract to the limbic system, and they continue to the cortex. These signals, which require only three relays on the way to the cortex, travel very quickly (Gunn *ibid*). Therefore, the combination of painful stimuli from A-delta fibers and the reacting motor system allows the patient to

---

17. These principals can be used with other pain, as well.

localize pain quickly and to act appropriately, such as by pulling the hand away from a hot fire.

C-afferent nociceptive messages travel up to the spinal cord and then to the brain more slowly than A-delta nociceptive messages, via fibers called the pleospino-reticulothalamic tract. On the way up, these signals, which enter at lamina I and II and travel to lamina V, VII and VIII, must pass several relays. At lamina I and V the fibers cross to the contralateral side and integrate with other levels (Willard *ibid;* Gunn *ibid*). The complexity of the C-fiber nociceptive signals probably leads to the phenomenon of referred pain.

By contrast, the majority of the information from the mechanoreceptors (A-beta fibers) is transmitted directly and quickly to the brain stem via posterior fibers (Gunn *ibid*). All of these messages are modified and are managed by the brain through the descending fiber systems. Some of the responses are voluntary; some are not.

*Types Of Localization*

Cyriax divides pain localization into three types:

• Shifting pain.

— Results from a shifting of a lesion, such as the shifting of a disc fragment, as may be seen in back pain that changes from one side to the other.

• Expanding pain.

— Increases the reference area as the local pain intensifies. When this pattern develops, one must consider serious conditions such as cancer.

• Referred pain.

— Originates in a fixed location. As it intensifies, its area of reference (but not its local pain) increases.

**Referred Pain**

Segmentation begins during embryological development. The ventral somite eventually differentiates into *dermatomes*, *myotomes*, and *sclerotomes*. The projection of these segments is one factor that determines the extent of pain reference. Since individual differences occur (probably due to developmental differences, post-traumatic rootlet anastomosis, and other causes), it is impossible to draw accurate maps of these distributions and therefore impossible to draw absolutely accurate referred pain maps. Kellgren (1938), Whitty (1967) and Hackett (1958) have demonstrated that when ligaments, musculature, and zygapophyseal joints are stimulated by chemicals, both local and referred pain occur, in both segmental and nonmanagement patterns. The embryonic segmental derivations of the viscera are summarized on Table 2-3 on page 622 in appendix B.

The deeper the origin of pain, the more difficulty the patient has localizing it, hence, patients have difficulty localizing soft tissue pain that is deeper than skin level. Usually such pain is referred from structures the patient does not recognize. This referred phenomenon is thought to be due to the organization of the nervous system. Therefore, for accurate and tissue-specific diagnosis the practitioner must have a clear understanding of the concepts of referred pain and the conditions that stimulate it.

Fundamental to the concept of referred pain is an understanding that the human body's interrelated parts influence each other mechanically and neurally. The tensegritous interdependency (mechanical chain) of the body's parts can make diagnosis difficult, because an injured tissue can cause a cascade of dysfunctions or reactions in other tissues. For example, an upslip of the innominate on the sacrum (at the SI joint) can result in mechanical tension on the sacrotuberous ligament, which can refer pain to the heel. Or when the shoulder joint is inflamed, the practitioner commonly finds secondary myofascial trigger points, muscle spasms and other compensatory misreactions, all of which can cause their own symptoms and signs. If the practitioner does not know the possible pain patterns and does not recognize the primary tissues at fault, he is likely to focus on the secondary manifestations and undoubtedly will chase his tail.

The presentation of referred pain patterns is summarized in table Table 2-8 on page 96. Figure 2-6 and Figure 2-7 on page 81 show the myotomes, sclerotomes and dermatomes.

### Theories of Referred Pain

Referred pain has been explained as errors occurring in the spinal cord or perceptual errors in the sensory cortex (Ombregt, Bisschop, ter Veer and de Velde 1995).

SPINAL CORD THEORIES. Melzack and Wall (1965) and Bonica (1990) attribute the false sense of pain localization to the organization of nociceptive afferent (pain sensory nerves) systems in the spinal cord. For example, spinal cord neurons in cats with knee input have been shown to converge with input from muscles in the thigh and skin in the lower leg, and therefore, can activate pain in the knee and in the thigh. Electrophysiological studies in animals have demonstrated convergence of nociceptor input from deep and cutaneous tissues into the same somatosensory spinal neurons (Cervero et al. 1992). Viscerosomatic convergence may be involved in RSD of an upper limb following an episode of cardiac pain (Bonica *ibid*).

MaCkenzie (1989) has described an "irritable focus" created by visceral afferents in the spinal cord so that other, segmentally somatic inputs could produce referred pain.

Sinclair et al. (1948) suggested that bifurcation (division) of axons of some primary sensory neurons, that innervate both somatic and visceral targets, leads to confusion about the source of the afferent activity, and explains the segmental nature of referred sensations.

SENSORY CORTEX ERROR. The *convergence-projection* theory states that since nociceptive sensory afferent fibers innervating both the visceral and somatic structures, enter the spine at the same level, and converge on the same dorsal horn transmission cells, pain from either one can be perceived as originating from the same level. Furthermore, since the brain is more used to receiving stimulation from somatic structures it tends to "dislocate" pain of visceral origin to somatic structures (Ruch and Patton 1965). As seen in cardiac infarct with radiating arm pain.

Hackett, Hemwall, and Montgomery. (1991) posit that ligament and tendon relaxation produces a hypersensitive state in these tissues. Subsequently, normal tension causes a barrage of afferent, somatic, proprioceptive, and sensory impulses to the posterior spinal root ganglions. From the ganglia, some impulses are conducted to the brain and are perceived as local pain. Others create exteroceptive impulses,[18] which also enter consciousness as superficial pain in a pattern associated with the sensory distribution from the same spinal segment. Hackett's proposed mechanism is similar to the *convergence-facilitation hypothesis* (Ruch 1965) which states that skin nociceptors that normally do not initiate pain will do so when "facilitated" by sensory impulses from deep structures.

Lewis (1942) proposed that interactions at supraspinal levels lead to referred pain and phenomenon.

EXTRASEGMENTAL REFERENCE. Cyriax believed that the dura mater does not follow the "rules" of segmental reference, and posited that pressure from the spinal disc is responsible for most pains that show these nonsegmental pain patterns. Extrasegmental pain may represent sclerotomal

---

18. Sensory receptors that get activated from stimuli that originate from outside the body.

*Table 2-8.* PAIN PRESENTATION

| PATTERN | PRESENTATION PATTERN | ORIGIN OF PATTERN |
|---|---|---|
| MYOTOMAL | Muscle Pain, Ache<br>Tightness<br>Tenderness | Muscles innervated by a spinal root<br>• The area of reference of those muscles |
| SCLEROTOMAL | Deep, Dull Ache<br>or<br>Piercing pain, numb-like sensation that is difficult to localize | Connective tissue structures and bone innervated by a spinal root<br>• The area of reference from connective tissue |
| DERMATOMAL | Paresthesia<br>— prickling<br>— tingling<br>— numbness<br>— heightened sensitivity | Superficial sensation innervated by a spinal root<br>• The area of reference from nerves felt on the skin |

reference (referred pain down the sclerotome or connective tissue innervated by a spinal nerve) and not necessarily dural reference. Orthopaedic medicine specialist Thomas Dorman has suggested that these pain references have ligamentous origin (Dorman 1991). New information shows that this type of referred pain may be due to chemical irritation of the dura and nerve roots and not just physical pressure. Moreover, many painful disc pathologies are due only to internal disc tears, which only show on special MRI studies.

According to Cyriax, extrasegmental pain reference:

• Of cervical origin may be perceived all the way from the head to the mid-thorax.

• From mid- and low-thoracic lesions may radiate to the base of the neck.

• From the low lumbar levels may reach the lower thorax (posteriorly), the lower abdomen, the upper buttocks, the sacrum and the coccyx. It does not extend to the upper limbs or hands, although often it reaches down to the lower limbs and ankles, but not the feet.

Cyriax believed that, as a rule, pain is referred only distally and never crosses the midline. The author has reservations about this concept as an absolute rule, because at times, when tissue is stimulated with a needle, the patient perceives pain proximally, or even contralaterally. More recent anatomical research supports these observations. This is especially true if deep scars are present, and is probably due to rootlet development. It is known now that the ventral and dorsal horns and the sympathetic system communicate with each other, and that the function of one may transform into the function of the other in chronic dysfunction (Willard 1994). In these cases, messages may cross midline. Clinically, however, the above guideline is useful.

REFERRED TENDERNESS. Cyriax considers these disc pressures to be the cause of referred tenderness (myofascial trigger points) within these regions. He posits that, when these trigger points are pressed forcefully, the patient identifies the pressure as the source of his pain. Cyriax regards this type of referred tenderness as a major obstacle to diagnosis of the true nature of these conditions, and adds that these spots can be either moved around or eliminated by manipulation. Scmorl and Junghanns (1968) and Dvorak (1990) also find that secondary muscle pain is often caused by vertebral dysfunction—not just by disc dysfunction—and that it will improve when the vertebral dysfunction is treated.

Referred tenderness and hyperalgesia (tissue sensitivity) has been shown to involve both peripheral and central mechanisms (Meyer, Campbell and Raja 1994). Referred tenderness and hyperalgesia may result from sensitization of secondary dorsal horn neurons or from a decreased threshold of primary peripheral afferents —with pain resulting from normal input of mechanoreceptor afferents (Cohen at el. 1993; 1992).

### Factors that Influence Referred Pain

Factors significant in the patient's perception of referred pain are:

- The more tenacious the incitation (painful lesion), the less likely the patient will be able to localize it, and the more likely the patient will feel it distally.

- The more superficially the lesion lies, the more precisely the patient can localize it.

- The deeper the lesion (excluding bone), the less accurately the patient localizes it.

- Pain is likely to be referred from muscles, tendons, bursas, ligaments and joint capsules in a way that the patient cannot identify the origin.

- Pain from bone hardly ever radiates. However, pain from the periosteum does radiate.

- The more distal the lesion, the more accurate the patient's perception regarding its origin. Pain that arises in the wrist or ankles commonly refers an ache to the forearm or leg, but rarely enough to mislead the patient as to its source.

The practitioner should always suspect that pain is referred, especially if local function is not disturbed, or if it affects large areas and is felt with great intensity.

Local anesthesia is the most effective way to confirm the location of the suspected lesion. Local acupuncture can be of some use in trying to reproduce the symptoms. However, it does not reproduce or eliminate the pain as reliably as local anesthesia does.

# Assessing Pain

Because pain perception is subjective, relative intensity of pain is difficult to measure. There is a growing trend to try to measure and quantify the results of the physical examination, during which patients tend to report more subjective findings than objective ones. Several methods are available to help the practitioner assess the patient's pain—none of which are flawless.

## Patient Drawing

The practitioner can begin the patient interview by reviewing a pain drawing done by the patient, and he may want to evaluate the drawing using the Wiltse's point evaluation method. Such drawings contain a great deal of general information that can assist the practitioner in the diagnosis of the patient's complaint (Figure 2-11 on page 100).

### Wiltse's Point Evaluation Method

A patient's pain drawing can be helpful in differentiating between organic and nonorganic pain. The practitioner can assign a "score" using a point method from seven categories, as described by Wiltse (Kirkaldy-Willis and Burton 1992). For each category, a score of one point (one irregularity) indicates a "normal" score; a score of five points or more indicates a strong psychological component to the patient's pain. The scoring categories are:

- Writing (anywhere) on the drawing.

- Nonphysiological pain pattern.
- More than one type of pain.
- Involvement of both upper and lower areas of the body.
- Markings outside of body contours.
- Unspecified symbols.

CORRELATION WITH OTHER PAIN ASSESSMENT METHODS. Nonorganic drawings have been shown to correlate with elevated hypochondriasis and hysteria scores on the MMPI; higher hospitalization rate and chronicity; and high scores on the McGill Pain Questionnaire (Tait et al. 1990).

## Dolorimeter

One means of quantifying a subjective examination is a dolorimeter (pressure meter), which measures in units called *dols*. Examples of dolorimeter readings are (Bonica *ibid*):

- Childbirth: 10.5 dols.
- Migraine:    5 dols.
- Toothache: 2 dols.

Aspirin may help pain under 2 dols.

## Visual Analog Scale (VAS)

The Visual Analog Scale (VAS), also called the Pain Visual Analog Scale (PVAS), is a common method of pain measurement. A subjective estimate of pain intensity, the VAS consists of an unmarked, 10 cm line labeled at one end as "no pain" and at the other as "unbearable pain" (Merskey 1973). The patient conveys the intensity of his pain by marking a line between the two extremes (Figure 2-11 on page 100).

## West Haven-yale Multidimensional Pain Inventory (MPI)

The West Haven-Yale Multidimensional Pain Inventory (MPI or MHYMPI), a multi-

dimensional pain inventory developed by Kerns, Turk and Rudy, is intended to supplement behavioral and psychophysiological observations and was specifically developed for evaluation of chronic pain patients (Kerns, Turk and Rudy 1985). It classifies patients as dysfunctional, interpersonally distressed, or adaptive-coper. The MPI provides information in nine clinical scales including:

- Pain dimensions and severity, including:
  - interference by pain on various functions.
  - role of significant others.
  - pain severity, and mood.
- Specific responses of significant others.
- Functional activities.

This test was compared with the Minnesota Multiphasic Personality Inventory (MMPI) and was shown to be much more useful for chronic pain patients (Berstein, Jaremoko, and Hinkley 1995).

## McGill Pain Questionnaire

The McGill Pain Questionnaire (MPQ), developed by Melzack, uses classes of words that have been determined to represent affective (mood), sensory and cognitive components of pain experience. The MPQ is able to separate sensory, affective, and evaluative dimensions providing assessment of different qualities of pain. The questionnaire provides three kinds of pain detail:

- Intensity of pain.
- Number of words chosen in each category.
- Pain rating index.

This questionnaire has been the subject of many studies that have confirmed its validity and reliability (Bradley, Prokop and Gentry et al 1981).

## Minnesota Multiphasic Personality Inventory (MMPI)

The Minnesota Multiphasic Personality Inventory (MMPI) is the most thoroughly researched of the personality inventories in both psychopathology and pain management. Studies by Bradley et al. showed that MMPI profiles of pain patients consistently clustered into categories:

- Depression.
- Somatization.
- Hypochondriasis.
- Manipulative reactions.

They found that chronic pain patients are not homogenous in personality makeup.

These patients bring to the pain situation their own unique, pre-illness personalities that can either contribute to or inhibit the clinical pain picture (Bradley, Prokop and Margolis et al 1978). The utility of the MMPI, the most commonly used inventory scale, has been questioned (Main and Spanswick 1995).

Other indexes that are used in the assessment of pain include; the Oswestry Low Back Index (Fairbank et al. 1980), Millon Behavioral Health Inventory (Gatchel RJ, et al. 1986), the Neck Disability Index (Vernon and Mior 1991), and the Roland Morris Scale and Illness Behavior Questionnaire (Roland and Morris 1983).

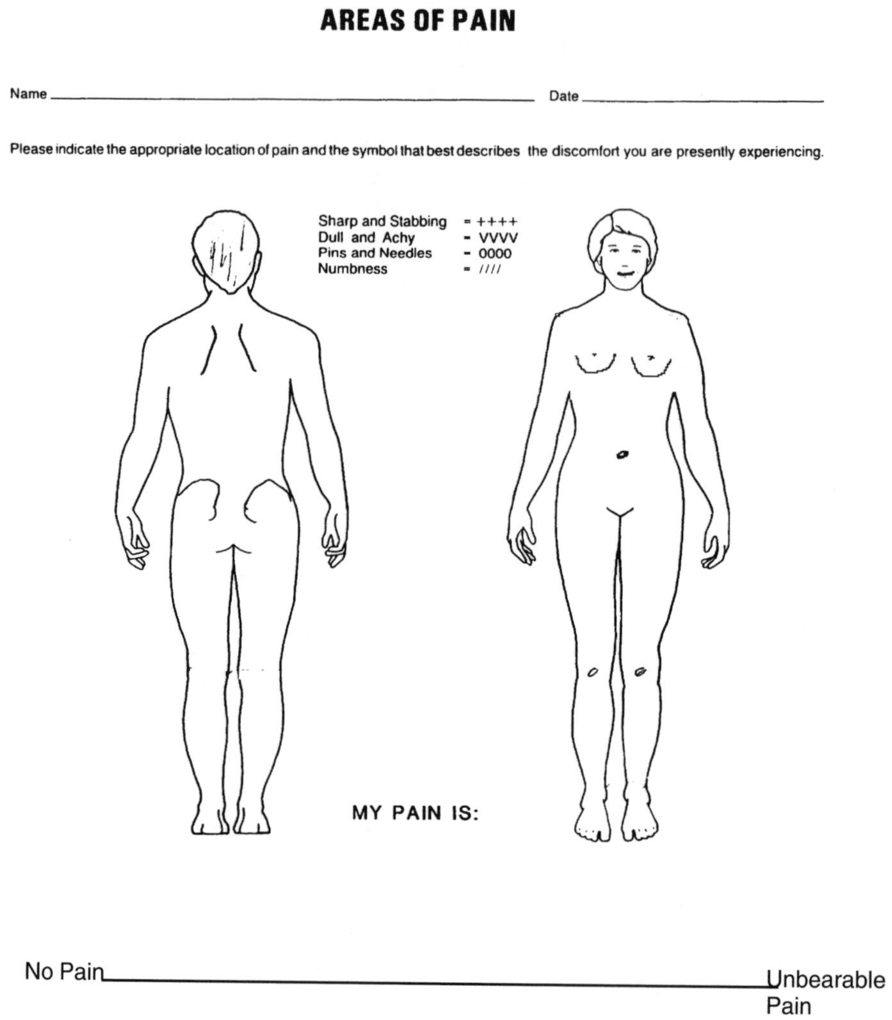

# AREAS OF PAIN

Name _____ Date _____

Please indicate the appropriate location of pain and the symbol that best describes the discomfort you are presently experiencing.

Sharp and Stabbing = ++++
Dull and Achy = VVVV
Pins and Needles = 0000
Numbness = ////

MY PAIN IS:

No Pain _____ Unbearable Pain

*Figure 2-11:* Pain drawing and visual analog scale (VAS).

# Chapter 3: *Musculoskeletal Medicine*

Musculoskeletal disorders can be understood and related by various methods. In OM most musculoskeletal conditions, unless due to direct forces (trauma) or indirect forces (strains), are caused (or allowed) by endogenous and deficiency factors. These processes allow exogenous factors to either invade the system or cause internal disharmony, which can give rise to blockage of the channels (painful obstruction, Bi syndromes), tissue damage, fatigue and/or pain. Therefore, in OM most types of musculoskeletal pain (unless due to trauma) are secondary. Emphasis is on the systemic, rather than the anatomical source of pain.

Soft tissue disorders fall within the domain of Painful Obstruction and Hit (martial art, bone setting, trauma) medicine. This chapter describes basic concepts of OM and BIOMEDICAL musculoskeletal disorders.

## OM Pathology & Etiology

Independent factors such as sprains, falls and collisions can cause acute soft tissue damage. Trauma damages the channels and collaterals, blocks Qi and Blood circulation, and induces hematomas, pain and localized dysfunction. Alternatively, deficiency allows for invasion of external pathogenic influences which also block Qi and Blood circulation. If the damage is not treated effectively immediately, further damage can occur due to blockage and malnourishment that leads to chronic soft tissue dysfunction and:

- Blood stasis.

- Tissue hyperplasia.

- Adhesions.

- Atrophy.

Continual overuse of any musculoskeletal structure, especially a weight-bearing joint, can cause chronic dysfunction due to increased metabolic need for Qi and Blood. Chronic lesions are characterized by:

- Fatigability of the affected structure.

- Stagnation of Qi and Blood.

- Diminishing strength.

- Inactivity.

- Pain.

# Organic Influences on Musculoskeletal Structure

An important consideration in soft tissue damage and painful obstruction disorders, is whether organic causes are affecting the musculoskeletal structure. The statements in Table 3-1, all from classic OM literature, illustrate the significance OM attributes to internal functions in soft tissue damage.

In acute musculoskeletal disorders attention to the Organ systems is usually secondary (to channels) and often is limited to the Tai Yang level. The Lungs, which together with Defensive Qi and Sinews channels control the *Exterior* (skin and muscles) are treated when external factors (Wind, Heat, Cold or Damp) are involved.

During chronic stages the Liver and its connection to Blood, sinews and muscular strength, the Spleen/pancreas and their connection to muscular texture, mass (flesh), Blood formation and Dampness, and the Kidneys and their connection to Essence (marrow) and bones are addressed often. The Lungs, together with Defensive and Nutritive Qi disharmony, are treated often in cases of chronic muscular pain and painful obstruction Bi syndromes.

*Table 3-1.* **OM LITERATURE: INTERNAL FUNCTIONS IN SOFT TISSUE DAMAGE**

| STATEMENT | PUBLICATION | SECTION |
|---|---|---|
| For External Factors to invade, there must be a preexisting deficiency. | Divine Pivot | |
| [Attributes inability to turn or bend to the Kidney.] [...Also, the] lumbar region is the Fu (organ) of the Kidney. | Precise Explanation of Pulse in Familiar Conversations | |
| The Kidney dominates the lower back and feet. Lower back pain is caused by overtaxing of Kidney energy. [This allows] overexertion (strain) to damage the channels and collaterals. | General Treatise on the Causes of Symptoms of Disease | Symptoms and Signs of Back Pain |
| When the Yang aspect of the body is damaged, the patient has difficulty flexing his back. When the Yin aspect of body is damaged, the patient has difficulty extending his back. If both Yin and Yang are damaged, the patient has difficulty in both flexion and extension. | General Treatise on the Causes of Symptoms of Disease | |
| Frequent attacks of Wind, Cold and Damp accompanied by traumatic impairment cause: <br>• Blood stagnation <br>• hard mass <br>• damage to Tendons <br>...In addition, disharmony of Qi and Blood allows for invasion of Wind, Cold and Damp. | Golden Mirror of Original Medicine | Important Notes on Orthopedics |
| If soft tissue damage is accompanied by Bi (Wind, Cold, Wet): <br>• Internal dysfunction such as Qi Blood deficiency is present. <br>or <br>• Organ Emptiness is present. | All Above References | |

# Painful Obstruction Bi Syndromes

In OM, Bi syndromes (painful obstruction syndromes) are used to describe the majority of muscular and bony disorders. Characteristically these Bi syndromes are manifested as pain, soreness, numbness, and impaired movement. The classic book *Canon of Internal Medicine/ Simple Questions* devotes an entire chapter to Bi syndromes where painful obstruction is mostly related to external pathogenic factors; Wind, Cold and Dampness. Later both external and internal Heat and deficiency syndromes were included. In *Simple Questions* Bi syndromes affecting the sinews and bones also were described as difficult to cure, suggesting that Bi syndromes presented a clinical challenge at the time.[1]

Painful obstruction and pathogenic factors, affect Qi and Blood (Nutritive and Defensive Qi) circulation, and with time results in the disruption of nourishment to the sinews—numbness and weakness ensues. Painful obstruction syndromes affect mainly the channels. However, if not effectively treated, painful obstruction can affect the Organs and even become fatal. For example, unresolved Bi syndrome can affect the Heart (Heart Bi) and cause symptoms of irritability with epigastric throbbing ("below the Heart" CV 14, Heart Alarm (Mu) point), rebellious Qi (rising of Qi, panting and pressure in the chest) and fear, as commonly seen with heart disease. In the classic *Canon of Internal Medicine/Simple Questions* it says:

> The five Yin organs are related to the five tissues where a chronic disease can settle in. In bone Bi syndrome the pathogenic factor reaches the kidneys; in sinew Bi syndrome it reaches the liver; in blood vessel Bi syndrome it reaches the heart; in muscle

Bi syndrome it reaches the spleen; and in skin Bi syndrome it reaches the lungs.

Organ Bi and polyarthralgia syndromes may correspond to biomedical disorders such as, rheumatic fever, rheumatoid arthritis, gout, and lyme disease.[2]

Theoretically, a painful obstruction (Bi) disorder is caused by exposure to adverse environmental conditions such as dampness, cold or wind. Characteristically it has a slow and progressive onset and begin with symptoms associated with external Wind, Cold and Damp (superficial syndromes)—or viral and infectious like syndromes. Clinically however, patients with arthritic or other pain syndromes almost never convey such a history. This may be due to lack of awareness or may be explained by the theory of latent pathogenic factors. *(Biomedical: Lately infectious agents, other than acute bacterial infections, have been associated with rheumatoid (RA), lyme and possibly osteo arthritis. For example, epidemiologic findings support the idea that HTLV-I infection is a risk factor for RA, and suggest that approximately 13% of the cases of RA in females living in Nagasaki are associated with HTLV-I infection [Eguchi, Origuchi, Takashima, Iwata, Katamine and Nagataki 1996.], Minocycline—an antibiotic—can be effective in about 50% of patients with RA if started early in the course of the Disease [O'Dell 1998],)*

Painful obstructive disorders have been further elaborated throughout the history of OM and were given different names such as: Wind Bi, Cold/Painful Bi, Hot Bi, Fixed/Damp Bi, Inflexible Bi, Bone Bi, Sinew Bi, Muscle Bi, Blood Bi, Skin Bi, and several Deficient type Bi syndromes.

Bi syndromes tend to develop in patients with constitutional weakness. Patients with Yang deficiency constitution are susceptible to the effects of windy, cold and damp environments and tend to develop Cold-Damp Bi syndromes. Patients with Yang fullness or deficiency Yin con-

---

1. In this authors' experience treatment of musculoskeletal disorders utilizing principles from the management of Bi syndromes are of only limited value. A more tissue specific approach is preferable.

2. Polyarthralgia is a variety of conditions which can result in multiple joint pain, swelling and possibly joint deformity

stitution are susceptible to the effects of windy, damp, and warm environments and tend to develop Damp-Heat Bi syndromes.

## Treatment

Treatment of painful obstruction syndromes is aimed at expelling pathogenic factors and mobilizing the stagnant Qi and Blood in the channels. Since deficiency is usually at the root, nourishing the Blood, harmonizing the Defensive and Nutritive Qi and warming the Yang are often integrated.

## Wasting Syndromes

Painful obstruction can lead to the development of a wasting syndrome (Wei-atrophy)—by obstructive depletion of Essence, Blood, Nutritive Qi and Yin Organs. Wei syndromes, characterized by decreased muscular mass and strength, are seen in diseases such as multiple sclerosis and flaccid paralysis (from motor-neuron disease or peripheral neuronal disorders), and in muscular atrophy from primary muscular disorders such as myasthenia gravis and viral infections such as poliomyelitis, and from strokes.

The classic *Simple Questions* describes five types of wasting syndromes, one for each of the Yin organs and its related tissue. Wasting syndromes were mostly attributed to Heat damaging the body Yin fluids, and were probably ascertained from disorders such as polio and infantile paralysis which often begin with a high fever.

In the classic *Simple Questions* wasting syndromes were also associated with Yang Ming Dampness. A discussion on paralysis (in the same text) shows a complex sense of lower extremity paralysis *(Biomedical: innervation?)*.

The Yellow Emperor asked:

Why is it maintained that only the Yang Ming should be used to treat paralysis?

Qi Po answered: The Yang ming is the sea of the five viscera and the six bowels; it is in charge of moistening the ancestral tendon.[3] The ancestral tendon is in charge of the lumbar bones and the function of the lumbar joints. The Chong channel is the sea of the channels and vessels, it is in charge of irrigating the rivers and valleys [of the sinews], and it meets with the Yang Ming in the ancestral tendon. The Yin and Yang meet in the ancestral tendon, and they travel upward along the abdomen to meet at the Qi Jie (Qi fairway) where the Yang Ming is the master. All these channels belong to the Girdle channel and are linked with the Governing channel [spinal system]. For this reason, when Yang Ming is empty, the ancestral tendon will be relaxed, the Girdle channel cannot draw together, and the person will suffer paralysis of the legs with an inability to walk.

As wasting syndromes evolve, deficiency becomes predominant and tonification of the Spleen/pancreas, Stomach, Liver and Kidney is appropriate. Retained pathogenic factors can result in a combined deficiency/excess syndrome.

Wasting syndromes of insidious onset such as myasthenia gravis, muscular dystrophy and multiple sclerosis are attributed often to endogenous and independent causes such as; excessive sex, overwork, irregular diet, trauma and unbalanced emotions.

These factors can also lead to sudden paralysis as seen in Wind Strike *(Biomedical: strokes)*.

### Treatment

Treatment is based on the type and stage of the syndrome.

---

3. Ancestral tendon usually refers to the penis or in this case the perineum and pelvic floor.

# OM: Classification of Soft Tissues

## Joints

Joints are formed by soft tissues and bones. They are classified as being part of the channel and Kidney systems and therefore are on the Exterior and Interior energy level. Joints are important in circulation and storage of Qi and Blood and are the place where Qi enters and exits the Interior (especially at the Sea points). Joints rely on nourishment from Blood, Fluids and Essence and are therefore influenced by Interior factors.

Blockage of circulation often occurs at the joint level due to excessive or lack of physical movement or invasion of external pathogenic factors both of which can result in a Painful Obstruction Syndrome (Bi).

## Sinews (Jin)

Sinews (Jin) in OM cover a wide range of tissues. Jin as been translated erroneously as tendons. Table 3-2 lists the Biomedical terminology for anatomical areas encompassed by the OM definition of "Sinews."

Table 3-2. **OM Sinews**

| |
|---|
| Fascia |
| Tendons |
| Ligaments |
| Subcutaneous Tissue |
| Aspects of Muscles |
| Joint Capsules |
| Cartilage |

Table 3-3. **Qing Dynasty Classification of Soft Tissue Damage**

| Qing Dynasty: Soft Tissue Damage |
|---|
| Sinew Rigidity |
| Sinew Flaccidity |
| Sinew Deviation |
| Sinew Laceration |
| Sinew Contusion |
| Sinew Slippage |
| Sinew Enlargement |
| Sinew Turned Over |
| Sinew Coldness |
| Sinew Heat |

The sinews (Jin) are often related to the functional parts of contractile units and in particular the tendons which are controlled by the Liver and Blood. According to the *Divine Pivot*:

> When there is an abundance of Blood, the sinews are solid and strong; when there is a deficiency of Blood, the sinews are weak.

In the classic *Simple Questions* the Liver is said to govern the sinews. Table 3-3 summarizes Sinews disorders as classified in the Qing dynasty.

## Flesh (Rou)

Muscle mass is mostly related to flesh (Rou) and according to the classic *Simple Questions* is under the control of the Spleen. The Spleen/pancreas, by its function of transportation and transformation provide for; the shape/mass, form and (possibly) tone of muscles, subcutaneous tissue and fascial mass. Therefore, good muscle tone, strength and shape are dependent on both the Liver and Spleen/pancreas health.

Contemporary OM classifies soft tissue damage by (Table 3-4 on page 106) the type of force responsible for the pathology and the pathology of the damaged tissue.

The principal symptoms of soft tissue damage are: Pain, Ecchymosis and Joint

*Table 3-4.* CONTEMPORARY CLASSIFICATION OF SOFT TISSUE DAMAGE

| CAUSE AND LOCATION | PATHOLOGY OF DAMAGED TISSUE | STAGE |
|---|---|---|
| Strain/Sprain<br>Injury due to indirect (intrinsic) forces such as:<br>• sudden movement<br>• heavy lifting<br>Occurs mostly in:<br>• periarticular fascia<br>• ligaments<br>• muscles<br>• tendons | Blood Stasis<br>Mild impairment of collateral circulation within:<br>• fascia<br>• tendons<br>• muscles<br>Includes mild laceration of tissues that does not lead to dysfunction | Acute stage 1-10th day<br>Middle stage 4th-14th day<br>Late stage 14th day-4 weeks |
| Contusion<br>Injury from external force (trauma)<br>Characterized by damage directly under injuring force to:<br>• subcutaneous tissue<br>• muscles<br>• tendons | Altered Position of Torn Tissue<br>Malpositioned tissues accompanied by Blood stasis, swelling, loss of normal function<br>Affected tissues may include:<br>• muscles<br>• tendons<br>• ligaments | Chronic<br>Constitutionally strong patient with effective treatment, unlikely to progress to chronic stage<br>Severe injury, tissue severed, or patient's Original Qi weak likely to progress to chronic stage, characterized by:<br>• muscular rigidity/flaccidity<br>• local skin paleness<br>• swelling and/or tissue hyperplasia |

dysfunction. Table 3-5 on page 107 describes the three main stages of soft tissue damage (early, middle and late), and the chronic stage, which is atypical.

## Differential Diagnosis

When diagnosing the acute and chronic stages, the practitioner must palpate carefully for maximum tenderness and tissue texture. Often these painful sites are at the location of the lesion. This is particularly important in the chronic stage,[4] because frequently the area has abnormal and scarred tissues and acupuncture points that can be treated. In addition, the practitioner should evaluate how well the involved structures are functioning.[5]

*Acute Damage*

If the patient presents with acute soft tissue injury, the practitioner should first exclude other medical conditions that might appear to be traumatic in nature or which allow such damage (such as latent toxin/cancer resulting in bone fracture). For example, Heat Bi *(Biomedical: rheumatoid arthritis)* and Wet Heat Multiple Abscesses *(Biomedical: gonococcal arthritis)* may present similarly to acute traumatic disorders; however, ordinarily Heat Bi and Wet Heat Multiple Abscesses do not have a history of trauma, and usually hematomas are not present. With fractures that are due to cancer, a history of mild trauma is common.

General symptoms such as a fever that is not allayed by perspiration; malaise; and/or poor appetite are common both in acute trauma and in internal medical conditions. These should be evaluated carefully, using modern lab work, if needed.

*Chronic Conditions*

If the patient presents with a suspected chronic condition, the practitioner should exclude the possibility of Latent Toxin *(Bio-*

---

4. This contrasts with Orthopaedic Medicine, in which local tenderness is considered less important during the chronic stage.

5. Channels and Collaterals are responsible for neurological and motor function.

*medical: such as cancer)* and Latent Heat-Toxin infections *(Biomedical: such as tuberculosis)* that, in early stages, can be mistaken easily for musculoskeletal conditions.

The practitioner should watch the general condition of the patient carefully, and may use both modern and traditional diagnostic techniques. Because many low-grade tumors and infections are elusive, the best clues come from observing the patient.

Table 3-6 on page 108 lists some complications that arise from soft tissue damage secondary pathologies.

Table 3-7 on page 109 summarizes pain in OM.

*Table 3-5.* **STAGES OF SOFT TISSUE DAMAGE**

| EARLY STAGE | MIDDLE STAGE | LATE STAGE | CHRONIC STAGE |
|---|---|---|---|
| First 2-3 days. | Begins 4-14 days after mild-to-moderate or severe injury. | Begins about 2 weeks after injury. Usually results from severe trauma or a weakness. | Atypical. Usually due to secondary factors, e.g., improper previous treatment, continuing weakness/ deficiency. |
| Characterized by<br>• severe pain<br>• local Blood stasis<br>• swelling<br>• dysfunction | Characterized by<br>• reduced swelling<br>• absorption of Blood stasis<br>• greenish-purplish color of ecchymotic Blood<br>• slightly warm skin<br>• pain reduced greatly | Characterized by<br>• change of ecchymotic color to yellow-brown<br>• symptoms reduced greatly<br>• Dysfunctions may not be noticeable | Characterized by (Usually)<br>• persistent, mild swelling<br>• development of adhesions & scars<br>• dull pain (ache)<br>• sluggish movement of affected parts |
| Recovery<br>Mild<br>Goes to middle stage. | Recovery<br>Mild-to-Moderate<br>Treated correctly, should heal 1-2 weeks. | Recovery<br>Expected within 5 weeks of injury, if did not heal by second week of treatment Some patients progress to chronic. | Recovery<br>Mild<br>Similar to middle stage. |
| Severe<br>Goes to middle stage, but middle stage is more prolonged. | Severe<br>By day 14 patient should be improved noticeably, with partial recovery of functions. | | Severe<br>May be prolonged. Symptoms may vary greatly by location. |

*Table 3-6.* COMPLICATIONS OF SOFT TISSUE SECONDARY PATHOLOGIES

| | |
|---|---|
| **LACERATION OF BONE FRAGMENT** | Caused by physical force exerted on tendon-periosteal junction. Palpability depends on location. |
| **DAMAGE TO CHANNELS (NERVES AND THEIR ENERVATED STRUCTURES)** | Identified by analyzing<br>• joint movements<br>• loss of sensation<br>• presence of marked muscle contraction<br>Modern neurological knowledge useful in this evaluation. |
| **CONGEALED BLOOD (OSSIFICATION)** | Nontreatment of traumatic injury and Blood stasis can lead to<br>• channel blockage<br>• insufficiency of tissues nourishment<br>Tissues can react by hardening, resulting in dysfunction, pain aggravation and formation of osseous lesions. |
| **CONGEALED DAMPNESS (INTER-ARTICULAR FREE BODY)** | Cartilage damage accompanied by other soft-tissue inflammation (Wind-Damp or Wind-Heat).<br>Can lead to ossification of these tissues which become interarticular free bodies. |
| **PROLIFERATED BI SYNDROMES (OSSEOUS ARTHRITIS)** | Inflamed tissue also may transform into "hardness" spurs that attach to joint surface. (Spurs usually develop along stressful paths.) |

*Table 5-7.* **PAIN IN ORIENTAL MEDICINE**

| | PAIN FELT | TEMPERATURE | SKIN/ TONGUE COLOR | AGGRAVATED BY | OTHER SYMPTOMS |
|---|---|---|---|---|---|
| Cold Pain | Usually local May be intense, may be worse at night, better during the day | Tissue/patient cold | White/ pale/ pale purple | Cold | Tissues contracted, muscles tight or spasmed |
| | Treatment: Spicy warm herbs, hot acupuncture, moxa, friction, warming massage | | | | |
| Hot Pain | Often radiates May be throbbing | Tissue/patient warm | Red | Heat | Tissues/ muscles may be flaccid or atrophied |
| | Treatment Cooling herbs, cooling acupuncture and bleeding, cooling massage | | | | |
| Damp Pain | Local, usually not radiating, often lower body Patient affected area usually feel(s) heavy | Patient/affected area usually feel(s) heavy | Yellow | Weather change | Tissues feel damp |
| | Treatment Eliminate damp herbs, cooling or warming per symptoms (Damp-Heat/Damp-Cold/Wind-Damp); acupuncture with cupping/moxa; circulating draining massage. | | | | |
| Wind Pain | Movement, radiation Often upper body, Often sudden onset | Hot/cold | Cyan/ green Normal | Exposure to wind | Muscle may twitch |
| | Treatment Spicy dispersing herb, sedating acupuncture, cupping, plucking massage | | | | |
| Blood Stasis | Fixed location; Often stabbing or paresthesia May be throbbing | Hot/cold | Dark/dry lusterles s/purple | Immobility/ Sleep | Often worse at night; Common with injury; Common in women and elderly |
| | Treatment Quickening Blood/Transforming Stasis, bleeding, vigorous massage | | | | |
| Qi Stagnation | Often at disease onset; distention/pulsating, nonfixed, poorly localized | Normal | Normal | Wind and Emotions Immobility | Frequently related to emotional factors; often subcostal tenderness and pain |
| | Treatment Qi-regulating and Qi-moving herbs, sedating acupuncture, cupping, vibrating massage | | | | |
| Qi/Blood Deficiency | Usually in chronic stage, dull, achy, area weak, often poorly localized | Normal or cold | Normal or pale | Fatigue | Pain worse in afternoon Possibly at night |
| | Treatment Tonify Qi and Blood, Vitalize Qi and Blood (mildly), Warm the channels | | | | |

# *Important Tissues: Biomedical Perspective*

The following are basic descriptions of the makeup and function of several important tissues. The understanding of basic biomedical concepts helps explain many of the treatments proposed in this text.

## Joints

Joints, the structural foundation of locomotion, are complex structures that can function only by an intricate integration of compression, tension, locomotive and proprioceptive elements (Figure 3-2).

### Connective Tissue

All elements in a joint complex contain connective tissue. Connective tissue (which includes cartilage and bone) develops from the mesenchyme, which arises largely from the mesodermal somites and the somatic and splanchnic mesoderm.[6] Ordinarily, connective tissue consists mostly of fibroblast cells;[7] the rest are mast cells,[8] macrophages,[9] plasma cells, pigment cells, lymphocytes and leukocytes.[10] *Fibroblasts* are involved in the production of fibrous elements and nonfibrous ground substance of connective tissue. The fibrous components are collagen

and elastin (Ombregt et al. *ibid*). Collagen is the most abundant protein in the body and is a component of all types of connective tissue. It tends to have great tensile strength, because of its triple helix configuration, but it is relatively nonelastic. It can be stretched only about 4% or so before it ruptures or is subjected to irreversible hysteresis (loss of elasticity). The biochemical configuration of collagen is highly dependent on the incorporation of the amino acid proline and requires vitamin C for normal production (Bates and Levene 1969).

Elastin can stretch 150% of its original length. There are 11 types of collagen found in connective tissue. Each type is genetically determined and differs in the chemical nature of the polypeptide chains that form the tropocollagen molecules found in the collagen fiber (Bogduk and Twomey *ibid*).[11]

*Nonfibrous ground substance* (Figure 3-1) is composed of proteoglycans, which are polysaccharide molecules—six to 60 glycoaminoglycans (GAGs), (also referred to as mucopolysaccharides)—bound to protein chains in covalent complexes (sugar amine bound together by a polymer). Within cartilage there are two main types of GAGs, chondroitin-4-sulfate and chondroitin-6-sulfate. All GAGs (Hascall and Hascall 1981) contain sulfate ester moieties which are required for normal GAG synthesis. Found in the extracellular matrix of connective tissue, proteoglycans can bind to a high proportion of water. In cartilage they are bound to hyaluronic acid chains to form a proteoglycans aggregate (Bogduk and Twomey *ibid*).

The primary function of GAG's is to provide flexibility and serve as a lubricant

---

6. Embryonic tissues.

7. Fibroblast is an undifferentiated cell in the connective tissue that gives rise to various precursor cells, such as the chondroblast, collagenoblast, and osteoblast, that form the fibrous, binding, and supporting tissue of the body.

8. Mast cell is a constituent of connective tissue containing large basophilic granules that contain heparin, serotonin, bradykinin, and histamine.

9. Macrophage is any phagocytic cell of the reticuloedothelial system including histocyte in loose connective tissue.

---

10. Leukocyte is a white blood cell. Five types of leukocytes are classified by the presence or absence of granules in the cytoplasm of the cell. The agranulocytes are lymphocytes and monocytes. The granulocytes are neutrophils, basophils, and eosinophils.

11. Polypeptide is a chain of amino acids joined by a peptide bond. It is heavier than a single molecule peptide but lighter than a molecule of protein.

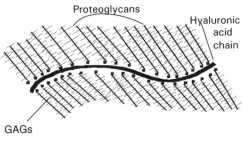

Figure 3-1:    Ground substance.

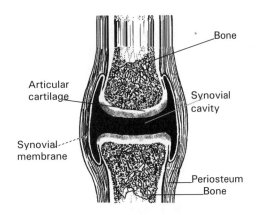

Figure 3-2:    Synovial Joint.

between adjacent collagen fibers and maintain interfiber distance by their negative electric charge (Bogduk and Twomey *ibid*).

### Cartilage

Cartilage, a non-vascular tissue, is comprised of a variety of fibrous connective tissues in which the matrix (intracellular substance of a tissue) is abundant and firm. Table 3-8 on page 112 lists the types of cartilage, based on their structure. Due to complex processes within the chondrocytes (cartilage cells), articular cartilage undergoes constant degeneration and regeneration. The joint's environment, including the synovial fluid, is important in the degeneration and regeneration cycle (Bonica *ibid*). *(OM: Tai Chi exercises, which are designed to open and close the joints, are believed to aid in the regenerative process).*

### Synovium

The synovium is a colorless, viscous fluid that lubricates and nourishes the joint, including the avascular articular cartilage. The inner surface of the joint capsule is lined with several synovial layers. Innervated by sympathetic nerve fibers, these layers are abundant in capillaries, venules and lymphatic supply. The synovium plays a significant role in infection control and in production of hyaluronate, which gives synovial fluid its viscosity. Trauma and disease can change the viscosity so that it no longer circulates properly.

### Categories of Joints

Joints can be categorized as freely-movable (diarthrodial) hinges, such as the shoulder and the zygoapophyseal (facet) joints, or semi-movable (amphiarthrodial), such as the intervertebral joints and the symphysis pubis. The sacroiliac joint has characteristics of both (Bonica *ibid*).

**FREELY-MOVABLE JOINTS.** Freely-movable joints are synovial in structure, held together by a capsule of dense, fibrous tissue and ligaments. Additional support is provided by muscles, tendons and atmospheric pressure (the inner joint space has negative pressure). One example of this structure is the hip joint: the two surfaces can stay together even if the soft tissues around them are severed. However, if a small hole in the synovial sac develops and air penetrates, the hip joint loses this adherence.

Movable joints are kept stable, and mechanical forces are distributed by a system that combines elements of tension and compression from the capsule, ligaments, muscles, fascia and bone. This system allows joints to survive great mechanical stresses.

**SEMI-MOVABLE JOINTS.** Semi-movable joints, such as the vertebral bodies, are separated by a disc. The bony surface of the joint is covered by articular cartilage of type 2 collagen, which has significant tensile strength (Table 3-8.)

## Joint Neurophysiology

Synovial joints are supplied by mechanoreceptors and nociceptive receptors (pain-receiving free nerve endings). The joint capsule has four types of receptors.

### Joint Receptors

Joint receptors have myelinated and unmyelinated fibers that have several functions, some of which are inter-regulating. The characteristics of joint receptors are summarized in Table 3-9 on page 113 (Wyke 1979, 1977; Mitchell 1993).

*Table 3-8.* **TYPES OF CARTILAGE**

| GENERAL | Description | Non-vascular tissue made of a variety of fibrous connective tissues. Three types, depending on structure. |
|---|---|---|
| **ELASTIC CARTILAGE** | Location | Ligamenta flava, ear and larynx |
| | Elasticity | More pliant than other cartilage |
| | Color | Yellow |
| **HYALINE CARTILAGE** | Location | Comprises the costal, nasal and articular cartilages on ends of bones |
| | Elasticity | Considerable |
| | Color | Often bluish |
| | Notes | The most abundant cartilage in the adult body |
| | | • Contains 80% H2O, which is bound by the negatively-charged proteoglycans |
| | | • High H2O content results in swelling of cartilage, allowing it to absorb mechanical forces |
| | | • Sustained pressure can result in plastic deformation |
| | | • Avascular |
| | | • Does not have a nerve supply |
| **FIBROCARTILAGE** | Location | Intervertebral discs of vertebral column Symphysis pubis A few other joints |
| | Elasticity | More elastic than hyaline but less than elastic cartilage |
| | Color | Whitish |
| | Notes | Appears as a transition between tendons or ligaments or bones Subject to hysteresis |

Table 3-9. JOINT CAPSULE RECEPTORS

| TYPE I | Functions | Proprioception, pain suppression, tonic reflexogenic effect on muscles, report tension of joint capsule outer layer |
|---|---|---|
| | Size | Small (6-9 $\mu$m) |
| | Myelinated | Yes |
| | Location | Joint capsule outer layer |
| | Most Active | At initiation and at end of range of motion |
| | Notes | Static and dynamic mechanoreceptors, low threshold, slow adapting |
| TYPE II | Functions | Phasic reflexogenic effect on muscle, pain suppression |
| | Size | Medium (9-12 $\mu$m) |
| | Myelinated | Yes |
| | Location | At deeper layers of capsule and articular fat pads |
| | Most Active | Mid-range of motion |
| | Notes | Dynamic mechanoreceptors, low threshold, very slow adapting |
| TYPE III | Function | Probably proprioception |
| | Size | Large (13-17 $\mu$m) |
| | Myelinated | Yes |
| | Location | Typical receptors of ligaments and tendons that insert close to, but not in, joint capsule |
| | Most Active | Probably in extremes of motion |
| | Notes | High-threshold mechanoreceptor, very slow adapting, more receptive to load than to degree of stretch |
| TYPE IV | Functions | Nociception, tonic reflexogenic effect on muscles, respiratory and cardiovascular reflexogenic effect |
| | Size | Very small (2-5 $\mu$m) |
| | Myelinated | Myelinated and unmyelinated |
| | Location | Throughout joint capsule, walls of articular blood vessels and articular fat pads |
| | Notes | High threshold, nonadaptive |

## Biomechanics of the Spinal Joints

Movement in the spine is produced by the coordinated action of nerves, muscles and levers. Elastic energy stored in the fascia and ligaments also provides momentum (spring). Prime mover muscles (agonists) initiate and carry out movement, whereas antagonist muscles often control and modify it (Lindh 1980). Spinal movements are always a combination of the actions of several segments, and sidebending is always coupled with rotation and translation. During active gait, the spine responds mostly passively to the primary propellants the lower extremity and pelvic system.

The spinal column is comprised of a series of vertebrae and joints that are capable of different motions at various levels. These are mainly determined by the facets and their angulation. Vertebral movements are described by three basic ways:

1. The relationship of a superior vertebra to the corresponding inferior vertebra. For example, in flexion the superior vertebra rotates and glides forward in relation to the inferior vertebra.

2. The direction of movement of the anterior aspect of a vertebra. For example, in rotation to the right, the anterior aspect rotates right and the

posterior aspect (spinous process) moves to the left.

**3.** Rotation around an axis, or translation (gliding) along an axis.

this kind of description specifies the horizontal (X), vertical (Y), or anteroposterior (Z) axis, within which the vertebral body moves.

For example, in flexion the superior vertebra rotates around a horizontal (X) axis and translates forward in relation to the lower vertebra along the anteroposterior (Z) axis (Panjabi and White *ibid*).

Movement characteristics of the spine are summarized in Table 3-10. Table 3-11 describes the three types of coupled movements. (see radiology chapter 4 as well).

*Table 3-10.* **MOVEMENT CHARACTERISTICS**

| MOVEMENT | CHARACTERISTICS |
|---|---|
| FLEXION | Posterior aspect of the spine becomes increasingly convex |
| | Spaces between vertebrae increase posteriorly |
| | Spaces at the anterior aspect decrease |
| | Superior vertebra glides forward on adjoining inferior |
| | Nucleus pulposus shifts backward |
| EXTENSION | Convexity increases anteriorly |
| | Superior vertebra glides backward in relation to inferior |
| | Nucleus pulposus shifts forward |
| SIDEBENDING | Sidebending always with coupled rotation |
| | "coupling" occur in same or opposite direction |
| | Nucleus pulposus shifts toward convexity |

*Table 3-11.* COUPLING OF VERTEBRAL MOVEMENT, FRYETTE LAWS

| DYSFUNCTION | DESCRIPTIONS |
|---|---|
| **NEUTRAL** | Bending to one side is coupled<br>  • with rotation to the opposite side<br>    — occurs in lumbar and thoracic spine, not in the cervical spine except in OA joint, if normal spine curvature is maintained<br>In "neutral" mechanics the spine is relatively stable<br>  • injuries occur less frequently |
| **NONNEUTRAL** | Refers to vertebral motions with the facets engaged<br>Side bending coupled with<br>  • rotation to same side<br>  • results in less stability than neutral spine mechanics<br>  • found in cervical, thoracic and lumbar spine<br>  • results in increased injury risk |
| **RESTRICTIVE** | Movement in one direction<br>  • reduces motion all other directions<br>  • used for localizing manipulation techniques |

# Muscles

Skeletal muscles make up about 40% of body weight. They are comprised of 75% water, 20% protein and 5% inorganic material, organic "extractives," and carbohydrates (Ombregt, Bisschop, ter Veer, and Van de Velde 1995). Muscles are well-vascularized, allowing them to recover from injuries relatively faster than tissues that have a smaller blood supply.

## Muscle Fibers

Muscles are composed of muscle fibers bound together by connective tissue. A single skeletal muscle cell is a thin cylinder, 10-100 microns in diameter that can extend up to 4cm in length. Skeletal muscle fibers may extend the entire length of the muscle and join with tendons at their ends. An electrically-polarized membrane surrounds each fiber. If the membrane becomes temporarily depolarized, the muscle fiber contracts.

Muscle fibers are composed of slender threads of *myofibril*. Each myofibril has two fine longitudinal fibrils, lying side by side, comprised of many regularly-overlapped, ultramicroscopic, thick and thin *myosin* and *actin* myofilaments that may extend the entire length of the muscle. A muscle fiber has about 1500 myosin filaments and 300 actin filaments, which are large protein molecules responsible for muscle contraction. Myofibrils are embedded in connective tissue that transmits the pull of the muscle cells during contraction.

Myosin is the thicker of the filaments and is twice the size of the thin filament Actin. Muscle contraction is achieved by attractive forces between these filaments causing them to slide together (Chusid 1982), (Figure 3-3).

### Muscle Contraction

Three mechanisms that induce action potentials (electrical depolarization of muscles) lead to the initiation of muscle contraction:

• Stimulation by nerve fibers.

• Stimulation by hormones and local chemical agents.

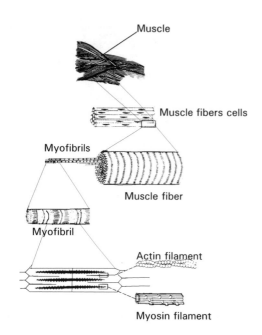

Muscle

Muscle fibers cells

Myofibrils

Muscle fiber

Myofibril

Actin filament

Myosin filament

*Figure 3-3:*   Fibrillar organization within skeletal muscle (after Bloom and Fawcett).

• Spontaneous electrical activity within the membrane itself.

Smooth muscles and heart muscles are stimulated by all three mechanisms; normally, skeletal (striated) muscles are stimulated only by nerve fibers (Chusid *ibid*).

## Muscle Functions

Muscles produce motion (acceleration, concentric action), stop motion (deceleration, isometric and eccentric action), and contribute to functions such as respiration, defecation and generation of body heat. Muscle health and function depend on the nervous, digestive, respiratory and circulatory systems to provide food (trophic factors) and oxygen, on the skin for protection and to help dissipate heat produced during muscle contraction, and on the kidney to excrete metabolic waste. Muscle contraction that does not involve muscle shortening (no movement) is called

*isometric* (constant length) contraction. Muscle contraction that involves movement of an object is known as *isotonic* (constant tension) contraction.

### Postural & Phasic Muscles.

Skeletal muscles are composed mainly of two fiber types: slow twitch (type I) and fast twitch (type II), summarized in Table 3-12. Table 3-13 on page 117 lists postural and phasic muscles.

**POSTURAL (TONIC) MUSCLES.** Postural muscles (also called *tonic*, or *red* muscles) have a significantly larger number of type I fibers than phasic muscles have. Type I fibers are more vascular and resistant to fatigue than type II fibers. Tonic muscles can withstand several hundred contractions before becoming fatigued. Often they are relatively deeper than phasic muscles. They tend to be monoarticular (span only one joint) and richly innervated (spindle-rich). They have relatively small motor units.

Tonic muscles are often the first muscles recruited during an involuntary reflex action such as maintaining posture. Since tonic muscles often span one joint and are prone to tightness (Mitchell 1993), they can perpetuate type II (non-neutral) somatic dysfunctions. These muscles are thought to have primary responsibility for countering the effects of gravity (e.g., for maintaining posture) and therefore are required to withstand work of long durations.[12]

**PHASIC MUSCLES.** Phasic muscles (*white* muscles), which consist predominantly of fast twitch (type II) fibers, are used for short periods when extra strength or quick response is needed. Phasic muscles often are relatively more superficial than tonic

12. However, since muscle function always is integrated with phasic muscles and other tissue, it is advisable not to consider muscle function in a reductionist fashion.

muscles, and they tend to be multi-articular (span several joints). Innervated by relatively large motor units, they are under voluntary reflex control. Because they are multi-articular, they perpetuate type I (neutral) somatic dysfunction (Mitchell 1993). According to Janda, these muscles are prone to weakness. When phasic muscles are contracted continuously (such as in reflex guarding), they become congested and sore.

*Table 3-12.* **MUSCLE FIBER TYPES AND MUSCLE TYPES**

| MUSCLE FIBER TYPES | |
|---|---|
| TYPE I — SLOW TWITCH | Strength training and interval training transform Type I into Type II |
| TYPE II — FAST TWITCH | Endurance training converts Type II to Type I. |
| **MUSCLE TYPES** | |
| TONIC (POSTURAL) | Have significantly larger number of Type I Fibers than phasic muscles<br>More vascular than Type II<br>More resistant to fatigue than the phasic muscle is<br>Can withstand several hundred contractions |
| PHASIC | Predominantly type II muscle fiber<br>Used for short periods when extra strength or quick response is needed |

*Table 3-13.* **POSTURAL AND PHASIC MUSCLES**

| POSTURAL MUSCLES (YIN) | PHASIC MUSCLES (YANG) |
|---|---|
| Suboccipital | Diagastrics |
| Masticatoris | Deltoids |
| Sternocleidomastoid (scm) | Scaleni/longus colli |
| Short, deep extensor muscles | Deep cervical flexors[a] |
| Upper trapezius | Lower/middle trapezius |
| Pectoralis | Lower stabilizers of scapula |
| Quadratus lumborum | Extensors of upper extremities |
| Psoas | Rectus abdominus[b] |
| Tensor fascia latae (TFL) | Gluteus medius |
| Rectus femoris | Gluteus maximus |
| Lower extremity adductors [sp] | Gluteus minimus |
| Hamstring | Tibialis anterior |
| Triceps surae | Vasti |

a. Jull, Janda 1987, Janda 1996.
b. The subject of whether the rectus abdominus obliques are phasic is controversial.

**TRANSFORMING MUSCLE FIBERS.** With training or electrical stimulation, muscle fibers can be transformed from one type to the other.

• Strength training and interval training transform type I-tonic to type II-phasic.

• Endurance training converts type II to type I (Dvorák 1990).

In the lumbar spine, both hypomobility and nerve root compression results in transformation of muscle fibers. These factors have been demonstrated histochemically (Jowett and Fidler 1975) to increase the proportion of slow twitch fibers, resulting in decreased dexterity.

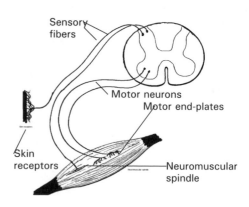

*Figure 3-4:*    A motor unit (After Crouch).

## Muscle Innervation

Skeletal muscle fiber is innervated both by efferent (motor) and afferent (sensory) nerves. Efferent axons arise from nerve cells located in the brainstem or the spinal cord. These nerve cells are called motor neurons or, somatic efferents. Motor neuron axons are myelinated. They are the largest-diameter axons in the body and therefore are fast-conducting. A large number of muscle nerve fibers are sensory in function (Sherrington has estimated at least 40%).

A motor neuron and the muscle fibers it innervates is called a *motor unit* (Figure 3-4). The region of the muscle membrane together with the terminal portion of the axon is known as the *motor end plate.* The junction that includes the axon terminal and the motor end plate is known as a *neuromuscular junction.*

Muscles have three major types of receptors (Chusid *ibid*):

• Muscle spindles — annulospiral ending, nuclear bag region and flower-spray endings.

• Golgi tendon organs.

• Free nerve endings.

## *Muscle Spindles*

Muscle spindles are specialized mechanoreceptive contractile fiber units containing *intrafusal fibers* surrounded by connective tissue. Muscle spindles are arranged in parallel to *extrafusal fibers,* which are the regular contractile fibers that provide the muscle's contractile force. The ends of muscle spindle capsules are attached to tendons at either end of the muscle, or to the sides of adjacent, extrafusal fibers. These fusiform (spindle-shaped) structures are several millimeters long and are found throughout the muscle, with a higher concentration (Richmond and Abrahams 1979) around the slow twitch fibers. Muscles responsible for fine and precise motor movements, such as tonic (postural) muscles, have a considerably higher concentration of spindles.

Muscle spindle stimulation by acupuncture is probably the most important aspects of this treatment technique in myofascial pain.

**NUCLEAR BAG REGION.** The two ends of each muscle spindle are contractile. The middle portion or receptor portion of a muscle spindle, the *nuclear bag region* (Figure 3-5), is noncontractile. Wrapped around the muscle spindle fibers in a complex manner

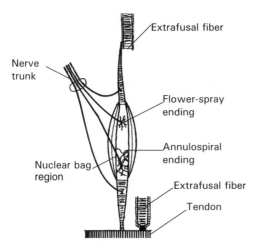

*Figure 3-5:* Muscle spindle (after Ganong).

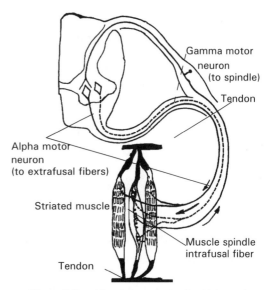

*Figure 3-6:* Muscle innervation by Alpha and Gamma motor neurons (after Waxman and deGroot 1995).

are two types of sensory endings that are found in the muscle spindle. These are the nuclear bag that contains *annulospiral endings* (primary endings), which are continuous with rapidly-conducting afferent (sensory) nerves, and *Flower-Spray Endings* (secondary endings) found on either side of the annulospiral endings, which are receptors for the smaller myelinated fibers (Waxman and deGroot 1995).

**MUSCLE SPINDLE FUNCTION.** The primary function of intrafusal fibers (spindle, nuclear bag and flower-spray endings)— which serve as the sensory organ of muscles—is to register changes in muscle length (the static response) and rate of change in muscle length (the dynamic response), both of which regulate muscle tone and help to protect the muscle from tearing. Muscle spindles are responsible for the stretch reflex and for muscle tone, which is essential for maintaining posture, and therefore is commonly involved in myofascial pain syndromes.

The receptors in the nuclear bag region, which adapt rapidly to changes in muscle length, velocity, and acceleration of contraction, serve the stretch reflex. Also responsive to stretch, flower-spray endings produce increased flexor and decreased extensor motor neuron activity (Waxman and deGroot 1995).

The arrangement and number of spindles—for example, the fact that a muscle with the tendency to tightness has many spindles—helps explain Janda's clinical observation that postural muscles tend to become short, whereas phasic muscles tend to become weak.

**GAMMA MOTOR NERVES.** *Gamma* motor (efferent) nerves, which supply motor innervation to the muscle spindles, comprise the small motor neuron system whose cell bodies are located in the ventral horn (spinal cord). These nerves are distributed to the motor end-plate on the contractile ends of the intrafusal fibers (muscle spindles).

Gamma motor nerves set the gain or resting tone of muscle spindles which increase the muscle's sensitivity to overall stretch. The gamma motor system is regulated by descending activity from a number of areas in the brain (Waxman and deGroot *ibid*).

**ALPHA MOTOR NERVES.** *Alpha* motor nerves

supply the regular contractile, extrafusal, muscle fibers (not the spindle). Alpha motor nerves arise from large anterior horn neurons (spinal cord), called alpha motor neurons. When alpha motor neurons fire, action potential in their axons propagate via the ventral roots and peripheral nerves to the motor end-plate were they excite the muscle (Waxman and deGroot *ibid*), (Figure 3-6).

### Golgi Tendon Organs

The Golgi tendon organs, which lie in series with the muscle fibers, serve as inhibitors of muscle spindles and contractile forces in the muscle. When tension at the muscle tendon fiber approaches a dangerous level, the Golgi tendon organs limit muscle contraction automatically, by:

• Reacting to tension in the extrafusal muscle which mass-activate Golgi receptors.

• Sending impulses to the spinal cord, which in turn excites inhibitory interneurons that relax the muscle.

Golgi tendon organs have a much higher threshold than do muscle spindles, and therefore do not over-control the muscle. The nerve fibers of Golgi tendon organs, which are myelinated, are believed to synapse in the ventral horn of the spinal cord with inhibitory interneurons (Renshaw cells) that terminate directly on alpha motor neurons of the same muscle. Therefore, Renshaw cells appear to be part of local feedback circuits that prevent overactivity in alpha motor neurons (Waxman and deGroot *ibid*).

### Free Nerve Endings

The third group of muscle nerve structures are the free nerve endings, which are associated mostly with blood vessels and pain receptors. Deep palpation and stimulation of free nerve endings can produce muscle pain.

### Sympathetic Innervation

Earlier researchers thought that skeletal muscles did not have sympathetic innervation (except for the blood vessels). Now direct sympathetic innervation to the intrafusal fibers of muscle spindles are known, and the fact that sympathetic stimulation causes muscle tension is recognized (Baker and Banks 1986). Muscle paralysis of animals that have been injected with curare (a plant alkaloid that induces paralysis of muscle by selective action on the myoneural junction) can be blocked by alpha-adrenergic antagonists, which act on sympathetic neurons. This sympathetic innervation has been demonstrated physiologically and anatomically (Passatrore, Filppi and Grassi 1985; Bridgman and Eldred 1981; Santini and Ibata, 1971; Baker and Daito 1981).

## Tendons

Tendons are fibrous connective tissues that attach muscles to bones and other structures. Their collagenous fibers are arranged fairly regularly. Tendons appear white because they are relatively avascular and therefore have a poor blood supply.

Collagen represents about 60-80% of the total dry weight of a tendon. Although tendons contain no or little elastin fibers (maximum of 2%), they nevertheless are slightly stretchable. The slight, rope-like interweaving pattern of collagen fibers allows for some elongation, which can mitigate pull at the tendon insertion. In a normal state tendons consist of 30% collagen and about 2% elastin embedded in an extracellular matrix containing 68% water (Ombregt, Bisschop, ter Veer and de Velde 1995).

Tendons are constructed by groups of fibers, each of which is composed of several fibrils, which form fascicles surrounded by the endotendon. The endotendon is an areolar connective tissue sheath (small space) that houses the nerves and blood vessels. The endotendon is enclosed by the epitendon and outer most layer is the paratendon. Tendons appear to receive only afferent (sensory) nerve supply (Brown 1995).

In most cases tendons attach to the skeleton. The tendon of the muscle that attaches to the less movable or proximal structure is called the *tendon of origin*. The tendon that attaches to the more movable or distal part is called *tendon of insertion*. Frequently the origin of a muscle is attached directly to the periosteum of a bone without an intervening tendon, but usually the insertion is tendinous.

Tendons can vary in shape from short and stocky to long and slender. Some tendons are broad sheets of connective tissues called *aponeuroses*.

# Fascia

Fascia is made of collagen and elastic fibers, ground substance and cellular elements. As with other types of connective tissue, fascia is susceptible to hysteresis.[13]

Fascia is continuous throughout the body and can provide support to muscles, joints, vessels, nerves and organs. Fascia functions as a tension member within the somatic frame. As muscles broaden they stretch the fascia that surrounds them, and this in turn provides support and protection to the muscle. The stretching of fascia distributes some of the load, as fascia is continuous throughout the body, and stores elastic energy. Fascia is susceptible to plastic deformation and (Greenman *ibid*) and is therefore thought to have a "memory"[14].

---

13. Although less so because of high elastic fiber content.

14. Fascia can maintain a distorted shape for a long time and often during myofascial release the patient will recall an old injury.

# Ligaments

Ligaments are bands or sheets of strong, fibrous, connective tissue. Their main function is to connect the articular ends of bones, forming support for the joints. They often brace cartilages and organs, and they provide support for the connecting muscles and fasciae of other structures as well.

Hinge joints such as the elbow or fingers need collateral ligaments to support the relatively lax joint capsule. Ligaments facilitate motion (by release of stored elastic energy) and limit motion, as well.

Ligaments get their tensile strength from collagen, which comprises 70-80% of the structure's dry weight. The ligament's elastin fibers, about 4% of its dry weight, give the ligament its elastic quality (Ombregt, Bisschop, ter Veer and Van de Velde 1995).

Structurally, ligaments are similar to tendons, however the collagenous fibers of ligaments are not arranged as regularly as those of tendons. Because ligaments are innervated richly by both mechanoreceptors and sensory receptors, they are a frequent source of pain. This is seen (and recognized) regularly in acute sprains. However, ligaments also are a common source of chronic pain in patients who may or may not have a history of acute trauma (Dorman *ibid*).

# The Spine

The usual spine is composed of 7 cervical, 12 thoracic, 5 lumbar and 5 fused sacral vertebrae. The spinal column has four anatomical curves: the lumbar and cervical lordosis which have a forward convexity, and the structures adjoining them, the thoracic and sacrococcygeal areas which are kyphotic with a backward convexity. Normal spinal curvatures develop through embryology and into adulthood. In the uterus, in order to conform to the uterine walls, the spine is convex posteriorly in its entirety—hence all posterior convexities are called primary curves. When a baby turns onto his abdomen and begins to look up the cervical lordotic curve develops. Lumbar lordosis develops into adulthood, probably beginning when the baby begins to crawl on all four limbs. The lordotic lumbar and cervical curves with their posterior concavity are called secondary curves.

Stability, as well as posture, is maintained mainly by ligamentous structures, and muscles and their fascias. In man, the forces of weightbearing at the spinal vertebrae increase progressively from the cervical to the lumbar spine, therefore the size of the discs increases. The curvatures of the spine provided by the discs, and other structures, allow for regional weightbearing capabilities, by preloading tension components of the spine.

Pain in the spine may arise from all structures containing free nerve endings, such as muscles, fascia, ligaments, including the posterior longitudinal ligament and the anterior longintudinal ligament, annulus fibrosus, periosteum of vertebral bodies, posterior arches, facets, dura mater, blood vessels and spinal cord (Hrisch et al. 1964). Pain often arises from sacroiliac structures as well.

## Ligaments of the Spine

Ligaments provide stability to the entire spine as well as being important in proprioceptive functions.

### The Anterior and Posterior Longitudinal Ligaments

The anterior and posterior longitudinal ligaments secure the vertebral bodies to one another and provide protection for the disc and cord. They are both extrinsically and intrinsically innervated (Willard *ibid*).

THE ANTERIOR LONGITUDINAL LIGAMENT. The anterior longitudinal ligament (ALL) is a broad, strong band of fibers that runs from the axis of the cervical vertebra to the sacrum. The ligament is narrower in the cervical region and widens inferiorly, the greatest dimension and strength being in the lumbar spine. The ligament is made up of dense longitudinal fibers that are tightly adherent to the discs and to the margins of the vertebral bodies (Bogduk and Twomey *ibid*).

THE POSTERIOR LONGITUDINAL LIGAMENT. The posterior longitudinal ligament (PLL) also runs along the posterior surfaces of the vertebral bodies, from the axis of the neck to the sacrum. Unlike the ALL, the PLL is relatively narrower in the lumbar spine than in the rest of the spine. This unfortunate arrangement is one possible reason that disc lesions in the lumbar spine are more common than in any other region (Cyriax *ibid*). The longitudinal fibers of the PLL are denser and more compact than those of the ALL (Bogduk and Twomey *ibid*).

### Ligaments of the Posterior Arch

The ligaments of the posterior vertebral arches also are important for stability, and provide elastic energy during movements.

THE INTERSPINOUS AND INTERTRANSVERSE LIGAMENTS. The interspinous ligaments are thin and membranous in composition, binding adjacent spinous processes. The intertransverse ligaments connect adjacent transverse processes. They are contiguous with the deep muscles of the back, especially in the thoracic spine (Bogduk and Twomey *ibid*). Tenderness of the interspinous ligaments is a good indicator of a dysfunctional vertebral level.

THE SUPRASPINOUS LIGAMENTS. The supraspinous ligaments connect the apices of the vertebra, providing stability and acting as a counterforce to flexion of the spine as well as assisting in the restoration of posture from the flexed to erect posture (elastic energy/springing). The supraspinous ligament becomes progressively less organized and in some individuals may not extend inferiorly to L4 (Bogduk and Twomey, *ibid*).

The interspinous and supraspinous ligaments act as force tranducers, translating the tension of the thoracolumbar fascia to the lumbar vertebra (Willard 1995).

**THE LIGAMENTA FLAVA.** The ligamenta flava (or yellow ligament) is more elastic than other ligaments in the spine—allowing separation of the lamina during flexion. They connect adjacent laminae of the vertebral bodies and function to restore the spinal column to a neutral position. The ligamenta flava are thickest and strongest in the lumbar spine.

NOTE: More details on ligaments are presented in appropriate sections of the book.

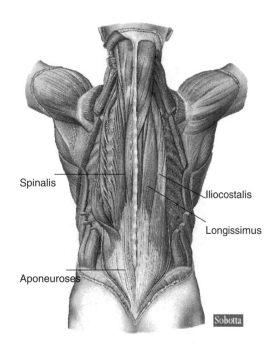

*Figure 3-7:*    Posterior muscles.

## Muscles of the Spine

Muscle actions are coupled always with those of other muscles and fasciae to distribute loads, increase stability, have concentric and eccentric functions (agonist/antagonist) and for storage of energy.

### Flexor and Extensor Muscles of the Spine

Functionally muscles affecting the spine can be divided into two major groups, the flexors and the extensors. However, flexion extension and stability of the spine and pelvis is dependent also on other associated muscles and their fascias, such as the abdominal, glutei, hamstrings and latissimus dorsi.

### Posterior Muscles

The posterior muscles affecting the spine are known collectively as the extensors. The extensors stretch from the head, shoulder, and trunk down to the sacrum and pelvis. The extensor muscles occupy

the broad gutters posterior to the vertebral bodies and transverse processes (TrPr's) on each side of the spine. These can be divided into three groups (Bogduk Twomey *ibid*).

### Superficial Group

**THE ERECTOR SPINAE.** The erector spinae is the most superficial group which arises from the iliac crest and sacrum through a strong aponeuroses (a flat fibrous sheet of connective tissue).

The erector spinae are composed of three columns (Figure 3-7).

• Spinalis and semispinalis.

— The most medial.

• Longissimus thoracis and capitis.

— Lateral to spinalis and semispinalis.

• Iliocostalis.

— Most lateral.

NOTE: The iliocostalis and longissimus arise from the illial crest and thoracolumbar fascia, but with the exception of a few

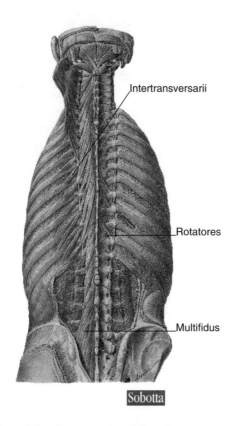

*Figure 3-8:*    Deep muscles of the spine.

medial fibers from the longissimus, do not attach to the lumbar vertebrae.

The sacral connection of the erector spinae can pull the sacrum forward inducing nutation in the SI joints, and tensing ligaments such as the interosseous and sacrotuberous (Vleeming et al, 1995).

**THORACOLUMBAR FASCIA.** A strong fascia, known as the thoracolumbar fascia, envelops the entire erector spinae in the lumbar spine. This fascia is connected anteriorly to the TrPr's and is continuous with the abdominal fascia, thus forming a tube around the spine. When the erector spinae broaden during extension the thoracolumbar fascia tightens, and with contributions from the latissimus dorsi, multifidus, gluteus maximus and biceps femoris, the spine is extended (Vleeming et al. *ibid*).

*Deep Muscle Group.*

**THE TRANSVEROSPINALIS.** The deep muscle group is collectively called the transvesospinalis, laying deeply to the erector spinae and running along most of the spine (Figure 3-8). These extensive muscles cross each other in different layers to construct a system of supporting trusses. When these are weak on one side of the spine, losing their lateral supporting function, or are in spasm, a functional retroscoliosis can result—as found in vertebral and pelvic dysfunctions.

The deep group include the:

• Rotatores.

• Intertransversarii.

• Multifidus.

**THE MULTIFIDUS.** The multifidus muscles have significant attachments to;

• Spinous process, interspinous ligaments, laminae, and articular capsules of the vertebra.

— In the lumbar spine to the medial, intermediate and lateral sacral crests, the sacropelvic surface of the ilium, and the thoracolumbar fascia.

The connection to the sacroiliac joints and ligaments integrate the multifidus into the ligamentous support system of the sacroiliac joints (Willard *1995*). Bogduk and Twomey (*ibid*) noted that out of the dorsal muscles only the multifidus could contribute significantly to extension of the lumbar spine, the thoracolumbar fascia and other contributing muscles also aid in extension.

*The Anterior Muscles*

The anterior muscles, or flexors, also are important in spinal function and stability. The anterior prevertebral musculature lies in close proximity to the vertebra and thus mechanically is disadvantaged, especially in the lumbar and thoracic spines. Flexion therefore must also be assisted by other muscles.

**FLEXOR MUSCLES**. In the lumbar spine the psoas (which is more a trunk flexor), and the abdominal muscles function as the major flexors.

In the cervical spine the paravertebral muscles of the neck do function as primary flexors. The flexors of the cervical spine are:

- Longus cervicis, longus capitis and the scalenes.
- The SCM and other muscles also assist with flexion of the neck.

NOTE: The psoas and scalenes often are dysfunctionally coupled. (more specific information is provided in the appropriate section).

In the cervical spine the longus colli and dorsal neck muscles are complementary and the longus colli counteracts the lordosis increment related to the weight of the head and to the contraction of the dorsal neck muscles. The longus coli and posterior cervical muscles form a sleeve which encloses and stabilizes the cervical spine in all positions of the head (Mayoux et al. 1994).

**STABILITY AND MUSCLE FUNCTION/DYSFUNCTION**. Myofascial structures are essential for load transfer, and according to Vleeming, force closure of the ilia on the sacrum—contributing to general stability of the spine and the lumbosacral regions. Forces between the spine and legs are transferred through the thoracolumbar fascia, both ipsilaterally and contralaterally. Electromyographic studies during isokinetic lifting and trunk bending movement demonstrate that the erector spinae, latissimus dorsi, abdominal and gluteus maximus muscles act in parallel and simultaneously —showing that these constitute a complex system. The muscular functions of the latissimus dorsi, contralateral gluteus and hamstrings are coupled, as well.

Together the above muscles and transverse and internal oblique abdominal mus-

cles as well as psoas major, all contribute to transferring forces and to stability of the SI joints by "force closure"—preventing shear of these joints (Vleeming, Stoechart and Snijers 1994).

## The Anterior Vertebral Column

The anterior vertebral column is composed of the vertebral bodies and discs. From a reductionist view the anterior column is the major resilient weight bearing and shock absorbing structure of the motion segment (two adjacent vertebra).

## Intervertebral Disc

The intervertebral disc lying in the center of the anterior spinal column is one of the larger avascular structures in the body. It is therefore liable to develop chronicity once injured—possibly making this pathoanatomically the weakest part of the motion segment (Bonica *ibid*). The disc is radiotranslucent therefore inadequately evaluated by X-ray. The discs make up about 1/4 of the length of the entire spine and are roughly 1/5 to 1/3 as thick as the neighboring vertebral body. In the lumbar spine the discs encompass about 30% of the length of the column in comparison to 20-25% in the thoracic and cervical spine. With weight bearing the discs shrink and dehydrate, and at night they usually rehydrate and regain their thickness.

In the cervical spine the discs are relatively thicker than in the thoracic spine, broader posteriorly and higher anteriorly. This is perhaps to accommodate the excessive strains on the disc from extensive cervical movements. In the thoracic spine the discs are relatively thin, probably due to the stability provided by the rib cage. In the lumbar spine the discs are quite large as they bear considerable strain, even though rotation and sidebending is restricted by the bony and articular arrangements (Bogduk and Twomey *ibid*).

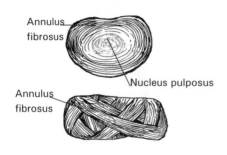

Annulus fibrosus

Nucleus pulposus

Annulus fibrosus

*Figure 3-9:*   Intervertebral disc.

Even with this lumbar architecture and minimal rotation, lumbar disc ruptures are quite common.

### Nourishment of Discs

In adults, the disc receives virtually all its nutrition by diffusion through the vertebral end plates and peripheral vessels. Therefore, motion of the vertebral column is important in maintaining disc health (Brown 1995), (see spinal stretch for exercise to nourish the spine chapter 9). Smoking inhibits the nutrition to the disc and may explain why patients who smoke often develop chronicity (Holm and Nachemson 1988; Battié et al. 1991).

### Disc Anatomy

The discs are made of:

• An external capsule of fibrocartilage (annulus fibrosus).

• A soft nucleus pulposus in the center (Figure 3-9).

### Annulus Fibrosus

The annulus fibrosus is made up of 20 concentric collar-like rings (lamellae) of fibers that crisscross each other to increase their strength and accommodate torsion movements of the spine. The thickness of each

lamellae increases from the nucleus outward (Farfan 1973). Its dry collagen mass is 60%-70% (Ombregt, Bisschop, ter Veer and Van de Velde 1995). The annulus fibrosus, because of its fiber arrangement, has a low injury tolerance to shearing, translation and displacement forces (Kopell and Thompson 1976). The annulus fibers contribute to torque resistance and when deferentially removed, at appropriate angles, rotation increases by $2°$ (Krismer, Haid, Rabal 1996).

Traditionally, the discs were not thought to contain nerves. However, the peripheral posterior aspect of the annulus fibrosus is innervated by nerve fibers from the sinuvertebral nerve. The lateral aspect of the annulus fibrosus is innervated peripherally by the anterior rami and gray rami communicantes. Chronic inflammation can cause an increase in the number of these pain fibers (Bogduk, Tynan and Wilson 1981; Bogduk, Windsor and Inglis 1988).

### Nucleus Pulposus

The nucleus is approximately 85% water and it's metabolism is anaerobic with oxygen concentration being as little as 5%-10% of that at the surface (Holm 1981). The dry mass of collagen is 10%-20% (Ombregt, Bisschop, ter Veer and Van de Velde 1995). The pressure within the nucleus pulposus keeps the annulus fibers taut and prevents the disc space from collapsing and therefore has the highest proteoglycan content in the body (Brown 1995). This allows for rotary, translatory and rocking movements between adjacent vertebrae. With aging the disc becomes less elastic and the nucleus dries up, reducing the likelihood of the nucleus to rupture.

## The Posterior Column

The posterior arch (column) of a vertebra is united by a thick pedicle to the vertebral body. The arch is created by:

- Connection of the spinous process.
- Laminae.
- Transverse processes (TrPrs).

### The Facet Joint (zygoapophyseal Joints)

Connecting two adjacent vertebrae are facets (zygoapophyseal joint or articular processes) which arise from the vertebral pedicle. The triangular posterior vertebral column is believed to have minimal weightbearing function. Adams and Hutton noted that about 20% of the entire load of a motion segment is taken up by the facet joints (Brown 1995)—although the tensegrity model postulates that loads are distributed throughout. By their architectural design the facets govern motion available in a vertebral segment and limit mechanical range of the discs. When the lumbar facet joints are removed, in "normal" cadaveric spines, rotation increases by 2° (Krismer, Haid and Rabl 1996).[15]

The role of facet joints in pain has been controversial. For example, osteopathic schools emphasize the facet's essential contribution to vertebral motions. When a dysfunction interferes with their opening or closing, normal motion may be altered leading to mechanical strains and pain. Cyriax, on the other hand, challenged this. Firstly, because he could not devise a system of examination to distinguish a "syndrome", and secondly because he claimed that two parallel surfaces cannot become blocked. Lately Bogduk (*ibid*) has shown the facets to be a common source of pain.

#### Facet Anatomy & Innervation

The facets are a true synovial joint and have a capsule that is well innervated from the dorsal rami. There is diffuse overlapping innervation to the lumbar facets from

3 root levels. This may explain part of the controversy, as it leads to poor localization and highly variable pain (Brown 1995).

Up to now we have looked at various elements, and subelements constructing the human body, from a reductionist point of view. The following section by Stephen M. Levin M.D. challenges these reductionist views and points out that all subsystems of the musculoskeletal system are united, are part of a metasystem that is independent and interdependent at the same time. Although there may be local and specific variations the underlying principles cannot be violated (*OM: Yin Yang principals*). This systemic view is consistent with many manual therapy concepts and OM.

# A Systems Science Model For Biomechanical Construction [16]

When given an apparently complex problem engineers search for the simplest elements of the problem, finding a solution, and extrapolate to the whole, more complex design. This usually serves us well, as most constructions in the non-biologic world are **Lego Set** ™ constructions built up block by block to completion of a preexisting design. This method has been adopted by bioengineers to explain biologic mechanics. The design used by most bioengineers to calculate the mechanical forces in vertebrates is the skyscraper (Schultz 1983) with the girders acting as the skeleton and the soft tissue draped like the curtain walls on the building. The simplest elements of the skyscraper model are the pillar, beam and lever.

But skyscrapers are immobile, unidirectional, gravity dependent structures

---

15. When both the facets and appropriate annular fibers are removed rotation increased by 7.6°.

16. This section is written by Stephen Levin MD.

that mechanically are Newtonian, Hookian and linear (Gordon 1988) in their behavior with high energy requirements. The forces necessary to stabilize a human would be bone breaking, muscle ripping and energy depleting if we were constructed like a skyscraper (Gracovetsky 1988). Much like the creationist's concept of biologic organisms, skyscrapers do not evolve but must be conceived as a whole. The design is from the top down. They are obligatorily vertically oriented and rigid, with rigid joints, otherwise they would collapse. In the skyscraper body frame analogy, apparently obvious similes do not work well. Any brick mason will tell us that stacked building blocks cannot function as a horizontal beam in a building. Neither can stacked vertebral blocks function as a spinal beam in a quadruped or a biped bending over. Nor do blocks, pillars and beams model the spineless worm, the soaring eagle, the swimming eel or the writhing snake.

Biologic structures are self generating and evolutionary (Gordon 1988). They must be structurally and functionally independent at each instant of their development. There are no temporary scaffolds that nature uses to support the emerging organism. The design is from the bottom up with a functioning lesser structure evolving into a more complex being. Organic chemistry is structural chemistry. Subcellular structures must exist as *structures* before they are integrated into a cell. A cell must have its' own stable construct before it joins with other cells. When removed from the organism organelles and organs are not amorphous blobs on the dissecting table but have individually stable forms of their own. The joints, intracellular or interstructural, are flexible. The structures must overcome the mechanical paradox of being able to convert from rigid to highly flexible and back again within an instant. It is apparent that over time biologic structures evolved that are self-generating, self-replicating, hierarchical, low energy consuming, stable (even with flexible joints), ominidirectional and able to

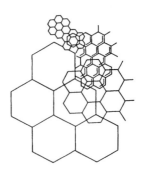

*Figure 3-10:* A self-generating hierarchy of hexagons.

function independent of gravity. They are instantly rigid or flexible depending on their needs. The structural components are, for the most part, nonlinear, non-Hookian, and non-Newtonian (Gordon 1978) in their, mechanical behavior with low energy requirements.

A system scientist seeks a more global, holistic and deductive solution than do other engineers. All subsystems are part of a metasystem that are independent and interdependent at the same time. Although there may be local and species specific variations the underlying principles cannot be violated. A subsystem that is incompatible with the metasystem cannot exist. Biologic structures must build themselves. Any "scaffolding" must itself be a functioning organelle before it evolves. An "ear" may not start out as an "ear" but it started as some functioning organ. Like an evolving beehive, (Figure 3-10) each cell packs into place in a self-generating, hierarchical, energy efficient pattern that is structurally stable at every step. The mechanical laws of beehive construction such as close packing, triangulation and unidirectional stability are universal and apply to biologic construction as well.

Thompson (1969) proposed a truss model as the support concept in biologic modeling. He suggests that trusses (Figure 3-11) can be analogous models for struc-

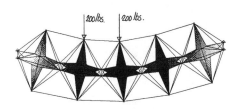

*Figure 3-12:* Load applied to a three dimensional truss.

tural support in vertebrates. Trusses have clear advantages over skyscraper, post and lintel construction as structural support systems for biologic tissue. They have flexible, even frictionless hinges, with no bending moments about the joint. The support elements are in tension and compression only. Loads applied at any point are distributed about the truss, as tension or compression (Figure 12 on page 129).

In post and beam construction the load is locally loaded and creates leverage. There are no levers in a truss and the load is distributed through the structure. A truss, is fully triangulated, and is inherently stable and cannot be deformed without producing large deformations of individual members. Since only trusses are

inherently stable with freely moving hinges, it follows that any structure having freely moving hinges, and that is structurally stable, must be a truss. Vertebrates, meeting those criteria, must therefore be constucted as trusses.

When the tension elements of a truss are wires or ropes or soft tissues, ligaments etc., the truss usually becomes unidirectional. The element that is under tension will be under compression when turned topsy turvy. The tension elements of the body (the soft tissues — fascia, muscles, ligaments, and connective tissue) have largely been ignored as construction members of the body frame and have been viewed only as the motors.

In loading a truss the elements that are in tension can be replaced by flexible materials, such as ropes, wires, or in biologic systems, ligaments, muscles, and fascia. However, soft tissue can only function as tension elements and the truss would will only function when oriented in one direction. There is a class of trusses, termed "tensegrity" (Fuller 1975) structures that are omnidirectional so that the tension elements always function in tension, no matter what the direction of applied force. A wire cycle wheel is a familiar example of a tensegrity structure. The compression elements in tensegrity structures "float" in a tension network just as the hub of a wire wheel is suspended in a tension network of spokes.

To conceive an evolution metasystem construction of tensegrity trusses that can be linked in a hierarchical construction, starting at the smallest subcellular component and have the potential, like the beehive, to build itself, the structure would be one integrated tensegrity truss that evolved from infinitely smaller trusses that could be, like the beehive cell, both structurally independent and interdependent at the same time. Fuller (*ibid*) and Snelson (1965) described the truss that fits these requirements, the tensegrity icosahedron (Figure 3-13).

The tensegrity icosahedron is a naturally occurring, fully triangulated, three-

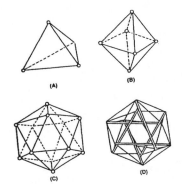

*Figure 3-11:* Three-dimensional trusses. (A) Tetrahedron; Four faces. (B) Octahedron; eight faces. (C) Icosahedron; Twenty faces. (D)

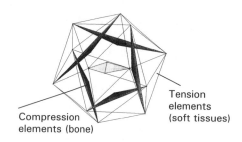

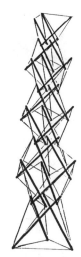

*Figure 3-13:* Tensegrity icosahedron compression elements suspended within tension elements.

*Figure 3-14:* A tensegrity column (by Kenneth Snelson, with permission of the artist).

dimensional truss that is omnidirectional, gravity independent, flexible hinged structure who's mechanical behavior is non-linear, non-Newtonian and non-Hookian. Fuller and Snelson independently use this truss to build structures. Fuller's familiar geodesic dome is an example, and Snelson (*ibid*) has used it for artistic sculptures that can be seen around the world. Naturally occurring examples that have already been recognized are the self-generating fullerenes (carbon$_{60}$ organic molecules) (Kroto 1988), viruses (Wildy and Home 1963), clethrins (de Duve 1984), cells (Wang, Butler and Ingber 1993) radiolaria (Haeckel 1887), pollen grains, and dandelion balls (Levin 1986 et al.).

Because of its ability to fill space (Brandmuller 1992) and from self organizing systems with stable carbon molecules (*ibid*), the icosahedron seems to be the space truss most suitable for biologic structures. The tensegrity icosahedron, first conceived by Kenneth Snelson (1965), with the outer shell composed of tension elements separated by compression elements suspended within the tension network, appears to be the most if not the only suitable structure that can model the endoskeleton of cells (*ibid*) or multicellular organisms that evolve from those cells. Icosahedron trusses are omnidirectional and once constructed, tension elements are always loaded in tension, and compres-

sion elements are always loaded in compression, no matter what the point of application or direction for load. Icosahedra are stable even with frictionless hinges and at the same time can easily be altered in shape or stiffness merely by shortening or lengthening one or several tension elements. The icosahedron can be linked in an infinite variety of sizes or shapes in a modular or hierarchical pattern with the tension elements, the muscles, ligaments, and fascia, forming a continuous interconnecting network, and with the compression elements, the bones, suspended within that network. The structure would always maintain the characteristics of a single icosahedron so that a shaft, such as a spine, may be built that is omnidirectional and can function equally well in tension or compression with the internal stresses always distributed in tension or compression with no bending moments and, therefore, lowest energy costs (Figure 3-14).

A unique property of a tension icosahedron, as a structure, is that it has a "J" shaped, non-linear, stress-strain curve when loaded, so that as a structure the icosahedron seems to be a non-linear dynamical system unto itself (Figure 3-15).

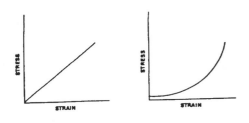

*Figure 3-15:* Linear and nonlinear stress-strain curves.

The icosahedron space truss has been shown to be present in biologic structures at the cellular, subcellular, and multicellular levels. In the spine, each subsystem (the vertebra, the disc, the soft tissues), would be subsystems of the spine metasystem. Each would function as an icosahedron independently and as part of the larger system, as in the beehive analogy. In a non-linear dynamical system, an icosahedron would be a stable "attractor" (Gleick 1988) or the underlying form of least energy that the non-linear system seems to be seeking.

The icosahedron space truss spine model is a universal modular hierarchical system that has the widest application with the least energy cost. As the simplest and least energy consuming system, it becomes the metasystem to which all other systems and subsystems must be judged and if they are not simpler, more adaptable, and less energy consuming, rejected. Since this system always works with the least energy requirements there would be no benefit to nature for spines to function sometimes as post, sometimes as a beam, sometimes as a truss, or to function differently for different species, conforming to the minimal inventory-maximum diversity concept of Pierce (Pearce 1978) as well as evolutionary theory.

The icosahedron space truss model could be extended to incorporate other anatomic and physiologic systems. For example, as a "pump" the icosahedron functions remarkably like cardiac and respiratory models, which themselves have been shown to be non-linear dynamical systems, and so may be an even more fundamental metasystem for biologic modeling. As suggested by Kroto (1988) the Icosahedron template is "mysterious, ubiquitous, and all powerful."

As this model is universally adaptable to all biologic constructs and mimics function and form it is proposed as the metasystem model for biologic constructs, from viruses to vertebrates, including their systems and subsystems.

This property is not demonstrated in mechanical systems such as post and lintel construction or lever construction or when using cubic or any other polyhedral shapes. J shaped, non-linear, stress-strain curves seem to be the sine quanon of biologic tissue (Gordon 1988). This property has been demonstrated in bone, muscle, disc, fascia, nerve, composite biologic structures (White and Panjabi 1978), and in just about any biologic tissue studied.

## Summary

It seems sensible to use a structure that has analogous mechanical properties to biologic tissue when biologic modeling. Viewed as a model for the spine of man or any vertebrate species, the tension icosahedron space truss, with the bones acting as the compressive elements and the soft tissues as the tension elements, even with multiple joints, will be stable in any position, vertical or horizontal, any posture from ramrod straight to sigmoid curve, or any position or configuration in between. Shortening on a soft tissue element has a rippling effect through the structure. Movement is created and a new, instantly stable, shape is achieved. It is highly mobile, omnidirectional, and low energy consuming. It is a unique structure that when used as a biologic model the constructs would conform to the natural laws of least energy, laws of mechanics, and the apparent peculiarities of biologic tissues.

# *Biomedical Disorders*

The following is a basic review of biomedical musculoskeletal disorders.

## Joint Disorders

In this book the term joint dysfunction—commonly occurring in the spine—is used to describe the loss of intrinsic motions, joint play or function in the joint complex without obvious pathology. In chronic cases, soft tissues are more extensively involved and joint dysfunction is more likely to reoccur (due to instability).

Joint receptors (more so than tendon or muscle receptors) are slow adaptive or nonadaptive. Therefore, their effects can be long-lasting both in their ability to maintain dysfunction and to have a therapeutic effect (Brown 1996). These subtle dysfunctions can often last for a long time, unnecessarily (since they respond to treatment), causing pain and disability. Manual therapy can affect these receptors and result in immediate relief of pain—at least temporarily. Relapses can be challenging to the practitioner. Ligamentous insufficiency is often the cause.

### Classifications of Joint Dysfunctions

Joint dysfunctions can be divided into those caused by internal or intrinsic forces and external or extrinsic forces (trauma).

#### *Intrinsic Joint Disorders*

Proper functioning of a joint relies on diverse factors. Pain and dysfunction can result from interactions among many of these factors. Often with unguarded movements, a common cause of intrinsic joint disorder, the driving factor is not that the tissues were injured, or the joint has underlying pathology, but rather, a lack of some kind of preparatory integration resulting in muscle guarding, spasm and leading to joint dysfunction. This sudden resetting of muscular tension, and length, can result in the joint losing normal motion and becoming restricted. This occurs often not when forces are extreme, but when the patient makes a simple movement absentmindedly or moves from a poor postural position and fails to make preparatory integration. Ligamentous insufficiency can be, in more chronic cases, an underlying perpetuating factor.

#### Extrinsic Causes

Extrinsic injuries are due to traumas. With traumatic injury a small soft tissue tear can influence joint tensegrity.[17] There may be abnormal load distribution, pain, muscle guarding and shortening with loss of motion.

#### Degree of Joint Dysfunction

Joint restrictions occur within the normal physiologic range of the joint. One or more vectors of motion are reduced. Dysfunctions range in degree from slight restriction to mild "subluxation."

#### *Subluxation*

Subluxations (nonphysiologic dysfunction) result in minor structural changes (minor dislocation) to the joint complex and therefore are not a pure dysfunction, (as by definition some tissue pathology occurs). If a subluxation is extreme, a dislocation occurs and is accompanied by significant structural damage, such as traumatic synovitis and capsular rupture (Garrick 1990). Subluxations can become chronic and lead to further loosening of

---

17. Tension integrity.

the capsule and other ligaments resulting in recurrent dislocations.

## *Hypermobile Joints*

Hypermobile joints tend to be more susceptible to developing chronic pain due to ligament sprains, recurrent injury, joint effusions, tendinitis, and early osteoarthritis (Wynne-Davis 1971; Beighton Grahame and Brode 1983).

## *Hypomobile Joints*

Hypomobile joints tend to be more susceptible to muscle strains, tendinitis resulting from overuse, and pinched nerve syndromes (Wynne-Davis 1971; Beighton Grahame and Brode 1983).

**SPINAL JOINTS**. Most joint dysfunctions in the spine are either caused by, or influence, the zygoapophyseal (facet) joints. Involvement of the vertebral facets can alter normal motion and load distribution —although other structures, especially muscles, are probably involved as well. Changes in load distribution can result also from internal derangement within a disc or facet meniscus from excessive forces. This can alter facet function, ligament tension, and may lead to joint dysfunction without obvious signs of pathology (Wynne-Davis 1986). Hypersensitivity of the joint's type III and IV nociceptors can develop with dysfunction (especially with inflammation) causing hypersensitivity to mechanical stimuli (Willard *ibid*).

Lewit (1991,1987), (Table 3-14) identified specific relationships between joint dysfunctions and muscular symptoms, which he called chain reactions.

## Three Phases of Degeneration

Kirkaldy-Willis and Burton (1992) described three phases to the joint degenerative process. These are; dysfunction, instability, and stabilization. Many of the

treatment principles presented in this text are designed to address the consequences of these degenerative processes.

## *Dysfunction*

The dysfunction phase is illustrated by a patient who usually has transient pain that responds well to manual therapies. Pathological tissue alterations are relatively minor and by and large the patient presents with a joint or soft tissue pain that is difficult to document. These patients may have suffered a minor trauma or strain, often due to a lack of good physical condition or unfamiliar activity.

**SYMPTOMS AND SIGNS**. The patient presents with acute, subacute or chronic pain. The pain usually is unilateral but may refer in a myotomal or sclerotomal distribution. Pain often is relieved by rest. Patients may or may or may not have a postural component to their pain and usually show signs of muscle strain. Abnormal motions at the affected joint usually are detectable.

If the muscle joint complex or posture is not corrected, soft tissue stress may result in pathological change such as, anoxia of muscle tissue with fibrotic deformations, joint restriction with consequence of immobility, and increased stress on the ligaments. This process then leads to the second phase, the instability phase.

## *Instability*

Here the patient still presents with similar symptoms; however, chronicity is the rule. Patients respond only temporarily to manual therapies. The prolonged dysfunction, poor physiologic posture, immobility, lack of activity, genetic and other individualized factors result in both mechanical and cellular stress on ligaments and other tissues. Ligaments lose their elastic character and joint stability is lost. This results in an increasing rate of degeneration at the joint complex.

*Table 3-14.* **CHAIN REACTIONS OF JOINTS AND MUSCLES,** LEWIT 1987

| JOINTS | MUSCLES |
|---|---|
| Co/C1 | Suboccipitals, sternocleidomastoid (SCM), upper trapezius (masticatories, submandibular) |
| C1/C2 | SCM, levator scapulae, upper trapezius |
| C2/C3 | SCM, levator scapulae, upper trapezius |
| C3/C6 | Upper trapezius, cervical erector spinae, (supinator, wrist extensor, biceps) |
| C6/T3 | SCM, upper or middle trapezius, scaleni (subscapularis) |
| T3/T10 | Pectoralis, thoracic erector spinae, serratus anterior (subscapularis) |
| T10/L2 | Quadratus lumborum, psoas, abdominals, thoracolumbar erector spinae |
| L2/L3 | Gluteus medius |
| L4/L5 | Piriformis, hamstring, lumbar erector spinae, adductors |
| L5/S1 | Iliacus, lumbar erector spinae, hamstrings, adductors |
| SI JOINT | Gluteus maximus, piriformis, iliacus, adductors, hamstrings, contralateral gluteus medius |
| COCCYX | Levator ani, gluteus maximus, piriformis (iliacus) |
| HIP | Adductors |

**SYMPTOMS AND SIGNS.** Signs of hypermobility and ligamentous pain are becoming more pronounced. Patients are often weak and often report a "giving way" or "catching" of the affected region.

*Stabilization*

In this phase patients often report that a previous severe condition is becoming less painful and that they feel increasingly stiff. Aging causes the ligaments to shrink. Joints develop other ways to stabilize (degenerative spondylosis).

**SYMPTOMS AND SIGNS.** Unless degenerative deformations lead to compression phenomenon or neuropathic sensitization develops, patients often report feeling less incapacitated.

**Prolonged Joint Immobilization**

Prolonged joint immobilization can lead to capsular adhesions and decreased ligamentous stress tolerance (Binkley and Peat 1986) and even demineralization (CT 1987;

Videman at al. 1979). Synovial joints exhibit a 30-40% reduction in concentrations of glycosaminoglycans (GAG) and water content. Loss of the water volume increases friction among the microfibrils and increases the potential for abnormal cross-linking or adhesion formation (Akeson, Amie and Woo 1980) and increasing joint compression (Ombregt, Bisschop, ter Veer and Van de Velde 1995). Other effects of immobilization are increased accumulation of metabolic by-products, and muscular atrophy with increase in the relative amounts of connective tissue, and neuromuscular discoordination.

The insertion sites of ligaments, tendons and joint capsules have relatively little vascular supply. Stress and normal joint motion are critical in maintaining tissue integrity at the insertion sites (Noyes et al. 1974).

By definition joint dysfunction results in partial joint immobilization (loss of motion) and therefore may lead to some of the pathologies discussed above. Joint dysfunction is often painful, which in itself can result in protective behavior and further immobilization, and therefore should be treated.

## Somatic Dysfunction

Somatic dysfunction is an osteopathic term that describes impaired or altered function of related components of the somatic system (skeletal, arthodial, and myofascial structures) and related lymphatic, vascular and neural elements. Somatic dysfunction in the past has been called "osteopathic lesion" (H-ICDA. ED. 3, 1978).

Although not a "diagnosis" in the regular medical sense, somatic dysfunction describes in a broad sense, the multiple effects of mechanical dysfunctions such as joint dysfunction of the spinal column, pelvis, or extremities which may produce limited motion, associated muscular involvement, autonomic reactions such as edema, referred symptoms and pain (Greenman *ibid*).

FACILITATED SEGMENT. Many of the concepts in "somatic dysfunction" came about from work done by IM Korr and colleagues in the early forties and fifties. Through a variety of experiments including pseudomotor activity as measured by skin resistance, thermography and EMG activity, they studied the" osteopathic lesion" and showed a complex reaction, mainly via sympathetic nervous system facilitation, which can develop when a mechanical dysfunction is present (Peterson 1979).

In 1940 Buchthal and Clemmeson noted that a state of enduring muscular excitation in the spinal extensors can be seen in dysfunctional spines. Denslow and colleagues reported such activity to represent chronic segmental facilitation of motor pathways, (Denslow, Korr and Krems 1947) which were mostly present in transitional spinal segments:

• Occipital-atlanto.

• Cervical- Thoracic.

• Thoracic- Lumbar.

• Lumbar -sacral.

— All of the above are areas were vertebral dysfunctions are found most often.

In 1662 Korr, Wright and Thomas reported that various types of insult including, *disturbed postures* and *injections* resulted in accentuation and increased facilitation of preexisting facilitated segments. Korr noted that pressure, percussion and other stimulation to the spinous processes of a dysfunctional segment results in increased electromyographic activity of the corresponding segment. Similar stimulation to spinous processes of normal segments does not result in such increased activity. Interestingly however, stimulation of adjacent "normal" spinal processes may result in increased activity in the dysfunctional segment ("cross talk"). Percussion of spinous processes is a useful clinical tool for diagnosing somatic dysfunction.

Another important observation by Korr is a relationship between visceral disease and changes of skin resistance. This reduction of skin electro-resistance shows a segmental relationship to the organ involved. Korr reports that in one patient who has been observed for some time, an area of low skin resistance, at the appropriate segments, appeared 3 weeks prior to a coronary occlusion. This reinforced the concept of viscerosomatic and somatovisceral reflexes and possible cycles of dysfunction and pain.

There are many acupuncture systems and instruments which use this phenomenon in the diagnosis and treatment of visceral disorders, via the evaluation of skin impedance and stimulation to the skin.

## Joint Pathology

Joint pathology is generally divided into inflammatory and non-inflammatory arthritis.

## Degenerative Joint Disease

Osteoarthritis (OA), or degenerative joint disease (DJD) is non-inflammatory condition based on radiographic findings characterized by the destruction of articular cartilage, overgrowth of bone with lipping and spur formation, and impaired function. The symptoms of OA are characteristically use-related joint pain and stiffness after inactivity (posain).[18] Contrary to popular belief, mild to moderate osteoarthritis often is not painful, as hyaline cartilage and synovium do not contain nerve endings (Wyke 1981). Degeneration of the joint complex is common with aging and genetic factors play a major role (Harper and Nuki 1980). If the capsule shrinks and keeps the joint stable, then the patient will most likely be pain free and show a capsular pattern of movement limitation with a hard end feel (Cyriax *ibid*). This condition may be referred to as *osteoarthrosis* (non-inflammatory DJD).

It seems that chronic inflammation of the synovium is an important feature in the pathology and pain production in osteoarthritis, when arthrosis becomes painful. The affects of synovial inflammation probably stimulate pain receptors in the synovial blood vessels, the joint capsule, the fat pads, the collateral ligaments, and the adjacent muscles (Baldry 1993).

Osteoarthritis probably is painful only when:

- Active inflammation occurs.

- Nociceptors become oversensitive due to chronic dysfunction and inflammatory mediators.

- There is an increase of nociceptor rootlets.

- When some mechanoreceptors or sympathetic receptors convert and function as nociceptors.

- There is instability.

18. Positional pain.

In the advanced stages, when the cartilage is eroded, this condition can become very painful and joint replacement may be necessary. When degenerative joint disease is accompanied by lax ligaments, a common occurrence, the ligaments themselves may be painful and proper treatment to them may resolve the pain (Dorman *ibid*).

### THE MAIN JOINTS AFFECTED BY OA INCLUDE:

- Small joints of the hands (mainly the distal interphalangeal joints and thumb base).

- Hips.

- Knees.

- Rarely the shoulders and ankles.

- Often the facet joints of the lumbar and cervical spine are effected.

Regeneration of cartilage, in rabbits, has been reported with electrical stimulation (Beker and Selden 1985). However, this author is not aware of any such evidence in humans. Anecdotal observations have suggested that prolotherapy can cause regeneration of cartilage, (because of some clinical success), but to date no study has proven this claim. Recently, surgical scraping and drilling into cartilage have been used to try to regenerate cartilage with variable success. Tissue grafting as been used in early OA, as well. It has also been suggested that glucosamine sulfate can help produce cartilage regeneration, but human studies are scarce.

## Monoarthritis

Inflammation of a single joint most often is due to injury. Crystalline disease such as gout, can also cause a monoarthritis, often of the big toe. Rheumatoid arthritis can begin in one joint as well. Other conditions, such as acute exacerbation of degenerative arthritis and rarely primary neoplasm of the joint, can present acutely as monoarthritis (Garrick and Ebb 1990).

## Oligoarthritis/Polyarthritis

When multiple joints are inflamed (oligoarthritis) and painful the cause is usually systemic. The leading possibilities are viral illnesses (hepatitis, mononucleosis and rubella) gonococcal infections, rheumatoid arthritis and related illnesses. Occasionally a patient may have generalized exacerbations of generalized degenerative arthritis (Garrick and Ebb 1990).

## Traumatic or Acute Arthritis

"Traumatic arthritis" or what Cyriax also calls steroid sensitive arthritis may follow injury to any joint, but is more common in joints with some degree of pre-existing osteoarthritis. In such damaged joints the trauma may be minor and the patient may not be able to recall a cause. The clue to "traumatic arthritis" is pain of sudden onset in a middle-aged or elderly patient presenting with a capsular pattern (Cyriax *ibid*).

With a single acutely inflamed joint (monoarthritis), even if traumatic, the possibility of infection must be considered (a joint tap and fluid analyses may be necessary). An infected joint must be treated aggressively in order to avoid serious disability. If the soft tissue over a joint shows signs of infection one never needles the soft tissue through to the joint capsule, as this can *infect the joint* (Unless tapping the joint).

## Osteopathic Joint Dysfunctions

Vertebral and pelvic dysfunctions can be divided into subluxation, neutral and nonneutral vertebral, sacroiliac and iliosacral dysfunctions. The distinction between sacroiliac and iliosacral (the same joint) pertains to the behavior of the sacrum between the ilia during spinal movements, and to iliosacral motions in response to lower limb movements.

## Subluxations

Subluxation, non-physiologic dysfunctions (movement greater than normal joint motions), are fairly common in the pelvic joints. Subluxations in the lumbar spine, although described in older chiropractic literature, are very rare unless they are part of spondylolisthesis. Pelvic shears, if not treated, can last indefinitely and often are very painful. Bizarre displacement of bony landmarks are seen often and can be quite confusing when analyzing for somatic dysfunction (Mitchell 1993).

Subluxation must be treated with manual techniques (manipulation), except possibly in cases of pubic shears that can, at times, respond to acupuncture.

## Vertebral Dysfunctions

In the lumbar, thoracic and cervical spine, one can find restrictions of flexion and extension that often are due to *nonneutral* (Type II) *dysfunctions* called FRS and ERS. FRS (side) is a positional term that describes a segment as flexed, rotated and sidebent to one side. The side is marked in parentheses. For example, if a segment is described as FRS(rt), it is flexed, rotated and sidebent to the right. Therefore, the restricted movements and often provocation of pain will be in the opposite directions, i.e. extension, rotation and sidebending to the left. Usually (Bourdillon and Day 1992) the total range of extension and flexion (in the sagittal plane) will be reduced. Figure 16 on page 138 shows an evaluation technique for FRS dysfunctions.

The opposite is true for ERS(rt), where the restricted motions and often the provocation of pain would be flexion, rotation and sidebending to the left. The spinous process and the supraspinous ligament would be tender. The Transverse processes (TrPrs) and/or the articular capsule often are very tender (Bourdillon and Day *ibid*). Figure 3-17 shows an evaluation technique to assess for ERS dysfunction. Figure 3-18 shows a segment with flexion and left sidebending restriction.

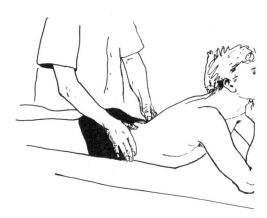

*Figure 3-16:* Evaluation of vertebral extension. Both spinous processes should translate posteriorly. If one side does not there is FRS dysfunction.

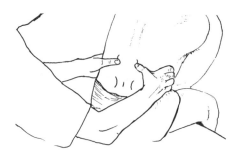

*Figure 3-17:* Evaluation of vertebral flexion. Both spinous processes should translate forward equally. If one side does not there is ERS dysfunction.

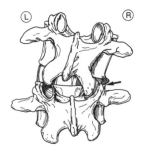

*Figure 3-18:* Flexion restriction, right facet does not open— FRS (rt) (Reprinted with permission Dorman and Ravin 1991).

In the lumbar and thoracic spines (not found in the cervical spine) the practitioner finds often *neutral* (Type I) *group dysfunction*. Neutral group dysfunctions are usually a compensatory reaction to a non-neutral dysfunction (Greenman *ibid*). Described as NR(side), the N represents neutral, the R represents rotation with the direction written in parentheses, sidebending is to the opposite side of rotation. Motion is restricted toward the convex side of the group, and rotation is restricted in the opposite direction. The total range of flexion and extension (sagittal plane) will usually be reduced (Bourdillon and Day 1992). Neutral group dysfunctions (Mitchell 1993) are maintained by multiarticular muscles that span several joints.

Neutral restriction of single motion segments (rotated and sidebent to opposite sides) can occur as well and are more commonly diagnosed with passive tests. Table 6 on page 626 appendix B summarize osteopathic joint dysfunctions.

### Pelvic Dysfunction

In the pelvis osteopathic dysfunctions are divided into iliosacral and sacroiliac dysfunctions. Table 3-5 on page 624, and Table 3-4 on page 623 in appendix B summarizes osteopathic pelvic dysfunction.

# Ligamentous Disorders

Normal ligaments usually are not tender when palpated. If they are injured or are stretched due to joint dysfunction they can become sensitive and painful. The pain of acute ligament sprains (tears) usually is felt several minutes or hours after the injury, as swelling *(OM: blockage)* develops. This delay in pain is commonly seen with disc annular ruptures and whiplash injuries. In chronic pain patients, ligament laxity and partial tears are frequent sources of pain.

Ligamentous laxity and insufficiency may result from:

- Injuries (acute overstretch).
- Poor physiologic posture or structure.
- Muscular weakness that leads to stresses on the ligaments.
- Loss of mobility at one aspect of a joint resulting in other parts of the joint being overstressed. Or other joints elsewhere being stressed.
- Degenerative joint processes that cause diminished joint volume.
  - Resulting in a relative increase of ligament length (the ligament is too long to hold the joint tightly because the joint volume is decreased, as commonly seen in degenerative disc disease).

Ligaments are especially susceptible to hysteresis and tissue creep, particularly when fatigued. Hysteresis or elastic energy loss after prolonged or repetitive loading can become permanent and result in an increase of tissue length, called "set". Set can easily occur if a ligament is stretched 4% behind the point of which all crimp or slack is removed. Hysteresis can affect:

- Joint capsules.
- Annulus fibrosus.
- All other ligaments (Bogduk and Twomey 1991).

When the above structures are fatigued they are more vulnerable to injury from inconsequential or unexpected activity. Following tissue fatigue and hysteresis the mechanoreceptors and proprioceptors compensate and adaptation occurs—in order to minimize the risk of tissue failure. Type I and II afferents habituate to stimuli and therefore may not continue to discharge, if hysteresis or tissue fatigue is chronic. This common occurrence may eventually lead to partial or complete inability of tissues to accommodate, and therefore leave the ligament vulnerable to injury. Sensitization, or the reduction of transmission threshold, and

dorsal horn responses to Type I and II mechanoreceptive sensory input as though it was painful input may result (Liebenson 1996).

## Symptoms

Ligamentous pain may be felt locally or distally, and in various patterns. Hackett et al. (1991) has mapped many of these reference patterns and describes them in his book.

### Posain & Nulliness

The hallmark of ligament pain is positional pain (for which Dorman has coined the term "posain"). Posain is the experience of increased pain when any position is held for a long period, such as sitting, standing in one position. Another important symptom of ligamentous laxity and insufficiency is the referral of a numb-like ache, which Dorman calls "nulliness". Nulliness is commonly mistaken for neurogenic symptoms, such as sciatica or carpal tunnel syndrome.

Ligamentous pain is aggravated by activity that strains the ligament, and is alleviated by rest. Often ligamentous pain is worse in the morning, due to posain. Injured ligaments are tender to pressure. Frequently, the pain can be reproduced by needle insertion, and is abolished by application of a local anesthetic. Injured and loose ligaments generally present clinically as hypermobile or unstable joints. *Further stretching of such ligaments should be avoided.*

### Instability & Ligamentous Insufficiency

Clinical instability is a common cause of ongoing pain refractory to treatment. Ligamentous laxity may result from trauma, repeated injuries (including excessive therapeutic manipulation) and degenerative changes. Increased spinal mobility has been shown to correlate with increased low back difficulties (Biering-Sonrenson 1984). In patients with idiopathic low back pain, spinal flexibility was inversely correlated with functional recovery (Lankhost et al. 1985). Patients with congenital hypermobility often develop muscle tightness around hypermobile joints, as an attempt to stabilize the joint. This tightness is associated with muscle weakness and vigorous stretching often results in increased pain and the development of trigger points (Brown 1995).

Clinical signs of lumbar and pelvic instability include (Dorman (*ibid*); Basmajian and Nyberg (*ibid*); Paris (*ibid*):

* Posain and morning ache that recurs later in the day after fatigue and stress.

* Catching and "giving way".

* Shaking of the lumbar spine on forward bending.

* More difficulty in returning to an upright position than in going into flexion (often needing assistance by grasping the thighs).

* Increased occurrence of bony subluxation.

* Involuntary muscle guarding.

* Abnormal lumbosacral rhythm (tendency to maintain lumbar lordosis during flexion).

* Increased pain when maintaining extreme range of motion.

* With spondylolisthesis (a forward slip of a part or a whole vertebra), sometimes a visible step-off, can be seen in the lumbar spine when the patient is standing, but may become reduced when the patient lies down.

* With instability of the sacroiliac joint the patients report at times a sudden giving way or sudden falls.

    — Dorman has named this phenomenon the "slipping clutch syndrome" (Dorman 1994).

## Neurogenic Inflammation

When ligaments are lax, the joint is more likely to shift from its normal position resulting in even more stresses on the richly innervated ligaments.

Recent research using immune-histochemical techniques suggest that when ligaments, and other connective tissue in the spine that receive a supply of small diameter fibers, (typical of pain and sympathetic receptors) are irritated, an initiation of "neurogenic inflammation" occurs. Neurogenic inflammation results from release of neuropeptides that interact with fibroblasts, mast cells and immune cells in the surrounding connective tissues (Levine et al. 1993). Neurogenic inflammation is thought to be a major factor in degenerative diseases and back pain chronicity (Garrett et al 1992; Weinstein 1992).

## Treatment

Ligamentous insufficiency is best treated in a global manner using manual therapies to address joint dysfunctions, periosteal acupuncture or prolotherapy to induce ligamentous hypertrophy, exercise to strengthen stretch and educate muscles, herbal and nutritional medication to correct metabolic and possible constitutional deficiencies.

## Sprains

Sprains describe injuries to ligaments. Sprains characteristically are due to some sort of extrinsic force placed on the joint, that moves the ligaments beyond the limits of the physiologic barrier. Therefore, when a sprain occurs some degree of subluxation will usually result. Treatment of subluxations is necessary if the joint is to regain full function.

*Grading of Sprains*

Sprains, like strains, are graded from mild to severe,

- Mild or Grade I Sprains, result in no detectable lengthening of the ligament and therefore no obvious abnormal laxity of the joint.
  - however, the joint is dysfunctional and possibly slightly subluxed, joint play is abnormal.
- Moderate or Grade II Sprains, are distinguished by lengthening or partial tearing of the ligaments, and are almost always associated with some degree of subluxation.
  - the joint may be hypermobile, but joint stability is mostly retained.
- Severe or Grade III Sprains, result in a complete loss of joint stability.
  - the distinguishing factor on examination is the end feel which lacks the normal capsular or leathery end feel.

Often with sprains the patient is aware of the injury immediately as it occurs. However, since symptoms often are delayed, the patient may continue with his activities and miss the opportunity to minimize bleeding and swelling. Pain from severe (grade III) sprains may disappear within minutes and be disproportionately mild. Mild sprains often remain painful for a long time, especially when left untreated (Garrick Ebb 1990).

# Myofascial Disorders

Most musculoskeletal disorders are accompanied by myofascial alterations, which may not require direct treatment—because "myofascial syndromes" often are secondary to other dysfunctions. Since muscles almost always react to painful stimuli with so-called spasm, the practitioner must assess the significance of this reaction.

Muscle responses range from contracture "spasm" and hypertonicity, to atrophy and hypotonicity. Striated muscle reactions (spasm, tension) serve to identify the lesion and amplify the experience of pain, and therefore are important diagnostically. Contractile unit disorders usually are characterized by increased muscle tone, accompanied by diminished plasticity and flexibility anywhere within the musculotendinous body. Pathology or dysfunction can affect the entire muscle or just a few longitudinal bundles. The muscle then becomes painful (Myalgia). If the spasm is allowed to continue fibromyositis (fibrositis), may develop. This is a pathological condition in which the elastic fibers in the muscle are lost and do not regenerate and it can lead to permanent contractures (Dvorák *ibid*).

Myalgia can be secondary to conditions such as viral infections where tissue texture changes often are lacking. Long-term myalgia due to neuropathy, spasm or guarding may lead to accumulation of waste products locally. When this develops, the muscles lose elasticity, become edematous, and often feel firm and doughy.

## Causes of Contractile Unit Pain

Contractile unit pain (muscles and attachments) may be due to:

- Direct injury or infection.
- Secondary infections in other associated areas.
- Reflexively due to somatic dysfunctions, most often;
  - Ligament and joint disorders.
  - Neurological dysfunctions such as chronic or acute injury to nerves, Gunn's "neuropathic pain" due to mild denervation.
- Other conditions:
  - Reflex sympathetic dystrophy.
  - Hypothyroidism.
  - Malignancy.

— Polymyalgia rheumatica.

— Osteomalacia.

— Osteoarthritis.

— Initial stage of various connective tissue diseases.

— Visceral disorders.

— Nutritional deficiencies.

— Sleep disorders.

— Psychological disorders.

— Parkinson's disease.

## Muscle Functioning & Anatomical Changes in Chronic Disorders

With chronic dysfunctions and pain, muscles have been shown to have changed characteristics. In chronic low back pain populations, EMG recordings have shown abnormalities (Wolf and Basmajian 1979).

Muscle fiber physiology in patients with chronic cervical dysfunction has been shown to transform in the direction from "slow oxidative to "fast glycolytic" (Unlig, Weber and Grob 1995). In patients with chronic low back pain histologic evidence of type I fiber hypertrophy on the symptomatic side, and type II fiber atrophy bilaterally, were documented by Fitzmaurice et al. (1992). In patients with acute low back pain unilateral wasting has been documented in the multifidus muscle by Hide et al. (1994). They further showed that atrophy was isolated to one dysfunctional segment and was not thought to be disuse related.

It is clear from these and other studies that muscle activity and form is affected in chronic pain sufferers. Of course this does not elucidate the underlying cause or if muscles are a source of pain.

## Muscle Spasms

Muscle "spasm" is defined as an involuntary sudden movement or muscular contraction that prevents lengthening of the muscles involved. Spasm often is due to pain stimuli to the lower motor neuron system. Spasms may be tonic (sustained) or clonic (alternating with relaxation). There is increased electrical activity in the muscle. However, many practitioners, clinically, consider muscle spasm as increased tension without significant muscle shortening and electrical activity, which is more properly called tension. Travell and Simons (*ibid*) suggest that this occurrence of taut muscle bands is the result of sustained intrinsic activation of the contractile mechanisms of the muscle fibers, without motor unit action potential stimulation (electrical activity).

### Early & Late Spasms

Muscle spasms can be divided into early and late spasms. Early muscle spasm occurs at the beginning of the range of motion, almost as soon as movement is initiated, and is associated with inflammation. Late spasm occurs at or near the end of the range of movement and is due to joint dysfunction, most often caused by instability of the joint.

**MUSCLE TENSION.** Excessive skeletal muscle tension may arise from limbic system dysfunction and may result in pain (Janda 1991). The limbic system is thought to be involved with abnormal behavior including depression, irritability, anxiety and sleep disorders with associated muscle tension and tenderness. Chronic tension may develop into "spasm" and may cause pain that is felt as sharp and well localized, or as a dull ache which is not as well localized. The pain is affected by muscle activity and associated frequently with both deep and superficial tenderness and tightness. Long standing tension can lead to tendinitis and fibrosis (Gunn *ibid;* Dvořák *ibid*).

Tight muscles may be stronger or weaker than normal, depending on the amount of tension. According to Janda (1993) moderately tight muscles are stronger than normal, but pronounced tightness leads to "tightness weakness". Maintaining a fixed position for a long duration often causes muscle tension, stiffness and pain (ligamentous or tendinous source should always be considered). Patients should be encouraged to move frequently and vary their activity, especially if they have to use the same movements repeatedly.

Increased tension, tone and vasoconstriction in the muscle or tendon may result in relative hypoxia, accumulation of metabolites, abnormal growth of connective tissue and degenerative changes, all of which may lead to fatigue, stress atrophy, and tissue weakening (Brown 1995). The resulting increase in motor unit recruitment leads to altered patterns of muscle contraction and increased vulnerability to injury. The injured muscles in turn remain even more vulnerable to dysfunction and pain. They are often shortened, especially after immobilization or protective behavior, and therefore, restoration of normal muscular function and length is important.

A sedentary life-style can result in overuse of postural muscles—and overloading of ligaments—encouraging the development of tightness. Tense muscles should always be stretched before activity or strengthening is attempted. Stretching tight muscles may result in improved strength of the inhibited antagonistic muscles (Janda *ibid*).

**MUSCLE SPASM IN ARTHRITIC JOINTS.** The source of pain in the arthritic joint has not been definitively established. Muscle spasm is probably a protective reaction to stretching of a painful joint capsule. The capsule, not the muscle, may be the major source of pain. This is evident in joints where no muscle spans the joint such as, acromioclavicular, sternoclavicular and sacroiliac joints. When these are stretched the joints are as painful as other arthritic joints that are under muscle control (Cyriax *ibid*). When arthritic joints are at rest the muscles usually are relatively relaxed and spring into spasm when the joint capsule is stretched or under load. This is called *involuntary muscle guarding*. In contrast, *voluntary muscle guarding* is seen in chronic unstable joints where muscle hypertrophy develops. Here the muscles appear bulky and "spasmed" both during weightbearing and non-weightbearing positions, often on the side opposite the instability (Paris *ibid*).

Cyriax identified the "*capsular pattern*," a limitation of movement, specific to each joint, that occurs as a reaction to arthritis and capsulitis. This pattern results from a reflexive protective spasm of muscles guarding the joint (involuntary guarding), which occurs upon initiation of passive or active movement in a particular direction. In later stages the contracted capsule can restrict movement in the identical specific vectors that were initially inhibited by spasm.

**MUSCLE SPASM IN BURSITIS.** Although movement is limited in a particular direction, there is usually no franc muscle spasm in cases of bursitis. The limitation is voluntary (pain avoidance) in that the patient limits the motion in response to pain but is actually capable of further movement (Cyriax *ibid*). Characteristically however, tender motor points will be palpable, and treatment of them may render an effective response (Gunn *ibid*).

**MUSCLE SPASM IN INTERNAL DERANGEMENT.** Blockage of movement caused by internal derangement usually is due to a combination of mechanical reasons and muscle spasm (Cyriax *ibid*).

**MUSCLE SPASM IN NERVE ROOT COMPRESSION.** Muscle spasm associated with the spine often serves to protect the nerve roots. Irritation of the nerve root, not the muscle is probably the direct cause of pain. In lumbar disc disease this can be demonstrated clearly by increased leg pain during neck flexion, which pulls on the nerve root but does not affect the leg muscles. And also, epidural anesthesia will allow for increased range in the straight leg raise test (Cyriax *ibid*).

**MUSCLE SPASM AND THE DURA MATER.** In

conditions that affect the dura mater, muscle spasm functions to protect the dura. In meningitis, the muscle spasm holds the neck in extension, as this keeps the dura in its shortest position. In the lumbar region, protective spasms of the hamstring muscles guard the theca from getting pulled via the sciatic nerve or keep the patient deviated so that pressure is minimized at the nerve (Cyriax *ibid*).

**MUSCLE SPASM IN DISLOCATION AND FRACTURE.** In the case of dislocation and fracture, muscles go into constant spasm. This may prevent reduction without first administering anesthesia (Cyriax *ibid*).

**MUSCLE SPASM IN MUSCLE AND TENDON RUPTURE.** When a partial rupture of the muscle belly or tendon occurs, the torn fibers go into spasm, leaving the unaffected fibers in a normal state. Therefore, function is affected only partially. With complete tendon rupture, the muscle belly usually does not go into spasm (Cyriax *ibid*), however, contractures may develop with time.

**PERMANENT MUSCLE SPASM / CONTRACTURE.** Schmidt has shown that nociceptive afferent stimulation via a gamma loop (viscous cycle) can affect skeletal muscles significantly, and that it can lead to permanent elevation of muscle tone. Therefore, even though muscle spasm and tension may be secondary at first, the muscle can develop intrinsic dysfunction that remains independently of the original cause. The cycle (Fassbender 1980) of nociceptive (painful) stimulation and chronic contractile unit dysfunction requires treatment to avoid the long term sequelae of muscle damage and hypertrophy.

## Muscle Weakness

Muscle weakness is one of the major causes of musculoskeletal disorders. Lack of muscle strength or balance can lead to excessive loads on the ligamentous structures supporting joints, which may degenerate and increase joint dysfunctions. Kraus showed that the majority of low back pain sufferers, in whom no "pathology" was identified, fail six basic tests for minimal muscular fitness (Bonica *ibid*).

Exercise programs are widely recommended to prevent the development of spinal pathology, to decrease pain, and to increase function. In some long-term follow up studies exercise was shown to effectively relieve 60-80% of patients who had low back pain (Kraus 1988). However, patient compliance and motivation are often problematic.

### Muscle Paralysis

Muscle paralysis can be due to upper or lower motor neuron lesions,[19] or may be due to intrinsic muscle diseases. Paralyzed muscles display decreased strength and altered tone in the affected muscle. They may be hypotonic (flaccid) or hypertonic (spastic), depending on the location of the lesion. Interruption of a spinal lower motor neuron,[20] or cells of the anterior horn, nerve roots or peripheral nerves, interferes with the circuit to the muscle. The muscle loses normal innervation.

**FLACCID PARALYSIS.** Korr found that nerves and neuromuscular synapses supply trophic (nourishing) substances to muscles. When a nerve is deactivated it loses this nourishing function, which can lead to muscle atrophy. Denervated muscles lose the normal tone, control and tendon reflexes, and this condition is called flaccid paralysis—as may be seen in carpal tunnel syndrome, disc disease, poliomyelitis, etc.

**SPASTIC PARALYSIS.** Interruption of upper motor neuron signals (suprasegmental)

---

19. Multiple sclerosis, strokes, brain tumors and Parkinson's are examples of upper motor neuron disorders.

20. Poliomyelitis, amyotrophic lateral sclerosis (ALS) are examples of lower motor neuron disease.

also diminishes muscle control, but without damaging the lower motor neurons. Innervation and nourishment of the muscle remains uninterrupted. Therefore, the muscle still receives input from the ventral horn motor neurons. Although voluntary control over the muscle is lost (brain messages lost), the muscle still has intrinsic tone and can become spasmed. This is called spastic paralysis. Tendon reflexes can still be elicited, as the cord is intact, and are hyperactive (because of decreased regulation from descending brain, i.e. upper motor neuron fibers). The muscle resists passive stretching. Clonus may be seen.

Acupuncture has been shown to effectively treat patients with symptoms related to sequela of strokes and muscle weakness (Li and Jin 1994). In a study done at Boston University acupuncture was effective in a specific type of stroke, and resulted in significant savings in patients care (Naeser, et al. 1994).

## Muscle Strain

Muscle strain (Table 3-15 on page 148) is used to describe injuries to the musculotendinous unit (contractile unit). Strains can occur anywhere within the contractile unit; in the tendon body, the tenoperiosteal junction, at the musculotendinous junction, or at the muscle belly.

### Causes of Muscle Strain

Strains occur usually due to intrinsic tension within the musculotendinous unit, most commonly when tension is suddenly and actively increased. This can occur with excessive muscle effort, such as in weight lifting. Strains may be due to overstretching, as well. Increase in tension can result from abrupt contraction of antagonistic (eccentric contraction) muscles and tendons, causing muscle fibers to fail before the muscle lengthens. Tension in the contractile unit is greatest during deceleration (eccentric action), requiring the muscle to

have some ability to lengthen at the same time it maintains the tension. Muscle stiffness with decreased ability to lengthen during deceleration is a common cause of strain. Another cause of strain, which in part may also depend on muscle flexibility, is a sudden interruption of motion during activity—occurring frequently during sport activities (Garric and Ebb 1990).

TENDON AVULSION. Tendon avulsion is a strain-type fracture, which results from a tendon and its bony attachment tearing loose from the surrounding bone. Such fractures vary in size from a small flake that is barely visible, (as occasionally seen with tennis elbow) to the large avulsions (many centimeters in length) seen when the hamstring origin avulses a portion of the ischial tuberosity (Garric and Ebb *ibid*).

GRADING OF STRAINS. Strains are graded in severity as mild, moderate, or severe.

- Mild / grade I strains are generally viewed as microscopic disruptions resulting in no defect in the unit on examination.

- Moderate / grade II strains involve significant but not complete disruptions of the musculotendinous unit.

- Severe / grade III strains are complete ruptures of the contractile unit.

According to Garric and Ebb (1990) mild, moderate and severe strains, occur most commonly at the musculotendinous junction. This author finds that strains occur more often and are liable to develop chronicity, at the tendon-periosteal junction.[21]

MUSCLE CONTUSION. Muscle contusions result from a direct impact to the muscle belly. This results in bleeding and swelling. Intramuscular bleeding can result in severe pain which may last for a long time, as it

---

21. Especially with repetitive strain disorders (degenerative strain).

may be difficult to disperse the blood.

**MYOSITIS OSSIFICANS.** Myositis ossificans is a benign condition which can result from trauma to muscle tissue or can be inherited. The condition is characterized by herotopic bone formation, which occurs after injury to muscle fibers, connective tissue, blood vessels and underlying periosteum (Gilmer and Anderson 1959). It occurs most often in males aged between 15 and 30 years old. The patient usually suffers from pain at the affected muscle; the muscle is shortened and resists stretching, and a mass often is palpable. This condition does not respond to conservative treatment, although the administration of diphosphonates may prevent the deposits of bone. Traumatic myositis ossificans may resolve on its own in the course of two years (Ombregt, Bisschop, ter Veer and Van de Velde 1995).

### Tendinitis & Tendon Strains

Historically the term tendinitis has been used as a catch all term. There is however, mounting evidence that distinguishes between the acute traumatic inflammatory type and the more insidious process of chronic tendon degeneration. The rate of collagen metabolism in tendons is relatively slow, and normally there is a balance between breakdown and synthesis. Degenerated tendons show decreased protein synthesis, replication, storage, and contractility. These changes can be due to ageing or repetitive use, and in sports injury can be due to immobilization which leads to cell atrophy. Additionally, degeneration may be due to decreased nutrition, diminished endocrine hormonal influences, and persistent inflammation (Brown 1995).

Blood supply to tendons is compromised at the sites of tendinous friction, torsion, or compression. Such areas are found particularly in the supraspinatus, achilles and tibialis posterior tendons. Many tendons have a "critical zone" at the junction between two groups of blood vessels which leads to poor vascular and oxygen supply. The insertion of a tendon into bone involves a gradual transition from tendon to fibrocartilage to lamellar bone. Very few blood vessels cross the tenoperiosteal junction (Brown 1995).

Tendinitis occurs at the tendinous attachments, tendon body or musculotendinous junction. The lesions may occur anywhere, but most commonly are found in the tenoperiosteal junction, which is the point of maximal mechanical tension with the poorest vascular supply (Noyes and Torvik et al 1974). Ruptures, however, seem to occur more often in the musculotendinous junction, especially in the achilles tendon (Garrick and Ebb 1990). A small rupture of several fibers can lead to a self-perpetuating inflammation because healing is constantly interrupted by use and re-injury. Adhesions can develop.

### *Tenosynovitis*

Some tendons are covered by a sheath that can get roughened and inflamed (tenosynovitis). In this condition crepitus (crackling sound or grating feeling) is elicited by passive motion. When a tendon sheath becomes severely inflamed without the finding of crepitus, the condition is called primary tenovaginitis.

Other causes such as infection or inflammatory disease should be excluded when tendinitis is suspected (Ombregt, Bisschop, ter Veer and Van de Velde 1995).

### Should Muscle Spasm be Treated

There is much controversy regarding the significance of muscle spasms and tension. According to Cyriax, Ongly, Dorman, and others muscle spasm (other than traumatic) and myofascial trigger points are mostly a secondary reflex condition which does not require direct treatment. They stress the role of discs, ligaments and tendons in musculoskeletal disorders and pain.

Ligaments and tendons are supporting structures, and are maximally affected by mechanical forces. They have a poor blood supply and therefore are susceptible to injury and the development of chronicity. These factors result in tissue damage and are seen as the overriding element responsible for chronic musculoskeletal pain. The above authors consider muscle tension, spasm and trigger points as manifestations secondary to ligamentous relaxation, tendinitis, joint dysfunction and subluxation. According to Cyriax, instead of treating muscles, the primary lesion should be addressed, and then muscle "spasms" and pain will resolve by themselves. It must be remembered, however, that if normal muscle function is affected, the balanced reflex action acting across joints, to provide support and to relieve load on the inert tissues, is lost and can result in inert tissue overload and damage (none-contractile tissues). Stability is then almost totally dependent on the ligaments which fall victim to creep and hysteresis.

Others believe muscles should be treated directly because, for example, the treatment may prevent the development of other lesions (such as tendinitis) that they see as secondary to muscle tension.

Gunn (1989) and Travell and Simons (1982) emphasize the role of muscles as causative factors in chronic disability and pain. Gunn states that:

> ... when pain is present, it is practically always accompanied by muscle shortening in peripheral and paraspinal muscles, spasm and/or contracture with tender painful focal areas in muscles, and autonomic and trophic manifestations of neuropathy. Muscle spasm and shortening is the key to musculoskeletal pain of neuropathic origins...

Cyriax (*ibid*), on the other hand, states

> ... In orthopedic disorders, the muscle spasm is secondary and is the result of, not the cause of, pain; it causes no symptoms of itself...The treatment of muscle spasm is

of the lesion to which it is secondary; it never of itself requires treatment in a lesion of moving parts...

Cyriax points out that muscle spasm is only rarely a source of pain. His supporting example is the effect epidural anesthesia has in disc disease, in which the anesthesia cannot reach the muscles, nevertheless reduces the pain and relaxes the muscle spasms. Cyriax also cites Conesa, who administered a muscle relaxant to treat spasmed stiff painful shoulders and obtained relaxation of the muscle without affecting the pain or range of motion.

Others point out that muscles that are in spasm ache due to production of metabolic by-products and the activation of stretch sensitive tissues. Sustained contraction of only 4% of the maximum voluntary contraction possible has been shown to lead to negative effects (Andersson 1990; Sato at el. 1984).

Gunn (1976, 1977) suggests that mild neuropathy can lead to muscle spasm (contracture/tension), shortening, and supersensitivity which can then lead to tendinitis, bursitis and joint restriction, treatment of which is effective. These conditions are accompanied often by sensory, motor and autonomic findings that suggest functional and/or pathological alterations in the peripheral nerves which also affect muscles (swelling, contracture, and hypersensitivity). Gunn (1989) suggests that dry needling of muscles which are affected by such nerve pathology can result in healing of the nerves and give long term relief from pain.

### Treatment

Treatment of contractile unit disorders may include stretching, neural-motor reeducation, massage, acupuncture/electroacupuncture, electrical stimulation (faradic, micro-current, interferential, high or low volt), coutertension positional release, muscle energy techniques, and medication. Acupuncture, via the release of

*Table 3-15.* **MUSCLE STRAIN**

| | |
|---|---|
| **INJURIES** | Can occur anywhere within contractile unit<br>  • In tendon body, tenoperiosteal junction, musculotendinous junction, or muscle belly<br>Usually due to intrinsic tension within unit<br>Strains graded in severity<br>  • Mild (grade I)<br>    — microscopic disruptions, little to no disruption signs<br>  • Moderate (grade II)<br>    — significant but not complete disruptions of unit<br>  • Severe (grade III)<br>    — complete ruptures of contractile unit |

growth factors, may be helpful in the late stage.

Strained muscles are often weak and tight. It is important to rehabilitate both of these aspects as stretching or strengthening alone often results in chronic dysfunction. Table 3-15 summarizes muscular strains.

# Fibromyalgia & Myofascial Pain Syndrome

Fibromyalgia (FM) syndrome must be distinguished from Myofascial Pain Syndrome (MPS). The first may be more of a systemic, medical disorder (possibly a component of chronic fatigue syndrome) and the latter a musculoskeletal (orthopedic) condition. This differentiation is important, since the prognosis of each of these is very different. Both MPS and FM may be caused by a variety of conditions which include; endocrine disorders, allergies, neoplasms, connective tissue diseases, infections, nutritional as well as joint and ligamentous dysfunctions.

## Fibromyalgia

According to a consensus document on FM—the Copenhagen Declaration—FM is a painful, non-articular condition predominantly involving muscles, and is the commonest cause of chronic widespread musculoskeletal pain. In FM the pain often is bilateral, variable and generalized. The pain cannot be explained by peripheral mechanisms only. The patient complains of fatigue, poor quality of sleep, morning stiffness and increased perception of effort. FM (Baldry *ibid*) is frequently associated with other medical conditions such as; irritable bowel syndrome, dysmenorrhea, headaches, and subjective sensation of joint swelling.

The prognosis of FM is much less favorable (than MPS) and patients often respond only temporarily to treatment. When complaints are "temporarily" limited to one or more sites of pain, successful treatment of those sites often is followed by another complaint located elsewhere. Reeves (1994) however, reported that prolotherapy was successful in treating more than 75% of his patients with "severe fibromyalgia." OM can be helpful.

### Mechanisms of FM

Animal studies (Mense 1990), have shown that activity in central nociceptive neurons, receiving input mainly from muscles, are under more central inhibitory control than central nociceptive neurons receiving inputs from skin. This central inhibition may explain why treatment to the CNS with antidepressants often is helpful in FM patients. Furthermore, a review article presented by Henriksson at the Second World Congress on MPS and FM states that there are, at present, a fairly large number of studies that indicate that FM patients have either a disturbance of pain modulation or a disturbed function of other regulatory systems. He further cites studies that implicate serotonin metabolism and deficiency, an increased substance P in CSF, and lower levels of cortisol,[22] epinephrine and norepinephrine following exercise in patients than in controls. Finally, he cites a few reports of immunological disturbances in FM, for example, a defect in the interleukin-2 pathway. Recently, information from PAT scans, has shown a dysfunctions in thalamic activity.

Some authors suggest that FM is a somatization syndrome due to depression. Recent research suggests otherwise (Stiles and Landro 1995). Their data showed that a cognitive dysfunction—reflecting a presumed compromise of the right hemisphere—which is present in major depression, is not found in primary FM. They concluded that this finding would suggest that primary FM and depression are different conditions.

### Differential Diagnosis

Several conditions can mimic fibromyalgia. Some examples include (Jacobsen, Samsoe and Lund 1993):

- Hypothyroidism.

- Widespread malignancy.

- Polymyalgia rheumatica.

- Osteomalacia.

- Generalized osteoarthritis.

- Early Parkinson's disease.

- Initial stage of various connective tissue diseases.

---

22. Licorice (Gan Cao) supplementation is often useful in these patients, especially before exercise.

### Diagnostic Criteria

The American College of Rheumatology criteria for the classification of *fibromyalgia* are;

1. History of widespread pain, extending into the sides of the body and pain above and below the waist.

2. Axial skeletal pain must be present. Low back pain is considered lower segment pain.

3. Pain must also be present in 11 of 18 tender sites on digital palpation of an approximate force of 4kg. These are:

   — At the suboccipital muscle insertions

   — Anterior aspects of the intertransverse spaces of C5-C7.

   — Midpoint of the upper border of the trapezius.

   — Origins of supraspinous above the scapula.

   — Upper lateral aspects of the second costochondral junction.

   — 2 cm distal to the lateral epicondyle.

   — The upper outer quadrants of the buttocks in the anterior fold of the gluteal muscle.

   — The posterior aspect of the trochanteric prominence of the greater trochanter.

   — Medial fat pad proximal to the joint line of the knee.

The diagnostic criteria suggested by (Yunus et al. 1981; Moldofsky et al. 1975) are:

- Widespread aching of more than 3 months duration.

- Cutaneous and subcutaneous sensitivity as demonstrated by skin roll.

- Morning fatigue stiffness with disturbed sleep.

- Absence of laboratory evidence of inflammation or muscle damage.

- Bilateral tender points in at least 6 areas.

## Fibromyalgia & OM

Because fibromyalgia presents with a varity of symptoms and fatigue is a common complaint, the disorder falls within OM internal medical classifications. Fibromyalgia may be best described by four OM clinical presentations.

1. Retention of pathogenic factors.

2. Latent pathogenic factors.

3. Pathogenic factors between the Interior and Exterior (Shao Yang).

4. Organic and internal disorders.

FM often begins following an infectious, or other medical disease which can lead to retained pathogenic factors. The main pathogenic factor seen clinically is Dampness. The more the myalgia, the more pathogenic Dampness or Phlegm. Dampness and Phlegm can result from:

- Improper treatment (or secondary to antibiotic therapy).

- Fever and Heat damaging the Fluids which congeal, thicken and do not flow.

  — this common clinical presentation can result in both Dampness and Yin deficiency.[23]

- Pathogenic factors damaging the Spleen/pancreas, disturbing the transforming and transporting functions of the Spleen.

- Prior weakness of the patient's Spleen/pancreas and a tendency to develop or retain Dampness.

- Pathogenic factors disturbing the Lung's descending function which normally direct Fluids to the Kidneys.

- Kidney Yang, Essence and True Qi deficiency.

23. A neutral herbal formula such as: Dioscoreae (Shan Yao), Pseudostellariae (Tai Zi Shen), Nelumbinis Nuciferae (Lian Zi), Atractylodis (Bai Zhu), Dolichoris Lablab (Bai Bian Dou), Amomi (Sha Ren), Coicis (Yi Ren), Poria (Fu Ling), Alismatis (Ze Xie),American Ginseng (Xi Yang Shen), should be used.

Latent Pathogenic Factors are seen most commonly in deficient patients that do not have a history of infectious disease. Insufficiency of the patient's True Qi, Kidney Qi and Essence result in pathogenic factors entering the Interior without the development of superficial symptoms (infectious symptoms). Later, symptoms of fatigue and muscle pain develop.

Pathogenic factors can be retained in the Shao Yang level (between the Exterior and Interior), especially in stressed patients. The patient is temporarily deficient (from stress) and therefore unable to dispel the external pathogenic factors. The main manifestation is alternating or combined symptoms of Heat and Cold.

Organic disorders, especially of the Spleen/pancreas and Kidney, can also result in symptoms of fatigue and muscle pain.

## Myofascial Pain Syndrome (MPS) & Trigger Points

MPS is a painful condition felt by some to be due to myofascial trigger point activation, either by direct causes or as a reactive mechanism to other dysfunctions. The pain of MPS is better localized than the pain from FM. The pain may be confined to a large area and involve several separate sites. However, it is often unilateral with a defined pattern of distribution. MPS is seen equally in males and females—whereas FM is more common in females. The patient is often awakened from sleep by pain, but chronic fatigue is not a common complaint. Tension headaches are a common associated symptom. Prognosis for MPS is very favorable and the condition responds well to techniques described later in this text.

## Myofascial Trigger Points (TPs)

Travell and Simons (1983) describe a myofascial trigger point (TP) as a small locus in the muscle that is strikingly different from its surroundings and is sensitive to mechanical stimulation. This kind of muscle trigger point must be distinguished from trigger points in nonmuscular tissue such as ligaments, fascia, bone, and skin.

**ACTIVE TRIGGER POINTS.** Trigger points can be either active or latent. Active trigger points are painful and symptomatic at the time of examination. When stimulated, they reproduce the patient's symptoms easily.

**LATENT TRIGGER POINTS.** Latent trigger points cause dysfunction but do not produce pain at the moment of examination. They have a higher threshold and require considerably more stimulation to elicit their typical reference. Sola and Kuitert (1955) found among 200 asymptomatic young adults that 54% had focal tenderness representing "latent myofascial trigger points." The prevalence of such tender areas, in both symptomatic and asymptomatic populations, resulted in a debate as to the significance of "myofascial pain syndromes" and myofascial trigger points.

**THE MAIN ACTIVATING FORCES OF TP ARE:**

**DIRECT CAUSES.**

*   Injury to muscles, tendons and/or joints.
*   Chronic stresses on muscles.
*   Lengthy periods of hypothermia.

**INDIRECT CAUSES**

*   Other trigger points.
*   Visceral disease.
*   Nutritional deficiency.
*   Arthritic joints.
*   Emotional stress.

**LATENT TRIGGER POINTS ACTIVATED BY:**

*   Overstretching, inactivity or momentary overtaxing of the involved muscle.

**OTHER CAUSES.**

*   Increased metabolic demands in short tight muscle may lead to ischemia and irritating metabolites.
*   Inhibition of antagonist muscle by over active tight agonist leading to fatigability and weakness.
*   Deconditioned muscles.[24]

**REFERRED PAIN FROM TP.** Pain referred from a myofascial TP does not follow a simple segmental pattern. Frequently, but not always, the pain occurs in the same dermatome, myotome or sclerotome of the TP. It usually does not include the entire segment, and often includes other segments (Travell and Simons *ibis*). Travell and Simons also report other symptoms, such as dizziness, tinnitus, localized vasoconstriction, perspiration and pilomotor activity, and positional pain (similar to posain from ligaments) associated with TPs. Travell and Simons have mapped and described each muscle trigger reference pattern in their book.

Travell and Simons concluded that since no EMG activity is found in taut bands associated with myofascial TPs, the muscle tightness cannot correctly be called spasm and does not involve motor unit activity. Galletti and Procacci (1966) have reported that a stellate ganglion block (anesthesia of a sympathetic ganglion in the neck) resolved pain and tenderness associated with active TPs in the deltoid. This suggests that the sympathetic nervous system affects TP activation. Gunn postulates that trigger points are supersensitive areas in the muscle secondary to intrinsic dysfunction within the neuromuscular complex—mostly due to neuropathic origin from degenerative disc disease. This may explain why trigger paints are so common as degenerative disc disease is (Miller, Schamtz and Scjultzis 1988) almost universal with aging.

---

24. lack of muscle conditioning and protective action can lead to some muscles becoming overactive while others are inhibited, resulting in joint stress and greater muscle fatigue.

A more recent study by Hubbard and Berkoff (1993), using a dual channel monopolar needle electromyogram (EMG), showed a 1 mm foci that sustained very high spontaneous EMG activity, and was stimulated by sympathetic fibers. Areas just 1 cm. adjacent to these foci were EMG silent. Another study by these researchers demonstrated muscle spindles in this 1 mm area. Injection of a medication that acts on sympathetic nerves was effective.

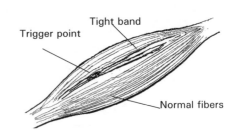

*Figure3- 19:* Trigger point.

**HISTOLOGICAL STUDIES.** Histological studies of muscles with trigger points both in MPS and FM have been inconclusive. Some studies reported negative findings, while others found changes (Glogowski and Wallraff 1951; Miehlke, Schulze and Eger 1950).

Hendriksson et al (1982) reported that muscle tissue biopsies from tender areas of patients with primary "fibromyalgia" show a "moth-eaten" appearance. He also reported that in these patients adenosine triphosphate (ATP) and phosphocreatine were reduced, lactate values were normal, and glycogen was below normal. He concluded that trigger points may be due to a primary metabolic disturbance or to an overload secondary to muscle tension.

Schroder and others reported that muscle biopsies in FM patients revealed moderate type II fiber atrophy. This type of atrophy, however, is also associated with disuse of striated muscles. The authors concluded that muscle biopsy does not contribute to the diagnosis of FM.

Lindman reported capillary structure irregularities in tender points in the trapezius muscle in both FM patients and controls. These irregularities were seen more commonly in the FM patients.

*Examination*

Examination for TP's reveals:

• Painful, shortened muscles, both on passive and active stretching.

• Strong isometric contraction, testing (resisted movements) may be painful, and muscles often appear weak.

• Cross-fiber palpation often evokes a "jump sign" and/or a local twitch.

*Treatment*

Travell and Simons (*ibid*) suggest stretch-and-spray, compression, puncture (injection or dry needling), nutritional supplementation and ultrasound as treatment methods. It must be reiterated that many times "trigger points" resolve spontaneously when joint dysfunction and ligamentous insufficiency are treated.

# Nerve Disorders

To one degree or another nerves are always affected in painful conditions.

## Neuropathic Pain

Neuropathic pain, which is less common than nociceptive pain, can be caused by trauma or disease evoked damage affecting the peripheral nerves, posterior roots, spinal cord or certain regions in the brain. In addition, one may see patients with similar or identical symptoms without detectable nerve damage, such as seen in post sprain reflex sympathetic dystrophy (RSD) (Bennett 1994).

Neuropathic pain usually results from prolonged damage to peripheral nerve tissue. Tasker (1991) proposed that the term "deafferenation pain" can be used for all conditions that are commonly called neuropathic pain. Effects of, and interaction with sympathetic nerves can occur with repetitive strain and ligamentous laxity, and can result in neuropathic pain. Viscerosomatic convergence may also be involved in reflex sympathetic dystrophy (RSD), as for example, occurs in the upper limb following an episode of cardiac pain (Bonica *ibid*). Sprouting of peripheral nerves after injury, although not always involving deafferenation, can result in convergence of low threshold mechanoreceptors and nociceptors leading to abnormal nociceptive output from mechanoreceptors (Willis 1993).

Neuropathic pain often is felt as continuous and burning like pain which is independent of posture or movement. It is extremely pressure and touch sensitive.

#### NEUROPATHIC PAIN IS COMMONLY SEEN WITH:

- Complex regional pain.

  Also called sympathetically maintained pain or reflex sympathetic dystrophy (RSD).

- Causalgia.

- Post-herpetic neuralgia.

- Stroke.

- Multiple sclerosis (MS).

- Spinal cord injury (Wall *ibid*).

Neuropathic pain from mild denervation is frequently associated with autonomic dysfunction such as (Gunn and Milbrandt 1978):

- Pilomotor reflex.

  Seen as goose flesh when the skin is exposed to cool air, in the dermatome with associated spondylosis.

- Vasomotor disturbances.

  Seen as vasoconstrictor action with pallor and cynotic skin.

- Sudomotor reflex.

  Seen as increased tendency to perspire.

- Trophic disturbances.

  Seen as trophedema.

Gunn (1992) suggests that neuropathic pain is common and can be due to spondylosis and "prespondylosis," with denervation supersensitivity due to nerve deafferenation.

## Neuritis

Neuritis or inflammation of a nerve (mononeuritis) or nerves (polyneuritis) may result from five general causes:

**1.** Mechanical causes: such as:

— Compression (the most common attended to by the orthopedic practitioner).
Pressure palsy may result from; discs, tumors, stenosis, casts, crutches or any prolonged pressure such as seen when alcoholics pass out leaning over an arm (saturday night palsy).

— Contusions and trauma.

— Violent or repetitive muscular activity or forcible overexertion of a joint.

— Hemorrhage into a nerve.

— Exposure to cold or radiation.

**2.** Toxic causes:

— Heavy metals such as; lead, strychnine, [25] arsenic, mercury, alcohol, carbon tetrachloride.

— Medications such as; hexobarbitol, sulfonamides, and vitamin B6.

**3.** Infections:

— Which may be localized and/or primary or secondary to:

25. Strychnine poisoning can occur when prescribing Semen Strychnotis, Ma Qian Zi, in large doses, or for prolonged periods (an herb used in OM for pain).

tetanus, tuberculosis, diptheria, malaria or various viral infections, such as Bell's palsy.

**4.** Metabolic causes:
— Nutritional deficiencies.
— Diabetes.
— Hypothyroidism.
— Toxemias of pregnancy.

**5.** Vascular or Collagen Vascular causes:
— Rheumatoid arthritis.
— Systemic lupus erythematosus.
— Sarcoidosis.
— Peripheral vascular disease.

## Pressure on Nerves

Pressure on nerve roots causes pain that the patient feels in all or any part of the relevant dermatome—depending on the severity of impairment. Pressure on a large nerve trunk usually is painless and results only in distal paresthesia ("pins and needles.") Paresthesia that results from pressure on a nerve root occurs while the pressure remains and stops when the pressure is removed. Paresthesia that results from pressure on a nerve trunk occurs when the pressure is removed, such as a leg "falling asleep." Paresthesias can also occur during pressure on small peripheral nerves, as seen in carpal tunnel syndrome for example. Prolonged pressure on nerves can result in nerve palsy and, depending on duration, may be irreversible.

*Paresthesia*

"Pins and needles" is an important symptom because it almost always implicates the nervous system. In primary disorders of peripheral nerves (intrinsic disorders) the pins and needles come and go without any relationship to movement (Cyriax *ibid*). Paresthesia or hyperalgesia, due to nerve injury, may be provoked by stroking the affected dermatome (in contrast to Dorman's nulliness, i.e., the numb-like sen-

sation felt distally due to ligament dysfunction, which is alleviated by stroking and massage).

The lesion or nerve pressure occurs almost always proximally to the area of paresthesia, numbness or pain. When the sensation of pins and needles is present but no movement evokes or aggravates the symptoms, a systemic or central nervous system involvement must be considered.

**NERVE ROOT COMPRESSION.** A nerve root with impaired mobility (such as from external pressure due to disc disease) may be painful and limited in range when stretched. For example, a straight leg raise (SLR) stretches the L4 - S2 nerve roots via the sciatic nerve, and can cause pain when these roots are entrapped.

Compression of nerve roots (radicular pain) is said to be classically accompanied by:

• Pain in the region supplied by the nerve.

• Radicular loss of sensitivity, according to the dermatome.

• Motor loss in muscles innervated by the corresponding roots.

• Deep tendon reflex changes.

NOTE: Tenderness is often present in the muscles of the entire myotome supplied by both the anterior and posterior rami, as the nerve root is often affected before it branches (Gunn *ibid*).

## Sympathetically Maintained Pain

Even though the observation is debatable, considerable evidence indicates that the sympathetic nervous system (SNS) is commonly involved in chronic pain and sympathetically maintained pain (also called complex regional pain and reflex sympathetic dystrophy). Apparently this involvement is due to post-injury nociceptor activity that is modulated by catecholamines, particularly norepinephrine (noradrenaline) (Wall *ibid*). Inflammatory mediators such as bradykinin, interleukin-8, prostaglandins and norepinephrine also have been shown to require the post-ganglionic sympathetic neuron for expression of hyperalgesia. Behavioral studies in rats point to a contribution of the sympathetic post-ganglionic terminals in the hyperalgesia of cutaneous inflammation and in the severity of arthritis (Levine and Taiwo 1994). Some researchers have postulated that norepinephrine and inflammatory mediators have an indirect effect through release of prostaglandins (Wall *ibid*).

As early as 1947, Korr described the contribution (including other than causalgia and reflex sympathetic dystrophy) the sympathetic nervous system makes to chronic pain. However, Korr's opinion remains disputed. Schott (1994) suggests that the clinical phenomena that imply sympathetic nerve involvement in pain might be attributed more satisfactorily to effects of neuropeptides that afferent C-fibers have released. Neither neurophysiological studies of nociceptors in rats nor psychophysical studies in humans have provided conclusive confirmation of the role of sympathetic efferents in inflammatory pain and hyperalgesia (Raja 1995). However, sympathetic innervation has been observed in most soft tissues and bones, including the vertebral bodies, discs, dura mater, and spinal ligaments (Ahmed et al. *ibid*). This finding supports the possibility of sympathetic contribution to pain.

### Sympathetic Hyperactivity

Chronic hyperactivity of the sympathetic pathways seems to be a prevailing theme in many conditions, including musculoskeletal dysfunctions. Clinically this can manifest as:

- Hyperhidrosis (excessive perspiration).

- Cold and wet skin.

- Vasospasm.

- Cyanosis.

- Edema.

In the early stage, the skin may be hot and dry, but not edematous. Depending on the severity of disorder, further trophic shifts may be seen, such as in skin thickness and texture, loss of hair, shortening of tendons, atrophy of muscles, osteoporosis and other degenerative changes in bone (Korr 1978).

Long-term sympathetic hyperactivity may be deleterious to certain sensitive tissues. At the very least, the result is vasoconstriction, and therefore reduced blood supply and nutrition to tissues. Some studies in animal models of neuropathic pain and clinical observations have confirmed these observations and point to a role the SNS plays in certain chronic pain states (Raja *ibid*). It has been suggested that emotional disturbances, because they influence the autonomic nervous system, may cause vasoconstriction in muscles and development of myofascial trigger points (Travell and Simons 1984).

Another important consequence of sympathetic hyperactivity is a reduced threshold of several types of receptors and sense organs that are influenced by sympathetic impulses. Many such afferent fibers may then exaggerate their discharge, causing them to report a greater intensity of stimulation than actually occurred. This can cause the patient to be hypersensitive (Willard *ibid*).

TREATMENT. Treatment of true neuropathic pain can be very difficult. All underlying conditions must be addressed. Acupuncture may be of some value (particularly in diabetic neuropathy, Abuaisha et al. 1998). Herbal therapy (both topical and oral) is of some value, as well. Pharmacological and injection therapy may provide some benefit.

# Disc Disorders

Pain in the low back usually starts after age 25 when early changes within the discs begin to develop, while similar changes in other structures of the vertebral column usually occur much later in life (Ramani 1985), although preceding muscular weakness and ligament laxity is probable and patients with herniated discs in the lumbar spine manifest a premature degeneration in the interspinous ligament (Yahia, Garzon, Strykowski and Rivard 1990). Studies in mice genetically predisposed to disc degeneration also suggest that the extracellular matrix components are often normal and that degeneration is due to abnormal extrinsic factors, such as paraspinal muscle weakness (Hopwood and Robinson 1973). Disc injuries may affect either the annulus alone, or both the annulus and the nucleus (Figure 3-20).

Disc pathology is the most common cause of nerve root impingement seen in the practitioner's office. In the past, many low back symptoms have been attributed to nerve compression by the disc. This has led to a large number of disc surgeries and was call by McNab the "disc dynasty" (Brown 1995). The new emphasis on biochemical pain from minor tears in the annulus fibrosus (due to torsional and compression injuries) may explain some of the elusive pain syndromes seen without mechanical pressure on the dura or nerve roots (Bogduk 1990), and may yet bring about a new disc dynasty. Several new techniques, including provocation CT discography, are being explored to elucidate these theories.

Many now think that the majority of chronic low back pain patients, refractory or only partially responsive to a treatment protocols, which include prolotherapy and manual therapy, are suffering from these types of disc lesions (Klein and Eek personal communication).

Various treatments have been tried for chemical disc pain, none of which have been very successful. It has been postulated that treatment with tetracycline may be effective as it can inhibit the enzymes responsible for abnormal disc pH (Klein 1995), however this does not seem to be born out clinically. Heating the discs has

been tried with little success and epidural and intradiscal DMSO injections are currently being studied. Longer periods of thermocoagulation directly at the annulus is being evaluated and may be helpful in about 50% of patients (Derby 1997).

## Disc Biochemistry

The biochemical role in patients with back pain due to disc disorders is increasingly receiving attention and importance. This may result in improved treatments as more knowledge accumulates.

### Glucosamiglycans

Herniated discs show a fall of total GAG (glucosaminglycans) and an increase in lower molecular weight sugar fractions of glycoproteins of the nucleus and annulus. There is also a premature appearance of proteins and non-collagenous protein in the nucleus. Age related disc degeneration results in a fall of total GAG's, as well (Brown 1995).

### Phospholipase A2 (PLA2)

Franson et al. (1992) demonstrated an increase in PLA 2 in prolapsed disc fragments. PLA2 is an enzyme that controls the liberation of arachidonic acid (important in the inflammatory cascade) from membranes. PLA2 in circulation is inflammatory itself—as it can cause inflammation when liberated. Expression of inflammatory mediators is achieved by PLA2 releasing fatty acids from lipid membranes. These can be converted to prostaglandins and leukotrienes, which are potent inflammatory mediators (Willburger and Wittenberg 1994).

PLA2 can be secreted by disc tears (which may be visualized only by special dye studies) making the disc and the immediate environment irritable—causing discitis. Willburger and Wittenberg suggest that since prostaglandin release from sequestrated disc is rather low, the inflammatory effect might actually be due to immunologic reactions, since nuclear material is a foreign substance in the circulatory system.

### Intradiscal pH

The intradiscal pH in symptomatic patients with disc pathology is often more acidic than in patients with similar radiological disc findings who are nonetheless asymptomatic (Mooney 1989). This change in pH can cause pain and may explain why some people with similar pathologies (as seen by MRI) have pain while others do not. Smoking lowers the intradiscal pH (Hambly and Moony 1992). Localized acidosis may explain segmental and non-segmental pain.

### Stages of Disc Injury

Disc injuries can be divided into four stages (MacNab 1977):

1. The first stage refers to a protrusion of the disc without rupture of the annulus.

   Also called disc bulge and internal derangement.

2. The second stage refers to ruptures in the annulus with expulsion of nuclear material and is termed disc prolapse.

3. The third stage is called extrusion/prolapse. Here the nuclear material reaches the epidural space.

4. The last stage is called sequestration and involves the separation of a disc fragment from the disc proper.

Disc bulge, rupture and extrusion are seen frequently, between 28-50%, in normal (asymptomatic) populations, and correlate poorly with clinical findings (Jensel et al. 1994; Rothman et al. 1984). This is probably due to differences in biochemical

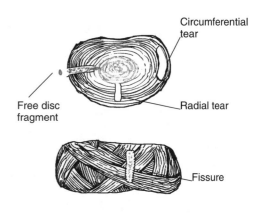

Figure3- 20: Disc tears.

reactions and inflammatory responses in different individuals.

### Disc Derangement

The first and second stage of disc disease (disc protrusion and disc bulge), are also called internal disc derangement or disruption (IDD). Disc derangements can be further divided into four stages by CT discography (Figure 3-21),

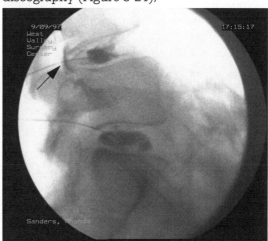

Figure3- 21: Two level discogram. Note the dye remains at the center of the disc at L5. At L4, note crescent shape dye print at the posterior annulus (arrow), indicating a fissure.

- *Grade 0.* In grade 0 the contrast medium is strictly confined to the nucleus with a normal perimeter.

- *Grade 1.* A disrupted nucleus extends into the inner third of the annulus.

- *Grade 2.* The nucleus enters the middle third of the annulus.

  Grade 2 may or may not be painful because the affected middle third of the annulus has an irregular nerve supply.

- *Grade 3.* The nuclear material has full access to the nerve endings in the outer third of the annulus and therefore produces pain.

- *Grade 4.* There is further annular disruption with vertical annular rupture — sometimes called fissures.

  Grade 4 annular disruptions show as high-intensity zones (HIZ) in the annulus with T2-weighted magnetic resonance images. These high intensity zones have been shown to have a high correlation (86%) with symptoms reproduced by provocation discography (Aprill and Bogduk 1992).

DIAGNOSIS OF DISC DERANGEMENT. The use of vibration may be a simple and useful tool in the diagnosis of internal disc derangements. Yrjama and Vanharanta (1994) report good correlation between sensitivity to vibration applied to the lumbar spinous processes by a standard electric toothbrush shaft (Braun) (with a blunt head instead of the brush) and provocation discography.

PATIENT EDUCATION. Disc derangements and extrusion are often preceded by one or more low back pain attacks and probably represent some degree of ligamentous laxity, segmental instability, and or other somatic dysfunction and restrictions. Therefore, patients with back pain should be educated about the possibility of developing acute disc disorder and what to do when they occur.

### Acute Disc Injury

Disc injuries occur generally when the patient performs an awkward or unguarded movement. Commonly, a sudden sensation that something "popped" in the back occurs, and sometimes an audible noise is heard. As patients usually have had a previous episode of back pain, the principals of McKenzie exercises (see chapter 5) should be taught to patients so that their early application may reduce the extent of herniation.

### Degenerative Disc Disease

Degenerative disc disease is almost universal with aging (Miller, Schamtz and Scjultz 1988) and is not necessarily symptomatic. Disc degeneration is demonstrated with equal incidence in subjects with or without pain (Nachemson 1992). Differentiating between patients that have stable or unstable segments is helpful. Nachemson, however, questions the reliability of segmental instability and isolated disc resorption as causative factors in low back pain. Smoking has been shown to increase the rate of disc degeneration (Battié et al. *ibid*; Helms and Machemson *ibid*).

Gunn (*ibid*) postulates that spondylosis/prespondylosis and degenerative disc disease are contributing factors to the unavoidable degenerative cascades that affect the nervous system. This leads to mild segmental denervation and neuropathic pain. Others suggest that the internal chemistry of the disc which is largely based on the relationship between mucopolysaccharides production and the water content in the disc may at times lead to pain. The water content is reduced with aging, and with degenerative disc disease and may be responsive to dysfunction and lack of normal motion. Dysfunction may lead to disruption of the disc chemistry and pH (Mooney *ibid*).

When discs degenerate, both function and regenerative qualities within the surrounding joint are affected, as normal motion is necessary for joint, soft tissue and disc nourishment. Disc degeneration has been shown to increase loads on the facets, and is associated with muscle weakness (Brown 1995).

## Symptoms & Treatment

Nerve compression from disc protrusions can lead to radiculopathy. However, to be a clinically significant mechanical nerve root compression by a disc (apart from internal disc derangements), there must be a true positive straight leg raise with dural tension signs, weakness of the appropriate muscles, loss of sensation and sluggish reflexes. An MRI finding without these signs can be misleading.

In the case of internal disc derangement and chemical discitis one may or may not see the above signs and symptoms of compression. Symptoms and signs will depend on the amount of swelling and chemical reaction. When the nuclear material is truly extruded and there is nerve root compromise, the patient may need surgery, but conservative treatment can be as effective as surgery in most cases. Surgical intervention for low back pain has been estimated to be helpful in only 1% of patients who have low back pain (Waddell 1987). Conservative treatment is effective even in patients who have radiculopathy (Saal and Saal 1989). In a follow-up of properly-selected patients who had disc herniations, at two years no difference in outcome was shown between patients who had been treated surgically and patients who had been treated conservatively (Weber 1983).

Epidural injection, or an oral steroid dose pack often are very helpful and can be combined with McKenzie exercises. All spinal dysfunctions and ligamentous laxity should be addressed. Acupuncture and herbs are used to address underlying constitutional weakness, and for analgesic affects.

# Facet Disorders

The role of facets in pain is controversial. Mooney and Roberston (1976) have shown that injection of the facets with hypertonic saline under specific radiographic control can lead to pain. The facet capsule can be sprained and probably elicit pain. Trauma from excessive stress to the joint and ligaments may cause them to pull tightly on the joint, leading to joint locking (Mennell 1952). With small ligamentous tearing, even greater restrictions may be seen (Turek 1984).

## Facet Meniscus

The facet joint contains a meniscus, or can develop one by damage to cartilage which remains attached to the external capsule. The process of meniscus formation is called intra-articular inclusion. A meniscus can probably get trapped and cause pain (like in the knee) (Bogduk *ibid*).

## PLA2 & Prostaglandins

PLA2 and prostaglandins, both of which are pro-inflammatory, can be released by the facet joint (Willburger and Wittenberg 1994). Prostaglandins can sensitize nociceptors making the joint more sensitive to pain from normal motions.

## Facet Degenerative Disease

The facets may develop marked osteoarthrosis, with possible ligamentous insufficiency, which may lead to pain and referred nulliness. This eventually leads to decreased efficiency of intervertebral joint and disc functions, increasing the possibility disc injury. Roaf (1977) suggested that degeneration of the facet joint results in reduced stability of the intervertebral disc and a decrease in the forces that can cause tears in the disc fibers. The removal of the lumbar facet joints in "normal" cadaveric spines increases rotation by 1.2° as compared to 2° when disc annular fibers are removed (Krismer, Haid and Rabl 1996).

The degenerative processes within the facet joint, like other synovial joints, can yield a synovial cyst that can emerge and create an extradural compression. This may cause a mechanical or chemical irritation of nerve endings (Brown 1995) Degenerative changes may also lead to foraminal stenosis.

### The Facet Syndrome

Sprain of the facet (facet syndrome) can lead to hemarthrosis and capsulitis of the facet. Symptoms usually consist of localized sharp pain with little or no radiation initially, involuntary muscle guarding, spasms and motion restriction. The pain is aggravated by all movements except flexion. Extension with side bending toward the painful side is especially painful (Kraft and Levinthal 1951).

When more than one segment is involved, a flattening of the normal spinal curve may be seen, more commonly in the thoracic and lumbar areas. Painful and tender muscle guarding with neutral vertebral dysfunctions often are evident above and below the restricted site (Helbig and Lees 1988). [26]

The criteria of facet syndrome diagnose consist of (Bonica *ibid*):

- Back, buttock and groin pain (or higher if in thoracic or cervical).

- Well-localized paraspinal tenderness.

- Pain reproduction with extension and rotation toward the painful side.

- Significant x-ray evidence of facet arthrosis.

- Strong correlation of pain relief by a facet block.

  Clinically, pain from the facet joints can often be indistinguishable from disc pain and can mislead the practitioner.

---

26. A group of vertebrae which are sidebent to one side and rotated to opposite sides.

### Types of Facet Dysfunction

Paris (1992) describes facet dysfunctions as painful and non-painful blocks.

**PAINFUL BLOCK.** A painful block is an acute condition which is initially felt as a sharp local pain, accompanied by simultaneous postural deviation. The onset of acute painful facet block and postural deviation is immediate, in contrast to disc lesions which take some time to lead to postural deviation.

**NOTE:** Clinically this presentation is more likely to be due to internal disc derangement or backward sacral torsions.

**A NONPAINFUL BLOCK.** A nonpainful block is also an acute condition in which the back is effectively stuck in a laterally deviated position (list) away from the blocked facet.

**NOTE:** Facet dysfunctions often accompany sacroiliac dysfunctions.

With internal derangement of the facets or discs, the joints most frequently lock in flexion. This typical antalgic posture can also be due to spasm of the psoas, spasm of deep aspect of the quadratus lumborum, extension spinal joint restrictions (see this chapter), and backward torsions of SI joint (see this chapter)

**TREATMENT.** Whether painful or not, facet disorders are treated with manual therapy. Thrust manipulation may result in a residual facet inflammation that should be treated accordingly. In the non-acute period the facet joint capsule and the surrounding ligaments can be needled to stabilize the joint (this may be difficult to perform accurately in the low back without fluoroscopic control). Steroid, Sarapin or proliferant injections may be needed.

# Periosteal Lesions

Periosteal lesions are common and can refer pain in a non-segmental distribution and to a sizable area (Kellgren 1949; Inman and Saunders 1944). Tears often appear in the periosteum—secondary to trauma or strains—where soft tissues are attached to bone. Vagler and Krauss describe periosteal changes in organic disease and treat them by massage.

## Treatment

Periosteal lesions can be treated by massage, periosteal acupuncture, electric stimulation, and if needed by injection.

# Scar Tissue

Prolonged immobilization of muscles or joints, injuries, infections and surgeries can all result in the formation of scar tissue. When joints are immobilized collagen fibers will be laid down in random and form scars. Scars can interfere with fascial load distribution, often adhering tissues that should move independently. Neural therapists consider scars as capable of neural irritation, constituting an "interference field" which may lead to numerous symptoms, including pain. Scar tissue formation (Wall and Gutnick 1974) may provoke pain mechanisms without involvement of the nociceptive system.

Stacher found scars to have higher skin resistance than adjacent, undamaged tissue. Scar tissue has a resistance of 120-500 kilo-ohms above that of the surrounding skin. Skin resistance in a "non-active scar" (i.e. not producing symptoms) is mostly uniform over the scar, whereas in an "active scar" there may be as much as 600-1500 kilo-ohms of variation.

Referred pain or numbness has been reported in skin and scar triggers, and the sensations are felt nearby or remotely. Travell and Simons (*ibid*) report burning, prickling and "lightning-like" jabs of pain from cutaneous scars.

## Treatment

Scars are treated by massage, myofascial release techniques, acupuncture needling and if needed by injection. The active scar is surrounded by needles which are inserted at the edge of the scar, at a distance of about 1 cm. apart. If the scar crosses a longitudinal acupuncture channel a point above, and below the scar, is added on the channel. An electrical stimulator or ion cord is connected to push the energy through the scar. The scar is then mobilized. For a highly symptomatic scar a topical application of Toad venom extract can be used as an anesthetic. If symptoms persist injection therapy with procaine may be necessary.

# Bursitis

Bursitis occurs when the synovial fluid, within the bursa, gets inflamed and leads to painful stimulation of nerve ending. The etiology of bursitis is unknown but can result from trauma, infections and inflammatory arthritis. Bursitis occurs most often in the shoulder but can be seen in several locations, including the knee, olecranon, retrocalcaneal, iliopsoas, trochanteric, ichial and bursa of the first metatarsal head (bunion), (Cyriax *ibid*).

## Treatment

Bursitis is treated by first addressing any accompanying joint dysfunction and myofascial pain and tension. Herbal therapy can be helpful. If needed the bursa can be injected.

# Inflammation

Inflammation is the means by which the body deals with insult and injury. Inflammation is a complicated and not fully understood communication between cellular and humoral elements.[27] Inflammation rids the body of foreign matter and disposes of damaged cells, and initiates wound healing. When inflammation affects a joint (such as in rheumatoid arthritis), the cartilage can be damaged by neutrophils[28] and lysosomal enzymes[29] that enter the area. This leads to a vicious cycle of repeated injury and persistent inflammation. Anti-inflationary drugs such as aspirin and other NSAIDs inhibit prostaglandin synthesis, which may affect inflammatory mediator production and cellular processes. Steroid hormones have been postulated to have a multitude of effects, probably the most significant in this context is the stabilization of lysosomal membranes (Ryan and Majno 1983).[30] Table 3-16 on page 165 summarizes inflammation.

## Chronic Inflammation

Chronic inflammation can evolve from acute inflammation, or occur without an acute phase. Histologically, chronic inflammation has two main features; the presence of granulation tissue,[31] and mononuclear predominance.[32] Mononuclear predominance can also be seen in the latter part of acute inflammation as mononuclear phagocytes[33] or macrophages.[34] In comparison to ordinary loose connective tissue, granulation tissue is more cellular and contains neutrophils, inflammatory cells and fibroblasts.[35] Granulation tissue is more vascular and has leaky capillaries. The formation of granulation tissue is the response of connective tissue and vessels to irritation.

In some forms of chronic inflammation other cell types appear, which suggests the development of immunologic reactions. These may include lymphocytes,[36] eosinophils and plasma cells.[37] In other forms where no immune response is present, the mononuclear cells are almost entirely macrophages. When inflammation is chronic, the vascular component, vasodilation and exudation is minimal and therefore, clinically manifests with less redness and heat (Ryan and Majno 1983).

It must be remembered that inflammation anywhere in the body can result in

27. Humoral response is one of the two forms of immunity that respond to antigens such as bacteria and foreign tissue. It is mediated by B-cell lymphocytes—marked by antibodies.

    Cellular immunity is dominated by T-cell lymphocytes. It is involved in resistance to infectious diseases, delayed hypersensitivity, resistance to cancer, autoimmune diseases, graft rejection and allergies.

28. Neutrophils are the circulating white blood cells essential for phagocytosis and proteolysis by which bacteria, cellular deris, and solid particles are removed and destroyed.

29. Enzymes with hydrolytic actions that function in intracellular digestive processes.

30. Cytoplasmic membrane-bound vesicle measuring 5-8 nm (primary lysosome) and containing a wide variety of glycoprotein hydrolytic enzymes.

31. Granulation tissue is any soft, pink, fleshy projection that forms during the healing process in a wound. It consists of capillaries surrounded by fibrous collagen.

32. Mononuclear cells are cells such as leukocytes, lymphocytes and monocytes, with round or oval nuclei.

33. Phagocyte is a cell that is able to surround, engulf and digest microorganisms and cellular debris.

34. Macrophage is any phagocytic cell of the reticuloedothelial system including histocyte in loose connective tissue.

35. Fibroblast is an undifferentiated cell in the connective tissue that gives rise to various precursor cells, such as the chondroblast, collagenoblast, and osteoblast, that form the fibrous, binding, and supporting tissue of the body.

36. Lymphocyte is a type of white blood cell that increases in number in response to infection.

37. Eosinophil is a granulocytic, bilobed leukocyte (white blood cell), that increases in number in response to allergy and in some parasitic infections.

musculoskeletal like pain, and may be caused by bacteria, viruses, parasites, fungi, spirochetes, and cardiovascular or autoimmune diseases.

## Wound Healing

Wound healing occurs in three overlapping phases (Banks 1991). The first phase has three major consequences; early wound strength secondary to crosslinking, removal of damaged tissue, and recruitment of fibroblasts.

- **First phase**. The first phase is the inflammatory phase, which can be divided into early and late stages.

  — *Early Inflammatory Stage*. The early inflammatory stage can last about 3 days during which cellular debris and humoral factors attract the initial influx of granulocytes. The first to appear are platelets[38] that secrete many chemical mediators of inflammation which result in the arachidonic acid cascade[39] and release of growth factors such as, platelet-derived growth factor (PDGF), platelet factor 4, insulin-like growth factor (IGF-1) and transforming growth factors.

  — *Late (Second) Stage*. In the second stage the monocytes and macrophages release polypeptide growth factors which activate the fibroblasts. The second stage of the first inflammatory phase lasts about 10 days.

- **Second Phase**. The second phase is the granulation tissue formation phase. It begins about two days after injury (overlapping with the first) and can last up to 6-8 weeks. The second phase is controlled by monocytes which are pluripo-

tential cells capable of essentially directing the complete sequence of events in this proliferative phase.

  — Monocytes begin to form mobilizing a soupy mixture of granulocytes and macrophages with infiltrating fibroblasts from granulation tissue. This is characteristic of a healing wound.
  Macrophages are capable of releasing numerous growth factors, chemotactants and proteolytic enzymes. They also can activate fibroblasts for tendon and ligament repair.

- **Third phase**. The third phase is the matrix formation or remodeling maturation phase. This phase is characterized by a trend toward decreased cellularity, decreased synthetic activity, increased organization of extracellular matrix, and more normal biochemical profile.

  — Fibroblasts remain to build a strong matrix of collagen. There is intrinsic healing as a result of endotendon fibroblast response.

  — Lasts about 6 months and the tensile strength of repaired ligaments reaches about 50%.[40] Full strength is only reached after 1-3 years. Collagen maturation and functional linear realignment are usually seen in about 2 months.

Cellular response after tendon laceration can be extrinsic or intrinsic. The extrinsic response is a proliferation and bridging of the injury by epithelial cells. Intrinsic healing is the result of an endotendon fibroblastic response (Brown 1995).

### Movement During the Healing Phase

Movement and activity are of primary importance in preserving homeostasis between collagen degradation and synthesis (Amiel and Woo 1981). Movement

---

38. Platelets are the smallest cells in the blood. They are essential for the coagulation of blood.

39. Arachidonic acid is an essential fatty acid that is a component of lecithin (esterified phospholipid) and a basic material for the biosynthesis of some prostaglandins.

40. For more information see acupuncture and dry needling chapter 5.

encourages collagen to be laid down in the correct anatomical arrangement and helps increase the production of ground substance and intermolecular cross-linking, therefore increasing the strength of the tissue. This occurs by improved vascular remodeling (in a longitudinal orientation), and by causing the orientation of fibroblasts and collagen to be laid in parallel to the fibers (Gelberman et al. 1989). Movement can also decrease the probability of the formation of abnormal adhesion and results in a more normal looking tissue rather than scar tissue (Dorman *ibid*). Movement also prevents the randomness of collagen fibers found in regular scar tissue. Movement during the granulation phase (about first 10 days) should not be too stressful on the healing tissue, as this can prevent normal healing.

### Factors that may Influence Healing

Healing can be influenced by smoking, collagen diseases, nutritional deficiency and some medications: (Brown, Orme and Richardson 1986; Battié et al 1991, and Lawson1989).

- Smoking can decrease fibrinolytic activity and nutritional supply to tissues including discs.
  This can lead to increased risk of poor healing and cause disc pathologies, surgical and fracture nonunions.
- Medications, especially anti-inflammatory medications.

- Collagen diseases such as Marfan's syndrome and Ehlers-Danlos syndrome.
- Nutritional deficiencies such as, vitamin C, B1, zinc, sulfur, copper, manganese, boron and proteins (see appendix A).

### Anti-Inflammatory Drugs

Non-steroidal anti-inflammatory drugs (NSAIDs) work by inhibiting the production of prostaglandins and thus may interfere with normal tissue repair. NSAIDs tend to be nonspecific and inhibit both helpful and non-helpful prostaglandins, hence can result in unwanted side-effects. NSAIDs use cause 20,000 *deaths* and cost $200,000,000 for treatment of side effects in the US., alone. It is estimated that 8% of the world adult population is prescribed an NSAID for a variety of conditions (Simon 1997). At least five studies, in both humans and animals, have reported that NSAIDs can lead to destruction of joints (Newman and Ling 1985; Shield 1993; Brooks, potter and Buchaman 1982; Ranningen and Langeland 1980; Brandt 1987). Hence, the harm/benefit ratio between the use or nonuse of anti-inflammatory medications is difficult to answer at this point. Inflammation is important for wound repair, but it can also lead to sensitization of nerves. Therefore, anti-inflammatory medication may have both beneficial and harmful affects. Long-term use should probably be avoided.

*Table 3-16.* INFLAMMATION AND WOUND HEALING

| | |
|---|---|
| **INFLAMMATION** | **Chemical and physical forces result in same initial inflammatory response**<br>    Cell degranulation, disruption of blood vessels, general cell damage,<br>  — leads to activation of variety of inflammatory mediators<br>**Chronic inflammation**<br>  — can evolve from acute inflammation<br>    occur without an acute phase<br>    vascular component, vasodilation and exudation is minimal<br>  — therefore, clinically manifests with less redness and heat.<br>    In some forms other cell types appear<br>    which suggests immunologic reactions<br>  — usually more pronounced redness and heat |
| **WOUND HEALING** | **Three phases**<br>1) 2 inflammatory stages<br>    divided into early and late stage<br>2) Granulation phase<br>3) Matrix formation and remodeling phase |

# Chapter 4: *Orthopedic Assessment*

This section presents concepts that are principally from western Orthopaedic Medicine.[1] Often integrated within OM, they can be important for assessment and treatment of musculoskeletal disorders.

## The Diagnostic Process

Before treating soft tissue lesions, the practitioner:

**1.** Interviews the patient for a history.

**2.** Examines the patient.

**3.** Assesses symptoms and signs.

**4.** Performs a differential diagnosis.

The accuracy of a diagnosis depends on a composite of the history and clinical findings, and on the practitioner's understanding of referred pain.[2] If a soft tissue lesion is seated deeply, discrepancies usu-

---

1. An updated Cyriax approach to soft tissue management. This approach integrates osteopathic concepts, as well.

2. Pain can be felt along the entire length or part of any structure that is innervated by the same spinal nerve (i.e. dermatome, sclerotome or myotome). Analogous to pain along a channel.

ally exist between the location of the pain and the location of the culprit lesion. Often the number of "objective signs" present is not sufficient to make a diagnosis, and the practitioner must correlate a set of subjective data.

### Determining the Origin of Symptoms

To determine the origin of a symptom or set of symptoms, a thorough screening and a full differential diagnosis are paramount. System-oriented schools such as OM and osteopathy perform screening examinations of the entire body. These approaches to examination hold that restrictions of motion are the primary origin of many painful conditions. In OM the restrictions are primarily of Qi, Blood and channel functions. In osteopathy, the presence of joint and soft tissue restrictions (which are expressed as channels, Qi and Blood in OM) are more important than the presence of pain and/or the provocation of pain by movement (Greenman 1989). Frequently osteopathy and OM consider the biomedical lesion to be an adaptation to motion and circulation restrictions.

## Evaluation Emphasis: Orthopaedic

In Orthopaedic Medicine the emphasis of evaluation is on joint and tissue *function and provocation of pain*, not tenderness. Palpation should be used only after identifying a suspected structure through selective tension methods (when possible) and through functional assessments.[1]

When the patient presents with a condition that affects moving parts of the body, some movement or posture must be capable of eliciting or aggravating the pain. The practitioner's task is to:

- Isolate the involved tissue by breaking complex movements into simplified elements.

- Test each element separately.

To demonstrate an abnormality, the practitioner must compare all tested structures with similar but unaffected structures. If the immediate location of pain is suspected to hold the culprit lesion, the practitioner must also demonstrate that this pain is not merely secondary to a painful movement (or referred) or normally sensitive tissue. This process, which is at the heart of selective tension, yields a nociceptive, lesion-oriented diagnosis.

The practitioner tests movement to assess for pain and limitations. The significance of pain and limitation and the significance of painless movement are equal, because they suggest different pathologies or dysfunctions. Since an involved structure cannot always be isolated, the practitioner must consider other information, such as analysis of several motions followed by deduction of the significance of the findings (Cyriax *ibid*).

## The Patient History

A comprehensive patient history is imperative for diagnosis of musculoskeletal conditions. In many instances a good history is sufficient for making a diagnosis, although (Mitchell 1995) the nature of somatic dysfunction and/or joint dysfunctions will not have been elucidated. The history can help the practitioner, not only in diagnosing the disease or dysfunction, but also in avoiding catastrophic mistakes.

The practitioner must learn, and continue developing, a crucial diagnostic skill: listening. The practitioner also must avoid asking leading questions because, in a subconscious effort to please the practitioner, many patients give the "expected" response.

Table 4-7 on page 627 through Table 4-12 on page 630 in appendix B are a summary list of inquiry topics for the patient history.

### *Age/Occupation Risk Factors*

Having recorded the patient's personal information, the practitioner notes the patient's sex and inquires about age, occupation and social history, including past occupations. Age and occupation can point to risk factors such as:

PATIENTS OVER 40 YEARS OF AGE.[2]
- Traumatic arthritis.
- Osteoporosis.
- Degenerative diseases.
- Osteomalacia.
- Cancer.
- Paget's disease.

YOUNGER PATIENTS.[3]
- Neurofibromatosis.

---

1. Cyriax's Orthopaedic Medicine, selective tension method, is very helpful for assessing the extremities but is limited for diagnosis of the spine.

2. Most of which are related to the OM Kidneys and Liver.

3. Most of which are related to OM Blood stagnation and pathogenic factors.

- Repetitive motion injury.
- Strains.
- Osteochondritis dissecans.
- Disc protrusions.

TRUCK DRIVERS AND OTHER PATIENTS EXPOSED TO VIBRATIONS.

- Disc disease.
- Deconditioning/postural syndromes.

### OPQRST *Pain/Complaint Inquiry*

The practitioner asks about the location of pain/complaint and whether the patient has suffered a trauma or other direct cause, and other questions that help focus on the possible source of the pain/complaint. Some practitioners use the "OPQRST" method of organizing their questions about pain/complaint:

**O**nset.

**P**rovoking or palliative factors.

**Q**uality and character of pain.

**R**adiation and referral of pain.

**S**ite of pain.

**T**iming of pain.

CHRONOLOGY AND PROGRESSION. The practitioner inquires about onset and past behavior of the symptoms, and the chronological progression of symptoms. For example, initially the patient feels pain close to the culprit lesion *(OM: Sinew channels)*. During later stages the pain is likely to be referred *(OM: pathology enters the Connecting and Main channels)*. So an account of where the pain started and to where it has progressed is helpful. In cases of trauma, the practitioner must be familiar with the forces affecting the patient, such as the direction of the trauma.

TIMING OF SYMPTOMS. Joints that have quickly filled with fluid or have suddenly swelled suggest the presence of bleeding and should be aspirated when possible. Whereas, in joints that fill up slowly the effusion is usually of serous fluid. Sprained ligaments develop pain progressively over several hours. Fractures, dislocations and internal derangements are painful at the onset. Muscle and tendon tears usually cause sudden pain during a particular movement. In repetitive micro trauma, such as overuse tendinitis however, the onset of pain is insidious. Pain following overuse often suggests tendinous disorders. Night pain, especially of insidious onset, suggests inflammation and serious conditions.

THE RELATIONSHIPS OF POSTURE, ACTIVITY, REST, AND EXERTION. The relationships of posture, activity, rest and exertion can provide important information. Ligament pain is commonly increased by inactivity and relieved by subsequent movement, although heavy work will exacerbates the pain. Rest will characteristically relieve pain due to joint dysfunction, in the absence of discrete pathology, and of overuse syndromes and disc disease.

Activity often aggravates the pain of vertebral (somatic) dysfunction, typically with certain movements being worse than others. Aggravation of pain by activity is seen with muscle strain, overuse syndromes and disc disease, as well. With pathological joints activity may initially alleviate pain but later will usually aggravate the pain.

EFFECT OF COUGHING: Pain aggravated by coughing, especially if the pain is felt in the upper limbs, suggests an intra-spinal (space occupying) lesion. A cough also can increase upper back pain from pleuritis, and from the SI joints, due to a momentary increase in intra-abdominal pressure which results in broadening of the SI joints.

PINS, NEEDLES AND BURNING. Pins and needles suggests nervous system involvement. But may also suggest metabolic or vascular involvement.

Vague tingling, "pins and needles" and numbness can be caused by a peripheral nerve, nerve root, nerve trunk, and central nervous system. "Pins and needles" in the feet are an early symptom of pressure on the spinal cord, and may be experienced before the plantar response becomes extensor (Babinski sign, see examination chapter 4). Tingling and numbness also can be caused by circulatory disturbances and diabetic neuropathy. In circulatory disturbances the limb often changes color. The proper differential diagnosis lies in understanding segmental references and performing a good patient history and examination.

Peripheral nerve lesions affect the integument supplied by that nerve—such as meralgia paresthetica a lesion of the lateral cutaneous nerve—which affects only the skin directly innervated by it.

Pain from a ligamentous source is frequently described as a vague numbness (nulliness), which in contrast to neurological tingling is alleviated by stroking of the structure. Stroking often aggravates neurological pain.

Central nervous system pain (upper motor neuron) is characterized by spontaneous burning or aching pain, hyperalgesia (excessive sensitivity to pain), dysesthesia (pins, needles, numbness, burning) and other abnormal sensations.

**TWINGES AND GIVING-WAY**. Twinges and giving-way often suggests instability, joint block (internal derangement), or tendinitis. Internal derangement of joints is suspected when there are symptoms of locking and sudden twinges, and a history of recurrence. When internal derangement affects a facet or intervertebral disc (IDD) the joint most frequently locks in flexion. This typical antalgic posture can also be due to spasm of the psoas and the deep aspect of the quadratus lumborum, FRS spinal and backward torsions of SI joint.

**PAINFUL TWINGES OCCUR IN FOUR DISORDERS:**

**1.** Loose body in the joint space.

**2.** Tendinitis, which frequently follows overuse.

— Often the patient describes a painful transitory loss of strength which may be due to mechanical stress on the lesion or due to adhesions.

**3.** Neurological origin, such as post-herpetic neuralgia and Morton's neuroma.

**4.** Joint instability.

— Often a momentary loss of strength accompanies the pain (Cyriax *ibid*).

**HISTORY, TRAVEL, DIET, SWELLING, PAIN AND PERSPIRATION**. A *history of heart* disease can suggest rheumatic disease. *Constitutional symptoms* such as weakness, fatigue, loss of weight and perspiring can be due to serious conditions.

*Perspiration* may suggest sympathetic nervous system involvement, pain or serious condition such as heart disease and lymphomas.[4]

*Rich diets* may cause gout and obesity which can result in musculoskeletal complaints.

*Recent travel* may suggest infections. Painful conditions of *ambiguous origin,* or of short duration, suggest a possible internal medical condition, but also common in orthopedic conditions.

The presence of *swelling* is indicative of an inflammatory process which can be from an autoimmune disorder.

The presence of a *rhythmic increase of abdominal pain* unrelated to movement, or severe pain felt ventrally, should raise suspicion of an internal medical disorder, especially when the abdominal pain is located at the same level as the back pain. When concomitant abdominal pain is at a level lower than the back pain, an orthopedic origin is more likely (Mennell 1964). Abdominal pain may be referred from the spine, thorax, pelvic organs and genitalia. Abdominal pain can be caused by both exogenous, endogenous and metabolic conditions, or by neurogenic disorders.[5]

---

4. Excessive perspiration or night sweat is often the first symptom in many serious medical condition especially lymphomas.

*Kidney, bladder, prostate and intestinal diseases* often cause low back pain. *Pelvic* and *rectal diseases* often give rise to sacral pain. Disorders of the *gallbladder, liver, heart, lung, pancreas, stomach, and ectopic pregnancy* often produce back and shoulder pain. Disorders of the *esophagus and heart* can refer pain to the neck, jaw, arm or back.

The use of the acronym CAUTION may be used to remind the practitioner of the symptoms and signs to look for when considering cancer:

**C**hanges in bowel and/or bladder habits.

**A** sore that does not heal.

**U**nusual bleeding or discharge.

**T**hickening or lumps in the breast or elsewhere.

**I**ndigestion or difficulty swallowing.

**O**bvious changes in a wart or a mole.

**N**agging cough or hoarseness.

MEDICAL CONDITIONS TO KEEP IN MIND. Neurofibromatosis (von Recklinghausen's disease), Schwannoma and other benign and malignant tumors, metabolic destructive lesions, vascular disorders, organic diseases, infections, depression and anxiety disorders should always be kept in mind.

In summary a comprehensive history is imperative in the diagnosis of musculoskeletal conditions and can both aid in the diagnosis as well as avoid catastrophic mistakes.

Table 4-12 on page 630 (appendix B) lists timing considerations for some symptoms and signs.

---

5.  For more details see Marcus A. *Acute Abdominal Syndromes Their Diagnosis & Treatment According to Combined Chinese-Western Medicine*, Blue Poppy Press, 1991.

# Examination

An understanding of several examination approaches can be helpful for making an accurate diagnosis. For example, when evaluating soft tissue lesions, the selective tension approach is most useful for identifying the anatomical source of pain (medical lesion or location of largest nociceptive output). Other examination techniques focus more on function. Evocation and interpretation of physical signs, an art that requires a considerable amount of practice, is best learned by apprenticeship. This section includes several examination methods.

One sequence used for a standard orthopedic examination is:

1. Vital signs.

2. Observation.

3. Palpation.

4. Percussion.

5. Auscultation.

6. Range of Motion/Movement Testing.

7. Orthopedic Testing.

8. Neurological Testing.

9. Examination of Related Areas.

10. Laboratory and Radiological Testing.

In this text, range of motion/movement testing is included in orthopedic testing. In Orthopaedic Medicine, palpation is done last, except for heat and swelling.

In this segment on examination, the term:

• *Motion* is used to describe manual medicine concepts of joint play and joint barriers.

• *Movement* is used to describe active movement.

• ROM can refer to either motion or movement, depending on the context.

# Vital Signs

The practitioner measures the patient's blood pressure, respiration, pulse, temperature, and weight.

# Observation

The observation process is predominately visual. Interpretive vocabulary is critical to the process, as well. To recognize whether a presentation is normal or abnormal, the practitioner must have a sufficient observational vocabulary. Visual observation is used to assess the patient gait and posture. To look for asymmetry, joint swelling and other deformities, and lastly, the patient reaction to questions and palpation is closely observed.

The theoretical central line of gravity (Figure 4-1) has been described as a plum line which passes from the mastoid process, just in front of the shoulder joint to a point in front of the knee, and on to a point in front of the ankle joint. Deviation from this plum line often is significant when making mechanical assessments even though minor postural deviation and minor leg length discrepancies do not seem to have any predictive benefit for neck and low back pain (Andersson 1991; Pope et al. 1985 and Dieck et al. 1985). In a failed back population however, Greenman (1992) did find a higher percent patients with leg length differences.

Direct and indirect vision serve as tools for different types of observation.

• Peripheral vision is best for assessing *movement*.

   For example, to compare general gait or bilateral movements of the respiratory rib cage, the practitioner gazes at the center of the patient's body and uses peripheral vision to assess symmetry.

• Central vision is effective for evaluating small vertical or horizontal planes (the

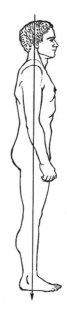

*Figure 4- 1:* Optimal posture.

practitioner's dominant eye is at a right angle to the plane being observed).

TO DETERMINE EYE DOMINANCE, THE PRACTITIONER:

**1.** (With arm extended) points across the room at an object such as a light switch.

**2.** Closes one eye.

   If the practitioner's finger still points at the object, that is the dominant eye.

Sometimes one eye is dominant for near vision and the other is dominant for far vision. Some individuals have eyes that are equally influential.

# Palpation

To assess by palpation, the practitioner must have:

• Good three-dimensional perception of anatomy.

• Knowledge of physiology.

- Ability to read the patient's expressions.
- Sensitive fingers.

When palpating, the practitioner checks mainly for:

- Asymmetry.
- Tissue texture abnormality.
- Temperature.
- Pain.

Palpatory vocabulary is essential for recognizing normal and abnormal findings. The most common mistake when palpating is applying excessive pressure. This leads to guarding, elicits tenderness in normal tissues, and distorts the practitioner's perception. Pressure must remain within normal physiological range for the tissue being assessed. Too much pressure results in a false interpretation.

## Palpating for Temperature & Swelling

Before beginning dynamic assessments, the practitioner uses the dorsum of the hand to detect variations in the patient's skin temperature.

## Palpating for Movement

When palpating for movement between adjacent bones, touching both bones simultaneously with one finger facilitates feeling the movement. When palpating bony structures, especially when trying to follow them during movement, the more sensitive technique is for the bone to come to the palpating finger (rather than the practitioner holding the bone to be palpated too firmly, when possible).

### Progression of Palpation

Palpation should progress layer-by-layer, "taking up slack" of each layer while proceeding inward, in this order:

1. About 2 cm above the skin, to sense the body's temperature radiation (*OM: Defensive Qi*).

2. Superficial tissues (skin), for thickness, moisture, ease of displacement (turgor) and tenderness.

3. Subcutaneous fasciae.

4. Intramuscular fasciae.

5. Muscular and tendinous tissues.

6. Joint capsules.

7. (When possible) bones.

(In Orthopaedic Medicine, the practitioner palpates first for temperature and swelling, identifies a possible lesion through selective tension and motion evaluations, and then palpates for tenderness all tissues that affect the region.)

## Palpation: Findings

A skilled practitioner can obtain a wealth of information from palpation. Tissue texture alteration, a semi-objective finding, is more important than pain and tenderness, subjective findings that can easily be misleading.

### Skin & Subcutaneous Mobility

Skin mobility should be part of any examination. Skin mobility, which can be evaluated by rolling a skin fold or stretching the skin, is performed along the entire length of the spine (*OM: along the UB and GV channels*), (Figure 4-2).

Frequently the skin roll points to dysfunctions that underlie a positive finding. Various authors have shown skin fold tenderness to corollate with musculoskeletal dysfunction and pathology (Baker 1951; Campbell 1983; Hirschberg Lynn and Ramsey 1994).

Signs often include changes in thickness of skin and subcutaneous tissues, with accompanying tenderness. Positive findings are common above a joint or dys-

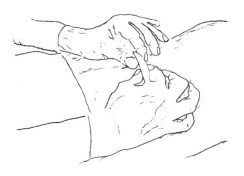

*Figure 4- 2:* Skin roll.

such as in skin mobility, moisture, appearance of skin pores, and hair loss might be present and may be segmental (dermatomally) in presentation. These changes can point to segmental dysfunctions, a "facilitated segment"[6] or a sympathetic system involvement.[7]

A light and quick touch over the skin often reveals increased friction at the level of the lesion (application of alcohol to the skin can dramatize this finding). In the spine, this process can be used to identify joint dysfunctions and the neurologic level (*OM: channels and Organs*) involved.

functional motion segment (adjacent vertebrae.) Unilateral findings are seen with vertebral (somatic) dysfunction. Bilateral and extensive findings can suggest a serious condition.

The skin roll is both diagnostic and therapeutic. To perform skin rolling, the practitioner grasps a skin fold between the thumb and index fingers and rolls the skin superiorly:

- Toward the neck.
- Over the center of the spine.
- At the sides of the vertebrae.

### Skin Overlying Active Lesions

Skin that overlies inflamed structures can be hypomobile and moist, and it may feel warm (*OM: Wet Heat disorders*). If the patient has a chronic disorder, trophic changes

### Asymmetries

Asymmetries may be seen, either during movement or with the patient still. They can point to:

- Congenital abnormalities (e.g., short leg).
- Compensatory changes (e.g., secondary rotoscoliosis due to sacral subluxation).
- Degenerative changes (e.g., facet degeneration).
- Functional disorders (e.g., facet locking and muscle spasm).

6.  "Facilitated segment" is a vicious cycle pain due to somatic/vertebral dysfunction (see chapter 2).

7.  Skin alterations in chronic patient often reflects OM Blood and Lung conditions. The distribution of the alteration points to the channel or Organ involved.

*Table 4-1.* **PALPATION OF CONTRACTILE TISSUES**

| LOCATION/TYPE OF TISSUE | TECHNIQUE/CONSIDERATION |
|---|---|
| TENOPERIOSTEAL JUNCTIONS | Carefully. They can be a site of trouble. |
| MUSCLE BELLY | Perpendicular to the muscle fibers, stroking the fibers gently as if they were the strings of a musical instrument. |
| WHEN SEEKING DEEP-LYING MUSCLES | Slowly and progressively deeper keeping overlying muscles relaxed. Begin perpendicular stroking only after reaching desired depth. |
| TENDER TENDONS | Along the direction of their inserting fibers. Perpendicularly when defining their borders. |

Although normal body development is not completely symmetrical (even the two sides of the sacrum are almost never symmetrical) the relationships among symptoms, function and symmetry become significant clinically, and are important for successful manipulation and some acupuncture techniques.

When the position of a joint is faulty, some ligaments are stretched permanently and some are shortened. Because ligaments are not designed to tolerate continuous stretching and are subject to hysteresis, they can elongate, weaken and become sensitive. If a joint is hypermobile, the ligaments may be palpably thin and long. In hypomobile joints, the ligaments may feel thick and short.

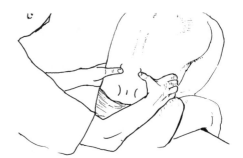

*Figure 4- 3:* Assessment of transverse processes forward translation when the spine is flexed.

### Excessive Warmth/Heat

Excessive warmth or heat means that an acute condition (acute inflammatory process) is active, or that a chronic condition is in an active flare-up (such as rheumatoid arthritis or subacute lumbago). Heat is palpable in the initial stages of torn tissue, e.g., superficial sprains and strains, hemarthrosis (blood in the joint) and broken bones (as long as they are superficial enough). In the initial stages of torn tissues, rest does not affect the resulting heat. With hemarthrosis the heat remains constant, and movement is extremely limited. If adhesions and/or loose bodies lie in an obstructive position, palpable heat follows exertion and abates quickly with rest (Cyriax *ibid*). Malignant tumors that are superficial may also produce local warmth.

### Excessive Cold

Cold skin may occur in an area affected by a nerve root palsy (*OM: blockage, Cold, deficiency or severing of channel and collaterals*). This is also true in conditions that affect vascular functions, such as reflex sympathetic dystrophy (RSD), intermittent claudication, facilitated segment and other conditions in which increased sympathetic tone

accompanies the disorder (such as chronic pain, anxiety). A cold foot that occurs only after exertion may suggest an iliac thrombosis. Heat or coldness of tissues, or subjective sensing of either, is an important aspect in selecting the appropriate OM herbal formula.

### Restrictions of Tissues or Movements

The practitioner can detect restrictions of tissues or movements by palpating structures during their arc of motion. By understanding vertebral motions and by following a pair of transverse processes, the practitioner may identify restrictions and design manipulations for restoring normal function (Figure 4-3).

### Palpation of Contractile Tissues

Following examination of the superficial integument, the practitioner palpates deeper fascia and muscles, looking for severed tissues, fibrotic changes (found in chronic conditions), taut muscular bands and trigger points. The practitioner palpates as indicated in Table 4-1 on page 174.

To determine whether tenderness lies in a superficial or deep structure, the practitioner can palpate the area during contraction and relaxation of the superficial muscle. Pain that is more pronounced when the muscles are tense suggests that the superficial muscle is at fault (*OM: Sinew channel*).

## TO DEMONSTRATE MUSCLE "SPASMS", THE PRACTITIONER FINDS:

- Indurated tissue that lies parallel to the uninvolved fibers.
- Thickening of spindle-shaped tissue.
- Pressure-evoked muscle twitch.
- Bundles that can be moved at right angles to the muscle fibers (Figure 4-4).

Objective tissue changes are more significant than elicitation of pain. The practitioner must establish the *source* of pain, because referred tenderness is a common phenomenon.

**PERIPHERAL PULSES.** The practitioner should also palpate peripheral pulses, because arterial pathology is a common cause of pain. (*OM: The pulses around Liv-3, St-43, K- 3, H-7, LU-9 and St-9 are assessed for their associated channels*).

## Percussion

Percussion of the abdomen and lungs is part of a general physical examination. Percussion of bone is part of the orthopedic examination. Findings of severe bone pain upon direct percussion suggests a fracture and/or cancer. Percussion of the spinous processes may help identify a facilitated segment (the muscles adjacent to the active segment become active when

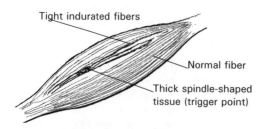

Tight indurated fibers

Normal fiber

Thick spindle-shaped tissue (trigger point)

*Figure 4- 4: "Muscle spasm" and trigger point.*

the spinous process is percussed).

## Auscultation

Auscultation of bowel and breath sounds is part of a general physical examination. Auscultation for a bruit in the arteries is important in musculoskeletal medicine, because arterial disease can be the cause of muscular like pain.

## Orthopedic Testing: Joints

To use the examination this text describes, the practitioner must understand the *joint barrier, joint play* and *end feel* aspects of joint assessment:

### Joint Barriers

Joint barriers are physiologic and anatomic barriers that the practitioner can see or sense. Joint barriers are described as:

- Anatomical (Total Range of Movement).
  - The extent of movement possible at a joint, from one anatomical barrier to the other, without injuring the joint. Movement beyond the anatomical barrier always results in injury.
- Physiologic.
  - The extent of active movement available in the joint (done by the patient).
- Elastic.
  - The next-level range of movement, available only by passive assessment (done by the practitioner). Thrust manipulations are active within the elastic barrier, in this "potential space."
  (*In OM the potential space at the elastic barrier is an areas where Qi force can be stored. Martial artists learn to control the opening and*

*closing [pumping] of these spaces to both cultivate and release energy).*

• Restrictive.

— A pathological barrier that interferes with the normal physiologic barrier. Usually this is found in one or more directions.

Techniques are designed to correct pathological barriers by moving the joint:

• Through the restrictive barrier (are called direct techniques).

• Away from the restrictive barrier (are called indirect techniques).

### Direction of Bind

The more the joint is moved from midline neutral toward the elastic barrier, the more tissue resistance (bind) the practitioner can feel. This resistance, called direction of bind, is due to soft tissue stretching.

### Direction of Ease

The farther from the elastic barrier toward the midline neutral (loose-packed position), the easier the movement becomes, or the less resistance felt. This concept is called direction of ease.

### Midline Neutral

Midline neutral is not necessarily located in the middle of the available active or passive range. Midline neutral is somewhere within the total range of movement or motion and can shift with dysfunction or pathology. Midline neutral can be different in different joints. Joint play is best appreciated at the midline neutral (loose-packed) position.

### Dysfunction

Dysfunction usually includes a mixture of some restricted movements and some full movements. The area of motion loss, as

defined by the restrictive barrier, becomes the new physiological barrier.

## Joint Play

Mennell describes joint play as a motion within a synovial joint, in which the motion is separate from, and cannot be initiated by, voluntary muscle contraction. Joint play consists of fine movement (less than 1/8-inch) in any plane the natural laxity of the joint capsule allows. The play available at each joint is the sum of all passive angular and translatory movements (such as x-y-z planes).

The range of joint play is the same for any given joint of the same kind (such as the shoulder, the wrist) with that type's characteristic end feel. Loss of joint play impairs function and is associated with pain.

Restoration of joint play is considered crucial for normal joint function. Familiarity with joint play is essential for the understanding of manual therapy techniques. Proper manipulation therapy is effective for restoring normal movement.

### Assessing Joint Play

Mennell has proposed nine rules for assessing joint play. The practitioner:

1. Must see that the patient is relaxed. To avoid painful movement, the patient's joint must be supported and protected.

2. Must be relaxed. The practitioner's grip must be comfortable for the patient.

3. Must isolate and examine one joint at a time (when possible).

4. Tests one movement at a time.

5. Holds one aspect of the joint stable while mobilizing the other.

6. Usually can ascertain the extent of normal joint play by examining the unaffected side.

**7.** Must stop the movement at any point that pain is elicited.

**8.** Must never use forced or abnormal movement.

**9.** (If the patient presents with obvious inflammation or disease) does not perform an examination of movement.

## End Feel

End feel is the characteristic sensation the practitioner perceives at the end of the patient's passive ROM. The best technique for establishing the cause of restriction is assessing the end feel; the results may even suggest a diagnosis. Several pathological conditions give rise to different end feels (Table 4-2 on page 179).

### Rubbery, Leathery

The normal end feel of the joint capsule when stretched is rubbery or leathery. In this state the sensation is like stretching a thick rubber band. This end feel can be found in non-acute arthritis or arthrosis (in the absence of significant muscle spasm and where the anatomical barrier is not engaged). *(OM: Normal end feel suggests that the Liver, Blood and Kidneys are essentially healthy)*.

### Boggy, Spongy

Boggy or spongy end feel occurs in the presence of edema. It also occurs in some early joint effusions in which movement of the joint comes to an abrupt stop but resistance fades slightly with sustained pressure. *(OM: This end feel suggests a diagnosis of Damp Heat and/or Phlegm)*.

### Hard

This end feel occurs when bone-to-bone contact causes the restrictive block or when adhesions cause the restriction. It can also occur when strong muscle spasms restrict movement at the joint. A hard end feel can be normal for some joints, such as elbow extension in which strong ligaments suddenly limit the range of motion in that vector. Muscle spasm, in severe active lesions such as inflammatory arthritis or fractures, can also give rise to a hard end feel. (The restriction may be in the capsular pattern). *(OM: A hard end feel suggests Sinew channel, Kidney, Essence, bone, and/or Blood stagnation and deficient disorders or congealed Phlegm and Blood)*.

### Abrupt, Hard Stop

This is a hard end feel which occurs rather abruptly following a smooth, frictionless movement, with some loss of end feel resiliency (normal rubbery sensation), and is associated concomitantly with increased range of motion. This end feel is seen often when the joint is hypermobile. (OM: Abrupt/hard stop suggest Spleen/pancreas, Divergent or Extra channels and/or Kidney, Essence and bone disorders).

### Springy Rebound

A springy end feel is found in the presence of internal derangement or a loose body in a joint. The sensation is as though something is pulling back at the end of the range of motion. Springy end feel is also encountered when a spinal joint is localized correctly before manipulation; however, in this situation the end feel is typically less springy than is felt with a loose body. *(OM: Springy rebound suggest Phlegm, Wet Heat, or "stone" [congealed Phlegm and Blood)*.

### Empty, Soft

An empty soft end feel occurs when the patient halts the movement because of severe pain before normal tissue resistance occurs (indicating that the physiologic or elastic barrier has not been reached). An empty soft end feel can be an indicator of

*Table 4-2.* **END FEEL**

| SENSATION | INDICATION | OM INDICATION |
|---|---|---|
| BOGGY, SPONGY | Edema<br>Early joint effusions | Wet Heat and/or Phlegm |
| HARD | Bone-to-bone contact causing a restrictive block<br>Adhesions<br>Strong muscle spasms<br>Capsular pattern<br>Can be seen in hypermobile joints | Spleen/pancreas<br>Divergent or Extra channels<br>and/or Kidney/bone disorder |
| RUBBERY OR LEATHERY | Normal examination of joint capsule when stretched<br>Non-acute arthritis or arthrosis | Liver, Blood and Kidneys are healthy |
| SPRINGY REBOUND | Internal derangement<br>Loose body | Phlegm<br>Wet Heat<br>or "Stone" (congealed Phlegm and Blood) |
| EMPTY, SOFT | Acute or serious diseases<br>Psychosomatic causes | Wet Heat abscess<br>Latent Heat and or Toxin<br>Trauma |

acute or serious diseases that must be ruled out, such as an extra-articular abscess, acute bursitis or cancer. Psychosomatic causes should be considered, as well. *(OM: Empty/soft end feel suggests Wet Heat abscess, Latent Heat and/or Toxin, and trauma).*

## Selective Tension

Selective tension the heart of the Cyriax approach to Orthopaedic Medicine, is a process by which the practitioner isolates and tests tissues for pathology. This method is very helpful for identifying lesions in the extremities. Table 4-3 on page 180 summarizes the four aspects of a selective tension examination.

During the examination both active (patient initiated) and passive (practitioner initiated) motion/movements can be painful. Since the active assessment stresses both contractile and inert structures, and the passive assessment stresses mostly inert structures, the significance of these examinations does not come to light until after the resisted movement tests are performed.

### Active Movement

The end points of active movements are due to the "physiological barrier." Active movements indicate:

- Ability and willingness of the patient to perform the movement.
- Range of movement possible.
- Degree of muscular strength.
- Direction of painful movements.
- *(Function of Sinews channels, Spleen/pancreas and/or Liver condition).*

The practitioner uses active movement to observe the ergonomics of function and the presence of functional substitution and compensations. This kind of assessment serves as a screening tool that may indicate the area of dysfunction quickly. The practitioner compares the results with the results of the passive motion and resisted movement examinations.

### Passive Motion

Evaluation of passive range of motion tests elastic and anatomical barriers (end feel) and the state of the **inert tissues** of a joint The:

- Capsule and ligaments.

- Bursae.

- Fasciae.

- Bony aspects of a joint.

- Nerve roots.

- Dura.

Passive testing can provide useful information about individual joints, and it may indicate the nature and stage of pathology (such as acuteness, inflammatory nature, restriction and/or elasticity).

When evaluating the passive ROM and end feel, the sequence in which the pain and limitations occur should be noted. Every joint has a unique end feel, e.g.:

- Elbow extension is limited by strong ligament tension that feels like bone-to-bone contact at full extension, which yields a hard end feel.

- Elbow (full) flexion is limited by soft tissue approximation (the biceps muscles), which yields a soft end feel.

*(Passive testing also provides information on OM's: Divergent and Extra channels, Pathological factors, Kidney, Essence, and/or Liver condition.)*

### Assessment of Passive Motions

For passive motion assessment, the patient must be relaxed. This state eliminates conscious control and muscular effort by the patient and makes it possible for the practitioner to evaluate the end feel at the joint.

- The practitioner mobilizes the joint through all vectors of movement, paying special attention to end feel and noting abnormalities. For each joint, the practitioner must be familiar with the normal degrees of movement. Comparison with a similar but unaffected joint is useful for identifying variations specific to the patient. At times, to assess a painful arc, the practitioner must complete passive motions even though the patient feels pain and/or resists.

*Table 4-3.* **EVALUATION USING SELECTIVE TENSION**

| MOTION TESTED | TARGET |
|---|---|
| **ACTIVE RANGE OF MOVEMENT AND ASSOCIATED SENSATIONS** | Ability / willingness of patient<br>Degree of muscular strength<br>Direction of painful movements |
| **RESISTED MOVEMENTS (ISOMETRIC CONTRACTIONS)** | Evaluation of contractile units |
| **PAINFUL ARC** | Seen in pinchable lesions |
| **PASSIVE RANGE AND SENSATIONS** | Evaluation of elastic and anatomical barriers<br>State of inert tissues |

*Table 4-4.* PASSIVE TESTING

| SYMPTOM/SIGN | INDICATION |
| --- | --- |
| **PAIN AT EXTREME RANGE** | |
| | Often caused by stretching of affected tissues. Also can be caused by the squeezing of tissues, such as the bursa between two surfaces (e.g., subdeltoid bursa by the acromion and humerus, the achilles between the tibia and calcaneus on full passive plantar flexion). |
| | Tendinitis |
| | • Usually the patient has full passive range of motion unless: |
| | — the inflammation has started spreading to the capsule |
| | — or |
| | — pain restricts movement |
| | Found commonly in joints in which the tendon contributes to formation of the capsule (such as the shoulder) or where stretching of the lesion is painful, as in some muscular and musculotendinous lesions. |
| **SUDDEN HALT** | |
| **SHORT OF FULL RANGE** | Most likely caused by a bony block and/or adhesion of soft tissues. Bony end feel is found in the presence of arthrosis and in joints that have bone spurs. |
| **FULL PASSIVE RANGE** | |
| **WITHOUT ACTIVE MOVEMENT** | Full passive range of motion with inability to perform one or more movements actively suggests loss of muscle function due to either mechanical or neurological causes. |
| **HYPERMOBILITY** | |
| Evidenced as excessive range of motion | Can occur: |
| | • following injury, especially in joints not under muscular control, such as acromioclavicular, sternoclavicular, sacroiliac, sacrococcygeal, symphysis pubis and knee |
| | • if ligaments around a joint are loose due to degeneration |
| | • if joint space is decreased, such as with loss of disc height |
| | • in presence of several connective tissue disorders, such as: |
| | — Marfan's syndrome (patient taller than average with arm span greater than height) |
| | — Ehlers-Danlos syndrome (skin excessively pliable) |
| | Asymptomatic hypermobility can be a normal variant. |
| **IMMOBILE JOINT** | |
| | May be secondary to severe muscle spasm, septic arthritis, or fibrous or bony ankylosis. |

*Types of Limitations*

During passive assessment, limitations of movement and motion can be in the capsular pattern or the noncapsular pattern.

- A *capsular pattern* is found in conditions that affect the entire joint, such as arthritis or capsular irritation.

- A *noncapsular pattern,* also called a partial articular pattern, is found with ligamentous adhesions, internal derangements, vertebral dysfunctions and extra-articular lesions.

Table 4-4 on page 181 summarizes the indications suggested by some symptoms and signs found in passive testing.

## Contractile Unit Testing

Testing of a contractile unit (a muscle and its attachment) requires isolation of the muscle. Therefore, the practitioner who is assessing muscle strength must have an understanding of muscle function.

Testing of individual muscles is useful for evaluating peripheral nerves, spinal nerves, and contractile unit functions and their disorders. Resisted movements (isometric muscle contractions), which help the practitioner assess the contractile unit, may provoke pain and/or demonstrate weakness.

To prevent movement during isometric (resisted muscle) testing, the test is performed with the joint in mid-range and stabilized. This stabilization is achieved by positioning the joint during the examination by the practitioner.[8]

Testing can involve:

- Isometric contraction with resisted muscle testing (resistance against a movement performed by the practitioner).

- Isotonic/active motion performed against resistance, gravity, or modified gravity.

A measure of muscle strength should be charted periodically. Several grading scales are available for documenting muscle strength. Table 3-5 provides a simple grading scale for active movements. Table 4-6 on page 184 summarizes findings of contractile unit tests.

---

8.  A minimal amount of movement is inevitable.

*Table 4-5.* **CONTRACTILE UNIT TESTING**

| LETTER | GRADE  | INDICATES |
|--------|--------|-----------|
| N      | Normal | A complete range of movement against maximal resistance |
| G      | Good   | Complete ROM against moderated resistance |
| F      | Fair   | Complete ROM against gravity |
| P      | Poor   | Complete ROM with gravity eliminated |
| T      | Trace  | Evidence of some muscle contractility but no joint motion |
| 0      | Zero   | No palpable contraction |

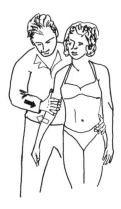

*Figure 4- 5:* Resisted muscle testing, shoulder abduction.

### Resisted Movement Testing

When testing isometric contraction (resisted movement), (Figure 4-5), the practitioner encourages the patient to pull or push with maximal effort while the practitioner applies enough counterforce to prevent motion. Although the practitioner cannot eliminate movement of the joint completely, this kind of motion should be kept to a minimum. Some inert tissues are stimulated by the resisted motion and minor shear movements may occur (thereby stimulating noncontractile tissues), but such instances usually are minimal.

To obtain useful information, the practitioner must isolate the muscle that is to be tested. If several resisted motions are painful, or if incompatible movements hurt, the pain is unlikely to be of contractile structure origin.

In the presence of arthritis and conditions that affect inert structures, resisted movements generally are painless. However, the resisted movements can be painful if a lesion lies directly under or near the muscle, and, during muscle contraction, the muscle contraction or broadening stimulates that lesion. The lesions affected most commonly from this kind of second-ary stimulation are bursae, abscesses and inflamed lymphatic glands.

Sometimes during an examination, even though resisted motions are painless, discomfort occurs when the patient relaxes the muscle tension. This can occur if the tested muscle has lesions or if a joint is unstable, such as a shoulder that has an unstable acromioclavicular or gleno-humeral joint. When a joint is unstable, pain may be felt when the patient "lets go" and presents with any of several types of muscle contractions.

When testing resisted movements, the practitioner makes note of abnormal sensations, both when the muscle is contracted and when the muscle is relaxed. The practitioner may need to repeat resisted movement tests several times in order to elicit pain from a minor lesion, especially in stronger patients. To facilitate the eliciting of pain, the practitioner can place the muscle in a position that is mechanically disadvantaged, with the joint at other than mid-range. This may help demonstrate minor lesions that are not detected using regular examination techniques.

## Common Patterns of Passive & Resisted Movements

Passive and resisted examinations are highly effective for determining the source of musculoskeletal pathology, which often presents in common patterns.

### Capsular Pattern

The capsular pattern (Cyriax *ibid*) is a specific standard, (for each joint e.g. shoulders), of range of motion restrictions seen when the joint is pathological. The capsular pattern is a limitation (to a relative degree) of specific movements in specific directions when a joint has arthritis or the entire capsule is inflamed.

In the presence of a capsular pattern:

• Some movement will have some degree of limitation.

*Table 4-6.* **CONTRACTILE UNIT TESTING: FINDINGS** (Cyriax *ibid*)

| A FINDING THAT IS | SUGGESTS |
| --- | --- |
| STRONG AND PAINFUL | Minor contractile lesion |
| WEAK AND PAINLESS | Complete rupture of muscle or tendon (more often a nervous system disorder) |
| WEAK AND PAINFUL | Possible major disorder, sepsis, cancer, fracture |
| PAIN ON ALL RESISTED MOTIONS | Underlying general sensitivity, a mental state, or a severe condition |
| PAIN FOLLOWING SUSTAINED OR REPETITIVE CONTRACTIONS | Intermittent claudication, tendinitis (seen in strong patients) |
| PAINLESS | Arthritis, conditions affecting inert structures |

- All movements may be limited, but to different degrees.
- Arthritis or capsulitis of each joint has its own pattern of limitation.

When active and passive movements elicit pain in the same direction, and if the discomfort emerges near or at the limit of range, and if resisted movements are painless, the lesion is likely to be of an inert structure. This pattern occurs with arthritis, capsulitis, bursitis and instability. The entire joint is affected only if the limitations are in the specific capsular pattern for that joint. Bursitis does not cause a capsular pattern.

In the initial stages of arthritis, a patient might not present with the entire capsular pattern. In such a case the movement may be limited in only one predictable direction (such as lateral rotation in the shoulder).

In lesions of recent onset, muscle spasm usually is responsible for a limited ROM, whereas more established lesions cause restriction through contraction of the joint capsule, as well. When secondary adhesions form, the limitation may change and become a noncapsular pattern (Cyriax *ibid*).

### Noncapsular Pattern

When a patient presents with limitation of movement that is not in a capsular pattern (i.e., there is only a partial articular pattern), the responsible lesion does not involve the whole joint. These conditions may be due to internal derangement, vertebral dysfunctions, ligamentous adhesions and dysfunctions, or extra-articular lesions. In the presence of ligamentous adhesions and extra-articular lesions, the patient feels pain when the adhesion or lesion is stretched. Therefore, some movements can be painful while others are not (Cyriax *ibid*).

### Internal Derangement

Internal derangement is found when a loose fragment blocks some aspect of the joint. The onset is often sudden and may give rise to pain and limitation of movement in the direction that engages the block. Typically only one direction of movement is limited and painful. The restriction may be disproportionate in one direction. This occurs commonly when a partially-torn anterior horn of the meniscus blocks the knee joint, blocking extension markedly but with little flexion restriction.

The joints that are prone to developing a loose body are the vertebral facet, the knee, jaw, and spinal vertebral column. Joints that develop a loose body less frequently are the hip, elbow and tarsal joints (Cyriax *ibid*).

## Extra-Articular Lesions

Extra-articular lesions are suspected when only one direction of movement is grossly limited but all other movements are full and painless. This state can be found in the presence of bursitis, partly torn muscles or other contractile lesions, and in situations in which a particular movement stimulates a cyst or other lesion (Cyriax *ibid*).

## Painful Arc

Painful arc refers to pain that the patient feels during part of the active or passive movement, but that abates as the movement continues; or that the patient feels only during part of the arc of motion. A painful arc implies the presence of a compressible lesion (Cyriax *ibid*).

# Neurological Testing

Reflexes are inborn stimulus-response mechanisms that can be classified according to the level of their representation in the central nervous system.

The clinically important reflexes are:

- Superficial (skin and mucous membrane).
- Deep (myotonic).
- Visceral (organic).
- Pathological (abnormal).

The essential neural portion of a reflex includes a sensory neuron and a motor neuron (other structures are involved, as well). In orthopedics, the superficial, deep, and/or pathological reflexes provide an indication of the state of the nerves and of the nerve roots that supply the reflex. The reflexes also provide information on the status of the upper motor neuron system.[9]

Table 4-7 on page 186 summarizes the reflexes.

## Deep Reflexes

The deep reflexes, also called the deep tendon reflexes, are the most commonly assessed reflexes in western musculoskeletal medicine.

With practice, the practitioner can elicit deep tendon reflexes (jerks) from almost any tendon. Table 4-8 on page 187 lists the most common tendon reflexes

## Superficial Reflexes

Table 4-9 on page 188 describes the superficial reflexes, subdivided here as mucous membrane reflexes (which are not highly relevant in orthopedics) and skin reflexes (which may be considered in orthopedics).

## Visceral Reflexes

The visceral reflexes are considered only occasionally in the musculoskeletal patient (generally after trauma). Table 4-10 on page 189 lists the visceral reflexes.

## Pathological Reflexes

Medical science has identified numerous pathological reflexes such as Babinski (Figure 4-6 on page 189), and Huntington's. A review of all of these reflexes is not within the scope of this text; however, several that are applicable clinically are mentioned in corresponding sections.

---

9.Neurons of the upper motor neuron system contribute to the formation of the pyramidal (corticospinal) and corticobulbar tracts, which may be affected by trauma and by vascular, neoplastic and other diseases. Lesions often result in hyperactive reflexes.

*Table 4-7.* **REFLEXES: SUMMARY** (Bates *ibid*)

---

### DESCRIPTION

Inborn stimulus-response mechanisms
Essential neural portion of a reflex includes both a sensory neuron and a motor neuron
Classified according to level of representation in central nervous system

### CLINICALLY IMPORTANT TYPES

Superficial (skin and mucous membrane)
Deep (myotonic) (in orthopedics, the most commonly-considered)
Visceral (organic)
Pathologic (abnormal)
In orthopedics, superficial, deep, and/or pathological reflexes are examined for:

- state of the nerves and roots that supply the reflex

- status of upper motor neuron system

### COMMON GRADING SYSTEM

0 Absent
1 Diminished
2 Average
3 Exaggerated
4 Clonus (causing repeated jerks)
Distinction is made as to whether reflexes are normal, weak (absent or diminished), or excessive (exaggerated or clonus)

**Diminished or Absent Reflexes**

- Diminished or absent reflexes can result from any lesion that interrupts the reflex arc or nerve root, or in the presence of peripheral nerve disease and cerebellar disease

**Excessive Reflexes**

- Excessive reflexes are seen when lesions of either the cortex or the pyramidal tract (descending cortical tract or upper motor neuron) result in decreased inhibition of normal reflexes

    **Warning.** Hyperactive reflexes can also be seen in the presence of strychnine poisoning and in some functional disorders. This must be remembered when prescribing Semen Strychnotis (Ma Qian Zi)

*Table 4-8.* **THE DEEP REFLEXES** (Bates *ibid*)

| REFLEX | DESCRIPTION | NERVE TESTED |
|---|---|---|
| MAXILLARY | Jaw reflex<br>A sudden closing of the jaw upon striking the middle of the chin when the mouth is slightly open | Cranial V |
| BICEPS | Flexion of the elbow when the biceps tendon is tapped | C5-6 |
| BRACHIORADIALIS | Flexion of the elbow and/or pronation of the forearm when the tendon or musculotendinous junction is tapped | C5-6 |
| TRICEPS | Extension of the elbow when the triceps tendon is tapped | C7-8 |
| PERIOSTEORADIAL | Flexion and supination of the forearm when the styloid process of the radius is tapped | C6-8 |
| PERIOSTEOULNAR | Extension and ulnar abduction of the wrist when the styloid process of the ulna is tapped | C6-8 |
| PATELLAR<br>(KNEE JERK) | Extension of the knee when the patellar tendon is tapped | L3-4<br>L 2-4 |
| HAMSTRINGS<br>SEMIMEMBRANOSUS,<br>BICEPS FEMORIS | Flexion of the knee when the hamstrings tendon is tapped | L5-S1<br><br>S1-2 |
| TIBIALIS<br>POSTERO-PLANTAR | Flexion and inversion of the foot when the tibialis posterior tendon behind the medial malleolus is tapped | L 4-5 |
| ACHILLES TENDON | Plantar flexion of the foot when the achilles tendon is tapped | S1-2 |

*Table 4-9.* **THE SUPERFICIAL REFLEXES** (Bates *ibid*)

| REFLEX | LEVEL TESTED | DESCRIPTION |
|---|---|---|
| Mucous Membrane Reflexes (Not commonly relevant in orthopedics) | | |
| Corneal | N5 | Conjunctival |
| Nasal | N1 | Smell |
| Pharyngeal | N9-10 | Gag |
| Uvular | N8 | Palatal |
| Skin Reflexes (Assessed occasionally in orthopedics) | | |
| Upper and Lower Abdominal | T8-12 | Tensing of muscles beneath the skin area. Stroking causes the umbilicus to move in the direction of the stimulated skin area. |
| Cremasteric | L1-2 | Elevation of the scrotum and testicle of the same side in response to stroking of the inner aspect of the thigh or the skin over Scapa's triangle. |
| Anal | L1-2 | Contraction of the sphincter ani in response to stroking of the perianal area, or upon inserting objects such as a gloved finger into the rectum. |
| Plantar | L4-S2 also upper motor | Plantar flexion of the toes upon stroking the lateral sole of the foot (known as Babinski sign.) |

*Table 4-10.* **THE VISCERAL REFLEXES** (Bates *ibid*)

| REFLEX | DESCRIPTION | NERVE TESTED |
|---|---|---|
| **OCULAR REFLEXES** | | |
| Light | Constriction of the pupil when light shines on the retina | Midbrain Cranial II, III |
| Accommodation | Group of three closely-associated reflexes that facilitate production of a sharp image on the corresponding points of the retina<br>When the eye looks at near-by objects, these reflexes are accompanied by constriction of the pupils | Central commissural connections that involve the occipital cortex and Cranial II, III |
| Ciliospinal | Dilation of the pupils when painful stimulation is applied to any sensory area, usually by pinching the neck | T1-2, Cervical sympathetic and sensory |
| Oculocardiac | Slowing of the heart rate produced by pressure over the eyeballs | Medulla, Cranial V and X |
| **OTHER VISCERAL REFLEXES** (PARTIAL LIST) | | |
| Carotid Sinus | Slowing of the heart and decrease in blood pressure (by vasodilation) due to pressure over the carotid sinus in the neck | Medulla, Cranial IX and X |
| Bulbocavernosus | Contraction of the bulbocavernosus muscles after:<br>• stroking the dorsum of the glans penis<br>• or<br>• pinching the skin of the penis | S2-4, pudendal, pelvic autonomic system |
| Bladder | Also called urinary reflex, vesicle reflex, micturation reflex<br>Contraction of the walls of the bladder and relaxation of the trigone and urethral sphincter in response to pressure within the bladder | pelvic autonomic system |
| Rectal | Impulse to defecate, caused by entrance of fecal matter into the rectum | pelvic autonomic system |

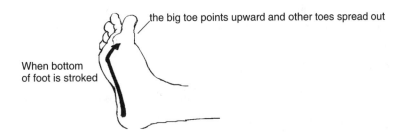

the big toe points upward and other toes spread out

When bottom of foot is stroked

*Figure 4- 6:* Positive Babinski sign.

# Screening Examination

The musculoskeletal screening has three objectives:

- Exclude a remote-area, orthopedic and neurological condition, that might be responsible for the presenting symptoms.

- Establish priorities.

- Find mechanical dysfunctions.

In general, screening examinations (general motion tests) are more sensitive for compensatory patterns than for detailed joint dysfunction. The practitioner must conduct further specific testing to identify joint dysfunctions. Since pain can result from abnormal adaptations and reaction to a primary dysfunction elsewhere, and since the primary dysfunction can be found anywhere, the screening examination helps the practitioner identify and be led to areas that require further investigation. Special attention is paid to the lower kinetic chain.

## Gait Analysis

The first step in the screen tests is a gait analysis (Figure 4-7). A patient's gait patterns can be very informative as to pathology in the lower extremities, the spine, and the central and peripheral nervous systems. Table 3-11 describes the most basic aspects of the gait examination.

*Table 4-11.* **GAIT ANALYSIS** (Hoppenfeld 1976)

| DEFINITION | | |
|---|---|---|
| | Sequence of motion that occurs between two consecutive heel strikes of the same leg.[a] | |
| **PHASE** | | |
| Stance | Heel strike | initial contact |
| | Flat foot | load response |
| | Single leg stance | mid-stance |
| | Heel-off | terminal stance |
| | Toe-off | pre-swing |
| Swing | Foot non-weightbearing and moving forward | |
| | Three segments: | |
| | • acceleration | in initial phase |
| | • mid-swing | legs parallel |
| | • terminal | during deceleration |
| | | (Swinging leg decelerates, allowing smooth landing of the foot) |
| Double-Leg | Parts of both feet in contact with ground. Occurs twice per gait cycle | |
| Single-Leg | Only one foot on the ground. Occurs twice per gait cycle | |

a. For a normal toe-off to occur, the patient must be able to flex the ankle, mid-foot and forefoot.

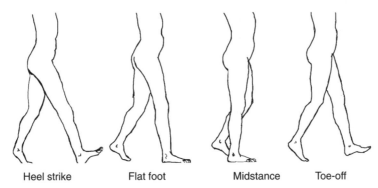

| Heel strike | Flat foot | Midstance | Toe-off |

*Figure 4-7:* Gait cycle.

The practitioner must pay particular attention to a few details concerning stance.

*Normal Gait*

Normal gait dimensions are:

- Distance between feet while standing is between 2-4 inches.

- Distance between feet while walking is between 2-4 inches.

- Stride length (length of one gait cycle) about 28-32 inches.

- Step (gait) length (equal on both sides) between 14-16 inches.

- Vertical pelvic shifts are symmetrical and approximately 2 inches.

- Lateral pelvic shifts are symmetrical and approximately 1 inch to the weight-bearing side.

- In the swing phase the pelvis rotates 40° forward. The opposite hip joint (which is in stance phase) acts as a fulcrum for this rotation.

Table 3-12 lists the locations the practitioner observes from front and back. Table 4-13 on page 192 lists the locations the practitioner observes from one side.

**WIDER-THAN-NORMAL STANCE.** A wider-than-normal stance may indicate a feeling of unsteadiness and poor balance, and could be due to brain and spinal cord lesions, peripheral neuropathy or inner ear disorders. Both stride and step length vary with the patient's age, size, fatigue, dysfunction and pathology.

**ABNORMAL GAIT.** Table 4-14 on page 193 describes five of the many abnormal gait patterns.

**GAIT OBSERVATION.** The practitioner begins the musculoskeletal screening by evaluating the patient's gait and other movements. Observation of gait from a distance, from where the pelvic, spinal and extremity movements can be seen more easily, can be helpful. Severity of pain can be detected readily by looking at the patient's movement pattern and amount of guarding. A patient who moves slowly and carefully is much more likely to have pain of severe musculoskeletal origin.

This examination is best performed from front, back and side, a combination that usually gives more succinct clues about the location of the dysfunction.

**MUSCULOSKELETAL SCREEN: GENERAL OBSERVATION.** Table 4-15 on page 193 through Table 4-17 on page 194 summarize general musculoskeletal observations.

*Table 4-12.* **GAIT OBSERVATION: FRONT AND BACK**

| LOCATION | OBSERVE FOR |
|---|---|
| Pelvic Area | Symmetry of laterality, height and rotation |
| Trunk | Swaying<br>Whether the upper trunk and extremities rotate to the opposite side of the pelvis and of the lower extremities |
| Lower Extremities | Bowing, varus or valgus |
| Feet | Base width, during gait and when still<br>Symmetry of stride, heel and toe strike, toe off |
| Ankle | Flexion<br>(The distal and proximal tibiofibular joints must function well for normal toe-off.) |
| Rearfoot<br>Midfoot<br>Forefoot | Whether the weight transfers from the heel to the lateral side of the foot and back across the metatarsal phalangeal joints to the great toe for push-off<br>Normal toe-off |
| Arms<br>Shoulder Girdle | Swing of the arms and behavior of the shoulder girdle |
| Patient's Footwear | Pattern of wear |

*Table 4-13.* **GAIT OBSERVATION: SIDE**

| LOCATION | OBSERVE FOR |
|---|---|
| Spine | Curves |
| General | Coordination of movements |
| Hip<br>Knee<br>Ankle<br>Mid-Foot<br>Fore-Foot | Ability to extend and flex |
| Gait | Gait length, Duration of gait cycle segments |

*Table 4-14.* **SOME ABNORMAL GAIT PATTERNS** (Hoppenfeld 1976; Mitchell 1995)

| PATTERN | DESCRIPTION | COMMENTS |
|---|---|---|
| **ANTALGIC** | The patient tries to avoid weightbearing or pressure on the affected site<br><br>A patient walking bare-foot on a rocky surface is a good example of an antalgic gait | • Generally a self-protective mechanism for pain avoidance<br>　— Results from spinal, hip, knee, ankle or foot lesion<br>• The patient might list away from the lesion, or positions the body in a way that minimizes pain<br>　— However, if a hip is painful, the patient might position the body weight over the painful hip vertically, decreasing the load on the femoral head<br>• The stance phase on the injured limb is shorter. The patient might try to support the affected area with one hand. The opposite arm might be outstretched, acting as a counterbalance |
| **ARTHROGENIC** | The patient's limb swings in a circular, cone-shaped arc (circumduction) around the affected joint | • Due to pathology of a single joint |
| **ATAXIC** | Seen in patients who have bad coordination or poor sensation. The patient may appear to be intoxicated | • Can be seen in patients who have cerebellar or peripheral/sensory lesions, and in patients who are intoxicated<br>　— Often in central nervous system lesions, all movements are exaggerated<br>　— In sensory or peripheral lesions the gait may be irregular, swaying and jerky. The patient may look down to see placement of feet |
| **SHORT LEG** | Lateral shift toward the short leg and a downward pelvic tilt with a possible limp-like gait | • Often patient compensates by rotating the innominate posteriorly on the long side and anteriorly on the short leg side (to equalize the leg length)<br>　— With a premature heel lift on the short leg side in mid-stance |
| **GLUTEUS MEDIUS**<br>(Trendelenburg) | Often results in an increase of lateral shift | • Usually seen in the presence of L-5 root lesions.<br>• The patient lists laterally to keep the center of gravity over the stance leg.<br>　— If the lesion is bilateral, the patient has a wobbling gate |
| **GLUTEUS MAXIMUS** | The patient moves the thorax posteriorly at heel strike in order to compensate for the weak gluteus maximus | • Often seen in patients who have a backward tilt (center of gravity moved posteriorly) and in patients who have S1 lesions |

*Table 4-15.* **GENERAL OBSERVATION: FRONT**

| LOCATION | OBSERVE FOR | |
|---|---|---|
| Pelvis | | Underwear is at the same level on both sides of the pelvis (help visually)<br>Muscle tone |
| Posture<br>(Customary,<br>relaxed) | Plumb Line | Head straight<br>Nose in line with the sternum and umbilicus<br>Shoulders, clavicles and upper limbs level and equal (dominant side might be slightly lower)<br>Arms equidistant from the trunk, and rotated equally<br>Hip bones (ilia), knees, head of fibula, malleoli and arches of the feet level and equal |
| Skin | | Evidence of segmental trophic changes<br>Cutaneous lesions and scars |

*Table 4-16.* **GENERAL OBSERVATION: FROM BEHIND**

| LOCATION | OBSERVE FOR |
|----------|-------------|
| SHOULDERS<br>SCAPULA | Levelness, scapular winging, muscle tone |
| SPINE | (Spinal curve) kinks, flat areas, scoliosis, step deformity, muscle tone |
| HIPS (ILIA)<br>BUTTOCKS<br>GLUTEAL FOLDS | Levelness, muscle tone |
| KNEES | Swelling, varus or valgus |
| ACHILLES TENDONS | Straightness, varus or valgus |
| SKIN | Evidence of segmental trophic changes<br>Cutaneous lesions and scars |

*Table 4-17.* **GENERAL OBSERVATIONS: FROM THE SIDE**

| LOCATION | OBSERVE FOR |
|----------|-------------|
| ENTIRE SIDE | Plumb line<br>Increased/decreased spinal curves<br>Step spinal deformity<br>Flat spinal segments |
| HEAD | Position |
| SCAPULA | Winging |
| SKIN | Evidence of segmental trophic changes<br>Cutaneous lesions and scars |

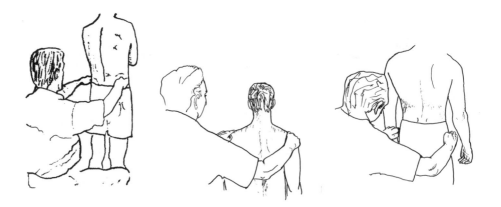

*Figure 4- 8:* Assessment of crest, shoulder and hip levelness.

## Screening: Movement, Postural & Muscles Length

The practitioner tests active movement with the patient in several positions.

**ACTIVE MOVEMENT, PATIENT STANDING.** The practitioner:

1. Tests trunk, lumbar and cervical sidebending, extension, rotation and flexion.

2. Observes for asymmetry.

3. Observes for increase or decrease of scoliosis, paravertebral asymmetry and muscle tone.

4. Performs a standing flexion test.

5. Repeats these observations with the patient sitting.

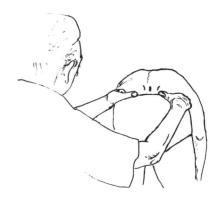

*Figure 4- 9:* Standing flexion test.

## Standing & Sitting Flexion Tests

The standing flexion test is used to evaluate iliosacral motion, the seated flexion test is used to evaluate sacroiliac motion. To perform a standing flexion test, the practitioner places two thumbs just at the inferior slope of the Posterior Superior Iliac Spine (PSIS), asks the patient to bend forward, and follows the movements of the PSIS. (If the ilia are not level, the practitioner places a book under the lower side). (Figure 4-9).

The upward movement of each PSIS should be equal. If either moves further or earlier, the iliosacral motion at that side is said to be restricted.

The practitioner repeats the same test with the patient seated (Figure 4-10).

**NOTE:** Testing the patient seated focuses the tests on the pelvis and spine, eliminating contribution from the lower extremities.

- If abnormal findings are decreased, the problem is less likely to come from the lower extremities and the iliosacral axis.

- If abnormal findings do not change or if they increase, the problem is more likely to originate in the pelvis or spine.

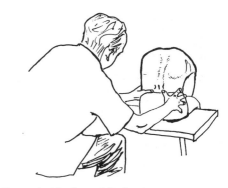

*Figure 4- 10:* Seated flexion test.

## Squat Test

To test the knees, hips, ankles and quadriceps muscle, the practitioner asks the patient to perform a squat. Any difficulty may reflect dysfunctions in these areas (Figure 4-11).

## Patient Prone

With the patient prone the practitioner:

1. Tests joint play in the spine by pushing on the transverse and spinous processes (Figure 4-12).

2. Tests uncompensated hip extension (psoas major muscle tension) by

stabilizing the patient's pelvis and lifting his thigh (Figure 4-13).

Hip extension should be equal on both side and end feel soft.

3. Tests for rectus femoris muscle tightness by flexing the patient knee (Figure 4-14).

Tightness results in early compensatory lifting of the patient's pelvis on the tested side. Tension should be equal on both sides.

**Patient Supine**

1. Performs a straight leg raise (SLR), and dural tension test (Figure 4-15).

2. Tests for hamstring muscle tightness by monitoring the opposite ASIS, noting how far the leg can be raised before the ASIS begins to move (Figure 4-16).

Tension should be equal on both sides. Leg raising of less then 45° indicates muscle tension.

3. Performs *Fabere Patrick's* maneuver to test the hips (flexion, abduction and external rotation) (Figure 4-17).

Normally the end feel is leathery and range equal on both sides.

4. Tests for uncompensated internal rotation at the hip (tension of the external rotators) by rotating the legs internally (Figure 4-18).

The end feel should be slightly springy and equal on both sides.

5. Tests for iliopsoas muscle tightness by having the standing patient bring his thigh to his chest, and then leaning backward onto the exam table (Figure 4-19).

Difficulty maintaining hip extension (the patient's lower leg tending to lift off the table) indicates a tight iliopsoas muscle.

A tight quadriceps muscle does not allow the lower knee to flex (while the patient is in this position). When knee flexion is reduced the hips compensate by flexing.

6. Tests for leg adductor tension using the same position used in the psoas tension test. But this time the patient's lower leg is abducted (Figure 4-20).

Abduction of less than 25° indicates excessive tension.

7. Tests for tensor fascia lata tension using the same position used in the psoas tension test. But this time the patient's lower leg is adducted (Figure 4-21).

Adduction of less than 15° indicates excessive tension.

8. Tests for upper trapezius tension by flexing and inclining the head contralaterally. Then from this position the shoulder girdle is pushed distally (Figure 4-22).

Normally the end feel is soft and equal on both sides. Hardness indicates excessive tension.

9. Tests for levator scapulae tension in a similar manner as upper trapezius, but this time the head is also rotated to the contralateral side. The practitioner's hand monitors the medial superior angle of the scapula (Figure 4-23).

Normally the end feel is soft and equal on both sides. Hardness indicates excessive tension.

10. Tests for sternocleidomastoid tension by first flexing the head maximally, then sidebending the neck to the opposite side, and while rotating the head to the same side extending the neck (Figure 4-24).

Normally the end feel is soft and equal in both sides. Hardness indicates excessive tension.

11. Tests for pectoralis major tension by moving the arm into abduction, making sure the trunk is stable (Figure 4-25).

Normally the arm should reach the horizontal.

## Patient on His Side

**1.** Tests for quadratus lumborum tension
by testing passive trunk sidebending.
(Figure 4-26).

   Normally tension is equal bilaterally.

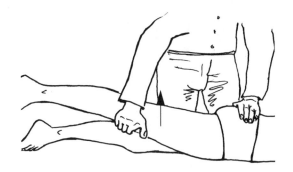

*Figure 4- 13:* Testing uncompensated hip
extension (psoas major).

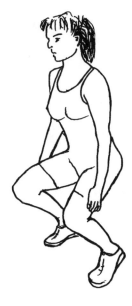

*Figure 4- 11:* Squat test.

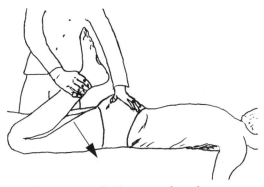

*Figure 4- 14:* Testing rectus femoris
tension.

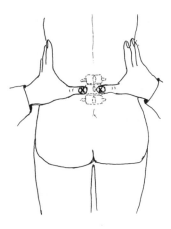

*Figure 4- 12:* Joint play assessment.

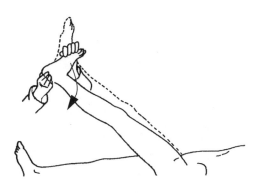

*Figure 4- 15:* Straight leg rase (doted line).
Dural tension test solid line.

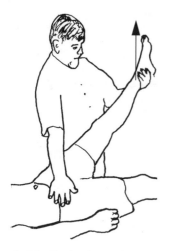

Figure 4- 16:   Testing hamstring tightness.

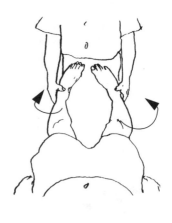

Figure 4- 18:   Testing uncompensated internal hip rotation.

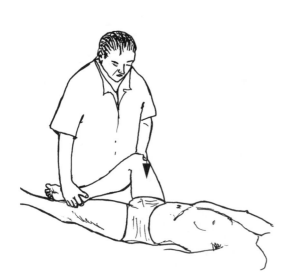

Figure 4- 17:   Fabere Patrick's test.

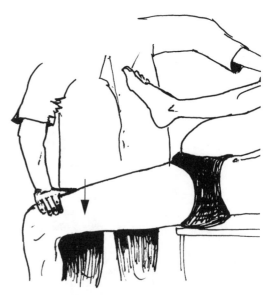

Figure 4- 19:   Testing iliopsoas tension.

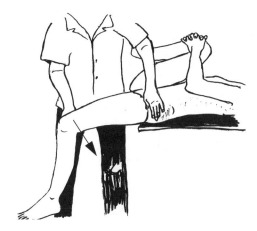

*Figure 4- 20:* Assessment of leg adductor tension.

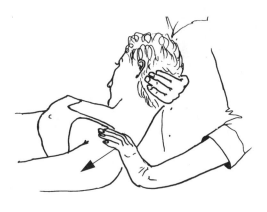

*Figure 4- 23:* Assessment of levator scapulae tension.

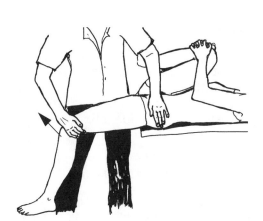

*Figure 4- 21:* Assessment of tensor fascia latae tension.

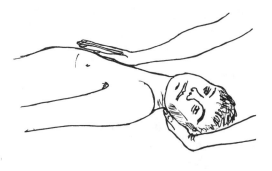

*Figure 4- 24:* Assessment of SCM tension.

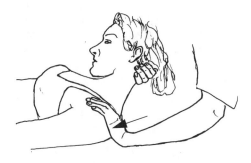

*Figure 4- 22:* Assessment of upper trapezius tension.

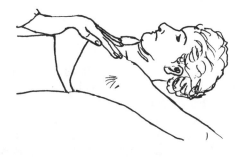

*Figure 4- 25:* Assessment of pectoralis major tension.

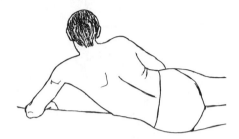

*Figure 4- 26:* Assessment of quadratus lumborum tension.

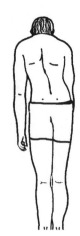

*Figure 4- 27:* Postural list.

## Screening Test Findings

The musculoskeletal screening can lead the practitioner to areas of dysfunction that are outside of the patient's complaint areas. Often these are primary and must be addressed.

### Width Between Patient's Legs

The width between the patient's legs are usually 2 to 4 inches. A wider stance can indicate that the patient has a feeling of instability. Stride inequality usually indicates lower limb dysfunction, but it may also be due to pain avoidance from symptoms in the head, neck or trunk (Hoppenfeld *ibid*; Mitchell *ibid*). A patient walking with a stiff spine, but with free pelvic superior shifts and rotational movements, is more likely to have a spinal lesion than a pelvic lesion.

### Decreased Lumbar Lordosis

Decreased lumbar lordosis suggests paravertebral muscle spasm (commonly due to backward sacral dysfunction), disc disease or other significantly painful lesions. Lordosis is increased with "sway back" (weak abdominal and psoas muscles, associated with Janda's pelvic crossed syndrome), spondylolisthesis, and anterior sacral dysfunctions.

### Antalgic Posture

Antalgic postures (typical lumbago list, or deviated away from pain) is commonly seen with psoas syndrome, disc lesions and backward sacral torsions. Or with extremity pain from the hip, knee or feet.

### Pelvic Tilt (Oblique Position)

A pelvic tilt due to shortening of the lower extremity can be detected as a "short leg gait." Here the patient shows a lateral shift toward the shorter leg and a downward pelvic tilt. These result in a limp-like gait, depending on the discrepancy between leg lengths. Patients may compensate for a short leg by rotating their innominates posteriorly on the long leg side and anteriorly on the short leg side. Such patients do not show a short leg gate; however, on the short leg side the heel lifts prematurely in mid-stance (Kuchera and Kuchera *ibid*; Mitchell *ibid*).

A pelvic twist often is associated with shortness of the piriformis and/or iliopsoas. Shortness of the thigh adductors and tightness of the quadratus lumborum and of the iliopsoas can lead to a functional short leg. Tightness of the piriformis makes the leg appear longer (Janda1996).

## Pelvic Lateral & Vertical Shifting

Pelvic lateral shifting (normally one inch or so) is to the weight bearing side. Vertical shift is highest in mid-stance and usually is about 2 inches, and may be increased on the side with pathology. Irregularities in hip shifting suggest anatomic asymmetries of the lumbar and pelvic joints (Hoppenfeld *ibid*; Mitchell *ibid*).

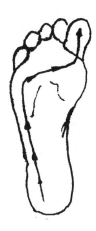

*Figure 4- 28:* Weight transfer across the foot during gait.

## Scoliosis

Scoliosis can be structural or functional. Abnormally high ilia, hips, unleveling of the sacral base or inequality in leg length can result in secondary scoliosis.

Hypertrophy at the thoracolumbar erector spinae, with/or without a scoliotic curve, often is due to lumbosacral instability and poor muscle tone.

## Rotated Leg

An internally or externally rotated leg usually is due to a rotation imbalance of the hips. A flexed knee and internally rotated foot (Dorman and Ravin 1991) may represent either a problem in the affected hip or pain from the posterior superficial SI ligaments—OM: *Tai Yang Sinew channel, Divergent channel and/or Yang Motility (Qiao) deficiency*. Bilateral toe-out (slew-foot) (Mitchell 1995) usually reflects poor trunk and head/neck posture.

A toed-out (push-off) phase of gait can result as a compensation to over pronated forefoot, hallux valgus with a flattened midtarsal joint, and forefoot and rearfoot varus. [10] OM: *Toe-out is often a result of Shao Yang channel and/or Yang Motility (Qiao) channel excess.*

The positions of the patellae relative to the position of the feet can call attention

to problems of the femur and knee, tibial torsions, and traumatic or degenerative displacements of the patella. OM: *Altered patellar position is mostly due to Shao Yang and Yang Ming Sinew channels disorders.*

## Alteration of Weight Transfer

Alteration of weight transfer across the sole of the foot is commonly due to somatic dysfunction (or ligamentous laxity) in tarsal articulations or rearfoot disorders (Mitchell 1985).

## Footwear

Problems of the foot sometimes can be seen as abnormal wear on the sole of the shoes. With foot varus, the inside of the sole frequently wears more quickly than the outside; with foot valgus, the outside of the sole can wear more quickly than the inside (OM: *Yang Motility (Qiao) deficiency, Yin Motility (Qiao) excess*). Some faster wear of the outside rear sole is normal, because at heal strike weightbearing takes place first on the outside, and moves up and across the front at toe-off. A "swirl" pattern (Mitchell 1995) may indicate excessive external

---

10. These dysfunctions often result in piriformis spasm.

rotator muscle tightness during the stance phase of the gait.

### Tilted Shoulders, Head, Upper Body

Tilted shoulders, head or upper body can be either primary, or secondary to lower trunk and limb dysfunctions and/or pathology. The shoulder on the dominant side usually is a little lower with a small tilt of the head to the same side.

Scapular winging can be seen in C5 palsy. Excessive head and neck movements could suggest impaired mobility in the lower spine or limbs. An unequal distance of the upper arms from the trunk can be seen with scoliosis.

An anteriorly protruded head can affect the entire musculoskeletal system and is usually due to weakness of the deep neck flexors and dominance or tightness of the sternocleidomastoid muscles; the pectoralis major is tight often, as well.

Tightness of the upper trapezius and levator scapulae can be observed on the neck and shoulder line; the contour may straighten.

### Cutaneous Trophic Changes

Cutaneous trophic changes such as loss of hair may occur in a segmental distribution (*or channel distribution*). Myofascial dysfunctions and a variety of symptoms such as local or referred pain, tingling and burning can result from scars. Muscle atrophy can be due to neuropathy or can be due to a primary muscle disease or from disuse.

## Universal Pattern

A common adaptation known as the universal pattern usually includes (Greenman 1996; Mitchell 1995):

- A slightly lower right shoulder with a slight tilt of the head to the right (in right handed people).

- Minimal scoliosis of the upper thoracic spine (convexity to the left).
- Slight forward rotation of the right innominates, commonly seen with a left-on-left sacral torsion.[11]
- Flattening of the right foot arch, somewhat more than in the left foot.
- Slight external rotation of the right leg.

The problems, dysfunctions and compensatory mechanisms that this section has described are multi-layered and complex. Treatment requires accurate diagnosis, which can take time. The practitioner should always perform a full examination, and the treatment approach should always be systematic. Some practitioners suggest that performing the examination before conducting the interview can reduce bias and help identify the root lesion.

## Laboratory Testing

Many musculoskeletal pains can be due to medical conditions that can be detected through laboratory testing. Therefore, laboratory tests can be especially prudent for patients that have chronic or acute pain of unknown origin.

The practitioner orders tests based on clinical presentations. For example, patients suffering from fatigue and generalized muscle pain (fibromyalgia) may be suffering from thyroid deficiency. Tests can include:

- Complete Blood Count (CBC) with differential count.
- SMAC 24 (a series of several tests).
- Sensitive Thyroid Stimulating Hormone (TSH).
- Urine Strip Analysis.
- (Men over 50) Prostate Specific Antigen (PSA).

---

11. A sacrum that is twisted and sidebent to the left.

In the presence of joint pain and/or swelling:

- CBC.
- Erythrocyte Sedimentation Rate (ESR).
- Rheumatoid Factor (RF).
- Antinuclear Antibodies (ANA).
- Uric Acid Level.
- Urinalysis.
- (Possibly) synovial fluid culture (aspiration of fluid to check for infections or crystalline disease).

The sections "Blood Tests," "Urine Tests" and "Some Additional Tests" contain brief descriptions of applicable tests.[12]

## Blood Tests

Blood tests are often used to exclude medical conditions that either are responsible for or are contributing to pain.

### Erythrocyte Sedimentation Rate (ESR)

Erythrocyte Sedimentation Rate (ESR), a nonspecific screening test, is an indicator of inflammatory processes that can be useful for diagnosing patients who have involvement of multiple areas from a systemic disease. For many of these conditions, this test also can be used to follow the level of activity.

The ESR increases with aging. Normal values vary with the specific techniques used and the laboratory that performs the test. ESR is a nonspecific marker. A persistent increase can be due to conditions other than those mentioned here.

**INCREASED ESR.** The ESR is increased in rheumatic fever, rheumatoid arthritis and the rheumatoid variants, systemic lupus erythematosus (SLE), polymyalgia rheumatica (PMR), temporal arteritis and acute infections.

---

12. For more information see Wallach (1978).

**EXTREMELY HIGH ESR.** Extremely high ESRs (greater than 100) can be found in temporal arteritis, tuberculosis and cancer.

**ESR NOT INCREASED.** The ESR is not increased in degenerative arthritis and in crystalline diseases such as gout, except during severe, acute attacks.

### Complete Blood Count (CBC)

Peripheral leukocytosis can be seen with acute infections. However, just as with the ESR, a normal white count (leukocyte) reading does not rule out the presence of infection.

**DECREASE IN WHITE BLOOD COUNT (WBC).** Decreased WBC can be seen in immune deficiency. An overwhelming infection can cause a decrease in the WBC as well.

**LOW RED BLOOD COUNT (RBC).** A finding of a low RBC, low hemoglobin (Hg) and a low hematocrit can be seen with anemias and can also be a clue to the presence of a systemic illness such as lupus erythematosus (SLE) and several neuropathies or internal bleeding.

**HIGH RBC.** A high RBC with high Hg and hematocrit is found in polycythemia.

**CBC WITH DIFFERENTIAL.** The differential of the cell types present can indicate the type of inflammation present (bacterial, viral or allergic).

### Rheumatoid Factor (RF)

Rheumatoid Factor tests for IgG antibodies in rheumatoid arthritis (RA). RF is negative in a fair number of patients who have rheumatoid arthritis, especially in early or mild stages. Usually the rheumatoid factor is negative in the presence of rheumatoid variants. The RF is positive in a significant percentage of patients who have systemic lupus erythematosus (SLE) and in patients who have some other conditions, such as syphilis.

## Antinuclear Antibodies (ANA)

Antinuclear Antibodies are antibodies to various nuclear constituents (such as DNA and nucleoproteins) found in patients who have autoimmune diseases such as lupus erythematosus (SLE). The test also can be positive in patients who have scleroderma or Sjogeren's syndrome, drug-induced, lupus-like syndromes, and in about one-fourth of patients who have RA.

## Uric Acid Level

The higher the uric acid level in the blood, the more likely the patient is to have attacks of gouty arthritis. Demonstration of a serum level of uric acid above defined normal limits, however, does not unequivocally prove that joint symptoms are due to gout.[13] Uric acid levels can be increased in cases of renal insufficiency and decreased in acute hepatitis.

## Serum Calcium

Serum calcium often increases in the presence of hyperparathyroidism and bone metastasis. Serum calcium can decrease in hypoparathyroidism and hyperthyroidism. Normal levels in children and adolescents are much higher than those in adults.

## Phosphorus

Phosphorus increases in the presence of hypoparathyroidism, severe kidney disease, acromegaly, and patients who have an excess of vitamin D. Phosphorus decreases in the presence of rickets, osteomalacia, malabsorption, and hyperparathyroidism. Normal levels in children and

---

13. Usually gout is diagnosed by the aspirate of synovial fluid that contains uric acid crystals.

adolescents are much higher than in adults.

## Alkaline Phosphatase

Alkaline Phosphatase is a phosphatase that increases with bone growth and disease, biliary and liver disease, and in Paget's Disease. Decreased levels can result in growth retardation in children. Normal levels in children and adolescents are much higher than in adults.

## Acid Phosphatase

Acid Phosphatase is a phosphatase that increases in the presence of metastatic prostate cancers. Normal levels in children and adolescents are much higher than in adults.

## Serum Glutamic-Oxaloacetic Transaminase (SGOT)

Serum Glutamic-Oxaloacetic Transaminase, an enzyme present in large amounts in muscle and liver tissue, is used primarily as an indicator of acute myocardial infarction and liver disease. SGOT is increased in cases of musculoskeletal disease, especially in the presence of muscular injury and dystrophies, and in heart and liver disease.

## Sensitive Thyroid Stimulating Hormone (TSH)

Sensitive Thyroid Stimulating Hormone, a test for thyroid function, reports an increased TSH level in hypothyroidism and a decreased TSH level in hyperthyroidism. Thyroid dysfunction is a common cause of myofascial pain syndromes.

## Prostate Specific Antigen (PSA)

Prostate Specific Antigen, which tests for prostate pathology, should be performed on men over 50 years of age, especially those who suffer from back pain. Manual palpation of the entire prostate is not possible and therefore, small early carcinomas might escape manual detection that can be discovered by abnormal levels of serum PSA. Prostate cancer can cause low back pain.

## HLA-B27 Antigen

HLA-B27 Antigen is a marker found in 90% of patients who have ankylosing spondylitis, and in about 70% of patients who have Reiter's syndrome, psoriatic spondylitis or enteropathic arthritis. HLA-B27 antigen can be present in normal samples, as well.

## Urine Tests

Urine tests can be helpful for assessing musculoskeletal disorders, especially back pain.

### Urine Dip Stick

The Urine Dip Stick Test is important especially for patients who have low back pain.

- In cases of urinary tract infection (UTI), the dip stick can be positive for white cells, nitrites, leukocyte esterase, and possibly protein.
- Kidney stones often present with blood in the urine.
- Diabetes presents with glucose in the urine.

The symptoms of these disorders can masquerade as musculoskeletal pain.

### Bence Jones Protein

An abnormal urinary or plasma protein that has unusual solubility attributes. Bence Jones Protein is found in patients who have multiple myeloma and osteosarcomas, and sometimes in patients who

have reticuloendothelial system diseases (RES).

### Osteomark – NTX

The Osteomark—NTX assay measures the urine levels of a compound linked to bone-breakdown (crossed-linked N-telopeptide of type I collagen). Hence, this test can be used to monitor the rate of bone loss and success of therapies used for osteoporosis.

# Additional Tests

Neurophysiologic studies provide a way to categorize muscle and nerve damage. They measure the integrity of the nerve muscle relationship and do not, by themselves, offer a specific etiologic diagnosis. Two tests that are very helpful in differentiating the possible causes of muscular weakness, numbness and paresthesias are electromyography (EMG) and Nerve Conduction Velocity (NCV) (Garrick and Ebb ibid).

### Electromyography (EMG)

Electromyography studies evaluate motor unit potentials. The physician:

1. Inserts thin electrode needles into specific muscles.
2. Observes the elicited motor unit potentials on an oscilloscope screen.

Many abnormal potentials and potential patterns are seen with denervation of the muscle. From the pattern of involvement of several muscles for which innervations are known, the specific location of the pathology can be surmised. Examples include root compression, compression of a specific peripheral nerve at a specific site, such as median nerve entrapment (carpel tunnel entrapment), or a polyneuropathy. Intrinsic muscular disease and myasthenia gravis present with very specific electromyographic patterns (Garrick and Ebb *ibid*).

### Nerve Conduction Velocity (NCV)

To measure Nerve Conduction Velocity, the physician:

1. Stimulates a peripheral nerve at a specific site.

2. Measures the time necessary for muscle action potentials to be transmitted distally.

3. Compares the time with the normal value listed for the age and sex of the patient.

A delay implies peripheral nerve compression somewhere along the nerve. This technique is especially useful for confirming a clinical impression of the location of nerve compression. Some polyneuropathies slow the conduction velocity, some do not. A comparison with normal nerve values helps differentiate these entities from compression neuropathies (Garrick and Ebb *ibid*).

# Imaging & Radiology [14]

## Medical Radiographic Imaging

Medical radiographic imaging remained relatively unchanged from the original way Roentgen did it until the 1960's. The use of X-rays was confined to X-ray machine emitting radiation and the image being recorded on photographic film. In the 1960's the development of more sensitive ways of detecting radiation became available. The development of nuclear medicine and computerized imaging

---

14. All Imaging information in the text is provided by Thomas Ravin MD.

began. Computerized axial tomograpy or CAT (CT) scanning combined this new way of detecting radiation that did not use film.

Musculoskeletal imaging can be done usually with plain X-ray imaging which has considerable advantages. X-rays use low doses of radiation and the cost to benefit ratio is high. MRI/CT can assist in the diagnosis of some musculoskeletal problems but they need to be correlated with the routine X-ray to be really useful.

The major emphasis in this text is on clinical methods which are low tech yet useful clinically. The use of radiology and other imaging techniques is ubiquitous and probably had detracted from clinical evaluation overall. The tendency to treat X-rays is a health hazard in the opinion of the authors. Judicious use of imaging can, however, support the soft tissue clinician.

### Safety of Imaging

Medical imaging has continued to raise some safety questions such as: what is this magnetic spectrum doing to the individual and is it fundamentally safe? The radiation doses created by modern X-ray equipment using modern film and film screen technology deliver doses which are very low and may not be much in excess of background levels. Of unknown impact on the body is MRI and ultrasound. Ultrasound can create some tissue warming at the frequency and doses used in the average human, but probably represent no significant threat to the body. The question as to whether MRI is free of harm is less well known. The effects on the human body of intense magnetic fields and multiple radio frequencies is hard to demonstrate. MRI is probably safe in the doses administered, but possible harm cannot be ignored.

It seems that all of these imaging techniques appear on the surface to be quite safe and their use in the holistic/complementary practice should not be denied over questions of safety, particularly when health needs are to be addressed. It should not be forgotten that even the lowest radiation doses may create some trauma to genetic material in the ovaries and testes. The impact of high intensity electromagnetic fields and radiation associated with many of these instruments lead one to approach the imaging modalities with some wariness, constantly keeping the risks versus the benefit ratio in mind. Modern imaging technology has made the risk to benefit ratios favorable, and particularly so in the extremities and axial skeleton in adults.

## Basic Principles.

An X-ray is ordered and labeled by the direction and relations the X-ray beam has to the patient. For example, a film labeled anterior-posterior view (AP), means that the X-ray beam is centered on the anterior portion of the part being filmed and the film is behind the patient. The lateral view has the central beam on the inside or medial aspect of the patient, with the film outside or lateral to the patient. The areas that are closer to the film show greater detail. So for example, to assess the spine an anterior-posterior view films is usually ordered (AP view, verses a PA). The films are displayed on the view box as though the practitioner is looking at the patient or the films right side on the viewers left. MRI, CT and ultrasound images are displayed the same way. If there are axial images (as though slicing a piece of salami) they appear as though the practitioner is looking from the feet to the head.

X-ray films are in fact negatives. The film which is exposed by radiation causes the silver crystals in the film to change shape and to stay on the film when it is developed. The unexposed portions of the film turn white. This results in denser tissues appearing more white than less dense tissues (bones appear whiter than soft tissue and air appears darkest). In order of depending degree of density are the following structures: metal, bone, soft tissue, water, fat, and air.

Basic imaging usually is ordered to exclude medical conditions such as cancers, infections (osteomyelitis) and metabolic and inflammatory bone diseases such as osteoporosis and ankylosing spondylitis. They should, therefore, be evaluated by a board certified radiologist to ensure that no subtle but significant pathology is missed. In acute trauma, films may show fractures and if the patient is short of breath the presence of pneumothorax.

With experience the radiologist can detect not only bony but also many important soft tissue changes, such as joint effusion, tendinous calcification, actopic bone or muscle, tissue displaced by a tumor, and the presence of air or foreign body.

In general the radiologist inspects for:

1. Overall size and shape of bone.

2. Local size and shape of bone.

3. Thickness of the cortex.

4. Trabecular pattern of the bone.

5. General density of the entire bone.

6. Local density of bone.

7. Margins of local lesions.

8. Any break in continuity of the bone.

9. Any periosteal change.

10. Any soft tissue change.

11. Relation among bones.

12. Thickness of the cartilage (joint space).

### Bony Architecture

The opacity of bones on X-ray varies. The apparent density of the bone depends in part on radiographic technique. Although appearances may suggest abnormalities of mineralization, it is known that these appearances often are misleading; hence it is wise to defer evaluation of mineralization to densitomery, dual photon absorptometry, single photon absorptometry, and CT scanning absorptometry. For osteoporosis to be evident on plain film, approximately 30-35% of the bone must be lost. These observations do not fall within the purview of soft tissue management.

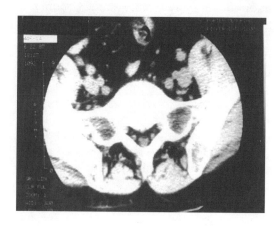

*Figure 4- 29:* CT scan of the pelvis.

### Limitations

Rentgenograms can not be focused like a light beam. They display a two-dimensional view of three-dimensional structures and there is superimposition of the several layers.

When joints are visualized, the joint space may be identifiable if the joint is seen end-on, and if the space is planar. When seen at an angle, curved joint spaces cannot be assessed reliably; hence, the assessment of degenerative joint disease is based primarily on associated phenomena such as osteophyte formation, the degree of subchondral bone sclerosis, subchondral cyst formation, and soft tissue swelling.

### Dynamic Studies

Ideally, imaging should reproduce abnormal physiological movement. Stress views and flexion/extension views are used in an attempt to visualize abnormalities at the end range of movement. Such views should be obtained with the patient just on the threshold of pain aggravation.

### Magnetic Resonance Imaging & Computer-Reconstructed Radiographic Tomography

Magnetic Resonance Imaging or MRI does not use X-ray to create the image (Figure 4-30). It uses radio signals created by nuclear polarity changing directions in strong magnetic fields and is analyzed in many different planes of the body, making it useful in many different areas. Since it does not use X-ray to create the images, it is a safe imaging technique near the eyes and gonads.

Computer-reconstructed radiogaphic tomography (CT) (Figure 4-29) and MRI

provide an enhanced scope of visualization of the interior of the body. The clarity of the pictures is seductive, but image reconstruction by computer is not analogous to photography. Adjustment in gain and other parameters can make and ablate appearances. Although the verisimilitude of precision is gracing these systems with a hallowed place in the contemporary medicolegal jungle, obtaining such images is nonetheless prudent and sometimes helpful—CT is best for imaging bones because the calcium absorbs X-ray, although the radiation exposure to the patient triples with CTs.

Radio waves that echo from magnetically charged protons, (like water molecules present in the soft tissues) are the source of MRI images, which, therefore, comprise the best technique for imaging these parts. When a practitioner wants to look at the bulging disc or the position of a nerve or tendon, MRI is best. The technique can help estimate any increase in water and occasionally also give some indirect information on how acute the process is.

Usually CT images are created in transverse sections. The stored information can be displayed as an image of cuts in other planes and even in three dimensions; however, there is loss of detail. In contrast,

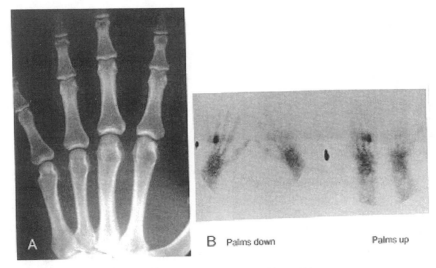

*Figure 4- 31:* Fracture positive on bone scan (B), negative on X-ray (A)

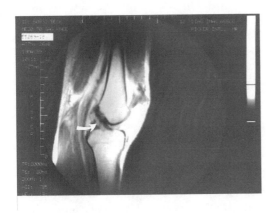

*Figure 4- 30:* MRI image of knee.

erated by radioactive decay of the atom's nuclear material. Nuclear medicine is a powerful tool for evaluating physiologic functions as the radiation dosage is small. The radioactive material can be attached to various molecules which go to various tissues in different amounts depending on health and sickness. Bone scanning, a nuclear medicine imaging technique, can be helpful in identifying lesion (cancers, fractures and metabolic diseases) which do not show on regular X-ray imaging.

with some planning, MRI studies can show any plane without loss of detail. This is an important advantage.

## Nuclear Medicine

Nuclear medicine is an imaging technique that takes advantage of the radiation gen-

### Bone Scans

In certain disease conditions the metabolism of bone is accelerated. The rate of incorporation of calcium phosphate taken from the circulating pool is increased. Tagging some of the circulating phosphate with a radioactive marker (technetium-99) leads to the concentration of some of the radioactivity at sites of increased metabolism and blood flow. These sites can be identified by obtaining a body scan of the radioactive emissions. Many conditions of bone show an increased uptake, hence the test is nonspecific but still sensitive.

After injuries, the clinician may want to exclude fractures and X-rays should be used first. Unfortunately fractures are not always seen. This applies particularly to hairline fractures of long bones and fractures in vertebrae that have other abnormalities or have had prior partial collapse, as well as the small bones of the wrist and ankle. The process that heals fractures involves an increased metabolism of bone, including the incorporation of pyrophosphate; therefore, even cryptic (hidden) fractures show up with bone scans.

In young patients, deposition of calcium and phosphate after a fracture begins promptly. Under the age of 65, acute fractures can be identified within 24 hours with 95% accuracy. Delays occur in persons who have slow metabolic rates caused by age and disease; however, within three days virtually all fractures show (Matin 1988; Rupani 1985).

Like hairline fractures, stress fractures are sometimes invisible on plain X-rays, and bone scanning can clinch a diagnosis. The cortex of certain bones consists of several layers; stress fractures typically involve only some layers. The amount of radioactive uptake, therefore, helps grade stress fractures as well (Matin 1979), (Figure 4-31).

Osteitis pubis, particularly in women, is sometimes visualized on bone scans better than on X-rays. Compression fractures of the vertebrae show an increased uptake for up to two years after injury (Daffner *ibid*). Most malignancies and myeloma occasionally can be identified with bone scans.

## Medical Ultrasound

Medical ultrasound was developed from a military tool refined in World War II for identifying submarines and is known as sonar. Ultrasound Imaging does not use X-ray to create the image. It uses sound waves which are sent into the body and the returning echoes are listened for, just as in sonar. The sound waves are then con-

verted into a visual image. Ultrasound, except for assessment of vascular circulation, is not commonly used in musculoskeletal medicine.

## Visceral Imaging

Visceral imaging spans the entire spectrum of imaging technology. The use of plain radiographic imaging of the viscera can be discussed briefly, but visceral imaging is the heart and sole of the newer imaging modalities, CT, MRI, ultrasound, and even nuclear medicine.

*Plain film* imaging of the chest is the standard by which all other imaging modalities are compared. Imaging of the chest for cardiac size and clarity of the lung fields has remained a standard of care for almost the entire 100 years of radiography. The routine chest X-ray is the gold standard for people with coughs, chest pain, and pleurisy.

Plain film imaging of the abdomen is also of value when looking for gas patterns or fluid levels as indicators of obstruction and large abdominal masses. These films have in many cases been supplemented by the use of other imaging technology particularly CT scanning which can better define the organs and nature of masses in the abdomen.

ULTRASOUND of the female pelvis is extremely safe and quite informative. The use of this in the evaluation of female pelvic pain and pregnancy is now the preferred technique over all others.

MAMMOGRAPHY, still being hotly debated, is perhaps the best single way of detecting early breast cancer. As with many costly screening tests, the cost of finding an individual tumor may never be rationalized, but in any individual it may be particularly helpful and valuable.

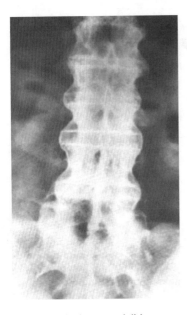

*Figure 9-32:* Ankylosing spondylitis.

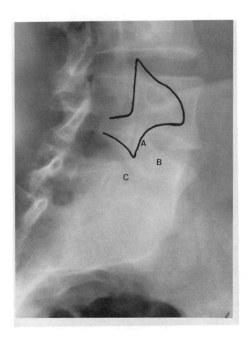

*Figure 4- 33:* Oblique views showing collar of on scotty dog.

# Imaging the Spine

Imaging of the spine (and feet) needs to be done standing or weight bearing and if done in any other way is of limited value. This cannot be over emphasized, as so often routine spine imaging is done non-weight bearing, and therefore little information is gained on mechanical disorders and joint dysfunction. Assessment of X-ray for possible causes of, and contributors to musculoskeletal dysfunctions and pain, should be undertaken by the holistic/complementary doctor. This type of analysis usually has not been done by the radiologist, and it is best done with knowledge of the clinical situation. Disc space narrowing and presence of somatic changes that impact function all need to be assessed on an individual basis. The use of X-ray imaging, particularly in the low back, is frequently misunderstood, but can be a powerful tool in therapeutic measures.

## Congenital Abnormalities

Many abnormalities, such as unequal leg length, unlevel sacral base, facet orientations, Ferguson's angle and kissing spinous processes, can only be shown by taking an X-ray. These abnormalities are clinically significant and may determine the appropriate treatment plan.

*Spondylolisthesis* which can be congenital in nature, but trauma seems to be the most common cause, can be demonstrated by several views. This lesion of the pars interarticularis can be identified on the AP and lateral X-ray. These views are relatively high in radiation and should be used sparingly and with forethought. The oblique image demonstrates the lesion and is identified as the "collar of the scotty dog." In degenerative spondylolisthesis the degree of anterior displacement is usually not more than about a fourth of the lower

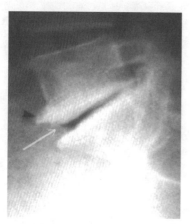

*Figure 4- 34:* Degenerated disc with vacuum phenomenon (white arrow). Note osteophyte formation (black arrow head).

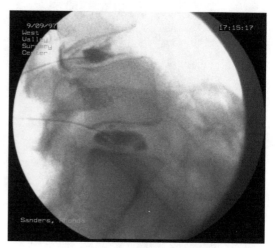

*Figure 4- 35:* Discography of L4-5 discs. Dye is injected into the nucleus of the disc. Pain and leaking are noted.

vertebral body width (first or second degree).

## Degenerative Disc & Joint Disease

Several degenerative processes can be demonstrated by X-ray in the spine and sacroiliac joints. Spondylosis or degenerative joint disease which can create abnormal joint mechanics is demonstrable by X-ray. The identification of the osteophytes adjacent to vertebral facets are evidence of persistent mechanical problems and are not directly correlated with pain. They are however often correlated with ligamentous laxity.

The sacroiliac joints are frequent sites of degenerative joint disease and instability. The presence of osteophytes, subarticular sclerosis (osteitis condesans) and joint space narrowing are indicative of abnormal joint mechanics. Increased movement in the sacroiliac joint causes an increase in bony architecture of the ilium—called osteitis condesans ilii. The earliest changes are a fuzziness of the subarticular bone and eventually the joint space becomes *narrower.*

The radiological assessment of disc space height is sometimes helpful. But the fact that the degree of degenerative disc disease does not correlate with pain makes this assessment of marginal value. The discs, which are made of fibrocartilaginous material, are radio-opaque and do not show an X-ray shadow. A *vacuum* sign can develop—due to collections of nitrogen gas in nuclear and annular fissures—and is seen with an incidence of 2 to 3% in the general population (Figure 4-34).

Assessment of disc disease is best done by MRI which can display the disc in sagittal and transverse planes. This allows for assessment of nerve root compromise and internal disc disruption, especially with a T2 image. Disc fissures can be demonstrated as high intensity zones (HIZ) on a T2 image, and by discography (Figure 4-35).

## Joint Dysfunction

Radiography of the spine can demonstrate persistent mechanical joint dysfunctions. Radiographic evaluation of the spine for somatic joint dysfunctions has remained a challenge since the first osteopaths began evaluating these structures by X-ray. The difficulty has been the correlation of the physical examination of a specific mechanical joint dysfunction with a specific radiographic finding. The problem has been that clinicians trained to assess joint function usually are not as adept at interpreting X-rays, and radiologists are not trained in assessing joint function. The clinician who takes the time to develop skills of reading X-rays for mechanical dysfunctions is rewarded by aiding his diagnosis and demonstrating the effects of treatments. To assess function by X-rays the films should be taken standing and in flexion, extension and sidebending.

Ideally the vertebrae are stacked in perfect geometric formation. Deviations from this ideal should be catalogued and evaluated in the quest for somatic dysfunction. Whether the spinous processes are aligned and whether they divide the spaces between the pedicles symmetrically should be assessed. If there is asymmetry, the relevant spinal level should be noted and the variations between the asymmetries surveyed. The presence of a lateral spinal curve or scoliosis indicates vertebral dysfunction. The nomenclature of the findings and ascription of clinical significance have progressed through a number of classifications, mostly in osteopathic circles. The present comments are based on Greenman's classification. The position of each vertebra is described in relation to the one below it. Motion is described as seen from above and in front of the vertebrae. This means that in rotation, the anterior surface of the vertebral body is used for definition rather than the posterior elements, which are available to palpation (Greenman *ibid*).

### Radiography of Vertebral Rotation

The spine functions as a unit. The short and long "Stays" regulating its interconnected movements consist of the intervertebral ligaments and joint capsules, the fascial sheets at all layers of the paravertebral muscles, and, in fact, the whole sausage of the trunk. Compensatory scoliosis—which seems to be reactive to a distant abnormality—occurs over at least three vertebrae and is often S-shaped and smooth. Vertebral intersegmental movements consist of side bending and rotation in opposite direction (Veldhuizen 1987). This is *type one scoliosis* (neutral dysfunction). An unlevel sacrum (sacral base) is one common cause (Nash 1969). The sacrum may be unlevel because of a geometric factor (i.e. leg-length discrepancy or asymlocation). The somatic dysfunction of the sacrum itself also can be classified.

The extent of scoliosis is commensurate with the amount of unleveling. The spinous processes rotate to the inside of the curve and the anterior surfaces face the outside of the curve. On lateral films the spinous processes fan out normally in flexion; the scoliosis is not seen. This type of scoliosis is usually secondary and does not cause back pain (Figure 4-36).

Rotation and sidebending of one vertebra on its fellow below *to the same side* is defined as a *type two somatic dysfunction* (nonneutral dysfunction). The findings are those of a *short-curve scoliosis* or a vertebral curve involving only two (or at most three) vertebrae. It is thought that type two somatic dysfunction is often caused by local factors, or at least local stiffness. The radiographic description of a type two lesion requires standing films, which should include erect anteroposterior and lateral films, taken in flexion and extension as well.

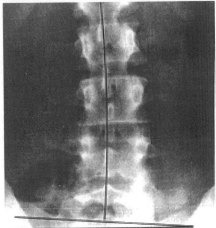

*Figure 4- 36:* Scoliosis from sacral base unleveling.

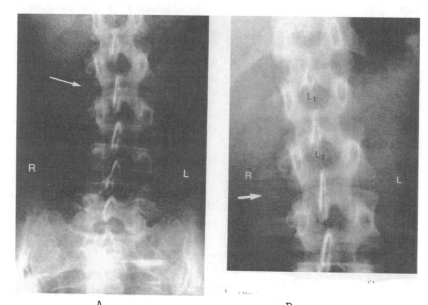

A                                    B

*Figure 4- 37:*   **A**; Type two dysfunction. The L2 vertebra is rotated right, side-bent right or "RSR". If the vertebra is stuck in flexion, the lesion is "flexed, rotated right, and side-bent right" Note right transverse processes are closer together and smaller. **B**; Anterior-posterior view of lumbar spine with the closed arrow pointing to the short curve scoliosis at L2-3.

An alteration in the AP curve (fanning of the spinous processes) is seen in flexion or extension, or both. The stuck joint prevents the adjacent vertebrae from moving into flexion or extension. (In the lumbar spine, flexion lesions are more common.

Because the vertebrae concerned retain a fixed position in side bending, they develop a two-segment *short-curve scoliosis* (Hayes 1989), as seen on the AP X-ray view.

The clinical description of type two somatic dysfunction is based on altered vertebral motion, as judged by palpation; the radiological description is based on still films, hence views at the extreme range of movement are needed (Figure 4-37).

In the radiographical analysis of type two somatic dysfunction the following should be noted:

- The way in which the concerned vertebrae are side bent and rotated.

- The response to flexion and extension.

The radiographic evaluation thus requires analysis of the spine vertebra by vertebra.

The position of the spinous process between the pedicles on the AP film defines rotation (Cobb 1958). The *bony appearance of the pedicles* can give clues about rotation as well.

The short-curve scoliosis is created because the lumbar vertebrae in the dysfunctional segment cannot rotate without side bending; therefore, the two transverse processes will *appear* to approximate each other on the concave side (Greenman *ibid*).

Objects are magnified in radiography the farther they are from the film. This can be used as a clue to vertebral rotation. If one transverse process *appears* larger, it is probably *farther* from the film (Figure 4-37).

In summary, in type two somatic dysfunction the radiographic findings might include:

1. A spinous process rotated out of the mid vertebral position.

2. Pedicles that appear to have different sizes or shapes.

3. Transverse processes on the inside of the curve spread farther apart and seeming larger.

4. Transverse processes on the outside of the curve spread farther apart and seeming larger.

5. A possible *flat spot* on the flexion/extension films (Figure 4-38).

### Changes on Magnetic Resonance Imaging & Computed Tomography

Type two somatic dysfunction might be suspected from the appearance of asymmetry in MRI and CT images. Since the upper vertebral body of the "short-curve scoliosis" is sidebent and rotated in the transverse plane, the changes will be reflected in the images. The rotation will appear to be a spinous process of the upper vertebra *not* in line with the rest of the spinous processes. The transverse processes will be inclined relative to the bottom of the film. The side bending will appear to be one transverse process, seeming to be more "imaged" than the other, or not equally sliced. Disc bulging may be seen posteriorly on the inside of the curve of the side bending. Zygoapophyseal joint asymmetry may be present in marked cases, and in chronic cases, osteoarthritis changes develop (Figure 4-39).

It is not possible to see changes with flexion and extension on MRI or CT because the gantry always is horizontal. The clinician will have noted if the patient has difficulty lying flat, but when the patient is made to lie as flat as possible for the study, a number of incidental observations may give graphic clues to the presence of type two somatic dysfunction. This dysfunction, as previously mentioned, causes side bending and rotation at one level, and because the patient may not be able to lie straight, the spine will not image symmetrically, the pelvic ring will be affected with asymlocation, and the coronal views might slice the sacrum tangentially. It should be remembered that the spine functions as a whole, including the pelvis. Through tensegrity the artificial straightening of the dysfunctional segment distorts the alignment of remote parts—in this case, the pelvis—which, although not weight-bearing, might be more easily repositioned in space.

It is a tautology that somatic dysfunction in the pelvic ring concerns the position of the three bones. It also concerns the position of the three bones within the trunk (as a sausage). This is why computer-assisted reconstitutions of the anatomical relationships in the supine torso can be a source of abundant information, which has so far remained untapped. For instance, the presence of an ilial upslip or downslip is reflected on the transverse images, one side appearing to be sliced lower than the other (Figure 4-40).

It so happens that type two somatic dysfunction is common at L4-L5 but is hard to evaluate on plain films. With MRI and CT images there are, however, many findings. (It is unlikely that these studies would be requisitioned for confirmation of somatic dysfunction in osteopathy or orthopedic medicine, but the images may be available through serendipity from the ubiquitous search for the opprobrious disc).

## Wrist Imaging

Lateral imaging of the wrist for the presence of ligamentous injuries is probably the most useful and powerful tool in diagnosing somatic joint dysfunctions and ligamentous laxity in all radiography. Other films of the wrist, including the radial and ulnar deviation views, also contain significant information regarding the presence of joint dysfunctions. This information should not be overlooked in any individual with upper extremity pain. Often a wrist dysfunction impacts both the elbow and the shoulder. Resolving pain complaints in these areas can become particularly diffi- cult unless wrist joint dysfunctions are treated.

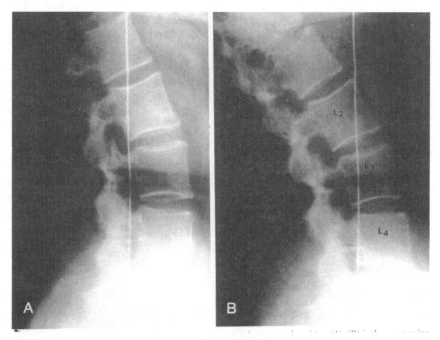

*Figure 4- 38:* Lateral standing view of lumbar spine in a neutral position (A). (B) is the same spine in extension. Note that most of the movement is from L3 and above. L4 vertebra moves only slightly and is therefore "fixed" in flexion.

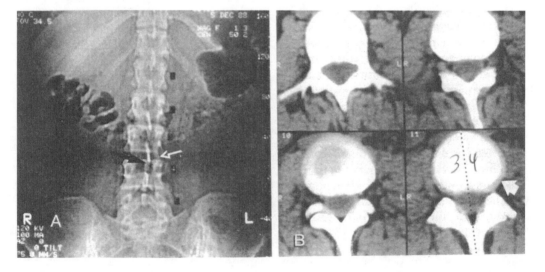

*Figure 4- 39:* A is an anterior-posterior computer reconstructed image showing a type II somatic dysfunction at L3-4. The L3 vertebra is side-bent left and rotated right. Black arrow points to a spinous process that is out of line, and the white arrow points to the disc space, which is compressed on the left side. In (B) note the disc bulging (white arrow). The vertebral bodies appear rotated and this is not an artifact but an essential observation. The dotted line is drawn on the long axis of the L3 vertebra and demonstrates the right rotation in axial plane.

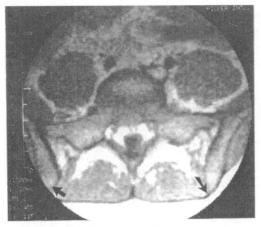

*Figure 4-40:* MRI scan with ilia cut unequally indicating sacral somatic dysfunction (even though the picture is centered on the disc). Note that the ilii (closed arrows) are unequal in size and are at different heights from the table top.

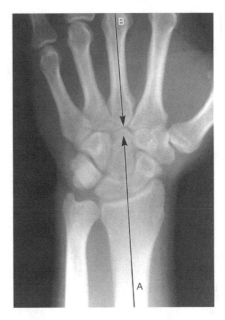

*Figure 4-41:* Wrist with normal alignment.

The lateral wrist film can demonstrate the presence of significant ligamentous injuries just by calculating the radio-scaphoid and the radio-lunate angles. The radio-scaphoid angle is a reflection of the integrity of the scapa-lunate ligament. Laxity of this ligament usually follows a fall with an outstretched hand and a dorsiflexed wrist. Injury to this ligament can have a significant impact on the dynamics of how the entire wrist works. The radio-lunate angle defines the relationship of the lunate to the radius and provides information regarding the status of the bony architecture of the entire wrist.

The posterior to anterior (PA) wrist films also contain important information on the presence of somatic joint dysfunctions, and again attention should be paid to the position of the scaphoid and the lunate (Figure 4-41). The scaphoid should appear to become bigger between radial and ulnar deviation. Lack of changes in its size is a significant finding and suggests the presence of joint dysfunctions of the wrist and possible ligamentous injury (For more information see chapter 10).

## Ankle Imaging

Ankle imaging is as equally important as wrist imaging. Sprained ankles, any inversion injury and almost any ankle injury is capable of creating a tremendous number of somatic dysfunctions and ligamentous injuries. Injuries to the ligament holding the tibia and fibula together (the syndesmosis) are frequent, particularly in sprained ankles. This slight widening of the ankle mortise creates a moderate amount of ankle instability that can sometimes be treated by conservative measures.

Also, since sprained ankles are so common and frequently create joint dysfunctions, assessment of the foot is particularly important. Assessment of foot imaging can best be done by looking at the lateral film for the cyma line. The cyma line is the combination of the curved linear line and the mid tarsal joint line. If this line is present and intact, there are no major foot faults or joint dysfunctions. If however, this line is broken, then either manipulative care, orthotics, injection or acupuncture therapy or at times surgery is indicated.

The lateral film is also capable of generating considerable information about other joint dysfunctions, including the talus and cuboid. During gate, the talus rotates medially and inferiorly to accommodate the tibia. This particular motion of the talus is controlled by powerful ligamentous structures. Injuries to these structures due to a sprained ankle frequently allow this bone to go into internal rotation and slight extension very early in the stance phase, and creates a very unstable foot. On the normal film, this bone should be horizontal. If tipped into a more vertical position, this is an indication of ligamentous laxity and talar instability which could also be interpreted as foot instability.

The cuboid is also quite important in identifying the presence of joint dysfunctions. When in an incorrect position, the cuboid can create a myriad of abnormalities. The correct position demonstrates a clear peroneus longus line, and the calcaneal-cuboid joint lines should align. When these two findings are present the bone is in good position and offers the foot considerable stability.

The cuboid which is the "keystone" of the lateral arch is frequently displaced in sprained ankles and other ankle and foot injuries. Think for a moment of all of the dysfunctions which are created by this single bone dysfunction. The peroneus longus is now being stretched. This causes it to fire early and longer than normal, causing "shin splints". A process of the cuboid lies above the long plantar nerve so when the bone rotates internally this process begins to stretch the nerve. This creates pain which is referred to the distal foot and can sometimes be mistaken for a Morton's neuroma. These foot dysfunctions (also common after motor vehicle injury) and pain crates a limp which can cause pain in the

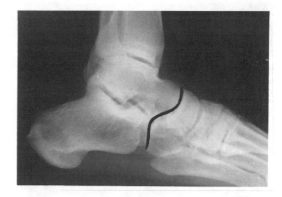

*Figure 4- 42:* Lateral view of foot with cyma line drawn on it.

neck, back and shoulder. (For more information see chapter 11).

**Knee Imaging**

The knee is frequently imaged by plain films, but generally only for identifying major dysfunctions and the presence of degenerative osteoarthritis (Figure 4-43). However, MRI of the knee has proven to be worthwhile (Figure 4-45). Assessment of the meniscus, anterior cruciate ligament, posterior cruciate ligament, the cartilaginous and bony structures adjacent to it can all be made using the MRI. Numerous "blind" areas on MRI of the knee occur but the only option is athroscopic evaluation which is much more invasive. MRI of the knee appears to be the least expensive and perhaps the best overall way to evaluate the knee.

Anterior knee pain, which is a frequent musculoskeletal complaint, can and often does leave radiographic "tracks". The Q angle of the femur and the tibia is an important measurement and is easy to evaluate on X-ray. The sunrise view of the patella is also helpful in the evaluation of anterior knee pain. Anterior knee pain can be due to many reasons that leave little or no radiographic changes, so the use of radiography should be used only after a

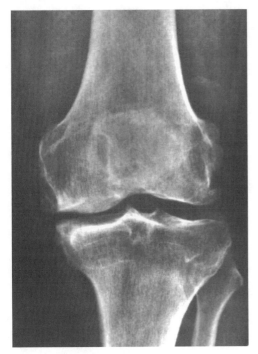

Figure 4- 43:  Degenerative joint disease of the knee.

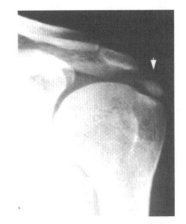

Figure 4- 44: Calcification of supraspinous tendon.

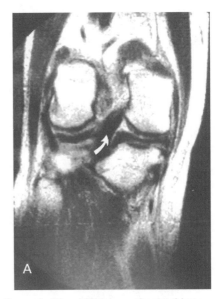

Figure 4- 45:  MRI image of normal knee.

careful physical evaluation is done. (For more information see chapter 11.)

## Shoulder & Elbow Imaging

The shoulder and elbow are frequently talked about as areas to be imaged by plain radiography. However the physical examination in these areas are so superb, and the imaging modalities relatively imprecise, that the X-rays usually are not needed (Figure 4-46). (For more information see chapter 10.)

In summery radiographic imaging can aid the clinician in determine the cause of musculoskeletal pain. Radiographic imaging is also vitally important in excluding other possible medical causes. More information on imaging accompanies following chapters.

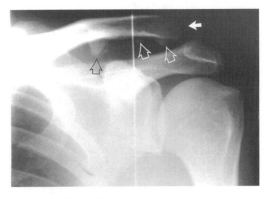

Figure 4- 46:   AP view of shoulder girdle with subluxed acrominoclavicular joint.

# Chapter 5: *Treatment Principles*

Oriental Medicine has many techniques that are useful for addressing both systemic and musculoskeletal disorders, and that are helpful in overall management of musculoskeletal disorders. Proper application of OM methods requires a full OM medical evaluation, several OM and acupuncture methods however, can be performed independently or with minimal knowledge of OM theory. This chapter reviews the treatment techniques used in this text, both OM and other methods.

## Complementary Orthopedics

Depending on the nature of the condition, OM and Complementary treatment of musculoskeletal disorders may include:

- Acupuncture/injection.
- Manual therapy/manipulation.
- Oral and topical herbal or other medications.
- Moxibustion.
- Cupping.
- Stabilization and other exercises.
- Nutritional therapy.
- Orthotics.

## Acupuncture & Dry Needling

For the purposes of this book:

**Acupuncture** is the practice of dry needling according to Oriental Medicine theories that have evolved throughout the development of Oriental medicine.

**Dry needling** is insertion of an acupuncture needle according to neuroanatomical concepts.[1]

The effects of acupuncture, including neurochemical, neurophysiologic, anti-inflammatory and circulatory, have been documented in detail in *The Neurochemical Basis of Pain Relief by Acupuncture* (Han 1987) and *The Vital Meridian A Modern Exploration of Acupuncture* (Bensoussan 1991). Acupuncture is most effective when used in conjunction with its related traditional systems, however, an understanding of energy flow, channel harmony and balance, and constitutional and Organ functions requires considerable training and experience. In this section both traditional and modern explanation of acupuncture (needles use) are included. This is done not only for the sake of understanding the mechanisms of acupuncture but also to provide practitioners with the tools to develop new techniques.

---

1. Although many "dry needling" techniques in this text are based on so called "neuroanatomical" concepts, they are supported by OM theory and needle techniques (see quote from *Simple Questions* on page 291).

## Purposes of Dry Needling

Dry needling is used to strengthen tendons and ligaments, stimulate Golgi receptors and muscle spindles, deactivate trigger points, treat overactive motor points, provide blood and growth factors to hemodynamically disturbed tissues (commonly seen in myofascial pain syndromes), reset motor points and neural control (possibly including replacement of oversensitive tissues with less sensitive microscars), and stimulate other reflex mechanisms.

### Strengthen Tendons & Ligaments

Needling may strengthen soft tissues such as tendons and ligaments by inducing a local inflammatory reaction:

- The mechanical trauma that results from needling may injure cells, including mast cells and vessels.

- Blood products (such as platelet growth factors and transforming growth factor beta) spill and activate healing.

- Amines and other mediators of inflammation are set free or are newly-formed locally, generating an acute inflammatory reaction.

- Plasma seeps into the tissues, possibly allowing blood to reach poorly-vascularized areas such as ligaments and tendons. After a delay of a few hours, the plasma begins to attract polymorphs. In the absence of significant bacterial infection, this leukocytic infiltration is mild and fades quickly.

- Macrophages migrate into the area of inflammation and work to remove red blood cells, fibrin, dead polymorphs and other cellular material. At the same time, with granulocytes, the macrophages work to activate fibroblasts.

- Local fibroblasts begin to hypertrophy and to generate collagen and elastic fibers. If foreign matter such as an injection of pomess (flower) solution is left in place, (or acupuncture suture burial—a TCM surgical technique) it causes a foreign matter response. This response, which includes invasion of giant cells and a strong fibrous reaction, adds strength to the tissue.

CAUTION: The healing process can be delayed and may be weakened: if the blood supply is poor, if the patient is poorly nourished (particularly in the presence of ascorbic acid and zinc deficiency), and if the patient is treated simultaneously with anti-inflammatory medications. Smocking can also affect healing.

### Stimulate Golgi Receptors & Muscle Spindles

Many acupuncture points are based on nerve arrangement. According to Gunn, two types are in muscles, principally in motor points and Golgi tendon organs (Gunn 1977). Rotation of a needle in hypertonic muscle tissues can tug on muscle fibers, not unlike the way thread rolls on a spool. This action seems to stimulate stretch-sensitive Golgi receptors and muscle spindles, which may account for the resulting muscle relaxation.

### Deactivate Trigger Points

Muscle needling may provide blood products and wash away sensitizing substances, brake fibrotic tissue that have entrapped nerve endings, and/or replace hyperactive nociceptors with nonpainful microscars. Travell has reported that active myofascial trigger points can be treated with "dry needling". This also results in muscle relaxation, which reduces mechanical stress on tissues such as tendons, thereby allowing more effective healing.

Jessen et al. (1989) remarks that, even in trigger point injection, the most important factor may not be the injected substance; rather, it may be the mechanical effects of needling on the abnormal tissue and interruption of the trigger point's mechanism, if one has developed.

## Treat Overactive Motor Points

Muscle motor points are points that are packed densely with sensory end-organs, causing muscle to be easily excitable and most liable to tenderness. In his writings on the relationship of motor points to acupuncture points and on their sensitivity to pain, Gunn (1976,1979) says that the practitioner can needle motor points to treat muscular pain and tension. The proposed mechanism is similar to that of needling techniques in other muscle tissues. Gunn postulates that growth factors released by injured cells and platelets also result in healing of mildly-demyelinated nerves.

## Provide Blood & Growth Factors

Chronic muscle tension and spasm can cause reduced oxygen and other nutrient supply. This, in turn, can result in a small area of abnormal function and ectopic muscle facilitation. Bleeding, which can be an effect of needling, can break microscars in these areas, and can provide blood and growth factors to facilitate healing.

## Alter Neural Control

Needling may alter neural control:

- By neurotransmitter and endorphin stimulation.

- By reflex action such as stimulation of inhibitory fibers by a fusimotor mechanism.

- By saturation of joint receptors.

## Stimulate Reflex Mechanisms

Needling cutaneous and other tissues can stimulate various spinal reflexes and serotinergic descending inhibitory systems (see chapter 2). Periosteal acupuncture techniques (Lawrence 1987) are believed to regulate sympathetic fibers in and around the periosteum, increasing blood circulation in the area.

# Acupuncture Mechanisms

Acupuncture points have been described as 2-8mm, cylindrical shaped, perforations within superficial fascia in which a neurovascular bundle runs (Heine 1988). They are intimately related to the distribution of nerve trunks, motor endplates and blood vessels (Dung 1984; Gunn *ibid;* Chan *1984*). Kellner (1966) has shown two types of acupoints, receptor and effector, by histological studies. Therefore, acupuncture effects are closely related to the nervous system and achieved by complex mechanisms which integrate peripheral, ascending, descending and higher centers in the nervous system.

The mechanisms of acupuncture's effects are thought to be largely neurochemical and neurophysiologic.

## Neurochemical Mechanisms

The fact that acupuncture analgesia can be transferred from a treated animal to a nontreated animal (Han 1992) by cross-circulation and CSF infusion to ventricles supports the hypothesis of a systemic neuropharmacologic effect.

## Opioid System

Early reports on the analgesic mechanism of acupuncture involved opioid systems.[1] In 1975, the year endorphins were discovered, David Mayer documented that acupuncture affects the opioid system in his demonstration that, in humans, naloxone can block acupuncture analgesia.[2] Naloxone has also been shown to block the analgesic effect of acupuncture on dental pain (the affects are influenced by dexamethasone levels), (Maver, Price and Rafii 1977).

---

1. These reports may have contributed to, and at least supported, the discovery of the endorphin systems (Han 1986).

2. Naloxone is a chemical that can block opioid receptors.

The newly discovered orphanin (opioid peptide) seems to have antagonistic effects on electroacupuncture analgesia (Han 1998).

The analgesic effects of acupuncture can be enhanced by D-phenylalanine and D-leucine, which enhance met-enkephalin degradation (Ehrenpreis 1985; Han 1991), or by bacitracin[3] (Zhang, Tang and Han 1981).[4] In a review, Pomeranz et al. (1977) concluded that acupuncture analgesia implicates the pituitary endorphins. They postulate that this is so, because placebo acupuncture is not as effective, the analgesic effect of acupuncture can be eliminated by ablation of the pituitary gland, and that naloxone is effective in blocking the analgesic effects of acupuncture.

### Non-Opioid Systems

Non-opioid systems are affected by acupuncture (see chapter 2 as well).

• Serotonin (5-HT), norepinephrine, GABA, calcium and magnesium ions, and secondary central cyclic nucleotides (Han 1987), and acetylcholine have been implicated in acupuncture analgesia (Guan, Yu, Wng and Liu 1986).

• Dopamine is implicated in inhibition of acupuncture analgesia (Patterson 1986).

• Anti-inflammatory effects have been elicited by stimulation of 17-hydroxy-corticosterone, ACTH and cortisol secretion (Ying 1976; Omura 1976; O'Connor 1981).

Inflammatory mediators can affect pain perception as beta-endorphin levels can be affected by ACTH. This is because ACTH can antagonize the enzyme cleavage from a large, precursor, pro-opiomelancortin (Smock and Fields

---

3. Bacitracin is a peptidase inhibitor (a D-amino acid), the injection of which results in increased neuropeptides.

4. Met-enkephalin degradation results in a net gain in opioid-like chemicals.

1980). Sin has summarized these anti-inflammatory effects of acupuncture (Sin 1984).

## Neurophysiologic & Other Mechanisms

Neurophysiologic mechanisms involve sensory nerves stimulated at the acupuncture point. The afferent systems seem to be important in acupuncture analgesia, and needle sensation (De Qi) is required for successful treatment of pain (Han *ibid*). Preacupuncture local anesthesia, of subcutaneous and muscle tissue, abolishes the needling sensation and acupuncture's analgesic effects (Chiang et al. 1973). This suggests that receptors within the muscle are responsible for the De Qi sensation, probably do to A-beta and A-delta fibers (Pomeranz and Paley 1979; Wang, Yao, Xian and Hou 1985).

Low threshold large diameter mechanoreceptors situated in the skin, muscles, tendons and joints are activated by innocuous stimuli that may activate the "gate control" mechanism. Acupuncture stimulates A-beta and A-delta (small and medium) fibers which enter the spinal cord and arrive at the medial and lateral portions of the dorsal horn. A-beta fibers terminate in the nucleus propius and in more ventral regions of the dorsal grey matter. A-delta fibers terminate in the marginal zones of the dorsal grey matter, the ventral portion of lamina II and throughout lamina III and inhibit dorsal horn cells at laminae I and V (Yaksh and Hammond 1982; Dorman and Gage 1982).

Analgesic effects that result from stimulation of small, myelinated fibers are transmitted both segmentally and bilaterally (Chiang et al. 1973, 1975). C-fibers do not seem to contribute significantly and application of capsicum, which selectively blocks C-fibers, does not affect acupuncture analgesia (Yu, Bao, Zhou and Han 1978).

## The Thalamus

The thalamus is thought to be the most important component responsible for the processing of pain impulses and/or integration of pain sensation. The centromedian nucleus of the thalamus, the rephe magnus nucleus, and the arcuate nucleus seem to be the main areas related to acupuncture analgesia (Zang 1980; Hamba and Toda 1988; Yin, Duanmu, Guo and Yu1984). Peripheral stimulation of an acupuncture point was observed to stimulate thalamic neurons with a similar pattern in a cat (Linzer and Van Atta 1975).

## Descending & Ascending Tracts

Innocuous stimulation of peripheral nerves may excite descending inhibitory serotinergic tracts that then can inhibit nociceptors (Bowsher 1991). The descending dorsolateral funiculus of the spinal cord seems to be involved in acupuncture analgesia. Lesions made at T1-T3 levels resulted in complete abolition of acupuncture analgesia (Shen, Tsai and Lan 1975). Lacerating the contralateral anterolateral columns eradicated the analgesic effect from stimulation of St-36, whereas, laceration of the dorsal column at the level of T-12-L1 or superficial lateral cordectomy did not affect acupuncture analgesia (Chiang et al. 1975). Cephalically, impulses produced by acupuncture analgesia are believed to be transmitted through the extralemniscal system, then to the thalamus and the sensory cortex.[5]

---

5. The lemniscus is a bundle of sensory fibers in the medulla and pons.

## Convergence of Visceral & Somatic Innervation

Experimental data that demonstrates the existence of convergence of visceral and somatic innervation in laminae V-VII may support the rationale for use of many manual and acupuncture therapies in somato-visceral and visceral-somatic pain. Electrical stimulation of the skin (acupuncture points) has been shown to influence nerves within gray matter (Selzer and Spencer 1969), and so may influence visceral function. Moreover, visceral pain has superficial receptive fields (irritation zones that can be mistaken for musculoskeletal pain) that can be activated by noxious and innocuous stimulation, and by muscle activity beneath the skin (Forman and Ohata 1980; Cervero 1982). Stimulation of acupuncture points at superficial receptive fields may provoke a reflex mechanism that may explain the empirical data about the effectiveness of acupuncture. Reflex mechanisms may also explain why the use of distal acupuncture points affects visceral pain.

## The Autonomic Nervous System

Most authors agree that acupuncture points posses lower skin impedance (Kho and Arnold 1997). Electrical skin resistance (impedance) can be demonstrated and measured using simple devices. Many diagnostic instruments used in acupuncture measure skin impedance for the purpose of diagnosing, treating, and following treatment results. Increased pseudomotor activity (increased perspiration from sympathetic activity) lowers skin impedance, which has been documented over injured areas and in segmental distributions (including from visceral disease), (Korr et al. 1962). Acupuncture diagnostic devices use this information in the selection of channels and points to be treated. However, the reliability of these instruments is questionable for various technical difficulties, and because the act of measuring (which passes an electrical charge through the skin) actually changes the impedance.[6]

Acupuncture points on the Urinary Bladder, upper Stomach and Large Intestine channels are in close proximity to the sympathetic ganglia, stimulation of which may affect the autonomic nervous system.

Using thermography, acupuncture's effect of increasing skin temperature locally, contralaterally, and in other regions has been documented (Lee and Ernst 1987, 1983; Ernst and Lee 1985). Ernst and colleagues have demonstrated long-lasting warming effects, as well. In some instances the temperature distribution was in a craniocaudal gradient, which they speculated was mediated by the reticular formation via the activation of diffuse noxious inhibitory controls on the convergent cells of the dorsal horn. Liao and Liao (1985) have demonstrated that stimulation of acupoint St-36 affected the leg of a stroke patient: producing a small temperature increase in the normal leg and a marked increase in both hands.

The circulatory effects and the decrease of hypersympathetic activity in pain patients is probably one of acupuncture's most important clinical effects.

---

6.  The instrument applies electrical charge across the skin in order to measure skin residence. This can change the properties and resistance of the skin. Some newer instruments may be more reliable.

## Immune Effects

Sabolovic and Michon have found stimulation of T and B lymphocytes by acupuncture (Sabolovic and Michon 1978). By influencing met-enkephalins, acupuncture can increase T lymphocyte rosette formation from human T lymphocytes (Wybran et al. 1979). Acupuncture has been shown to increase beta-globulins, gamma-globulins, lysozymes, agglutinins, opsonins and complement (Dragomirescu et al. 1961). Acupuncture influences beta-endorphins and met-enkephalins, both of which may enhance natural killer cell activity (Matthews et al. 1984).

## Electrical Effects

Several electrical and electromagnetic theories have been proposed. Robert Becker associated cellular polarity and DC currents with growth, healing and regeneration of tissues, including articular cartilage (Becker and Marino 1982; Becker 1972). Burr (1972) suggested that all events in the body generate electro-dynamic fields, The bioelectrical homeostasis and its relation to acupuncture was reviewed by Zukauskas et al. (1988) and Zhu Zong-Xiang (1981).

# *Acupuncture Therapeutic Systems & Techniques*

## Channel Therapies

The channels—the pathways that carry Qi, Blood and body fluids throughout the body—provide for the free flow of Yin and Yang, and serve as a conduit for communications between all parts of the body. The classic *Yellow Emperor* describes 365 acupuncture points on the Main channels that correspond with the number of days in the year. Over time the number of points has grown and now stands at several thousands. In practice however, individual clinicians probably use an average of a hundred points or so.

In this section, the term *channel therapy* is used to describe a variety of ways of treating the body via the channel system. The Major points, described below, can be used to activate the channels and are often sufficient to attain a clinical response.

### Channel Treatment Design

Treatment must always follow the individual condition of each patient. The major differential diagnosis questions, which always must be considered, are whether the disorder is Full or Empty and whether the patient's constitution is deficient or strong. These determine the appropriate technique. The channels can then be treated from the more superficial Sinews channels to the deep Main, Divergent and Extra channels according to the location of the disease and condition of the patient. A simple therapeutic program, or needling input, can be achieved by selecting the main activating points for the particular channel at the energetic level being affected. For example, early after injury or if the condition results from external

pathogenic factors, the Sinews channels can be used first. As, and if, the symptoms progress, or if there is bleeding and/or edema, treatment directed to the Connecting channels can be added, in order to prevent further progression of pathogenic factors and eliminate Blood stagnation. If symptoms begin to expand and involve larger areas the Main channels are integrated into the treatment plan. In late and chronic stages when significant tissue pathology is present, or if the patient is weak and has Organic involvement, the Divergent and Extra channels may be emphasized.

### *Electroacupuncture*

The use of electricity to augment the therapeutic effects of acupuncture has a long history. In 1765 a Japanese acupuncturist, Gennai Hiaga, reported the use of electrical stimulation on acupuncture needles. In 1825 the French physician, Chevlier Sarlndiere, described the application of an electric current applied to acupuncture needles to treat rheumatic conditions. Since the 1950s practitioners in the Orient have been using, and researching, the use of electroacupuncture extensively.

In musculoskeletal practice, electrical stimulation is used often with the appropriate electrode placed at the points that activate the applicable channel system. In general, the cathode (-) pole is considered to have a tonifying effect.[7] Often, for Sinews channel treatment the cathode (-) pole is used at the distal areas and the anode (+) pole is used on the proximal areas. Electrical stimulation can be used to facilitate circulation (tonify), or inhibit circulation (sedate) within the channel. To promote circulation the cathode (-) pole is used close to the origin of the channel (points with lower numbers) and the anode (+)

---

7.  Most acupuncture stimulators are biphasic and do not have true polarity. Some instruments have a modified wave which stimulates one pole for a longer duration (monopolar) and therefore have a polar bias. DC stimulation can result in burns and usually is not used.

pole down stream.[8] To sedate, the electrodes are switched and the anode (+) pole is used close to the origin of the channel. Electrical stimulation is used together with local or special function points to channel the energy to, and through the lesion.

Lower intensity stimulation of 2mA seems to be better than higher intensity stimulation (3mA) for the treatment of chronic pain from inflammation and neuropathic origin (Han 1998), (for more information see electrical stimulation chapter 5).

*Orthopedic Integration*

Acupuncture treatments also can be based on modern orthopedic evaluations, which enables the treatment to be more lesion specific. Functional and structural assessment are then used to determine which channel or local tissue is to be treated.

Channel (distal) therapy and local-needling therapy are dependent on palpatory findings. Tissue texture changes are highly significant in determining which channel or local tissue is affected and where the needle is to be placed. This contrasts with Orthopaedic Medicine, in which local tissue texture and tenderness are less important (see referred pain chapter 2). Therefore, when using Orthopaedic Medicine diagnostic information (which can yield a lesion-specific finding, i.e., a small lesion which is responsible for a wide range of symptoms and signs), needling input is very specific, and depends on provocation and functional testing, and is less dependent on local palpation for tenderness (in the area of symptoms).

When spinal joint dysfunctions reoccur frequently the channel that is associated with the level of dysfunction can be assessed and treated. For example, if frequent dysfunction occurs at L-5 the Large Intestine channel can be assessed and treated if appropriate,[9] especially for flexion restriction. For extension restrictions

the coupled Lung channel may be treated, as well.

*Energy Circulation*

Circulation of energy throughout the channel system is paramount for health, the loss of which leads to disease and pain. Without proper circulation the channels can become empty of Qi and Blood, or they can develop areas of stagnation and fullness. Because of the Yin and Yang laws of nature, a deficiency state must be accompanied by an accommodating excess. The opposite is true in the presence of excess. Both should be addressed.

**CHANNEL OBSTRUCTION.** In OM, all pain results from obstruction in the channels. As the old saying goes: "Tong ze bu tong; Bu tong ze tong." (If there is free flow, there is no pain; If there is no free flow, there is pain.) Therefore, mobilization of Qi and Blood (or the affected structure) is the treatment most likely to unblock the channels and treat pain.

The channel and subchannel therapies in this section can be performed without extensive OM diagnostic evaluation or extensive knowledge of specific acupuncture point functions. Although these methods are highly effective for musculoskeletal applications by themselves, without OM diagnostic and treatment techniques they are less effective for addressing root causes, and may result in only temporary improvement.

**CHANNEL ACTIVATION/DOWNWARD DRAINING.** Channel activation is probably the most common therapy used for many musculoskeletal disorders. The technique can be used by itself; or in conjunction with other methods. The practitioner:

1. Needles tender and abnormal points in and around the painful area.

---

8. DC electricity flows from the (-) to the (+) pole.

9. The back Shu (Transport) points of the Large Intestine is at L5.

**2.** Usually needles 1-2 points more downstream on the affected channels.

Most often the Accumulating, Connecting and/or Spring points are used.

**3.** Often combined with:

Command points to activate appropriate channel.

Well point to activate the Sinews channels. Reflex points (ear, wrist and ankle, etc.) to activate analgesia of affected area.

## Locating Points

Locating points is an acquired art. As with all physical medicine arts, it demands palpatory vocabulary and finger sensitivity.

Most often, acupuncture points are located on the body surface in depressions between muscles,[10] tendons and other soft tissues. Frequently these points have a different tissue sensibility. The depression may have a firm or soft texture, the area may feel damp or relatively dry. At times, heat or some type of vibration can be sensed just over the point. Pathological (congested) points (often non channel points i.e. Ashi or trigger points) may feel indurated and hard.

10. The word acupoint in Chinese means a hole or depression.

### Slide Finger Lightly Over Surface

One way for the practitioner to locate an acupuncture point is to slide a finger over the surface around the anatomical region where a point is said to be located, until feeling a depression. Little force should be used when making contact with the patient's skin, because the depression may present either as a physical trough or as a sudden loss of tissue elasticity. Acupuncture points are tender frequently.

### Subcutaneous Point

To assess the condition of acupuncture points at the subcutaneous level the practitioner presses the skin, taking up the slack between the skin and subcutaneous tissues, and moves the skin over the subcutaneous tissue. This may reveal indurated pathological areas and acupoints.

### Points Move

Textbooks describe the location of acupuncture points as "fixed," measured in body inches (*cuns*) from body landmarks that often are skin creases and/or bony, tendinous and muscular areas.[11] These point locations only serve as guides. Points move constantly, and personal variations occur. Figure 5-1 illustrates regional cun measurements.

11. A body inch (cun) is defined as the width of the patient's thumb, or as the distance between the ends of the patient's interphalangeal creases on the radial surface of the middle finger. The distance between the outer edge of the index finger and the outer edge of the little finger is said to be three inches.

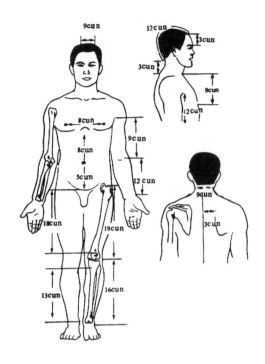

*Figure 5-1:*   Cun measurements.

## Principles for Selecting Techniques & Points

Creating a treatment plan is an intellectual and a tactile process. In general, the practitioner selects points and techniques that correspond to the condition. Sensitive points and channels are emphasized over theoretical points. The practitioner:

- Needles the appropriate level and reaches the lesion.

  — needles superficially for superficial syndromes (in muscle and skin) and when the patient reacts strongly to light pressure, or if the pulse is floating.

  — needles deeply if a lesion is deep (in a tendon or bone) and if the patient likes deep pressure or the pain

increases on deep pressure or the pulse is submerged.

- Needles superficially and uses bleeding techniques for Hot conditions.

  — if the pulse is quick, removes needle after obtaining Qi.

- Needles deeply and uses moxibustion for Cold and deficient conditions.

- Needles contralaterally in the spaces (valleys) between the muscles for pain of unfixed location and that moves around (Wind.)

- Bleeds the collaterals (superficial and deep blood vessels, Connecting points) and then needles St 36 for a chronic Painful Obstruction Disorder (Bi) that has been refractory to other treatments.

- Treats a single channel for acute disorders (may be sufficient). Treats several channels in chronic disorders.

- Chooses points that have a wide therapeutic range and activate multiple systems, such as P-6.

  — P-6 is the command point for the Yin Wei channel and regulates the Pericardium channel. It opens the chest, calms the spirit and regulates the autonomic nervous system.

  — Sp-6 connects the three leg Yin channels.

  — TB-8 connects the three arm Yang channels etc.

- Chooses extremity points for their dynamic and activating properties.

- Uses points unilaterally to vitalize Qi and Blood, thereby alleviating pain and facilitating movement.

- Uses points bilaterally to tonify and strengthen.

- Disperses indurated, hard and sensitive points.

- Tonifies or applies moxa on soft unresilient and depressed points.

- Treats men first on the left side and women on the right side. Or treats the side where the pulses are stronger first.

- Treats points generally from Yang to Yin, i.e., from the back to front, from top to bottom. The needles can be withdrawn in the same way.

However, in deficiency, needles from bottom up and front to back

— treats Alarm points first followed by back Shu points.

### Acute (Yang) Disorders

For acute (Yang) disorders such as for patients who have constant pain, inflammation (tenderness, swelling and warmth) and guarding, or for patients who have local pain and otherwise are strong and healthy, the practitioner uses acupuncture, electroacupuncture or ion cords

(Table 5-1). If points on Yang channels are strongly sedated it is a good idea to tonify a point on the paired Yin channels, in order to protect the patient vitality, especially in old and weak patients.

### Chronic (Yin) Disorders

For chronic disorders such as for patients who have intermittent pain, no obvious inflammation, pain mostly during some movement but not in others (dysfunction), and/or mild local tenderness that pressure seems to relieve, the practitioner uses acupuncture or electroacupuncture as indicated in Table 5-2.

*Table 5-1.* **ACUTE (YANG) DISORDERS**

| | |
|---|---|
| Acupuncture | The practitioner:<br>Uses many local needles at the site of pain (stronger stimulation or positive pole electrostimulation).<br>1. Applies a sedating needling technique.<br>2. Leaves the needles in place until local erythema diminishes.<br>3. Uses bleeding techniques. |
| Electroacupuncture | Indicated frequently. The practitioner:<br>Uses strong stimulation, usually at the connecting point, to activate the channel and drain the area.<br>• Applies the anode (+) pole locally and the cathode (-) pole distally<br>or<br>• Uses the cathode (-) pole locally to push energy through.<br>   (The frequency can be set to 100-200Hz, alternating with a low 2-4 Hz.) |
| Ion Cords | Can use ion cords to direct energy through the channel. Uses the open side of the diode locally. |

*Table 5-2.* **YIN DISORDERS**

| | |
|---|---|
| | The practitioner:<br>1. Uses few local needles, at the site of pain.<br>2. Applies a tonifying needling technique (mild stimulation, moxa or negative pole electrostimulation).<br>3. Leaves needles in place for no more then 10 minutes.<br>4. Uses moxa to warm and push the energy and blood through the channel. |
| Electroacupuncture | The practitioner:<br>• Uses mild stimulation: the cathode (-) pole locally, the anode (+) distally, at the source point to add local energy and open blockage of the channel.<br>or<br>• Uses mild stimulation: the cathode (-) pole distally, the anode (+) locally, to activate the channel. (Frequency can be set to 2 Hz, if needed, alternating with 75-100 Hz.) |

*Balancing of Yin & Yang*

In general, the goal of acupuncture is to harmonize (balance) the Yin and Yang. The balancing of Yin and Yang has several aspects, such as balancing top and bottom, left and right, anterior and posterior, Qi and Blood, etc. Balancing general areas of the body originated early (before the Five Phases theory) when numeric systems dominated Chinese philosophy (as used in Tong-Style acupuncture). Even numbers were considered Yin and odd numbers Yang. Numbers were assigned to different areas. Acupuncture points were chosen based on the number and location of symptoms.

**BALANCING TOP AND BOTTOM.** Points can be treated in a balanced fashion. For example, when treating tennis elbow, the practitioner can balance LI-11 with a contralateral needle at St-36. This combination (on similar energetic levels, both being on Yang Ming) can both strengthen the treatment and balance the top/bottom energetic imbalance (especially in chronic cases).

> NOTE: Some systems, Tong-style acupuncture for example, do not combine top and bottom points and consider it detrimental.

When using many points which are either on the upper or lower parts of the body, the practitioner may want to balance these with a point on the opposite level.

Balancing top and bottom is usually not necessary in acute conditions when mobilization of Qi is more important [at the moment]. Mobilization of Qi can be accomplished by choosing a point contralateral to the area of symptoms, vitalizing Qi and Blood through the affected area.

**BALANCING LEFT AND RIGHT.** Left and right imbalances are common, as both stagnation and deficiency can manifest on one side of the channel and result in a Yin Yang reaction. Disorders that affect the left side are considered Yang; disorders that affect the right side are considered Yin. Therefore, it is common to choose points on the left side for men (men are usually more Yang) and on the right side for women (women are usually more Yin).

In treatment of left/right imbalances, the Extra and Divergent channels are particularly useful—especially the Yang Motility (Qiao), Yin Motility (Qiao), Conception (CV) and Governing (Du) Extra channels. When treating men the practitioner can choose an extra channel command point on the left and its coupled point on the right. When treating women, the practitioner can choose an extra channel command point on the right and its coupled point on the left.

Needling sensitive points on one side and applying moxa on less sensitive points on the other side can be useful. Using a Yang channel on one side with a Yin pair on the other side is common, as excess in one often results in deficiency of the other. The ear point Master Oscillation is useful, as well.

**BALANCING ANTERIOR AND POSTERIOR.** To balance the dorsal and ventral aspects of the body, the Urinary Bladder and Governing (Du) channel can be treated first, followed by ventral/anterior channels. Treating back Shu (Transport) and Alarm (Mu) points and connecting them with an ion-cord or electrical stimulator is a good way to balance the anterior and posterior somatic aspects.

Treating the Connecting channels, which connect the exterior aspects of the channels with the interior aspects, also balances the ventral and dorsal aspects.

The Girdle (Dai) channel encircles the trunk and balances the ventral/dorsal, and top/bottom somatic aspects.

**BALANCING QI AND BLOOD.** To balance Qi and Blood the practitioner can combine points on channels that have more Qi with points on channels that have more Blood. Points on channels with more Blood may be bled when excessive, or moxa may be used to build the Blood when deficient. Adding a point on the Yang Ming channel makes it possible to balance both Qi and

Table 5-3. **CHANNEL QI/BLOOD BALANCE**

| Channels | Balance of Qi and Blood |
|---|---|
| Tai Yin LU and Sp | More Qi and Less Blood |
| Yang Ming LI and St | More Qi and More Blood |
| Shao Yin H and K | More Qi and Less Blood |
| Tai Yang UB and SI | Less Qi and More Blood |
| Jue Yin Liv and P | Less Qi and More Blood |
| Shao Yang GB and TW | More Qi and Less Blood |

Blood, as Yang Ming channels have more Qi and more Blood. Table 5-3 lists the channel's balance of Qi and Blood.

*Pain All Over*

Vague and defuse pain is most often due to Blood emptiness, together with Penetrating (Chong) channel disorders. Dampness and external Wind can be a cause, as well. Blood emptiness results in drying of Sinews and formation of Internal Wind. Symptoms are chronic and associated with paleness and dizziness. Treatment is aimed at tonifying the Qi and Blood, and subduing Wind. Point such as:

- St-36, 37, Sp-6, 10, 4, 21, LI-11, Lu-7, UB-11, 17, 20, GB-34, and 20 can be used.
- For Dampness St-40, Sp-9, 21, 6, CV-9, 12, GB-34 and P-6 can be used.
- For External Wind (sudden onset) GB-20, 31, 34, UB-62, 11, 16, LI-4 and TB-5 can be used.
- SP-21 which is the master of all the Connecting channels is used often for any of the above conditions.
- Sp-4 and P-6 are used to activate the Penetrating (Chong) channel, ie. Blood. Lu-7 and K-6 can be used as well.

**Frequency & Number of Treatments**

The ideal frequency of acupuncture treatment for musculoskeletal and other condi-tions has not yet been established. The half-life of acupuncture analgesia is 15 to 17 minutes in humans and 7.5-13 minutes in rabbits (Han 1986; Han Zhou and Xuan 1983 McLennan H, Gilfillan and Heap 1977). In other animal studies some analgesic effects last about 48 hours. An additional treatment after 48 hours has a cumulative effect (Han *ibid*). Other effects, such as circulatory often last for shorter durations, although long-term effects have been demonstrated, as well. It therefore makes sense to treat the patient every other day for the first few treatments and then reduce the frequency.

In China patients are frequently treated daily for long periods and perhaps this is the reason for the high success rates reported in the Chinese literature. It is possible that frequent treatments reinforces physiologic memory, as frequent sensory experiences can result in strengthening of synaptic connections.[12] When treating patients every day or every other day, it is better to alternate points, as overusing a point depletes its Qi and Blood (in animal studies daily treatment does not offer any advantage over treatment every other day).

Generally, patients show some improvement within four visits; however, some do not until 10 to 15 visits. Patients who do not show significant improvement

---

12. Long-term potentiation (LTP) is characterized by enhanced transmission at synapses that follow high-frequency stimulation (see chapter 2).

by the 15th treatment would probably not benefit from any further treatment.

NOTE: The above guidelines do not apply when techniques that rely on the regeneration of soft tissues (after strong periosteal acupuncture for ligaments and tendons) are used. In these cases it may take up to several months before the results can be assessed, as many patients report improvement two to three months later—even in difficult cases with chronic mild instabilities. The treatment course usually is 10-15 treatments.

## Adverse Effects & Complications

Complications from acupuncture are quite rare. The most common side effects are *drowsiness* and *fatigue* immediately following a treatment. These effects can be minimized by reducing the number of points and duration of treatment. Patients should be warned and if need be should take some time before driving or operating dangerous equipment. In rare cases, some patients experience an energizing effect that can result in a euphoric and almost manic state. These patients report difficulty sleeping after treatments. In these patients needling St-36, P-8, and moxa on K-1 at the end of the treatment session can prevent such complications.

### Vasovagal Reactions

Vasovagal reactions (light-headedness, fainting and nausea) are frequently encountered with new patients, especially when treating the upper body (GB-21). It is more common in slender and young patients and is rare in the elderly. Strong pressure on the lower abdomen is helpful and extract powder of Ginger made into tea quickly resolves any residual feelings of nausea and light-headedness.

### Bleeding & Bruising

Bleeding and bruising can result from deep and strong techniques (and may be induced on purpose). These are almost never severe or bothersome. A history of a bleeding disorder or use of anti-clotting medications may be a relative contraindication. Ginseng and Pseudoginseng (Tian Qi) can be prescribed for such patients to minimize the risk of bleeding with only minimal effect on thrombin time or blood viscosity.

### Serious Complications

More serious complications, such as *pneumothorax*, *punctured viscera* and *infections*, can occur. However, with proper technique these risks are minute. A Medline computer search at Copenhagen University's library of medicine, after deleting reports with inadequate or questionable descriptions and duplicate articles, showed 41 published reports of adverse effects attributed to acupuncture for the years 1980 through 1995. These were pneumothorax (most frequent), bacterial endocarditis, hepatitis, cardiac tamponade, and injury due to broken needle tips (Rosted 1996). Considering the sheer volume of acupuncture treatments performed in Europe per year, acupuncture can be considered extremely safe.

## Needling Techniques

Inserting and manipulating needles is a skill that demands practice. The insertion and manipulation can be performed in many ways, using techniques that vary according to tradition and personal preference. Although acupuncture is often thought of as the stimulation of specific points at or near the skin, the classic literature often referred to needling of anatomical tissues as well (see quote from *Simple Questions* page 291).

Even a beginner can achieve a painless insertion by using a guide (a hollow tube, usually supplied with the needles); the practitioner quickly taps the needle into the subcutaneous layer. After the needle is inserted, the practitioner can manipulate the needle until the De Qi is sensed.

### Obtaining De Qi

Obtaining De Qi is necessary for Chinese-style acupuncture treatment to succeed. The patient senses the arrival of Qi as a dull ache, tingling, warmth, chill, distention, electriclike movement, or other "strange" sensations. Japanese acupuncture systems often use sensationless (by patient) techniques, especially when tonifying or strengthening.

Generally, the practitioner first decides whether the desired stimulation is to be supplementing or dispersing, which determines the depth and direction of needle insertion. Stimulation continues until the practitioner feels the De Qi sensation as tissue resistance to needle manipulation (necessary with Japanese techniques as well), and until the patient indicates feeling the arrival of Qi. Normally, unless electricity or stronger stimulation is needed, once De Qi arrives no further needle stimulation is needed.

### Tonification & Sedation

Many techniques are available for achieving tonification and sedation. Throughout history the methods described have contradicted each other (O'Connor and Bensky 1981). In older texts consideration was given to the day of the month, patient's date of birth and respiratory cycles. For example, in the classic *Divine Pivot*, sedation/dispersion was contraindicated at the time of the new moon, and tonification/supplementation contraindicated when the moon was full.

Recently, a Japanese physician, Prof. Nishijo (Tanaka 1996), has suggested that superficial needling during exhalation, in a sitting subject, results in long-lasting parasympathetic activation evident in longlasting reduced heart rate (exhalation is a parasympathetic dominated phase of respiration; the heart rate slows down). This technique can be thought of as *tonification*. The sympathetic system is said to be activated by needling more deeply, with the patient lying down, and during both inhalation and exhalation (i.e., continues stimulation). Low-frequency, 1 Hz electro-stimulation can be added. The points used are said to be irrelevant.[13]

**TONIFICATION/SUPPLEMENTATION.** The most accepted guidelines for tonification are:

1. Use a thin needle.

2. Prepare the point by massaging in the direction of the channel.

3. Inserts the needle:
   Along the direction of channel flow.
   Slowly and as painlessly as possible.
   During exhalation.
   Superficially first, then
   more deeply only after obtaining Qi.

4. Leave the needle in position 0-15 minutes. Longer retention is possible, but the patient may become fatigued.

5. Withdraw the needles quickly (from the inferior to superior points), during inhalation.

6. Immediately apply pressure to the point to prevent Qi from escaping.

Electrical stimulation with the cathode (-) pole at the point can be used. (Place the anode (+) upstream on the channel).

**NOTE:** Japanese practitioners often emphasize painless and shallow techniques with little stimulation.

**SEDATION/DISPERSION.** The most accepted guidelines for sedation are:

1. Use a thicker needle.

2. Insert the needle:
   In the direction against the channel flow.
   Quickly and deeply.

---

13. This author finds this technique helpful, at times, in the treatment of painful disorders, using normal point selection.

During inhalation.

**3.** After obtaining De Qi, pull the needle out somewhat.

**4.** Leave the needle in position 10-45 minutes. (Stimulate stronger and longer than for tonification).

**5.** Withdraw the needle slowly (from superior to inferior points), during exhalation.

**6.** Do not apply pressure to the point (allow Qi to escape).

Electrical stimulation with the anode (+) pole at the point can be used. The cathode (-) can be placed up the channel.

### Point Injection (Fluid Acupuncture)

Point injection is a common modern OM technique used for both its systemic and local effects. Both modern pharmaceuticals and traditional herbs are injected.[14] The practitioner:

**1.** Selects a point in the vicinity of the lesion.

**2.** Injects directly into the lesion.

**3.** Injects Shu points to strengthen.
    For injection, commonly used medicines are:
    Radix Angelicae Sinensis (Dang Quai)
    Flos Carthami (Hong Hua)
    Radix Ligustici Wallichii (Chuan Xiang)
    Dextrose
    Procaine
    Steroids/Licorice.

### Prolotherapy

Prolotherapy is a biomedical technique that uses injections for the purpose of tightening and strengthening loose or weak ligaments, tendons, or joint capsules through the multiplication and activation of fibroblasts. The most common proliferant used is a 15% dextrose solution that when injected results in an osmotic gradient and cell dehydration.[15] The resulting inflammation activates a fibroblastic healing response. A before and after biopsy and strength studies show increased ligament size and strength (Dorman *ibid*).

# Main Channels

Treatments that use the 12 Main channels vary, depending on style and tradition and on the patient's condition. Points on the Main channels can be used in Five Transporting (Phases) treatments and in other channel therapies, as well.

The practitioner can select points on the Main channels based on the points':

- Traditional functions (e.g., strengthen the Spleen, eliminate Dampness, move the bowels).

- Physical location, channel therapy (Table 5-4 on page 237).

- Placement within the channel energetic flow (e.g., Well (Jing), Spring (Ying), Stream (Shu), River (Jing), Sea (He) points), (Table 5-6 on page 238).

- Main activating points (Well (Jing) points for Sinew channels, commend points of Extra channels, etc.).

- Five Phases theory (Table 5-16 on page 249).

- Experience points (page 250).

---

14. In China point injection is used commonly for treatment of musculoskeletal and other disorders.

15. Dextrose injected into ligaments and acupoints is used in modern TCM for similar conditions.

*Table 5-4.* QUALITIES OF QI WITHIN THE CHANNELS

| | |
|---|---|
| **WELL/JING** | Has *greatest* Yin-Yang *polarity* and the least amount of energy. Located at the nail area where each channel's Qi emerges. |
| **SPRING/YING** | As Qi begins to trickle and accumulate, it takes shape here, much as a gushing, babbling brook takes form. Here Qi *gains* a great deal of *momentum*, begins to surge; however, since the channel is still constricted in size, the Qi's transporting power is limited. |
| **STREAM/SHU** | Flow grows and becomes large enough to *carry* and *transport*. Continues to Jing (River) points. |
| **RIVER/JING** | Qi, channel size and momentum are great enough to *traverse* great *distances*. |
| **SEA/HE** | Finally the Qi arrives at the Sea/ He points, where the channel's Qi *unites* with the Qi of the associated *organ*. |

*Table 5-5.* MAIN CHANNELS: TONIFICATION AND SEDATION POINTS

| CHANNEL | TONIFICATION POINT | | SEDATION POINT | |
|---|---|---|---|---|
| Lung | Lu-9 | Earth | Lu-5 | Water |
| Large Intestine | LI-11 | Earth | LI-2 | Water |
| Stomach | St-41 | Fire | St-45 | Metal |
| Spleen | Sp-2 | Fire | Sp-5 | Metal |
| Heart | H-9 | Wood | H-7 | Wood |
| Small Intestine | SI-3 | Wood | SI-8 | Earth |
| Bladder | UB-67 | Metal | UB-65 | Wood |
| Kidney | K-7 | Metal | K-1 | Wood |
| Pericardium | PC-9 | Wood | PC-7 | Earth |
| Triple Warmer | TW/TH-3 | Wood | TW/TH-10 | Earth |
| Gall Bladder | GB-43 | Water | GB-38 | Fire |
| Liver | LIV-8 | Water | LIV-2 | Fire |

*Table 5-6.* **FIVE PHASIC POINTS: INFLUENCE**

| POINT | PHASIC QUALITY | CHANNELS | LOCATION | GOVERNS/AFFECTS |
|---|---|---|---|---|
| Well/ Jing | Wood---> Metal----> | Yin Yang | Finger/Toe Tips | • Visceral disease<br>• Fullness below heart<br>• Release of Fullness and Heat<br>• Restoration of consciousness<br>• Activation of Sinew channels<br>— body surface<br>— musculoskeletal disorders<br>— acute disorders |
| Spring/ Ying | Fire ----> Water---> | Yin Yang | Hands/ Foot | • Heat and Fullness (fever)<br>• Change in complexion (not just face)<br>• Disorders of the surface and channels<br>• Pain<br>Qi blood stagnation; accelerates and pushes Qi through channel[a] |
| Stream/ Shu | Earth----> (source-point)<br><br>Wood----> | Yin<br><br>Yang | Wrist/ Ankle | • Prolonged disease (energy begins to internalize)<br>• Diseases that come and go<br>• Bodily heaviness<br>• Joint pain<br>• Activation of defensive and original Qi (regulates Internal/External, Deficiency/Excess) |
| River/ Jing | Metal ----> Fire -----> | Yin Yang | Arm/Leg | • Diseases affecting the voice<br>• Dyspnea, asthma, cough<br>• Chills and fever (malaria)<br>• Structural and channel disorder, especially on extremity (helps nourish joints and sinews), paralysis or spasms<br>• Dampness of muscles, joints, bone |
| Sea/He | Water---- > Earth ----> | Yin Yang | Elbow/ Knee | • Bleeding<br>• Organ disease, especially stomach<br>• Regulates flow between Channels and Organs<br>• Irregular appetite<br>• Rebellious Qi (reflux) and diarrhea<br>• Deep-seated disorders<br>• Painful obstruction, spasm or paralysis |

a. Can be used instead of Well/Jing points.

# Connecting Channels

The Connecting channels (vessels) leave the Main channels at the Connecting (Luo) points (Table 5-7 on page 240). They are important clinically, especially when there is a need to re-route Qi from one channel to another, or when two channels are affected. Both can be accomplished by needling the Source point on the primary affected channel and its coupled Yin-Yang Connecting (Luo) point.[16] The source point is used on the channel which was affected first and the Connecting (Luo) on the channel affected later. This technique is also good for somatic pain originating from the Organ systems.

The practitioner can also reverse the Source and Connecting (Luo) points. For example, Excess or Stagnation of Qi or Blood in a channel (painful location or swelling along the channel) can be treated effectively by needling a point upstream and a point downstream of the lesion, and at the same time needling the Connecting (Luo) point and the Source point on the paired Yin-Yang channel. In chronic disorders local points can be tonified (by needle technique or addition of moxa) and the Connecting (Luo) point (most often on a Yang channel) is sedated. The paired Source point is tonified.

## Disorders of Circulation

The connecting channels are important in disorders of circulation. Swelling (Damp, Phlegm or Blood stasis), masses, spider veins, and changes in skin colorations are all signs of Connecting channel disorders. Often an area near dysfunctional articulations shows congested and dark blood vessels. The vessels and the Connecting (Luo) point are bled.

### External Pathogens

The Connecting channels also can be affected by invasion of Exterior pathogenic factors (Wind), giving rise to pain. Symptoms will manifest in the Connecting channels before entering the Main channels. For such conditions the practitioner needles the Connecting (Luo) point on the affected side. When pathogenic factors enter the Connecting channels, pain may begin to radiate.

Theoretically, incorrect treatment of the Connecting channel can result in further movement of pathogenic factors into the Main channel. In practice, however, this does not seem to occur.

### Painful Obstruction/Bi Syndromes

Correct treatment to the Connecting channels (vessels) is said to prevent further movement of pathogenic factors and therefore prevent the development of painful obstruction (Bi syndrome).[17] The Connecting channels are therefore important in preventing the development of chronicity and should be used early in the course of acute or subacute disorders.

### Treatment of Lesions Outside the Channels

The Connecting (Luo) points can be used to treat disorders that fall between the defined somatic arrangement of Yin and Yang channels, as well.

# Divergent Channels

The Divergent channels can be reached and activated through their Access points,

---

16. Also known as the guest host technique.

17. Ling Shu (Spiritual Axis).

*Table 5-7.* **CONNECTING/LUO POINTS**

| CHANNEL | CONNECTING/LUO POINTS |
| --- | --- |
| Lung | LU-7 |
| Pericardium (Master Heart) | PC-6 |
| Heart | H-5 |
| Spleen | Sp-4 |
| Liver | LIV-5 |
| Kidney | K-4 |
| Conception/Ren | CV-15 |
| Large Intestine | LI-6 |
| Triple Warmer/Heater | TW-5 |
| Small Intestine | SI-7 |
| Stomach | St-40 |
| Gall Bladder | GB-37 |
| Urinary Bladder | UB-58 |
| Governing | Gv-1 |
| Great Spleen Connection | Sp-21 |

both on the channel and on the paired Yin-Yang point. Treatment usually includes needling the Return point and a Directing/Focusing (local) point (Table 5-8 on page 241) to channel the energy to the injured area.

### Pathological Tissues

Since the Divergent channels connect directly to the Organs (and Original and Nourishing Qi), they are used to treat visceral and Yin (substance) disorders. Therefore, the Divergent channels are used to treat pathological (beyond dysfunction or energetic) conditions, or to reinforce the channel and Organ functions.

*Prevention of Chronicity*

The connection between the Divergent channels, and the Main and Sinews channels (Internal/External), can be used to prevent the materialization (becoming Yin/structural) of dysfunction and energetic disorders.[18] Therefore, the Divergent

channels may be used to prevent chronicity and in disorders of Shao Yang—between Internal and External. (The Connecting channels may be more appropriate if exogenous factors are involved).

*Other Uses*

The Divergent channels can be treated when Internal/External coupled (Organ/Channel) disorders are present, and in left right imbalances. When symptoms keep moving from one side to the other, the Divergent channel is used often, together with Yang Ming (Stomach and Large Intestine) channels.

## The Sinews Channels

The Sinews channels are best employed within the first 72 hours after injury, but

---

18. The Connecting (Luo) channels are used for the same purpose.

*Table 5-8.* **DIVERGENT CHANNELS**

| CHANNEL | ACCESS POINTS | | RETURN POINT |
|---|---|---|---|
| Lung<br>Large Intestine | Lu-1 | and LI-15 | LI-18 |
| Spleen<br>Stomach | Sp-12 | and St-30 | UB-1 or St-1 |
| Heart<br>Small Intestine | H-1 | and SI-10 | UB-1 or St-1 |
| Kidney<br>Urinary Bladder | Ki-10 | and UB-40 | UB-10 |
| Pericardium<br>Triple Warmer | P-1 | and TW-16 | GV-20 |
| Liver<br>Gall Bladder | LIV-12 | and GB-30 | GB-1 |

they can become the principal treatment up to two weeks after onset of injury. Sinews channels are used as an adjunct to other channel therapies at later stages as well. They are activated by the Well points, the most distal of the Main channel points. Most often, treatment is employed unilaterally on the painful side. When the Sinews channels are used to address more chronic dysfunctions of locomotion and gait, they are combined with the Main, Extra and Divergent channels.

**THE SINEWS CHANNELS CAN BE ACTIVATED BY:**

- Tapping the Well and first four painful (Ashi) or Main channel points quickly with a burning incense stick.

- Needling the Well points. Electrical stimulation can be used.

- Needling the termination points on the head or trunk:

    CV-2 or 3 for the **Yin-Leg** Sinew channel.

    SI-18 for the **Yang-Leg** Sinew channel.

    GB-22 for the **Yin-Arm** Sinew channel.

    GB-13 for the **Yang-Arm** Sinew channel.

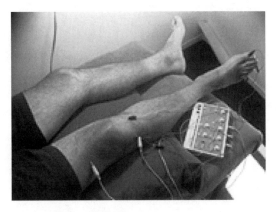

*Figure5- 2:* Sinews channels activated for the treatment of acute knee strain.

- Treating local points at the painful area (see chapter 6).

*Fullness*

Acute disorders often result in Sinews channel fullness. Local triggers (Ashi points) are carefully located and needled superficially. The related Main channel is tonified by use of moxa at the tonifying point. If after treatment the patient symptoms have moved, but not resolved, the process is repeated.

*Emptiness*

Chronic disorders often result in Sinews channel emptiness (Defensive Qi depleted). The pain is dull and poorly localized. Treatment emphasis is on moxa of local trigger (Ashi) points. Needling of local points is superficial and mild. The related Main channel may be sedated. If the pain follows a wide distribution the Connecting (Luo) point is used, as well.

# Extra Channels

The Extra channels (Table 5-9 on page 242) are used with various treatment methods, usually for chronic persistent disorders. Selection can be based on channel indication, by diagnosis of an abnormality, involvement of several channels, the abdominal pattern, and trajectory of the channel.

## Musculoskeletal Use

The decision to use Extra channels in musculoskeletal medicine can be based on a combination of the indication, topical organization and abdominal signs. For example, the Yang Linking (Wei) channel, which combines aspects of the UB, GB, ST, TW, SI and GV channels, is indicated for cervical pain with headache that radiates from the base of the head (GB-20) to the forehead or behind the ipsilateral eye.

This channel also is effective for musculoskeletal disorders that affect the sides of the body (unilateral) or that radiate to the side of the body, such as sacroiliac joint disorders radiating to the hip. The Yang and Yin Linking (Wei) channels together with the Girdle (Dai) channel can also be used for structural instability. The Extra channels should be used in all chronic disorders—especially in deficient patients (see page 38) .

*Channel Activation*

The Extra channels are activated by the superior and inferior Master (Meeting) points (of the paired Extra channel) and a Coupled point.[19] Four of the Master (Meeting) points also are Connecting (Luo) points of a Main channel. Each of the Extra channels also has an Activation point and a Departure point. Four Extra channels have lower Accumulating (Xi) points (Table 5-9).

---

19. Each Extra channel is coupled with another channel in a Yang-Yang and Yin-Yin relationship.

*Table 5-9.* **EXTRA CHANNELS (VESSELS)**

| VESSEL | MASTER)POINT | COUPLED POINT | ACTIVATING POINT | ACCUMULATING POINT |
|---|---|---|---|---|
| Governing | SI-3 | UB-62 | GV-1 | — |
| Conception | Lu-7 | Ki-61 | Ki-1 | — |
| Penetrating (Chong) | Sp-4 | PC-6 | Ki-3/St-30 | — |
| Girdle (Dai) | GB-41 | TW-5 | GB-26 | — |
| Yang Motility (Qiao) | UB-62 | SI-3 | UB-62 | UB-59 |
| Yin Motility (Qiao) | Ki-6 | Lu-7 | Ki-6 (Ki-8) | Ki-8 |
| Yin Linking (Wei) | PC-6 | Sp-4 | Ki-9 | Ki-9 |
| Yang Linking (Wei) | TW-5 | GB-41 | UB-63 | GB-35 |

# Point Gateways & General Treatment Methods

This section addresses some of the major point gateways used in OM to treat patients through the channel systems.

## Source Points

Source points are said to contain and release the Phasic (Elemental) quality of the Organ/Channel systems. They are the place in which the Original Qi resides within the channel. These points are used often, either when tapping into the Organ/channel's energetic quality, or when directing the energy of one channel—with the Connecting point—to its Yin-Yang pair.

## Entry & Exit Points

The idea of *continuous* energy circulation throughout the Main channel system originated in the *Spiritual Axis*. The Entry Point is where the channel Qi enters, the Exit point is where it exits. Entry and Exit point combinations may be used when other treatments have failed, and when the physical finding is an excessive pulse in a principal Main channel combined with a weak pulse in the next channel on the circadian flow.

Table 5-10 lists the Source, Entry and Exit points for the Main channels.

### Treatment Timing

Channel energy circulation, especially Ancestral Qi circulation, is said to take 24 hours and is stronger for a period of two hours at each channel. Symptoms that occur regularly at particular times are often considered to be consequences of this circadian energy system. Symptoms of excess may appear during peak hours (maximal energy), symptoms of deficiency may appear during peak-out (minimal energy) time of Qi flow (12 hours after the peak hour, so-called "mid-day mid-night" rule).

*Table 5-10.* **Source, Entry, Exit points**

| Main Channels | Source Points | Entry Points | Exit Points | Circadian Time | Tonification Points[a] | Sedation Points[b] |
|---|---|---|---|---|---|---|
| Lung | Lu-9 | Lu-1 | Lu-7 | 03 am - 05 am | Liv-8 | Lu-5 |
| Large Intestine | LI-4 | LI-4 | LI20 | 05 am - 07 am | Lu-9 | LI-2 |
| Stomach | St-42 | St-1 | St-42 | 07 am - 09 am | St-11 | St-45 |
| Spleen | Sp-3 | Sp-1 | Sp-21 | 09 am - 11 am | St-41 | Sp-5 |
| Heart | H-7 | H-1 | H-9 | 11 am - 01 pm | Sp-2 | H-7 |
| Small Intestine | SI-4 | SI-1 | SI-19 | 01 pm - 03 pm | H-9 | SI-8 |
| Urinary Bladder | UB 64 | UB-1 | UB-67 | 03 pm - 05 pm | SI-3 | UB-65 |
| Kidney | K-3 | K-1 | K-22 | 05 pm - 07 pm | UB-67 | K-1 |
| Pericardium | PC-7 | PC-1 | P/MH8 | 07 pm - 09 pm | K-7 | P-7 |
| Triple Warmer | TW-4 | TW-1 | TW-23 | 09 pm - 11 pm | P-9 | TW-10 |
| Gall Bladder | GB-40 | GB-1 | GB41 | 11 pm - 01 am | TW-3 | GB-38 |
| Liver | LIV-3 | LIV-1 | LIV-14 | 01 am - 03 am | GB-43 | Liv-2 |

a. These are special tonification points to be used at the channel's circadian time.

b. These are special sedation points to be used at the channel's circadian time.

When other types of treatment have failed, sometimes treatment during special times proves effective. The time most opportune to strengthen Qi is just after a channel peaks. The most opportune time to disperse Qi is during or prior to the peak period.

The energy circulation that follows this sequence travels from one Main channel to the next through the Entry and Exit points (page 243). The prescribed source, entry, exit, tonification and sedation points can be used at the appropriate time.[1]

## Accumulating/Cleft/Xi Points

The Accumulating (Cleft/Xi) points (Table 5-11) are areas in the channels where channel Qi and Blood concentrate and accumulate, usually in the middle half of the leg or forearm. There are 16 Accumulating points: one on each of the 12 Main

---

1.  In contrast to older theories, such as the five transporting points theory, in which energy in all of the channels flows proximately.

channels and one each on the Yin Motility, Yang Motility, Yin Linking and Yang Linking channels. On palpation, these points are felt easily as clefts or depressions in the muscle. The Accumulating points are tender often if a disease is acute; they are almost always tender when circulation in the channel is obstructed. These points can be used for both diagnosis and treatment. If channel stagnation is severe, they may become indurated.

Although the Accumulating points are used commonly in acute disorders and have been referred to as emergency points, they can be used in chronic disorders (and in weak patients) when accompanied by channel obstruction. The approach of using Accumulating points in deficient patients is similar to the attacking methods used in herbal medicine. The theory is that by the elimination of pathogenic factors, the patient's condition is strengthened.

As Accumulating points do not have a phasic property, they can be used to treat the channel without having any secondary Five-Phases related effects. They are used often in musculoskeletal pain.

*Table 5-11.* **ACCUMULATING POINTS**

| CHANNEL | ACCUMULATING (CLEFT, XI) POINTS |
| --- | --- |
| Lung | Lu-6 |
| Pericardium | PC-4 |
| Heart | H-6 |
| Large Intestine | LI-7 |
| Triple Warmer | TW-7 |
| Small Intestine | SI-6 |
| Stomach | St-34 |
| Gall Bladder | GB-36 |
| Urinary Bladder | UB-63 |
| Spleen | Sp-8 |
| Liver | LIV-6 |
| Kidney | K-5 |

*Table 5-12.* **INFLUENTIAL/MEETING POINTS**

| ASPECT INFLUENCED | POINT |
| --- | --- |
| Yin Organs | LIV-13 |
| Yang Organs | CV-12 |
| Qi | CV-17 |
| Blood | UB-17 |
| Sinews | GB-34 |
| Blood Vessels | Lu-9 |
| Bones | UB-11 |
| Marrow | GB-39 |

## Influential/Meeting Points

The Influential (Meeting) points (Table 5-12) are empirical points that have been found particularly effective for treatment of the tissue/energy they influence. They are used to access the broad sphere of each system they influence (e.g., GB-39 for marrow, brain, nervous, blood and bone).

## Back Shu (Transport) Points

Back Shu (Transport) points (Table 5-13 on page 247), (Figure 5-3), are located on the Urinary Bladder channel, from the third thoracic vertebra to the second sacral vertebra, through which the Qi of the Organs circulates. Organ disorders can cause tenderness reflexively at the back Shu points. Therefore, these points are used often to diagnose and treat Organic diseases.

The back Shu points corollate closely with spinal and autonomic innervation of somatic and visceral structures. Table 5-3 on page 622 lists the embryological segments, Table 5-2 on page 622 lists sympathetic segments.

The back Shu points are situated in depressions in the erector spinae muscles, about midway between the medial edge of the scapula and the midline. In musculoskeletal medicine the back Shu points are used in segmental and facet joint disorders and to affect the Organs, as well. Needles are best left in back Shu points for no more than 10-15 minutes to avoid fatiguing the patient. The Back Shu points, with their associated channels are used often to treat vertebral dysfunctions.

## Hua Tuo Jia Ji Points

Hua Tuo Jia Ji (paravertebral) points are located in the first paravertebral trough about 0.5 cun lateral to the Governing channel and level with the lower border of the spinous processes. These points overlie the intrinsic spinal muscles and facet joints and therefore are very useful in treatment of vertebral joint dysfunctions. They can be used for both diagnosis and treatment and often their use is based on the same principles as back Shu points.

## Alarm (Mu) Points

The Alarm (Mu) points (Table 5-13 on page 247), (Figure 5-3), are situated ventrally in the chest and abdomen, and are said to connect directly to the Organs and to reflect Organic health. As with the back Shu points, the Alarm (Mu) points become tender in reaction to Organic disease. Most are located in the appropriate somatic/neuralgic areas particular to the organ they represent.

The Alarm (Mu) points are used often for the treatment of Heat or Yang disorders. In combination with Sea (He) points the Alarm (Mu) points can be used to treat acute excesses, as well.

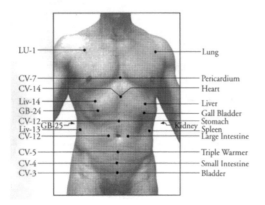

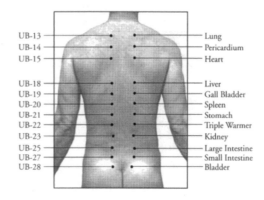

*Figure 5-3:*    Alarm (Mu) and Back Shu points.

**BACK SHU AND ALARM POINTS COMBINED.**
The Back Shu and Alarm points are combined often in treatment of Organic disorders and when balancing the dorsal and ventral channels. The Back Shu and Alarm points can be used to treat Defensive and Nutritive Qi (Wei and Ying) disharmony, as well. [2] Treating the back Shu and Alarm points for 5 minutes at the beginning of treatment can be very helpful for weak and fatigued patients. Connecting an electrical stimulator with the (-) pole at the Alarm (Mu) point and (+), pole at the back Shu point can facilitate the treatment (Figure 5-4). The appropriate Source point and moxa is added often.

---

2.  Commonly seen in musculoskeletal disorders with symptoms of changing pain, Heat (inflammation) and Cold (or alternating) and symptoms of hyper sympathetic tone—excessive perspiration. Use with a variation of Cinnamon Combination (Gui Zhi Tang+-) and Jade Windscreen Powder (Yu Ping Feng San).

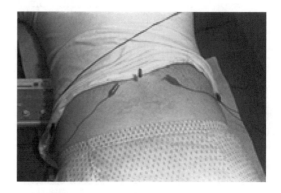

*Figure 5-4:*    Patient Kidneys strengthened by electroacupuncture with (-) pole on the Alarm points and (+) pole on the back Shu points. GV-4 is needled and Moxaed.

*Table 5-13.* **BACK SHU AND ALARM (MU) POINTS**

| ORGAN | BACK SHU (TRANSPORT) POINTS | ALARM (MU) POINTS | MANAKA ALARM (MU) POINTS[A] |
|---|---|---|---|
| Lung | UB-13 | Lu-1 | Lu-1 to Lu-2 |
| Pericardium | UB-14 | CV-17 | P-1 |
| Heart | UB-15 | CV-14 | CV-17 (Pericardium), K-23, Sides CV-14 |
| Liver | UB-18 | LIV-14 | LIV-14 to GB-26 |
| Gall Bladder | UB-19 | GB-24 | GB-24 to -29 |
| Spleen | UB-20 | LIV-13 | GB-26 to -21 |
| Stomach | UB-21 | CV-12 | CV-12 to St-21 |
| Triple Warmer | UB-22 | CV5 | St-25 Upper Warmer CV-17 Middle Warmer CV-12 Lower Warmer CV-5 |
| Kidney | UB-23 | GB-25 | K-16, occasionally GB-25 |
| Large Intestine | UB-25 | St-25 | St-27 or slightly lateral to St-27 |
| Small Intestine | UB-27 | CV-4 | St-26 or slightly medial to St-26 |
| Urinary Bladder | UB-28 | CV-3 | K-11 |

a. The late Dr. Manaka was a contemporary Japanese physician.

## Five Phases Points

Within each channel system resides a five-phasic and quality representation of energy that is concentrated at the associated phasic (transport, or command) point. These points are used to manipulate the channel's phasic qualities.

The Five Phasic points (Figure 5-5), also called the Five Element points or the Five Transporting points, are located on the extremities of the Main channels. They are used to treat specific energetic and disease processes, and to manipulate the phasic qualities of the Main channels and Organs. These Phasic points, which depict the growth of Qi from small and shallow to large and deep,[3] can be compared to the flow of a river from its origins to its merging with the sea. The Qualities of Qi evolve as the Qi travels down the channel (Table 5-10 on page 243). In all channels, the flow

of Qi from the Well points on the fingers and toes (first points) to the Sea points on the elbows and knees (last points) is in a proximal direction, from the extremities toward the torso. At the Sea point the Qi is said to merge (enter deeply) with the channel's associated organ Qi.

Each Main channel has a principal tonification point and a principal sedation point that can be used to supplement or drain *energy* from the channel, summarized in Table 5-11 on page 244. Table 5-12 on page 245 summarizes the locations and conditions influenced by the Five Phasic Points.

Each of the Five Phases (Transporting) points has, in its region of the channel, a characteristic quantity and quality of Qi, and a phasic/elemental quality. These five phases points are used to manipulate the channel's phasic quality and quantity. For example, in patients with abdominal pain due to Liver Spleen disharmony, the Wood point on the Spleen channel can be

3.  The theory of proximal flow of channel Qi predates the 24-hour Qi flow theory from one channel to the next which does not always flow in a proximal direction.

*Table 5-14.* **FIVE PHASES POINTS YANG CHANNELS.**

| CHANNEL | WELL (JING) METAL | SPRING (YING) WATER | STREAM (SHU) WOOD | RIVER (JING) FIRE | SEA (HE) EARTH |
|---|---|---|---|---|---|
| Large Intestine | LI-1 | LI-2 | LI-3 | LI-5 | LI-11 |
| Triple Warmer | TW-1 | TW-2 | TW-3 | TW-6 | TW-10 |
| Small Intestine | SI-1 | SI-2 | SI-3 | SI-5 | SI-8 |
| Stomach | St-45 | St-44 | St-43 | St-41 | St-36 |
| Gall Bladder | GB-44 | GB-43 | GB-41 | GB-38 | GB-34 |
| Bladder | UB-67 | UB-66 | UB-65 | UB-60 | UB-40 (54) |

*Table 5-15.* **FIVE PHASES POINTS YIN CHANNELS**

| CHANNEL | WELL (JING) WOOD | SPRING (YING) FIRE | STREAM (SHU) EARTH | RIVER (JING) METAL | SEA (HE) WATER |
|---|---|---|---|---|---|
| Lung | Lu-11 | Lu-10 | Lu-9 | Lu-8 | Lu-5 |
| Pericardium | P-9 | P-8 | P-7 | P-5 | P-3 |
| Heart | H-9 | H-8 | H-7 | H-4 | H-3 |
| Spleen | Sp-1 | Sp-2 | Sp-3 | Sp-5 | Sp-9 |
| Liver | Liv-1 | Liv-2 | Liv-3 | Liv-4 | Liv-8 |
| Kidney | K-1 | K-2 | K-3 | K-7 | K-10 |

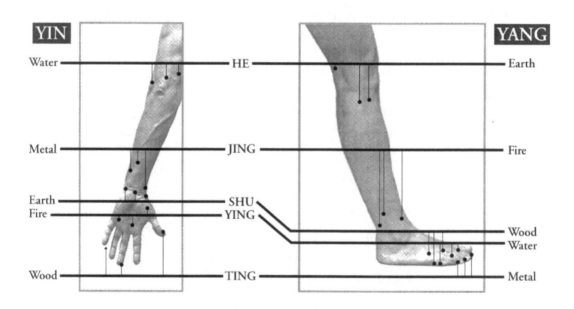

*Figure 5-5:* Five Phases points.

sedated while the Earth point on the Wood channel can be tonified.

In order to activate a phasic quality within the patient, the phasic point in the channel that is currently most active (in circadian circulation) can be stimulated. For example, to activate a Wood phasic quality in a patient seen between 9-11 am, the point Sp-1 (Wood point of Sp channel) can be stimulated.

Table 5-15 and Table 5-14 on page 248 list the Five Phases points for the Yang and Yin channels.

### Supplementing or Draining Energy: The Four Needle Technique

The Five Phases points are used also to supplement or drain energy through the Four Needle technique. This method uses the channel's sedating and tonification points and, on related channels, points that either supplement or deplete the intended channel. For each Organ/Channel system, regardless of whether the intention is to tonify or to sedate, two points are tonified and two are sedated. Table 5-16 and Table 5-17 on page 250 list the points used in the Four Needle sedation and tonification techniques.

## Group Connecting Points

The Group Connecting points are four points on the extremities where several channels intersect.

- P-5 connects all the arm Yin channels and therefore can be used in disorders of the Lungs, Heart, Pericardium and chest. P-6 is often substituted.

- TW-8 connects all the arm Yang channels. TW-8 is one of the forbidden points for needling and therefore many practitioners use TW-5 instead. It can be used in disorders of the Small Intestine, Large Intestine and Triple Warmer, and in arm, neck and shoulder disorders.

- Sp-6 connects all the leg Yin channels and therefore can be used in disorders of the Liver, Spleen and Kidney. This point is used often in weak and deficient patients.

GB-39 connects all the leg Yang channels and therefore can be used in disorders of the Gall Bladder, Urinary Bladder and Stomach. It is used often in disorders of the lower extremity and neck.

*Table 5-16.* FOUR NEEDLE TECHNIQUE SEDATION

| CHANNEL | SEDATING TECHNIQUE | | TONIFYING TECHNIQUE | |
|---|---|---|---|---|
| Lung | Lu-5 | K-10 | Lu-10 | H-8 |
| Large Intestine | LI-2 | UB-66 | LI-5 | SI-5 |
| Stomach | St-45 | LI-1 | St-43 | GB-41 |
| Spleen | Sp-5 | Lu-8 | Sp-1 | LIV-1 |
| Heart | H-7 | Sp-3 | H-3 | K-10 |
| Small Intestine | SI-8 | St-36 | SI-2 | UB-66 |
| Bladder | UB-65 | GB-41 | UB-54 | St-36 |
| Kidney | K-1 | LIV-1 | K-3 | Sp-3 |
| Pericardium | PC-7 | Sp-3 | PC-3 | K-10 |
| Triple Warmer | TW-10 | St-36 | TW-2 | UB-66 |
| Gall Bladder | GB-38 | SI-5 | GB-44 | LI-1 |
| Liver | LIV-2 | H-8 | LIV-4 | Lu-8 |

*Table 5-17.* FOUR NEEDLE TECHNIQUE TONIFICATION

| CHANNEL | TONIFYING TECHNIQUE | | SEDATING TECHNIQUE | |
|---|---|---|---|---|
| Lung | Lu-9 | Sp-3 | Lu-10 | H-8 |
| Large Intestine | LI-11 | St-36 | LI-5 | SI-5 |
| Stomach | St-41 | SI-5 | St-43 | GB-41 |
| Spleen | Sp-2 | H-8 | Sp-1 | LIV-1 |
| Heart | H-9 | LIV-1 | H-3 | K-10 |
| Small Intestine | SI-3 | GB-41 | SI-2 | UB-66 |
| Bladder | UB-67 | LI-1 | UB-54 | St-36 |
| Kidney | K-7 | Lu-8 | K-3 | Sp-3 |
| Pericardium | PC-9 | LIV-1 | PC-3 | K-10 |
| Triple Warmer | TW-3 | GB-41 | TW-2 | UB-66 |
| Gall Bladder | GB-43 | UB-66 | GB-44 | LI-1 |
| Liver | LIV-8 | K-10 | LIV-4 | Lu-8 |

## Commonly Used & Auxiliary Points

There are many acupuncture points that can be used in the treatment of musculoskeletal disorders. Table 5-18 summarizes the more commonly utilized.

Management of musculoskeletal disorders often requires attending to other systems and to mental states. Table 5-20 on page 253 summarizes points used for the endocrine system. Table 5-19 summarizes points for mental conditions. Table 5-27 on page 271 through Table 5-29 on page 273 present additional commonly used points in musculoskeletal medicine.

*Table 5-18.* COMMONLY USED POINTS IN MUSCULOSKELETAL DISORDERS

| POINTS | USES |
|---|---|
| SI-3 | Strengthens the spine and relaxes muscles |
| UB11-20 hua tou jia ji points at these levels | Lesions in the superficial and deep thoracic spine muscles Vertebral dysfunctions |
| UB-11 | Tightness of the upper spine Weakness in one or all bones and joints in body Trapezius, levator scapula and rhomboid disorders |
| UB-18 | Tightness and tension of the mid-back. General tightness |
| UB-20 | Pain and weakness of the thoracolumbar area Weakness of the extremities |
| UB-23 | Weak or stressed patient |
| UB-62 | Relaxes the muscle channels over the entire spine |
| GV-26 | Central pain and weakness of the spine |
| ST36 | Strengthens weak patients Strengthens all skeletal muscles |
| CV-6 | Weak patient, especially with a slipped disc |
| GV-4 | Exhausted weak patient |

*Table 5-18.* COMMONLY USED POINTS IN MUSCULOSKELETAL DISORDERS (CONTINUED)

| POINTS | USES (CONTINUED) |
|---|---|
| GB-34 (can use Beside Three Miles) | Fatigued muscles, and weakness of tendons, ligaments and bones<br>Pain in the lateral trunk |
| GB-41-TW-5 | Lateral trunk pain |
| GB-38 | Aches and pains throughout the body<br>Muscular spasm in general<br>Pain and stiffness of the neck<br>Pain and soreness in the calf and lateral aspect of the lower extremities |
| Liv-5 | Back stiffness with loss of flexion<br>Coldness<br>Aching and pain in the lower leg and feet and difficulty flexing the knee |
| Liv-3-2 | Spasms, cramps and pain especially in a neurotic patient |
| LI-15, LI-11 and LI-4. | Pain, numbness and weakness along LI muscle channel |
| GV-4, UB-23, K-3 and CV-4 | Supports the weak patient (Kidney deficiency) |
| Liv-3 and LI-4 | General bodily tension |
| UB-62 and SI-3 | Regulates muscular activity along the posterior and lateral aspect of the spine, especially in patients with flaccidity of the muscles of the medial aspect of the lower extremity and spasm of the lateral aspect<br>Strengthen the spine |
| LI-14, 11, 10. 4, SI-8,9, TW-5 | General "Controle Loop" for arm |
| GV-13, UB-10/GB-20, TW-15, LI-15, SI-9, UB-39 | General "Controle Loop" for cervical syndrome |
| SP-6, Liv-8, 12, St-36, GB-37, UB-58 | General "Controle Loop" for blood supply in the lower extremity |
| TW-22, 17, GB-17 | General "Controle Loop" for blood supply in the head |
| Sp-5, 6, 9, Liv-8, TW-4, 5 | General "Controle Loop" for connective tissue |
| GB-34, St-36, LI-10, 11, K-8, P-6, UB-23 | General "Controle Loop" for musculature |
| LI-14, 15, SI-9, 2, local points | General "Controle Loop" for shoulder |
| GV-4, UB-31, GB-30, 26,/27/28, UB-23, 50 | General "Controle Loop" for lumbago |
| TW-5, UB-23, 47, Liv-8, | General "Controle Loop" inflammation |
| Three nine miles (a combination of three points) 88.25-26-27 | Upper and/or lower back pain with leg pain or nulliness<br>Tightness of the iliotibial tract<br>Unilateral headache or back pain (for unilateral pain, needle contralaterally)<br>Vertebral hypertrophy |
| Correct tendons (a combination of two points) 77.01-02 and Upright scholar 77.03 | Central or bilateral upper back and/or neck pain<br>Disc pathology |
| Fire Complete 88.16 | Vertebral dysfunction and pathology with upper back, foot and heel pain |
| Two yellow 88.12, 88.14 and UB-40 (bleed) | Spondylitis (vertebral hypertrophy) |

*Table 5-19.* **COMMONLY USED POINTS: MENTAL CONDITIONS**

| INDICATIONS | POINT GROUP/MAJOR POINTS |
|---|---|
| Madness, psychosis, mania, "possession" | Ghost points<br>GV-26, Lu-11, Sp-1, P-7, UB-62, GV-16, St-6, CV-24, P-8, GV-23<br>CV-1 LI-11<br>Hai quan (bleed) |
| Excess above, Deficiency below<br>• Anger<br>• Irritability<br>• Insomnia<br>• Agitation<br>• Sharp headaches relieved by cold compress<br>  — Cold feet, nightly muscle cramp<br>  — weakness in legs, hemorrhoids<br>Deficiency above, Excess below<br>• Mental confusion<br>• Difficulty concentrating<br>• Loss of memory<br>• Sequelae to CVA<br>  — Hot feet<br>  — Strong physique | Windows of the Sky[a]<br>LI-18, St-9, Lu-3, TW-16,<br>UB-10<br>Minor Points:<br>SI-17, SI-16, CV-22, PC-1,<br>GV-16, SI-17, SI-16 |
| Insomnia, Thought Disorder, Agitation, Anger, Labile Depression, Any Mental Stress | H-7, Yin Teng, LI-4, LIV-3<br>Yin Teng, GV-20 with electrical stimulation<br>Ear: Shen Men, Tranquilizer/Valium, Internal secretion, Master Cerebral, Stress Control/Adrenal |
| General "controle loop" for depressive state | H-3, CV-6, UB-39 |
| General "controle loop" for exhaustion, mental and physical | CV-6, Liv-13, 3; CV-4, UB-39, GB-37 |
| General "controle loop" for sleep | UB-62, K-6 |

a. Windows of the Sky points are found as a group only in modern western texts. They are located in the neck area and most have the character for heaven (tian) in their name.

*Table 5-20.* **POINTS: ENDOCRINE DYSFUNCTIONS**

| POINTS: ENDOCRINE DYSFUNCTIONS | | | | | | |
| --- | --- | --- | --- | --- | --- | --- |
| **ADRENALS** | **PANCREAS** | **PARATHYROID** | **PITUITARY** | **OVARIES** | **TESTES** | **THYMUS** |
| K-7 | Sp-3 | UB-11 | CV-15 | K-13 | K-11 | Sp-2 |
| UB-47 | K-3 | UB-58 | CV-16 | UB-67 | CV-3 | |
| CV-10 | UB-20 | GB-30 | CV-19 | K-7 | CV-4 | |
| Sp-6 | TW-3 | St-36 | K-13 | GB-37 | CV-5 | |
| GV-6 | LIV-2 | GV-2 | Sp-6 | Sp-6 | UB-47 | |
| CV-6 | CV-3 | LIV-3 | K-11 | K-2 | St-30 | |
| CV-16 | | GV-15 | UB-47 | GV-4 | GV-3 | |
| P-7 | | UB-3 | GB-37 | LIV-3 | GV-4 | |
| | | P-7 | GB-5 | | UB-60 | |
| | | | UB-60 | | | |
| | | | CV-10 | | | |

# *Other Treatment Systems*

Several systems of acupuncture are helpful in the management of musculoskeletal disorders. This section describes some of the more commonly used systems.

## Abdominal Assessment

The model of abdominal examination, assessment and treatment that was developed mostly in Japan follows the basic principles found in the classic Chinese *Book of Difficulties*, the oldest book in which abdominal topography is mentioned (Matsumoto and Birch 1988). Chinese medicine considers the abdomen to be a location imprinted with the function and dysfunction of the entire system, i.e., it is a somatotropic area that reflects the health of the entire system.

The areas of the abdomen correspond to different channels and Organs. The practitioner uses several maps to interpret the findings of the examination. The fact that each map is slightly different invites criticism; however, the practitioner can use the physical findings (without an official diagnosis) and treat the abdomen directly to affect both local and distal disorders. Therefore, the differences in the maps are not critical.

Treatment of the abdomen frequently results in deep relaxation of the patient. It can be used at the end of musculoskeletal treatment, when this relaxing effect facilitates the integration of the newly established post-treatment sensory patterning, or at the beginning of treatment to prepare and relax the patient. Meridian balancing through evaluation of the pulse (page 257) can be incorporated at the same time.

## Status of Patient's Constitution

In OM, treatment techniques used in musculoskeletal disorders depend on the patient's constitution and local pathology. Diagnosis by abdominal palpation is particularly useful when determining the patient's constitution.

A healthy abdomen should be more relaxed and flaccid above the navel, whereas the area below the navel should be fuller, tighter and more resilient. The rectus abdominus muscles should not be rigid. If the abdomen is full and rounded with a wide costal arch, the patient is considered to be strong (Yang constitution). Presence of these normal signs suggests a strong patient who can be treated more aggressively.

If the abdomen (especially below the navel) is weak and flaccid, without resilience, and has a narrow costal arch, the patient is considered weak, especially in Kidney Qi (basic vital energy). This type of patient must be treated less aggressively, and the poor constitution must be addressed. If this does not occur, the treatment outcome is often poor. Both acupuncture and herbal medicines should be prescribed.

### *Yang Deficient Constitution*

Patients who are constitutionally Yang deficient tend to be flabby (fat/poor muscle tone); the abdominal muscles are poorly developed and the lower abdomen and flanks are cold. These patients fatigue easily and may be sensitive to cold. They may have a shallow, shiny or dark complexion, and their tongue tends to be pale and enlarged (with teeth marks).

### *Yin Deficient Constitution*

Patients who are constitutionally Yin deficient tend to be thin; the abdominal wall is thin, is often tight and weak, and may feel warm, especially the upper abdomen. The abdominal extensor muscles are floating and ticklish when pressed. These patients tend to have a nervous but weak disposition and tend to feel warmer, which can affect their sleep quality. Their complexion may be flushed, grayish or yellowish and the tongue thin and red.

### Lung Disorders

The condition of the Lung is palpated in the upper thoracic areas around Lu-1. If the skin is dry and the flesh is soft, or if the upper ribs can be easily seen or felt, the Lungs are deficient. Tenderness or indurations can be palpated at GB-20, GB-21, UB-13, UB-43, GV-12, Lu-1 and Lu-5.

### Heart Disorders

Heart disorders often result in palpatory findings in the epigastric region. The areas between CV-15 and CV-12 are assessed carefully. If there is a strong pulsation or the area is hard, the Heart is deficient. Tenderness or indurations may develop at CV-15, CV-14, UB-15, P-6, H-3 and H-6 in both excessive and deficient disorders.[4]

### Liver Disorders

Liver disorders can result in darkening of skin along the lower border of the costal arches, and in palpatory findings, especially on the right side. The areas on the sides of the abdomen anterior to GB-26 are assessed carefully. Lack of muscle tone in the flanks or in the subcostal areas, especially in the right Liv-13 area, reflect a Liver deficiency and may predispose the patient to a "stroke." Tenderness or induration can be palpated at GV-20, GV-22, CV-4, Sp-6 and Liv-8.

---

4. The Heart is considered the most Yang of the Yin Organs and therefore tends to develop disorders related to excess (and usually is not included in the basic deficiency patterns). However, some say the Heart should never be sedated, instead the Pericardium is treated (Miriam Lee personal communication).

### Spleen/pancreas Disorders

Spleen/pancreas disorders often result in a somewhat yellow skin along the lower border of the costal arches, and palpatory findings on the left side (early writings, however, state the opposite, with Liver changes palpable on the left and Spleen/Lung on the right). The area between CV-12 and CV-9 is assessed carefully. The Spleen/pancreas is deficient when this area feels mushy, when it feels bloated as though full of fluid, or if the patient is extremely ticklish. Tenderness or indurations can be palpated at CV-12, CV-14, Liv-13 and Sp-8.

### Kidney Disorders

Kidney disorders often result in the hypogastric area, around CV-6, being cold and depressed with a tight band of tension that can be palpated deeply. Excessive pulsation at this area results from Kidney deficiency. Tenderness and induration can be palpated at CV-7, CV-9, SI-19, UB-23, UB-52, and K-7.

### Blood Stagnation

Blood stagnation and stasis often result in palpable reactions in the lower left abdominal quadrant. The area may show discoloration, small spiderweb veins, or greenish-blue skin colors. The diaphragm is sensitive often. Liv-4 may be sensitive.

### Excess Dampness/Phlegm

Dampness often results in palpable changes and audible sounds, especially over and in the stomach and intestines. The abdominal wall and other tissues may feel soft and soggy. St-40 may be sensitive.

### Yin Linking (Wei) & Penetrating (Chong) Extra Channels

The findings of Liver disorders are also true for disorders of the Yin Linking and

Penetrating extra channels. Tenderness may be elicited at Liv-14, GB-24, Sp-21 and P-1.

### Yin Motility (Qiao) & Conception (Ren) Extra Channels

In disorders of the Yin Motility and Conception extra channels, the abdomen often is thin, and poor muscle tone may form a trough in the midline. Tightness may be found in the lumbar region. Tenderness may be elicited at K-11 trough 16, St-30 and LU-1 and 2.

### Yang Linking (Wei) & Girdle (Dai) Extra Channels

In disorders of the Yang Linking and Girdle extra channels, the ASIS area often has palpatory tenderness, especially on the left. Palpatory tenderness also can be found along the Girdle channel, from the navel to the lateral edge of the abdomen.

### Yang Motility (Qiao) & Governing (GV) Extra Channels

In disorders of the Yang Motility and Governing channels, palpatory tenderness may exist along the ASIS, K-11 and St-26. Tenderness also may be found at the PSIS, the posterior axilla region and the cervical vertebrae.

## Examination

In the Japanese system, the abdominal examination is performed with the patient supine and the legs straight (because only tension is assessed, no deep muscle relaxation is needed). The practitioner:

1. Prepares the patient by wiping the abdomen dry with a tissue.

2. Evaluates the area just above the abdomen, looking for radiating heat.

3. Assesses the entire abdomen (using a very light touch) for areas that have abnormally high levels of cold, moisture, hardness, or softness; indurations; depressions; excessive sensitivity to pain; and tickling or itching.

4. [Addition by the author] observes the direction of tissue preferences to drag (direction in which it is easier to pull skin).

5. Pushes the abdomen with medium firmness (just enough to take out the slack between the skin and the subcutaneous tissue) and moves the skin/fat over the subcutaneous tissue, feeling for tissue texture abnormalities such as softness or hardness, small lumps, or depressions. This technique (step 5) also can be used anywhere on the channel systems or on the musculoskeletal system to find dysfunctional acupuncture points or Ashi points.

Normal abdominal skin should be smooth and even in consistency. The abdominal wall should be soft and resilient. The skin should be neither excessively dry nor moist, and neither hot nor cold. Palpation should not elicit point tenderness or indurations, and strong pulses should not be present.

## Treatment

Following assessment, abdominal areas that have abnormal findings can be treated directly and without a "diagnostic interpretation." The practitioner:

1. Locates abnormal areas.

2. Assesses the tissue drag preference within the abnormal areas.

3. Inserts a needle shallowly in the direction of tissue resistance.

4. Leaves the needle in for 10 minutes.

In areas where a definite sense of depression is felt, moxa application is appropriate.

**SESSHOKU-SHIN TECHNIQUES.** Another, less specific treatment uses Sesshoku-Shin techniques. The practitioner:

1. Holds the needle between the thumb and first finger, such that the tip is exposed only slightly and the skin is stretched lightly by the other hand.

2. Stimulates the abdomen by tapping the skin lightly with the needle, crisscrossing the area until a faint redness appears on the skin.

This may elicit a reflex action in the desired channels.

# Meridian Therapy

Meridian therapy, a Japanese-style treatment, uses the radial pulse to evaluate and treat the relative strength and weakness of the Channel and Organ systems (Shudo and Brown 1990).

## Pulse Diagnosis

Pulse diagnosis, the heart of the OM assessment method, is a complex, highly subjective system of diagnosis. The practitioner assesses six positions of the radial artery pulse (near the wrist) for a minimum of 28 characteristics at three depths. Discussion of these techniques is not within the scope of this book.

A more simple version of pulse diagnosis, used with the Japanese Meridian Balancing system, is fairly easy to learn and is a good way to evaluate the patient's meridian/channel balance and energetic health. The practitioner evaluates the six positions of the pulse for relative deficiency or excess, which reflects the balance of the meridians (channels) and organs.

*Wrist Unit Measurement*

The area over the radial artery just above the wrist is divided into three positions: distal (called *inch*), middle (*bar*), and proximal (*cubit*). The location of these three positions is based on the unit measurement by which acupuncture measures distances and locations of points. The entire anterior aspect of the forearm between the cubital and carpal creases is considered to be 12 units (*cuns*).

• The proximal pulse is two units above the crease of the wrist.

• The middle position is located usually next to the radial eminence and is slightly proximal to the highest point of the radial eminence.

• The distal position is located halfway between the middle position and the crease of the wrist.

*Finger Placement*

The practitioner's finger placement and the patient's wrist position are extremely important for a correct reading. Any inconsistency between the two results in false interpretations. The practitioner's fingers should be arranged in a straight line on top of the patient's wrist positions, with the fingertips resting against the tendon of the flexor carpi radialis.

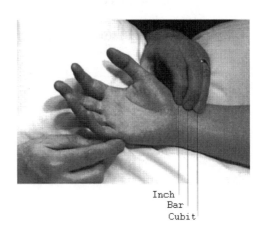

Inch
Bar
Cubit

*Figure 5-6:* Finger placement.

**THREE PALPATION POSITIONS**. The practitioner palpates the pulses on both wrists simultaneously. The beginner may find it easier to assess one position at a time, i.e., proximal, middle, and then distal, palpating each position at three levels: middle, superficial, and deep.

- At middle level the pulse is felt most strongly with medium pressure.
- At superficial level the pulse is barely palpable with very light pressure.
- At deep level the pulse just about disappears due to application of strong pressure.

The major qualities of the pulses can be assessed best at the middle level of pulses, where the Stomach Qi is evaluated. If the Stomach Qi pulse is very deficient (especially in the middle right position or Spleen pulse), the patient is said to be seriously ill.

*Strength & Size of Pulse*

The meridian balancing system emphasizes the relative strength and size of the pulse for diagnosis. Treatment is then applied to the "weakest Yin" (deep pulse) meridian/Organ system. The relative strength of the pulse at a similar position and the pulses on the control cycle (see Five Phases chapter 1) are assessed and should be equal in strength and size. A pulse that is weak at both the Yin and Yang levels is considered balanced, even though weak.

For the orthopedic patient, treating the most excessive Yang (superficial) pulse as well, is often helpful. Table 5-21 lists the Organs associated with the wrist pulses.

The points used for treatment vary. Generally, the Source points on the most deficient meridian are used first. After needle insertion, the practitioner rechecks the pulse to see whether a positive change has occurred. If the response is inadequate, either mild stimulation to the tonification point or use of the Four Needle techniques (Table 5-17 on page 250 and Table 5-16 on page 249) is recommended.

Excessive pulses should be treated by first draining the accumulation points, and then (if necessary) by applying the Four Needle technique.

*Table 5-21.* **PULSES: ORGAN ASSOCIATIONS**

| WRIST | POSITION | DEPTH | ORGANS |
|-------|----------|-------|--------|
| Left | Distal | Superficial | Small Intestine |
|  |  | Deep | Heart |
|  | Middle | Superficial | Gall Bladder |
|  |  | Deep | Liver |
|  | Proximal | Superficial | Bladder |
|  |  | Deep | Kidney |
| Right | Distal | Superficial | Large Intestines |
|  |  | Deep | Lung |
|  | Middle | Superficial | Stomach |
|  |  | Deep | Spleen |
|  | Proximal | Superficial | Triple Warmer |
|  |  | Deep | Pericardium |

# Auricular Therapy

Auricular therapy is very useful clinically and does not require knowledge of OM. As with abdominal diagnosis, auricular therapy draws on the concept that one part of the body can have a somatotropic system representation that can show dysfunctions of the entire body bioholographically.[5] The ear has origins that are mesodermal (innervated by cranial V), endodermal (cranial X) and ectodermal (C1, C2, C3) that may represent a bioreflex mechanism of embryonic tissues. Some research has demonstrated a possibility that the connection of the ear to cerebrospinal innervation and spinothalamic fibers in the reticular formation[6] is responsible for the diagnostic painful response seen in the ear (Helms *ibid*).

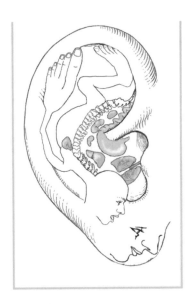

*Figure 5-7:*   French topographical map.

### Origins of Auricular Therapy

Auricular therapy was developed, not through OM, but by Dr. Paul Nogier, a French physician. In their own development of this type of therapy, the Chinese considered both Dr. Nogier's observations and a quotation from the *Simple Questions* and *Divine Pivot* that states that all the Yang channels pass through the ear and the Yin channels meet in the ear. Working in the mode of Dr. Nogier's research, the Chinese developed another topographical map that varies a little from the French map but is very similar.

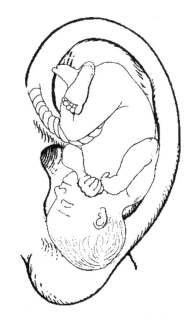

*Figure 5-8:*   Chinese topographical map.

### *Historic Uses of the Ear for Treatment*

Practitioners in other cultures, such as French folk healers, Persians, Egyptians and Greeks (Hippocrates), have used the

---

5.  Miniaturized areas representing reflexively the whole body, much in the way that a fragment of a hologram shows the entire hologram.

6.  The reticular formation is a modulating intersection that activates and inhibits cranial, spinal, somatic, visceral and autonomic impulses (see chapter 2).

ear to treat various diseases. A blind study at the UCLA pain clinic demonstrated a 92% concurrence in musculoskeletal injury diagnosis between medical and auricular diagnoses (Oleson et al. 1980).

## Examination

A careful inspection of the ear should precede any therapeutic procedure. Frequently, signs such as an edematous, inflamed area, pronounced superficial capillaries, flaking, dryness and discoloration are seen in reflex-auricular areas that reflect bodily pathology or dysfunction. Active areas usually are tender and have a lower skin impedance.

For auricular diagnosis, an electric skin resistance measuring device (point locator) is ideal. The practitioner:

1. Cleans the ear with alcohol and wipes the ear dry.

2. Uses a point locator probe to scan all areas, making sure the pressure used is uniform throughout.

3. Treats the area to correct the energetic signature.

Chronic, unresolved lesions frequently leave skin changes at their reflex auricular areas. These lesions are tender and often are edematous with superficial capillary clustering. Therefore, they have low skin resistance. Healed lesions often show an area in the ear that has increased electrical conductivity but is not tender.

controlling the exact site of insertion is more difficult. Also available are semi-permanent needles, magnets, metal balls and seeds that can be left in place for as long as one week.

### Points

Generally, points are selected on the ipsilateral ear over the reflex area that corresponds to the injured tissue (Figure 5-7). For the treatment to be effective, the point must be active. When treating pain, stimulation to the points at the back of the ear, directly behind the active point in the front, is helpful. Frequently several important points called Master points are used at the same time. Master points are used on the patient's dominant side (right ear in right-handed patient). Many Chinese practitioners needle men on the left and women on the right. Table 5-22 lists some uses for each Master point. Figure 5-11 illustrates commonly used Chinese points.

Auricular therapy is frequently combined with other channel therapies. Electrical stimulation can be connected between the affected area and the reflex area in the ear. Areas in the ear that have clusters of blood vessels can be bled.

## Treatment

The ear is made mostly of cartilage, and its blood supply is poor. Since the ear is physically close to the brain, it is imperative to use appropriate, clean techniques when needling ear points.

### Tools

The surface of the ear is very sensitive. A good needle technique is required to minimize pain. The ideal needle (½-inch, 34/36 gauge) can be inserted quickly with a twist of the fingers, allowing for minimal discomfort and maximum control (Figure 5-9). A guide tube may be used. However,

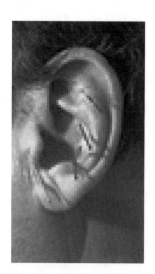

*Figure 5-9:*   Ear points needled

*Table 5-22.* **AURICULAR MASTER POINTS**

| NAME OF POINT | USE |
|---|---|
| Point Zero/Solar Plexus | Used often at beginning of treatment:<br>• to bring ear and entire body into homeostatic balance.<br>• to activate other ear points. |
| Shen Men/Spirit Gate | Used commonly:<br>• to treat anxiety and other psychiatric disorders.<br>• to treat pain.<br>• to regulate the nervous system.<br>Almost always active and tender. Can be used as a standard for impedance measurements.<br>Useful for anti-stress (adaptogenic) treatment. |
| Endocrine/Internal Secretions | Used often for weak, depleted patients.<br>Important for regulating hormonal system. |
| Sympathetic | Used:<br>• to regulate autonomic nervous system, blood circulation to limbs and temperature; and for pain control.<br>• commonly for musculoskeletal disorders. |
| Thalamus/Pain Control | Used to inhibit spinothalamic (pain) transmission. |
| Master Cerebral/ Psychosomatic | Used for chronic pain and psychosomatic disorders. |
| Master Sensorial/Eye | Used to treat distorted perceptions, both somatic and psychological. |
| Master Oscillation/ Cerebral Hemispheres | Used to treat problems of cerebral laterality (often found with dyslexia). If untreated, laterality problems can reduce auricular therapy effectiveness. |
| Tranquilizer/Valium/ Hypertension | Used:<br>• to relieve muscle tension, general tension.<br>• to sedate.<br>• to lower blood pressure. |
| Stress Control/Adrenal | Used to control stress by regulating the adrenal system. |

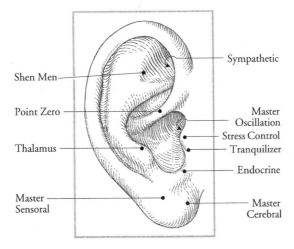

*Figure 5-10:* Master points

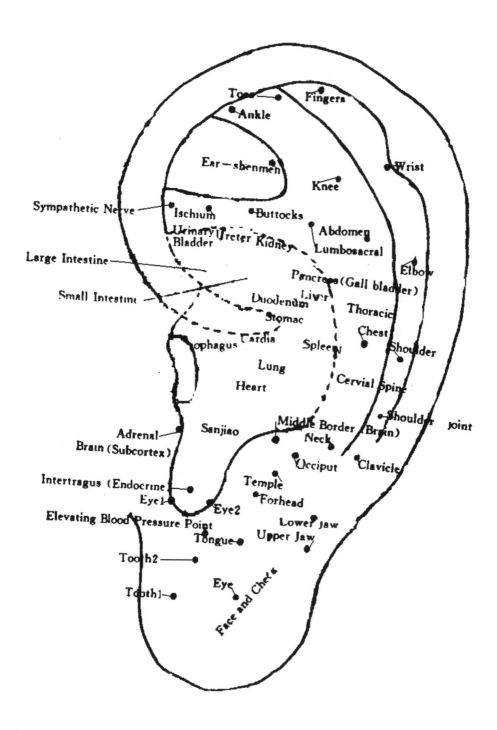

*Figure 5-11:* Commonly used (Chinese) auricular points.

# Wrist & Ankle Acupuncture

Wrist and Ankle Acupuncture (Zhang 1991) is a modern technique developed by a Chinese physician, Doctor Zhang Xinshu. Dr. Zhang's method incorporates longitudinal symptom patterns that are similar, but not identical to, the 12 OM cutaneous regions. The cutaneous regions are superficial areas on the skin (OM dermatomes) which are under the influence of the Main channels (Figure 5-12). The six wrist points (Table 5-23) and six ankle points (Table 5-24 on page 264) are located in the centers of their respective regions, a few points on the Yin side of the joint, a few on the Yang side and a few at the intersecting areas (Figure 5-13).

## Wrist Points

The wrist points, labeled *Upper 1 through Upper 6*, are in a circular shape located about two finger-breadths proximal to the wrist crease.

## Ankle Points

The points at the ankle, called *Lower 1 through Lower 6*, are located in an approximate circle, three finger-breadths proximal to the highest spot on the malleoli.

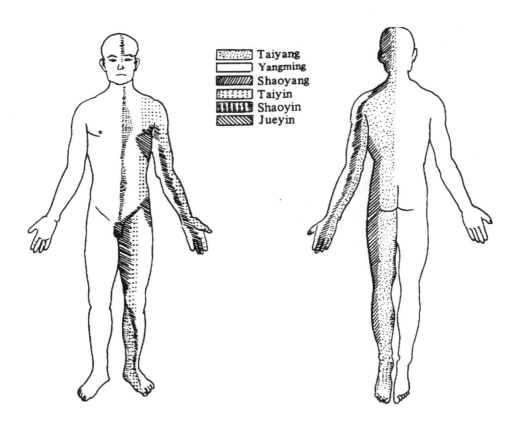

Taiyang
Yangming
Shaoyang
Taiyin
Shaoyin
Jueyin

*Figure 5-12:* OM dermatomes.

*Table 5-23.* **WRIST POINTS**

| POINT | LOCATION | USE |
|---|---|---|
| Upper 1 | Between ulna and tendon of flexor carpi ulnaris muscle. Found by sliding thumb along border of ulna until point is found in a depression between border of ulna and radial side of tendon. | Shao Yin distribution Very frequent |
| 2 | On ventral side of arm between tendons of palmaris longus and flexor carpi radialis muscles. Treatment may be blocked by a blood vessel. Needle insertion can be aimed proximally to avoid the vessel. | Jue Yin distribution Infrequent, for thoracic and rib dysfunctions, and for muscular headaches |
| 3 | On the ventral side of the arm on the border of the radius, between the radius and the radial artery. | Tai Yin distribution Seldom used |
| 4 | At the lateral surface of the radius. | Yang Ming distribution Sometimes, for cervical lesions |
| 5 | In center of dorsal side of forearm, midway between ulna and radius. | Shao yang distribution Very frequent |
| 6 | On dorsal side of forearm, 1cm medial to edge of ulna. | TaiYang distribution Frequent |

*Table 5-24.* **ANKLE POINTS**

| POINT | LOCATION | USE |
|---|---|---|
| Lower1 | Close to medial anterior border of tendocalcaneus muscle. | Shao Yin distribution Infrequent |
| 2 | On medial aspect of the leg at edge of tibia. | Tai Yin distribution Sometimes for SI, lumbosacral ligamentous, and L3 disc lesions. |
| 3 | 1cm medial to anterior crest of tibia. | Jue Yin distribution Seldom |
| 4 | Midway between anterior crest of tibia and anterior border of fibula. | Yang Ming distribution Frequent |
| 5 | On posterior border of fibula, in groove between border of fibula and tendon of peroneus longus muscle. | Shao Yang distribution Frequent |
| 6 | Close to lateral border of tendocalcaneus. | Tai Yang distribution Frequent |

## Selecting Foot & Ankle Points

Selection of points is based on the location of symptoms and signs (Table 5-23 -Table 5-25). When pain is unilateral, the practitioner needles the point on the affected side. When pain is at midline, or if it is on the side but location of the discomfort is difficult to ascertain, the practitioner needles the points bilaterally.

Wrist points are used for pain in the upper body; ankle points are used for pain in the lower parts. In motor impairment of the limbs (such as paralysis and tremor), Upper 5 is used for the upper limbs and Lower 4 is used for the lower limbs.

*Table 5-25.* **WRIST AND ANKLE POINTS: AREAS AND TYPES OF PAIN**

| AREA/TYPE OF PAIN | POINT TO BE NEEDLED |
|---|---|
| Unilateral | Affected side |
| Midline | Bilateral |
| Location difficult to distinguish | Bilateral |
| Upper body | Wrist |
| Lower body | Ankle |
| Upper limbs: motor Impairment (paralysis, tremor, etc.) | Upper 5 |
| Lower limbs: motor Impairment (paralysis, tremor, etc.) | Upper 4 |

### Needling Techniques in Wrist and Ankle Acupuncture

During wrist and ankle acupuncture, the needle penetrates only subcutaneously.[7] The practitioner:

1. Pulls the skin tight at the site of insertion.

2. Introduces a 4 cm, 32-gauge needle at a 30-degree angle, toward the painful site (usually proximally).

3. Inserts the needle until sensing the first loss of resistance.

4. Verifies that the depth of the needle is correct.

   If the practitioner were to let go of the needle, it should drop and lie flat on the skin surface. If the needle were not to lie flat, the needle would be either too deep or too shallow.

5. Advances the needle subcutaneously, about 3.5 cm. This should be painless.

6. (If the patient feels pain) adjusts the needle.

7. (Generally) asks the patient to mobilize the affected area.

8. Leaves the needles in about one-half hour. (In a few cases the needle can remain for as long as 24 hours).

---

7. Subcutaneous needling is used when treating superficial fascial layer restrictions as well.

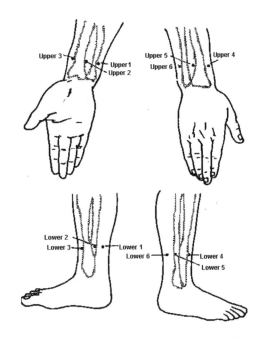

*Figure 5-13:* Wrist and ankle points.

## Tong-Style Acupuncture

Tong-style acupuncture is a specialized style that has been passed from person to person within the Tong family. It is an effective ancillary technique for management of musculoskeletal disorders.[8]

Tong-style is a simple system that involves little of the traditional theories. The principal points are on the Main channels. Non channel points are used, as well. (Tong-style points are included in applicable treatment sections.) Tong points are located within somatoreflex areas that correspond to specific Organ systems. These regions are unique to the Tong-style system (Figure 5-15).

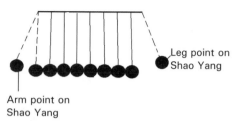

*Figure 5-14:* Energy activation.

## Activating a Wave Through the Channel System

The strengths of Tong-style acupuncture are its simplicity (as points are mainly selected on a regional basis) and its use of a minimal amount of points on unaffected areas. This results in little or no aggravation of symptoms and allows the patient to move the affected joint during treatment.

Commonly, to activate a wave through the channel system (Figure 5-14), the practitioner selects 1-4 points on the energy circulation channel system as far from the lesion as possible (as seen in Table 5-26 on page 268). The wave is said to result in a concentration of energy at the area of the lesion. (Unless the lesion is in the center of the body, needling of bilateral points is almost always considered inappropriate because this "results in a clash of energy," except when tonifying).

A second rational for choosing a contralateral point is that pain (Stagnation of Qi and Blood) in one side on the channel results in a Yin Yang reaction with emptiness and weakness at the opposite side.

## Locating the Points

In this method, the names of the Main channel points differ from (and have different functions than) the standard Main channel points; however, an understanding of the channel system (and early numeric systems) helps in determining the location to be needled. The practitioner finds the source of pain and needles at the same level of energy on the channel system as far away from the lesion as possible: if the pain is located on the ankle—Gall Bladder channel (Shao Yang)—the practitioner needles at the contralateral wrist (Shao Yang channel).[9]

### Commonly Used Tong-Points[10]

- Correct Straight Tendon (77.01) is located 3.5 cun superior from the base of the heel (Figure 5-15).

- Upright Straight Tendon (77.02) is located 2 cun above 77.01.

  — The two points are known as correct tendons and are mainly used for head and neck symptoms.

- Beside Three Miles (77.22) is located 1.5 cun lateral to St-36 on the GB line.

8.  The author, who studied Tong's acupuncture with renowned acupuncture physician Dr. Miriam Lee, finds Tong style an effective ancillary technique for management of musculoskeletal disorders.

9.  Although not a pure Tong-style application Dr. Lee often used this rationale to choose points.

10. Point Names and numbers are taken from Master Tong's Acupuncture Blue Poppy Press.

- Beside Below Three Miles (77.23) is located 2 cun below 77.22.
  - The two points are known as beside three miles and are used mainly for one sided complaints.
- Heaven Emperor Quasi (77.18) is located 4 cun below the knee joint, about 1.5 cun below (Sp-9) the medial epicondyle of the tibia.
- Earth Emperor (77.19) is located 7 cun above the medial malleolus on the Spleen line.
- Human Emperor (77.21) is located lateral to Sp-6 on the Kidney line.
  - 77.18 can be used for upper extremity pain, stiffness and weakness, especially of the shoulder.
  - The above three points are known as three emperors and are used mainly to treat Kidney weakness and back pain.
- Four Flowers Quasi (77.09) is located 10 cun below the inferior lateral edge of the lower border of the patella, 0.5 cun above St-38.
  - This point is used for head symptoms and ocular-headache.
- Four Flowers Below (77.11) is located 5 cun below 77.09.
- Bowel Intestine (77.12) is located 1.5 cun above 77.11.
  - These two points are used for proliferated Bi syndromes (generalized joint swelling).
- Passing Through Kidneys (88.09) is located at the superior medial angle of the patella.
  - This point is used for cold and painful lower extremities in men.
- Passing through Upper Back (88.11) is located 4 cun above the medial edge of the patella.
  - This point is used for shoulder pain and general swelling.
- Bright Yellow (88.12) is located at the midpoint of the midline of the medial aspect of the thigh.

- This point is used for low back tension from Liver disorders.
- Three Nine Miles (88.25-88.27). The first point is located in the midpoint of the midline on the lateral aspect of the thigh. The second is 1.5 cun horizontally anterior to the first. The second is 1.5 horizontally posterior to the first.
  - These points are used for musculoskeletal pains especially when the patient suffers from fear.
- Flower Bone Three (55.04) is located 2 cun posterior from the web between the third and fourth toes on the planter surface of the foot.
- Flower Bone Four (55.05) is located 1.5 cun posterior to the web between the fourth and fifth toes on the planter surface of the foot.
  - These two points are used for thoracic paravertebral pain, sciatica and for leg and foot numbness. They are especially useful for SI joint pain. The practitioner should mobilize the joint while the needles are in.
- Hand Five Gold (33.08) is located 6.5 cun above the pisiform and to the lateral side of the ulna.
- Hand Thousand Gold (33.09) is located 8 cun above the pisiform and to the lateral side of the ulna.
  - These two points are known as hand five thousand gold and are used for sciatica with UB channel distribution.
- Five Tigers (11.27) are located on the radial division between the palmar and dorsal surface of the phalange bone of the thumb. The five points are situated in equal distances on the shaft.
  - These points are used for ankle sprains and polyarthritis.
- Water Passing Through (1010.19) is located 0.4 cun inferior to the corner of the mouth.
- Water Gold (1010.20) is located 0.5 cun medial to 1010.19.
  - These two points are used for back pain aggravated by coughing with Kidney weakness.

- State Water (1010.25) are located on the sagittal midline on the back of the head, the first point is located at the external occipital protuberance. The second point is located 0.8 cun above the first.

— These two points are used for lower back pain, especially midline pain. And for weakness or numbness of the lower limbs.

*Table 5-26.* **LOCAL CONTRALATERAL POINT CONNECTIONS**

| JOINT/ AREA OF PAIN AND VICE VERSA | LOCAL AREA AND POINT | CONTRALATERAL AREA AND POINT | CONTRALATERAL JOINT/AREA OF PAIN AND VICE VERSA |
|---|---|---|---|
| Shoulder | LI-15 | St-31 | Hip |
| | SI-10 | UB-36 | |
| | TW-14 | GB-30 | |
| | LU-2 | SP-12 | |
| | H-1 | K-11 | |
| | P-2 | LIV-11 | |
| Elbow | LI-11 | ST-36 | Knee |
| | SI-8 | UB-40 (54) | |
| | TW-10 | GB-34 | |
| | LU-5 | SP-9 | |
| | H-3 | K-10 | |
| | P-3 | LIV-8 | |
| Wrist | LI-5 | ST-41 | Ankle |
| | SI-5 | UB-60 | |
| | TW-4 | GB-40 | |
| | LU-9 | SP-5 | |
| | H-6 | K-5 | |
| | P-7 | LIV-4 | |

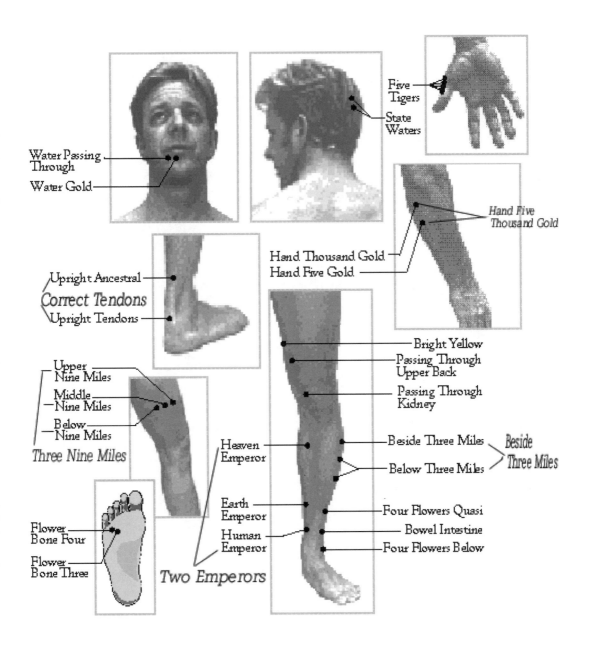

*Figure 5-15:* Commonly used orthopedic Tong-style points.

### Blood Vessel "Bleeding"

In addition to needling, Tong-style acupuncture frequently includes "bleeding" of blood vessels and Tong-style acupoints. Whereas Tong-style needling often is performed distally, Tong-style bleeding is performed locally. Points on the back (UB) channels are bled often.

Bleeding is used to vitalize Blood, and to clear Heat and other pathogenic influences. Clearing Heat and pathogenic influences by bleeding is done often for deficient patients (especially Lung related points on UB channels) and for lower extremity pain (UB-43). Bleeding is used in deficient patients, even though it is a sedating technique, because by eliminating pathogenic influences (which results in a decreased burden on the Organs), the patient is strengthened (by a method similar to the attacking method used in herbal medicine).

# Herbal Therapy

Herbal medicine has been the core of OM throughout its history. It was emperor Sheng Nung, around 2800 B.C., that is credited with the discovery and first systematic recording of the healing powers of plants, although his classic text did not appear until about 100 B.C. Since the time of the *Theses on Exogenous Febrile Diseases*, in the third century B.C., practitioners have been accustomed to using formulas or combination of herbs that were categorized in specific groups and assigned to specific disease states. These prescriptions address the patient's general condition and disease (so called root and stem). In OM, formulas are designed using four major categories of herbs. These are:

- Chief or King herb which is the main herb that is directed against the principal pattern discrimination or disease state.

- Minister or Deputy herbs which aid the chief in addressing the principal pattern, as well as serve as the main element directed against a concurrent pattern or disease.

- Assistant herbs which; reinforce the effect of the chief and/or minister; balance the effects of the chief and/or minister by having an opposite effect; and moderate or eliminate the toxicity of the chief or minister herbs.

- Guide or Envoy herbs which; direct the formula to the appropriate channel or region; harmonize and integrate the actions of the other herbs.

Although not all formulas contain all these elements it is this balanced approach, to formulation, which accounts for the low toxicity and side-effects seen with Chinese herbal therapy. The proper practice of Chinese herbal medicine requires a thorough understanding of OM theory. This text covers commonly used patent medicines and "experience" formulations designed to address defined orthopedic presentations.

Acupuncture points and herbs can be chosen based on the location and type of symptoms. Table 5-27 on page 271 through Table 5-28 on page 272 summarize points and herbs used commonly in musculoskeletal disorders. Table 29, "Commonly Used Classical and Patent Medicines Available Commercially for Musculoskeletal Pain Syndromes," on page 273 summarizes the most frequently used formulas and their indications.

*Table 5-27.* **HERBS AND POINTS BY TYPE OF PAIN**

| TYPE OF PAIN | HERBS | ACUPOINTS |
|---|---|---|
| Cold | Ephedra (Ma Huang), Cinnamon (Gui Zhi), Radix Angelicae (Bai Zhi), Asari (Xi Xin) Ginger (Sheng Jiang), Aconite (Fu Zi) | Moxa-GV-14, GV-4, CV-4 |
| Heat | Puerariae (Ge Gen), Gardeniae (Zhi Zi), Fel Bovus (Niu Dan), Moutan (Dan Pi), Caulis Lycii (Di Gu Teng) | LI-11, Sp-10, Liv-2, GV-14 |
| Wind | Siler (Fang Feng), Notopterygium (Qiang Huo), Kadsura (Hai Feng Teng), Lycii (Gou Qi Gan), Uncariae Cum Uncis (Gou Teng), Gastrodia (Tian Ma), Lumbricus (Di Long), Buthus Martensi (Quan Xie), Scolopendra (Wu Gong) | GB-20, GB-21, GB-31, UB-12 |
| Qi Stagnation | Cyprus (Xiang Fu), Saussurea (Mu Xiang), Lindera (Wu Yao), Corydalis (Yan Hu Suo), Curcuma (Yu Jin), Bupleurum (Chai Hu), Rosa (Mei Gui Hua) | Liv-3, Liv-14, UB-18, CV-17, Cv-6 |
| Blood Stasis | Corydalis (Yan Hu Suo), Red Peony (Chi Shao), Salvia (Dan Shen), Safflower (Hong Hua), Ligusticum (Chuan Xiong), Turmeric (Jiang Huang), Achyranthes (Niu Xi), Millettia (Ji Xue Teng) | UB-17, Sp-10, LI-4, LI-11, Liv-3, Liv-4, St-36 |
| Damp | Poria (Fu Ling), Coicis (Yi Yi Ren), Alismatis (Ze Xie), Atractylodes (Cang Zhu), Stephaniae (Fang Ji) | St-40, Sp-9, CV-9, UB-20, UB-21 |
| Wind-Damp-Heat | Gentianae (Qin Jiao), Erythrinae (Hai Tong Pi), Mori (Sang Zhi) | Combination of above points |
| Wind-Damp-Cold | Angelica pubescens (Du Huo), Clemetisis (Wei Ling Xian), Erythrinae (Hai Tong Pi), Chaenomelis (Mu Gua), Acanthopanacis (Wu Jia Pi), Caulis Piperis (Hai Feng Teng) | Combination of above points |
| Deficiency | **Qi**—Condonopsis, (Dang Shen), Astragalus (Huang Qi), Atractylodes (Bai Zhu), Poria (Fu Ling) | CV-6, Cv4- St-36, LI-11, LI-4, Sp-6, |
| | **Blood**—Angelica (Dang Gui), Prepared Rehmannia (Shu Di), Peony (Bai Shao), Ligusticum (Chuan Xiong), Lycium (Gou Qi Zi), Mulberry (Sang Shen) | Lu-7, UB-17, UB-18, Sp-10 |

*Table 5-28.* **HERBS AND POINTS BY PAIN LOCATION**

| LOCATION | HERBS | ACUPOINTS |
|---|---|---|
| Head | **General**—Ligusticum (Chuan Xiong) | Beside Three Miles |
| | **Supraorbital**—Angelica (Bai Zhi), Gypsum (Shi Gao) or Cimicifuga (Sheng Ma) | GV-23, UB-2, LI-4 |
| | **Orbilal**—Viticis (Man Jing Zi) | TW-5, GB-41 |
| | **Temporal**— Bupleurum (Chai Hu), Scutellaria (Huang Qin) | GB-20, GB-38, GB-43, Taiyang |
| | **Vertex**— Ligustici (Gao Ben), Asari (Xi Xin), or Evodia (Wu Zhu Yu) | GV-20, GB-20, UB-7, Liv-3, K-1 |
| | **Occipital**—Notopterygium (Qiang Huo), Ephedra (Ma Huang) | GB-20, UB-10, UB-60 SI-3 |
| Neck | Pueraria (Ge Gen), Notopterygium (Qiang Huo) | GB-20, GB-21, UB-10, SI-15, GV-14, Hua tuo jia ji points<br>Correct tendon, GB-39, TW-5, SI-3 |
| Shoulder | Turmeric (Jiang Huang) | LI-15, TW-14, SI-9<br>St-38, St-39, Beside Three Miles |
| Upper Limbs | Turmeric (Jiang Huang), Gentianae (Qing Jiao), Mori (Sang Zhi), Notopterygium (Qiang Huo), Siler (Fang Feng), Cinnamon (Gui Zhi), Clematis (Wei Ling Xian) | LI-15, LI-11, LI-4, TW-5, SI-6<br>GB-30, GB-34, GB-39, St-39, St-36 |
| Lower Limbs | Achyranthes (Niu Xi), Chaenomelis (Mu Gua), Angelica pubescens (Du Hou), Stephaniae (Fang Ji), Bombyx Batryticatus (Jiang Can) | GB-30, GB-34, GB-39, St-36<br>LI-15, SI-6,<br>UB-43 (bleed) |
| Lower Back | Ciboti (Gou Ji), Eucommia (Du Zhong), Dipsacus (Chuan Duan), Loranthus (Sang Ji Sheng) | UB-23, UB-52, UB-25, GV-4<br>Huatuojiaji points, Tender points<br>GV-26, UB-7, GV-20, State H20 |
| Foot/heel | Eucommia (Du Zhong), Dipsacus (Chuan Duan), Loranthus (Sang Ji Sheng) Deer Horn (Lu Rong) | K-3, K6, UB-60, Correct tendon,<br>P-7, P-7-1/2,<br>UB-43 (bleed) |

Table 5-29. COMMONLY USED CLASSICAL AND PATENT MEDICINES AVAILABLE COMMERCIALLY FOR MUSCULOSKELETAL
PAIN SYNDROMES

| MEDICINE | USE | DISEASE APPLICATION |
|---|---|---|
| Feng Shi Xiao Tong Wan Wind-Wet (Rheumatism) Reduce Pain Pills | Wind-Damp (Bi syndrome), weakness, pain | Fibromyalgia, myofascial pain syndromes, leg cramps |
| Xiao Juo Luo Dan Pill Minor Invigorate Collaterals Special Pill | Wind-Cold accumulation, Wind-Damp accumulation, pain | Joint pain and stiffness (especially lower body), paresthesia |
| Jiu Wei Qiang Huo Tong Nine Herb Tea with Notoptrygium | Wind-Cold Damp, acute lower back sprain, fever and chills without perspiring, headache or stiff neck, generalized aches/pains | Fibromyalgia, URI, acute sprain |
| Jia Wei Er Miao San Augmented Two-Marvel Pill | Damp-Heat, scanty yellow urine, atrophy of lower extremities, painful area feels hot (worse in rainy or hot weather), fidgetiness, thirst with no desire to drink | Rheumatoid arthritis, gouty arthritis, gonococcal arthritis, UTI, post-viral myofascial pain |
| Juan Bi Tang Remove Painful Obstruction Tea | Wind-Damp; Wind-Cold | Osteoarthritis, rheumatoid arthritis, gouty arthritis, bursitis, post viral myofascial pain |
| Lian Po Yin Coptis and Magnolia Bark Tea | Damp-Heat, sudden turmoil (vomiting and diarrhea), abdominal distention | Post-viral myofascial pain, fibromyalgia |
| Ping Wei San Calm the Stomach Powder | Dampness, distention fullness, loss of appetite, Fatigue | Post-viral myofascial pain, fibromyalgia |
| Chu Shi Wei Ling Tang Eliminate Damp Calm Stomach with Poria Tea | Damp-Heat, distention fullness, loss of appetite, fatigue | Post-viral myofascial pain, fibromyalgia, especially lower body |
| Yunnan Bai Yao Yunnan White Medicine | Bleeding, pain | Sprains, strains, trauma |
| Fu Yuan Huo Xue Tang Tang Kuei and Persica Tea (revive health by invigorating the Blood tea) | Blood stasis, traumatic injuries with chest and/or flank pain | Acute injuries, costochondritis |
| Tao Hong Si Wu Tong Four Substances Tea plus Tao Ren (persica) and Hong Hua (carthamus) | Blood Deficiency w/Blood Stasis, often used for women, lusterless complexion, generalized muscle tension and menstrual dysfunction | Neurogenic headache, fibromyalgia |
| Gu Zhe Cuo Shang San Broken Bones and Bruise Powder | Blood stasis, aids regeneration of bone and soft tissues | Fractures, lacerations, trauma |
| Yan Hu Suo Zhi Tong Pian Tetrahydropalmatine 50 mg. This product is a pharmaceutical extract | Strong analgesic, strong sedative | Severe pain |
| Huo Luo Xiao Ling Dan Fantastically Effective Pill to Invigorate the Collaterals | Blood stasis, analgesic | Fixed local stabbing pain (especially if increases at night), pain in various locations |
| Du Huo Ji Sang Wan Angelica Loranthus Pill | Wind-Damp accumulation, deficiency of Liver, Kidney, Qi and Blood | Chronic arthritis in elderly |

Table 5-29. COMMONLY USED CLASSICAL AND PATENT MEDICINES AVAILABLE COMMERCIALLY FOR MUSCULOSKELETAL PAIN SYNDROMES (CONTINUED)

| MEDICINE | USE | DISEASE APPLICATION |
|---|---|---|
| Jin Gui Shen Qi Wan<br>Rehmannia Eight F. (pill)<br>plus<br>Du Zhong (eucommia),<br>Gou Qi Zi (lycium fruit), and<br>Ba ji tian (morinda)<br>Yao Tong Pian (patent)<br>Back Pain Tablets | Kidney Yang Deficiency, cold sensation in lower body, edema in asthma, often used in geriatrics, strengthens the sinews | Diabetes, hypothyroid, arthritis, asthma, adrenal insufficiency, ligamentous insufficiency |
| Yao Tong Pian<br>Back Pain Tablets | Chronic low back pain with Kidney weakness, nocturia, weak knees | Adrenal insufficiency, ligamentous insufficiency, chronic low back pain |
| Jian Bu Hu Qian Wan<br>Healthy Steps Tiger Stealthily Pills | Congenital Weakness, Wei syndrome (wasting syndrome), paralysis | Sequelae of poliomyelitis, flaccid paralysis, muscular atrophy |
| Kang Gu Zeng Sheng Pian<br>Against Bony Hyperplasia | Liver and Kidney Weakness, Proliferated Bi syndrome | Bony hyperplasia, chronic joint pain |
| Zuo Gui Yin<br>Restore the Left (Kidney) decoction | Empty Kidney Yin | Chronic weakness, chronic low back pain |
| You Gui Wan<br>Restore the Right (Kidney) Pill | Empty Kidney Yang | Chronic weakness, Chronic low back pain |

# Other Techniques

Several techniques are used regularly in OM therapy. Among the more common are ion cord, cupping, scraping, moxibustion, electrical stimulation, laser therapy and manual therapy.

## Ion Cord Technique

An ion cord is a simple device made of electrical wire with a diode in the middle. It is used to direct the channel flow in one direction and influence cellular polarity. Japanese authors use ion cords frequently in treatment of Extra channels, burns and other conditions.

# Cupping

Used for centuries in both the East and the West, cupping is a method of increasing circulation by causing local congestion (often a hematoma) and fascial tissue stretch. Using a flame (Figure 5-16), a cupping instrument, or even a breast pump, the practitioner:

1. Creates a partial vacuum in a jar.

2. Applies the semi-evacuated cup to the patient's skin.

The suction draws up the underlying tissue, thereby stretching the fascia, forming blood stasis, and possibly drawing out interstitial fluid. The drawing out of interstitial fluid, which may result in blisters, is thought to increase circulation and to be otherwise therapeutic, especially in patients who have Bi syndrome from Wind-Damp.

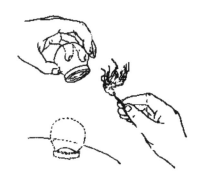

Figure 5-16: Cupping

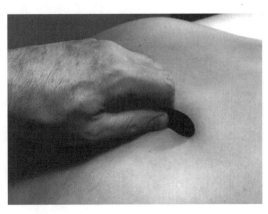

Figure 5-17: Scraping.

**3.** (To create further stretching) leaves the cups in place for 5-20 minutes and/or moves them up and down, i.e., the practitioner can:

Pull the cups upward, perpendicular to the affected area.

and/or

Pull the cups in a direction parallel to the affected area.

and/or

Slide the cups up and down the patient's skin (without breaking the vacuum).

Sliding the cups while the vacuum is maintained can be quite painful for the patient. The practitioner should do this only after having performed regular. cupping and pulling of cups several times.

vasodilation. This procedure, which has both diagnostic and therapeutic value, should be repeated (usually 1-6 sessions) until the skin no longer responds with quick bruising and prolonged erythema.

## Moxibustion

A common treatment for chronic musculoskeletal pain, moxibustion tonifies, warms and vitalizes Qi and Blood. The practitioner ignites a preparation of Artemisia Vulgaris and either places it directly over the point, holds it above the point or attaches it to a needle (Figure 5-18).

## Scraping

Scraping (Gua Sha) is a useful OM technique for reducing pain and loosening tight muscles. The practitioner applies a medicated oil (or any oil) to the skin and scrapes the area with a porcelain spoon or other instrument (Figure 5-17) until a skin erythema (redness)—or even a hematoma (bruise)—is created. Intense, prolonged redness, which occurs due to the so-called "red response," indicates an area of low

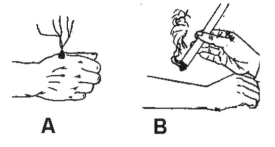

**A**          **B**

Figure 5-18: (A) Direct moxa, (B) Indirect moxa.

A good, whole-body moxa treatment that strengthens the constitution, increases circulation and helps Original and Nutritive Qi can be done at:

- St-36.
- Sp-6 and 10.
- CV-12 and 8.
- GV-14 and 12.
- UB-17, 18, 20, 23, 32 and 52.

These points can be either treated simultaneously in one session (or alternately in several sessions).

# Electrical Stimulation

Electrical stimulation is used frequently in treatments of musculoskeletal disorders, either by surface application or via acupuncture needles. Electrical stimulation has three basic biological effects: electrothermal, electrochemical and electrophysical. These effects can be seen locally (on a tissue/cellular level), systemically as well as segmentally.

## Local Effects

Locally, electrical stimulation can cause peripheral nerve excitation, alteration of enzymatic activity and alteration of protein synthesis (Owens and Malone 1983; Stanish, Valiant and Bonen, et al. 1982). Local contraction of muscles and an increase in venous blood and lymph circulation (a segmental effect) may: slow atrophy that has occurred due to denervated muscles, reduce swelling, and facilitate the healing process (Weiss, Kirsner and Eaglstein 1990; Bettany, Fish and Mendel 1988).

Electrical stimulation may:

- Influence the migratory, proliferative, functional capacity of fibroblasts.

- Speed repair of tendons and ligaments and improve their tensile strength.
- Influence bone regeneration (Bourguignon and Bourguignon 1978; Owoeye, Spielholx and Fetto, et al. 1987; Akai, Oda, Shiraski and Tateishi 1988; Brighton and Pollack 1986).

Local anodal (+) stimulation seems to result in greater tendon strength than cathodal (-) stimulation or no stimulation (non-treated control groups), (Owoeye, Spielholx and Fetto, et al. 1987).

## Systemic & Segmental Effects

Electrical stimulation can have analgesic effects, both systemic and segmental. Loss of presynaptic inhibition, such as occurs with Type I mechanoreceptors on Type IV nociceptors, facilitates the noxious input at the dorsal horn, allowing more pain signals to register in the brain (see chapter 2).

Electrostimulation and/or electroacupuncture can:

- Stimulate Type I inhibitory receptors and A delta fibers, thereby activating the gate control mechanism.
- Activate endogenous polypeptides and catecholamine-mediated analgesia.
- Affect joint mobility due to muscle group contraction.
- (Possibly) modulate internal organ activity due to somatovisceral reflex.

### Effects in the Vicinity of the Electrodes

Direct (monophasic) electrical stimulation has several effects in the immediate vicinity of the electrodes. (Table 5-30), (Shriber 1974).

The body's attempt to restore pH balance results in increased local circulation. An associated ion interchange occurs between the two electrodes. Electrophoresis (interchange of ions between the two poles, iontophoresis) can be used to deliver medication through the skin (Fig-

Table 5-30. ELECTRODE EFFECTS

| ANODE (+) | | CATHODE (-) | |
|---|---|---|---|
| Nerve excitability | decrease | Nerve excitability | increase |
| Acidity | increase | Alkalinity | increase |
| Fluid | decrease | Fluid | increase |
| Skin hardness | increase | Skin hardness | decrease |

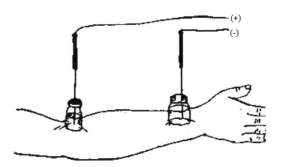

Figure 5-19: Combined electroacupuncture and iontophoresis.

ure 5-19). This increased circulation and the interchange of ions may contribute to reported acceleration of bone healing and regeneration of other tissues by electrical stimulation. Clinical use of biphasic (AC current), nonpolarized stimulation has been shown to cause collagen formation and osteogenesis, as well (Brodsky and Khalil 1988; *ibid*).

**IONTOPHORESIS.** Continuous, unidirectional (galvanic) current (DC) is the current of choice for iontophoresis. Other current forms, such as conventional pulsed high-voltage, sine wave, and interferential currents, are not as effective in iontophoresis. Due to the risks of electrical burns, from DC currents, the stimulation should be kept under 1 mA/cm$^2$. Also, because the caustic effects from alkalinity under the cathode (-) pole is greater than the acidic reaction under the anode (+) pole, the practitioner reduces the current under the cathode by increasing the cathode (-) elec-

trode size—it should be twice the size of the anode. The practitioner should also keep in mind that DC currents have anesthetic effects on the skin, and therefore the patient may not be aware of ensuing burns (Cummings 1991).

Table 5-31 summarizes common substances used in iontophoresis.

### Electrical Frequency

Many neurotransmitters and physiologic mediators have been implicated in the multiple electrostimulation and electroacupuncture effects. The frequency of electrical stimulation used appears to have specific effects summarized in Table 5-32.

Table 5-31. CLINICAL IONTOPHORESIS (Cummings 1991)

| ION | SOURCE | POLARITY | INDICATION |
|---|---|---|---|
| Acetate | Acetic Acid | Negative | Calcium deposits |
| Chloride | Sodium chloride | Negative | Scars and adhesions |
| Copper | Copper sulfate | Positive | Fungus infections |
| Dexamethasone | Decadron (brand name) | Positive | Inflammation |
| Hyoluronidase | Wyadase | Positive | Edema |
| Magnesium | Mag sulfate (Epsom salts) | Positive | Muscle spasm |
| Salicylate | Sodium salicylate | Positive | Edema |
| Tap water | | Alternating polarity | Hyperhydrosis |
| Xylocaine | Xylocaine | Positive | Pain |
| Zinc | Zinc oxide | Positive | Dermal wounds |

*Table 5-32.* **EFFECTS OF ELECTRICAL FREQUENCIES IN ELECTROSTIMULATION**

| SOURCE | FREQUENCY | INTENSITY | RESPONSE |
|---|---|---|---|
| Le Bars et al. 1979 | Low | High | Activation of A delta and C fibers |
| Cheng, Pomeranz 1979 | Low (2--6 Hz) | High | Tends to activate opioid systems[a], resulting in rapid-onset, short-lasting, noncumulative analgesia |
| Melzack, Wall 1965 Cheng, Pomeranz 1979 | High (200 Hz) | Low | Activation of thick, afferent fibers that may suppress nociception segmentally. Slow onset, long-lasting, cumulative analgesia, more serotonin mediated[b]. |
| Han *ibid,* Stuz and Pomeranz *ibid*. | Low (2 Hz) Medium (15 Hz) | | Activation of Beta-endorphins Activation of Methionin-enkephalin, Leucin-enkephalin and A, B dynorphin. |
| | High (100) | | Activation of dynorphin A and B |
| Shanghai Inst. of Physiology | Low (2 Hz) High (90 Hz) | | General, distal analgesia Segmental analgesia |

a. Blocked by naloxone, an opioid blocker.
b. Blocked by chlorophenylalanine a serotonin synthesis inhibitor.

# Laser Therapy

Lasers (Figure 5-20) are increasingly being used in the treatment of musculoskeletal disorders. The effect of low-energy laser stimulation has been reviewed by Sasford (1989). Low-energy laser stimulation has been shown to stimulate collagen formation, protein synthesis, cell granulation, neurotransmitter release, phagocytosis and prostaglandin synthesis, among other effects (Basford 1989).

Lasers have been shown effective in the treatment of carpal tunnel syndrome (Chen 1990; Naeser 1996) and many other musculoskeletal disorders.

The optical laser power used ranges between 5mW and 150mW and is in the infrared range. 5mW visible lasers may be used; however, their penetration is shallow and exposure time needs to be fairly long, about 3 minutes per 1 joule of energy. Each point is stimulated usually with 1-15 joules.

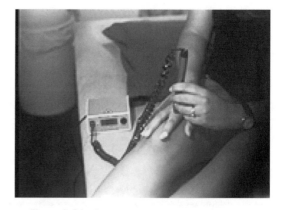

*Figure 5-20:* Patient self-treating with a laser.

# Massage/Manipulation

The following section covers both OM and non-OM treatment methods. The classic *Golden Book for Original Medicine* ("Important Notes on Orthopedics" section) tells us that manipulative massage was the main OM method of treating soft tissue disorders. Since then, generations of practitioners have achieved improvements and advances that, since the Communist Revolution, have been systematized and improved.

The Chinese characters that make up the words Tui-Na, or manual therapy (manipulative massage), are composed by the character for hand together with the characters for vertebra and unify. The Chinese characters that make up the word massage are composed by the character for hand together with the characters for safe and numbness. Hence the art of Tui-Na-Massage incorporates high-velocity manipulations and nonthrust techniques. Table 5-33 on page 280 introduces OM manual techniques for treating sinew disorders, summarized in Figure 5-21 through Figure 5-23.

Massage and many types of manipulation have been used in the treatment of musculoskeletal disorders since the beginning of time. Among different schools techniques often are similar. However, since the theories explaining pathophysiology vary considerably, so do the descriptions of similar techniques. The following section describes both OM, western Osteopathic and other techniques.

## Massage/Mobilizations without Impulse

Massage is widely used in the treatment of musculoskeletal disorders, and may have both palliative and curative affects. Massage techniques can be used also to prepare the tissues for additional specific joint thrust manipulation. Used in both the acute and chronic stages of injuries, massage has circulatory, mechanical and neurological effects. Massage can:

- Reduce swelling.
- Inhibit spasms.
- Circulate blood.
- Rupture adhesions.
- Flush out extravasated blood and damaged cells.

- Restore correct placement of tissues.
- Increase local metabolism.
- Reduce pain.

Schools of massage therapy have many similarities. In general, all OM massage techniques fall within the following three categories:

### Separating Adhesions & Breaking Scars

This method is used for both acute and chronic soft tissue injuries. The tissue is rubbed perpendicularly to the course of the fibers, which encourages muscle fibers to broaden as they contract, breaking microscopic adhesions that may be binding them together. The technique is useful for mobilizing scars and other tissues such as tendons and ligaments. It also has an analgesic effect.

Cross-fiber massage is used to prepare tissues for thrust manipulation, especially when used to rupture adhesions. When treating tendinitis (with cross-fiber massage) it is important that the patient avoid painful and aggravating activities until the lesion has healed. Cross-fiber massage can be used also as a prophylactic treatment in patients with recurrent strains or tendinitis. In general, the technique is applied for 10-20 minutes and repeated 3-5 times a week.

During the acute phase of sprain/strain injuries, cross-fiber massage can be used gently — beginning with one to two minutes and building up to 15 minutes — on a daily basis, to prevent scar formation. Friction (cross fiber) massage to a muscle belly should always be given with the muscle relaxed. Tendons with a sheath and ligaments are treated with the tissues in tension.

### Rearranging Displaced Tissue & Restoring Their Normal Function

To rearrange displaced tissues and restore their normal functions, force is applied along the fibers in a longitudinal direction.

This type of technique (effleurage) can be used to relax muscles and disperse edema and extravasated blood. Therapeutic passive movements also fall within this category, as well as many of the thrust manipulations used in OM.

### Inhibitory & Stimulatory Techniques

Inhibitory techniques are done by deep, steady pressure to acupuncture, Ashi (painful) points, muscle insertions and origins, etc. Inhibitory techniques are used mostly at the beginning or end of treatment for their analgesic effect, or as preparation for other techniques. *Stimulatory*

techniques, which are more vigorous, with quicker motions and pressures, are used mostly in chronic cases to improve circulation and activate the channels.

OM describes many massage techniques that fall within the above three categories such as pressing, rubbing, pushing, grasping, rolling, digging, plucking, kneading, dragging, abrading, rub-rolling, pinching, tweaking, flicking, knocking, patting, hammering, extending, bending, rotating, shaking, stretching, treading, holding and supporting. Table 5-34 on page 281 lists general precautions to exercise when using these methods.

*Table 5-33.* **REGULATING THE SINEWS**

| PRESSING | • Inhibitory or stimulatory |
| | • Used mostly on local and distal channel points and tissues |
| | • Stops bleeding, analgesic |
| CIRCULAR RUBBING | • Warming and vitalizing |
| | • Used in large areas or locally to mobilize Qi and Blood |
| PUSHING | • Inhibitory |
| | • Used locally on affected tissues |
| | • Rearranges soft tissues |
| | • Stops bleeding |
| GRASPING | • Dispersing |
| | • Usually used locally, but also can be used distally |
| | • Analgesic, Blood vitalizing |
| AUXILIARY METHODS | • Kneading |
| | • Splitting |
| | • Rubbing |
| | • Rolling |
| | • Rotation |
| | • Traction |
| | • Lifting |
| | • Tapping |
| | • Shaking |
| | • Moving |
| | • Tugging (pulling) |
| |   — promotes Blood circulation |
| |   — disperses Blood stagnation |
| |   — reduces swelling |
| |   — relaxes and activate Sinews |
| |   — loosens or break adhesions |
| |   — softens scars |
| |   — reduces pain |
| |   — restores normal location of displaced tissues/bones |

*Table 5-34.* **GENERAL CONSIDERATIONS FOR REGULATING SINEWS**

| | |
|---|---|
| **ACUTE CONDITIONS** | Use light (not necessarily superficial) manipulative techniques that reach dysfunctional tissues.<br>For chronic condition, use "heavy" manipulative techniques that are<br>• steady<br>• correct<br>• firm<br>• nonviolent |
| **SLIGHT JOINT DISLOCATIONS, DEVIATION OF SINEWS, TURNED OVER SINEWS (CONTRACTIONS)** | To relax and relocate displaced tissues safely, flex, extend, and rotate the joint to its physiological ROM.<br>Use Pushing methods to restore correct tissue location<br>High-velocity manipulation to gap joints restore correct location/function. |
| **ACUTE SOFT TISSUE INJURY WITH SWELLING AND INTERNAL BLEEDING** | Use pressing method, by thumbs or by palm of hand:<br>• helps stop further bleeding<br>• helps reduce swelling |

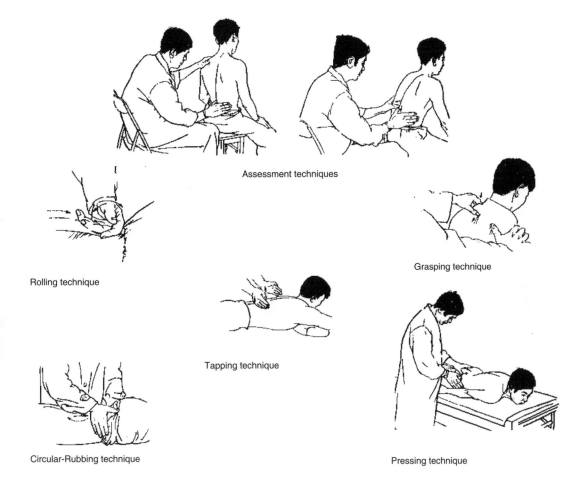

Assessment techniques

Rolling technique

Grasping technique

Tapping technique

Circular-Rubbing technique

Pressing technique

*Figure 5-21:* Traditional Chinese Tui-Na massage techniques.

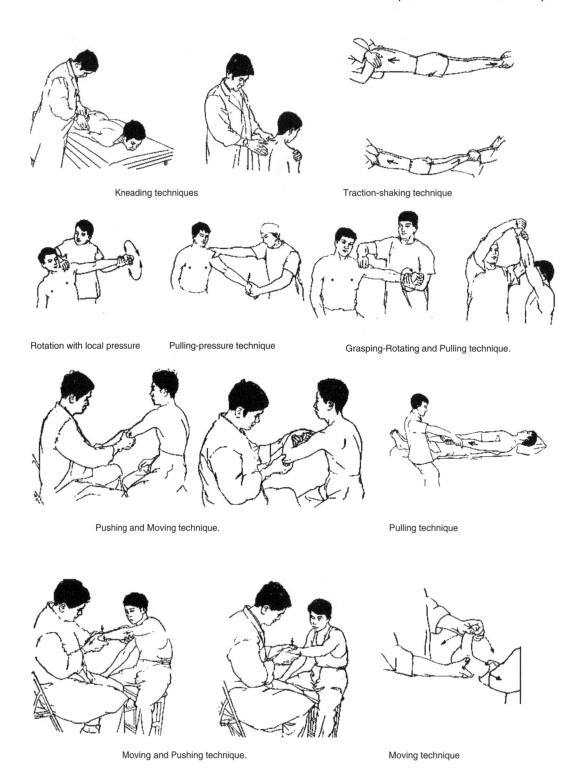

Kneading techniques

Traction-shaking technique

Rotation with local pressure          Pulling-pressure technique

Grasping-Rotating and Pulling technique.

Pushing and Moving technique.

Pulling technique

Moving and Pushing technique.

Moving technique

*Figure 5-22:* Traditional Chinese Tui-Na manual therapy techniques.

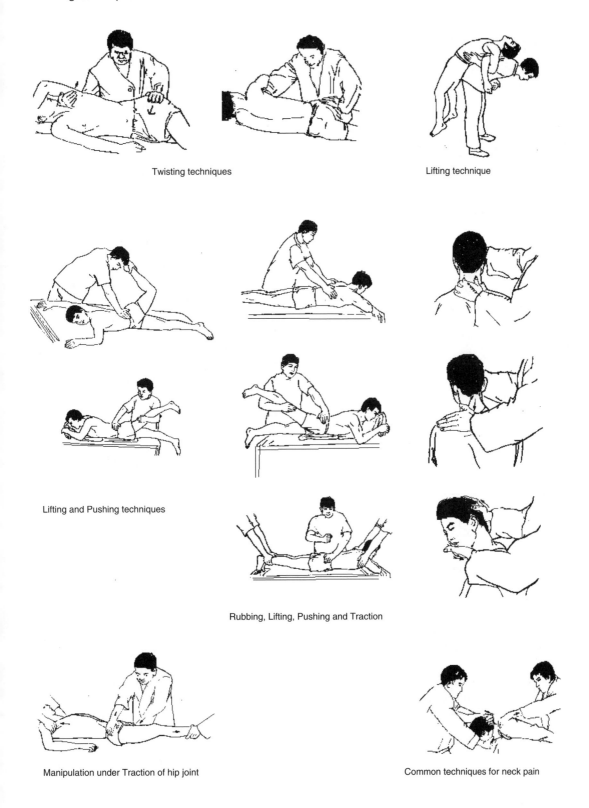

Twisting techniques

Lifting technique

Lifting and Pushing techniques

Rubbing, Lifting, Pushing and Traction

Manipulation under Traction of hip joint

Common techniques for neck pain

*Figure 5-23:* Traditional Chinese Tui-Na manual therapy techniques.

# Western Manual Therapies

## Osteopathic Manipulations Without Impulse

Western osteopathic techniques are extremely effective and often better tolerated by patients. The osteopathic literature describes three types of indirect methods (Greenman *ibid*):

- Balance and hold.
- Dynamic functional procedures.
- Countertension-positional-release (Strain-counterstrain ™ ).

And two types of direct methods:

- Muscle energy.
- Myofascial release.

### Balance & Hold

With balance and hold, motion at the joint is introduced in seven directions to identify:

- The point of maximal ease within each movement.
- The point of maximal ease within the respiration cycle.

After identifying these positions the patient is asked to hold them as long as possible. This procedure is repeated as many times as necessary to correct the dysfunction (Greenman *ibid*). Balance and hold is not elaborated upon in this text. However positioning of patients with these principles in mind is recommended when giving certain acupuncture treatments.

### Dynamic Functional Techniques

As the name implies, the practitioner uses dynamic functional techniques to try to restore normal function by means of motion. The joint is guided by applicable movements along a new path of increased ease to restore normal motion patterns. This process may reduce nociceptive and abnormal mechanoreceptive output, allowing the joint to relearn more normal behavior (Greenman *ibid*). Dynamic functional techniques are also not covered in this text.

### Release by Countertension-Positioning

Countertension positional release (strain-counterstrain ™ ) was developed by Larry Jones, DO., although apparently there are Ayurvedic writings from the third or fourth millennium which describe very similar techniques (Rex LB., DO., personal communication). Countertension-positional release is effective especially for muscle spasm with an accompanying exquisitely tender point, but can also be used to treat vertebral dysfunctions (Greenman *ibid*).

The mechanism by which this technique works may be that by keeping the muscle in a countertension position (shortened position) and slightly increasing tension on its antagonist, the sensory (afferent) input from proprioceptors is "shut down," effectively suppressing the local protective cord reflex and inducing muscle relaxation.

Countertension-positional release is performed by first identifying tender points anywhere in the muscular system (often located at acupuncture or trigger points) or at the prescribed Jones points. The patient is then positioned in such a way that discomfort and tenderness at these points are greatly reduced. The patient is then held, by the practitioner, in this position for around 90 seconds before slowly and passively being returned (without any patient effort) to normal position. Jones techniques are covered in the appropriate parts of the text.

*OM uses a supporting/stimulating method (treating Yin within Yang) which is somewhat similar to indirect osteopathic techniques. The joint is moved away from pain or toward the nonpainful barrier and held there while acupuncture points are stimulated (by massage) along the channel that affects the pathological (painful) side of the joint.*

## Muscle Energy

Osteopathic muscle energy technique was developed by Mitchell Sr. and uses postisometric relaxation,[11] reciprocal inhibition (Figure 5-24) and isotonic contraction to restore mobility to joints. Similar techniques are used by other systems and with different rationales.[12] Muscle energy techniques are both passive and active (requiring patient participation).

In the osteopathic model, which for the most part uses positional diagnosis, muscle energy is used most commonly to treat joint dysfunctions. Postisometric relaxation and reciprocal inhibition relax the affected muscles, resulting in the restoration of normal function.

Muscle energy is considered a direct technique, in that it addresses the restrictive barrier of a dysfunctional joint. For muscle energy to be effective, the joint barriers must be accurately engaged at the feather edge of their dysfunctional limits (i.e., not too far into barriers, joint must remain loose packed), in all three planes. This requires a great degree of palpatory skill by the practitioner. The most common mistake beginners make is to overpass the barrier and loose joint play. The beginner is encouraged to monitor the movement just above the spinal joint being treated (when localizing motion from above) and at the joint just below (when localizing from below).

The muscle contraction force made by the patient must be away from the restricted barrier and should be no more

than a few ounces when treating short muscle restrictors, such as in non-neutral (type II) vertebral dysfunction. There should be only moderate force when treating multisegmental muscles such as neutral group (type I) dysfunction—otherwise, muscle recruitment can reduce the effect (Mitchell 1985). The contraction is resisted by the practitioner to ensure that the muscle effort is isometric (no movement of the joint is allowed). This position is held for 4-6 seconds, after which the patient is instructed to completely let go. The joint is then moved to the edge of the newly gained restrictive barrier and the procedure is repeated 3-5 times.

Some techniques classified as muscle energy use both respiratory assistance and isotonic contraction of muscles. Muscle energy techniques can be used as the principal method for treating vertebral and pelvic dysfunctions are covered in the appropriate sections of the text.

Muscle energy (postisometric relaxation) can be used to stretch any shortened muscle, as well.

## Myofascial-Release

Myofascial-release techniques are relatively new additions to osteopathic treatments. However, similar techniques have been in use for a long time. Fascia often behaves as if it has a memory, as it is able to maintain tissue deformation for long periods. In myofascial-release techniques the practitioner applies pressure on the fascia in a specific direction while an activating force, such as deep breath, is initiated by the patient. This method re-educates the fascia back to the normal physiologic state (Greenman *ibid*). Myofascial-release per se is not covered in this text; however, a type of subcutaneous dry needling which has a similar effect is described. Many massage and cupping techniques are effective, as well.

---

11. The relaxation of a muscle after isotonic contraction.

12. The activation of antagonist muscles which then inhibit the agonist muscle.

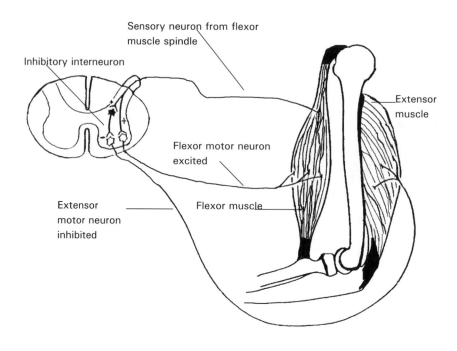

*Figure 5-24:* Reciprocal inhibition of motor neurons to the opposing muscle (After Lehmkuhl and Smith 1983).

# Manipulation with Impulse

Thrust techniques are commonly used in many traditional therapies around the world.

### Short Lever Techniques

Short lever techniques (Figure 5-25) are achieved by the practitioner's thrust directly on the joint being manipulated, without the use of a lever arm. Many OM manipulations are short lever and require significant physical strength. They are therefore of limited value and are not described in this text. In OM, short lever techniques are sometimes used in combi-

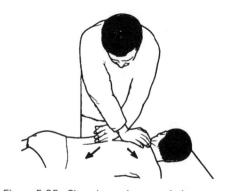

*Figure 5-25:* Short lever thrust technique.

nation with long lever techniques. They are used also by other therapies such as orthopaedic, osteopathic and chiropractic, especially in the thoracic spine.

## Long Lever Techniques

OM, Orthopaedic, osteopathic and other manual therapy styles widely use long lever thrust techniques (Figure 5-26). Parts of the body (leg, arm, hip, shoulder, trunk and spine) are used as lever arms to transmit the manipulator's force to the desired segment.

These manipulations are performed in order to increase the joint's range of motion, displace any structure blocking a joint space, and restore the normal location and function of a misaligned or dysfunctional joint. The joint usually is placed at its restrictive barriers (or away from pain), and an activation force is delivered via the lever arm. This type of manipulation gaps the two joint surfaces and allows them to spring back into a more physiologic position.

Joint specific techniques may be designed to gap or not gap the joint, and usually are directed through the restrictive barrier. Orthopaedic Medicine and some OM long lever techniques are less joint specific as compared to osteopathic techniques, which usually are also less forceful. OM, chiropractic, osteopathic, and some Orthopaedic techniques combine short lever with long lever techniques, which can increase localization. OM and Orthopaedic Medicine also commonly use manipulation techniques under traction (Figure 5-27).

Many theories attempt to explain the therapeutic action of high velocity short amplitude manipulation (thrust techniques), not all of which consider the direct "mechanical" action of the thrust. For example, high velocity short amplitude manipulation forcefully stretches hypertonic muscles against their muscle spindles, leading to a barrage of afferent impulses to the CNS. This may then, by reflex inhibition of gamma and alpha motor neurons, lead to re-adjustment of muscle tone and relaxation. Stimulation of mechanoreceptors may in turn shut down the "gate" by inhibiting small caliber nociceptors and may also result in reciprocal inhibition.

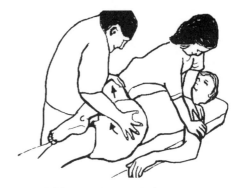

*Figure 5-26:* Long lever technique.

Many muscle energy techniques (non-thrust) are long lever methods directed at muscles that affect the restrictive barrier.

### Contraindication to Spinal Thrust Manipulations

Manipulations with impulse should not be used in patients with:

- Bleeding disorders or anticoagulant medications.
  May cause disastrous complications from bleeding.

- Rheumatoid disease, Reiter's syndrome and psoriatic arthritis.
  May result in ligamentous laxity and instability, especially in the cervical spine were the transverse ligament is affected often.

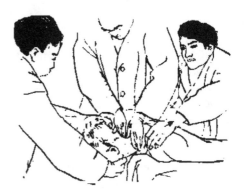

*Figure 5-27:* OM combined long and short lever technique under traction.

- Spinal cord compression is an absolute contraindicated to manipulation.
- Radicular pain with/without sensory, reflex and motor signs.
  Such patients rarely benefit from thrust techniques and often are made worse; thrust techniques are probably better avoided.
- Susceptibility to fractures from infections, osteoporosis, neoplastic disease etc.
- Hypermobility unless mild.
  Is a relative contraindication.

Applicable manipulations with impulse, i.e., thrust (both specific and nonspecific) are covered in the appropriate sections in the text.

# The McKenzie System

The McKenzie system uses loading strategies to evaluate and treat spinal disorders.

## Treatment with McKenzie System

McKenzie has developed a treatment system for disc derangements and other spinal disorders based on the patient's response to load strategies that either increase or decrease the patient's pain. He has originated the so-called "centralization phenomenon" which is based on the idea that pain originates often from tears within the annulus (McKenzie 1981; Donelson Silva and Murphy 1990) and in which the exercise goal is to centralize the pain; i.e., from peripheral (leg or arm) to central (low back and neck). By controlling posture and avoiding detrimental positions, the patient can promote a return of the nuclear material to the center of the disc.

In the McKenzie system spinal disorders are divided into postural syndrome, dysfunction syndrome, and derangement syndrome. Each of the syndromes responds differently to loading (Jacob and McKenzie 1995).

- The postural syndrome tends to exhibit delayed onset of symptoms in response to sustained static loading at end range. Symptoms can last for extended periods after loading is terminated.
  - The treatment approach is to avoid postures and loading strategies that bring the joints to end range. Stabilization exercises are helpful.
- The dysfunction syndrome tends to exhibit immediate onset of symptoms and mechanical responses at the restricted end range of the joint. Symptoms are reduce quickly when loading is terminated.
  - The treatment approach is frequent static or dynamic loading at or to the restricted end range.
- The derangement syndrome may exhibit immediate or delayed onset of symptoms following loading at the obstructed end range, at mechanically unimpeded end ranges, during motion, or with midrange static loading. Symptoms persist often and peripheralization increases when loading is terminated
  - The treatment strategy involves pursuing and avoiding certain loading tactics, as well as the order in which each is accomplished. Only movements and postures that result in centralization are used.

Disc derangements have been divided by McKenzie into posterior, anterior and lateral deviations.

### Posterior Deviations

Experiments on cadaverous lumbar motion segments have shown that lordotic postures create a concentration of vertical compressive stresses within the posterior annulus. These stresses can be particularly high following sustained "creep" loading, or following damage to an adjacent vertebra (Adems 1995), probably resulting in posterior deviations. Repetitive loading in a lordotic posture can lead to "hairpin bend" deformations of the lamellae within the posterior annulus, leading to a posterior bulge of the disc (Adams, Dolan and Hutton 1988), therefore leading to posterior deviations.

In posterior deviations, the most common type, the nucleus is shifted backward. Pain from posterior deviations increases with flexion and sitting. It decreases with extension and standing.

Examination for posterior deviation is positive when, after the patient flexes his or her spine 10 or more times, flexion increases *peripheral* pain. Subsequent extension movements should immediately decrease and *centralize* the pain. The evaluation is done weightbearing and non-weightbearing.

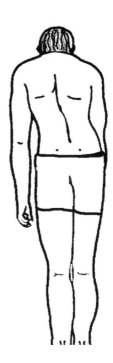

*Figure 5-28:* Typical posture of a patient who has a posterior-lateral deviation.

### Anterior Deviations

Anterior deviations are rare (about 10%) and are characterized usually by pain and peripheralization on extension and when standing, with reduction of pain and peripheralization when sitting. Anterior deviations are symptomatically very similar to facet syndromes.

Examination positive for anterior deviations is when repeated spinal extensions result in increased pain and peripheralization, and subsequent repeated flexion *centralizes* and reduces the pain, immediately.

### Lateral Deviations

Lateral deviations usually are combined with either posterior or anterior deviations. With the addition of lateral deviation, the patient has a side bending component and often presents with a postural list (Figure 5-28).

Examination positive for lateral deviation is found when lateral gliding to one side peripheralizes the pain, while gliding to the other side *centralizes* the pain. A flexion or extension component may be added for anterior or posterior deviations.

### Validity of Mckenzie System

The validity of the concepts of the McKenzie system have been evaluated by Aprill et al. (1995). Remarkably, the McKenzie evaluation and magnetic resonance imaging (MRI) and computed tomograpy (CT) discography showed an 83% agreement on the level of disc associated with pain provocation, 93% agreement on localization of painful tears within the disc, and 85% agreement on identifying whether the affected disc was contained or extruded.

# Chapter 6: *Treatment of Myofascial Tissues*

Treatment of myofascial tissues using protocols described here are often helpful. Treatment can begin with stimulation of the appropriate Sinews channel, by needling the channels' Well and termination points, followed by a layered acupuncture approach that directs treatment from superficial external layers, to deeper somatic tissues. In the classic *Simple Questions* the appropriate level to be needled is illustrated in the discussion on "Deep Punctures:"

> When disease is in the sinews.... needle the sinews, between the muscle layers without hitting the bone. When the disease is in the skin and muscles.... needle the big and small spaces, and needle deeply several times to generate heat. Take care not to injure the sinews and bone. When the disease is in the bones.... needle deeply, taking care not to injure the vessels nor the muscles. The needle path is through the big and small spaces. When the bones are warmed the disease ends. [1]

Acupuncture (and local dry needling) is therefore an art that requires practice. The practitioner must apply an exacting amount of stimulation. Too much can cause undue pain and injury and too little can render the treatment ineffective.

Muscle shortening and tension often respond to needling, either when treated directly or when the antagonists to the contracture are needled *(OM: Yin/Yang)*. Generally, contracted, shortened or spasmed muscles respond quickly to treatment, both qualitatively and symptomatically, usually resolving in 1-3 treatments. Relapse rates depend on the causative factor. Often periosteal acupuncture is necessary to obtain long-lasting results.

## Contractile Unit Disorders

Following examination of the superficial integument, palpation of deeper fascia and muscle is performed, looking for any altered tissue texture, such as superficial or deep nodules, tight bends or doughy muscle, severed tissues, fibrotic changes (often found in chronic conditions), restricted fascial layer motions, and trigger (Ashi) points. The tenoperiosteal junctions, often a site of trouble, should be palpated carefully. Palpation of the muscle belly should be perpendicular (cross-fiber) to the muscle fibers, gently stroking the fibers. When looking for deep-lying muscles, palpation should proceed by going deeper slowly and progressively, keeping overlying muscles relaxed. Stroking should begin only after the desired depth is reached. Tender tendons should be palpated along the direction of their inserting fibers, and they should be palpated perpendicularly to define their borders. To determine whether tenderness lies in superficial or deep structures, the practitioner can palpate the area during contraction and relaxation of the superficial muscle overlying the area. Pain that is more pronounced when the muscle is tense suggests that the superficial muscle is at fault.

---

1. This classical reference supports many of the needle techniques proposed in this text. It is clear that treatment was designed based on tissue pathology and needles inserted directly to the affected tissue and not just to "acupuncture points".

Muscle "spasms" and/or triggers manifest as indurated tissue lying parallel to the fibers involved, spindle-shaped tissue thickening, pressure-evoked muscle twitch, and bundles that can be moved at right angles to the muscle fibers.

Fascial layer motions can be assessed by gentle sheer movements applied by the practitioner, or by applying pressure over symmetrical areas and then asking patient to move the joints underlying the pressing hands. A restricted fascia will result in increased movement of the practitioner's hand on the affected side.

Objective tissue changes are more significant than elicitation of pain. The practitioner must establish the source of pain, because the location of pain may not correlate directly with the underlying condition that is responsible (referred tenderness is a common phenomenon).

## Locate Hyperactive Motor Points & Bands

Once dysfunctional muscles are identified (by review of the patient's history, pain drawings and functional assessments), the practitioner should locate all hyperactive motor points in the involved muscles. (Frequently the hyperactive motor points are the same as local acupuncture points). The practitioner:

• Palpates to identity tender areas (ashi points), trigger points in the areas where motor points are.

• Applies an electrical stimulator to the skin with sufficient voltage to cause a muscle contraction, but not strong enough to cause twitching in multiple locations when applied to none motor points.

If electrical stimulation is too painful, the intensity can be reduced.

(Even if the level of stimulation is insufficient to cause muscle contraction) asks the patient to identify the most sensitive areas.

Or:

— With impedance testing, uses a point locator to identify active skin over the points.

**NO MUSCLE TWITCH.** If electrical testing produces the sensations of increased electrical conduction, sensitivity or pain in the patient but no visual muscle twitch is seen, the area requires exploration with palpation and deep needling. This probe often yields a deep-seated muscle lesion or hardened tissue, and probably represents an area that has increased endplate activity (high internal electrical stimulation of muscle, resulting in spasm).

## Needle Hyperactive Motor/Trigger/Ashi Points

### TREATMENT 1

Once the hyperactive points are located, the practitioner:

**1.** Marks the points.

**2.** Activates the appropriate Sinews channel.

**3.** Uses a thin-gauge, #30-38 needle to needle them.

**4.** (Initially) uses the needle to lightly stimulate the outer, subcutaneous tissues at the site. Inserts the needle farther, first in the direction that shows superficial tissue drag-resistance.

This process may elicit muscle twitches, possibly through abnormal sympathetic pathways. The needling stimulates A-delta and large-caliber fibers, activating Wall and Melzack's "gate" and descending pathways. Through normal feedback mechanisms, the pain threshold increases and causes relaxation of the muscle, both of which make the rest of the treatment (if needed) more comfortable for the patient.

**NOTE:** Often this treatment is sufficient for obtaining a clinical response and trigger deactivation. If some positive affect is achieved this process is repeated in the next few sessions.

If needed:

5. Advances the needle slightly, paying attention to needle feel.

   The practitioner proceeds slowly to avoid the possibility of the patient feeling great pain or reaction.

6. (If a muscle twitch occurs quickly) rotates the needle slightly to the left, and no further stimulation is needed at that site.

## TREATMENT 2

If the patient does not respond to treatment within a few days, the practitioner:

1. Treats the same locations again, stimulating the points more vigorously to cause several twitches.

2. Rotates the needle gently counterclockwise, until feeling a slight tug on the fibers, and then pulls gently on the needle. Often this elicits a deep or referred ache and several more muscle twitches. (This is done in order to put the muscle fibers under tension, hence stimulating the spindle apparatus).

3. Leaves the needle in place 1-5 minutes.

4. (When the muscle relaxes) removes the needle gently.

## TREATMENT 3

If the patient does not improve following the second session, the practitioner:

1. Needles the active lesions even more vigorously, to cause local bleeding.

   This bleeding releases growth factors, thereby treating hemodynamically-disturbed areas and possibly transforming some overactive muscle fibers into nonpainful microscar tissue.

(To avoid adhesions, the practitioner should incorporate movement and cross-fiber massage).

2. (If hard-like tissue is found) needles throughout the tissue, gently rotating the needle back and forth no more than 1/8-turn, until feeling a "letting go" of the tissue and no resistance to the needle remains.

   Or:

3. Use triangle (bleeding) needle or scalpel to cause more extensive bleeding.

**POSITIONING OF PATIENT.** Patient positioning is very important when treating contracted muscles. It:

• Allows the practitioner to reach otherwise unreachable areas.

• Facilitates joint movement in the desired direction.

Also, if the patient is in proper position, the shortening of the fibers by the rotation of the needle will be more likely to result in muscle relaxation and less likely to cause post treatment flare or spasm.

When needles are retained for long periods the patient should be positioned comfortably such that the injured area has minimal nociceptive input (muscle in the treated area should be at maximum relaxation and comfort).

## Tendinous Lesions

If muscular dysfunction and pain are due to tendon relaxation or inflammation, the practitioner:

1. (For inflammation) needles the tendon-periosteal junction, using a thin needle (gauge 34-38) locally around the tendon but not through it.

   Needling through it may lead to unnecessary inflammation and pain.

2. Advances needle insertion slowly and takes several seconds to reach the

periosteum, paying constant attention to needle feel in order to prevent unnecessary injury and muscular reaction.

3. (Once the periosteum is reached) gently pecks the periosteum.

4. (Either) withdraws the needle or connects a unipolar electrical stimulator with the anode (+) pole placed locally at the injured tendon, and the cathode (-) held by the patient or connected to a motor point, an ear point corresponding to the muscle, or a distal point on the Sinews channel that passes through the muscle (most often Accumulation point).

Stimulation is maintained for one to five minutes only. Biphasic (AC) current or positioning of the cathode (-) just distally to the injured site can be used, as well.

NOTE: Cross fiber massage can be applied before or after the treatment.

*Tendon Insufficiency*

For tendon insufficiency, the tendon-periosteal junction is needled more vigorously and/or the anode (+) is connected locally and the cathode (-) just distally (some patients respond better to local cathode (-) application). The treatment lasts 30-60 minutes (or longer). Bipolar (AC) current can be used, as well.

## Subcutaneous Fascia

Fascial restrictions can be treated with subcutaneous needling, guiding the needle in the restricted direction. Several insertions and withdrawals, in a fanlike distribution, may be needed to release the restrictions. Often this is all that is needed.

Using light palpation, the practitioner may encounter hard or soft nodules in fascial layers that should be needled (especially in the sacroiliac areas). Often, needling these nodules causes sharp local pain and referred pain to the areas of the patient's complaints. Cross-fiber massage is integrated to separate the nodules from surrounding tissues. In addition, either a bleeding and cupping technique or a moving cup technique is effective and can be incorporated.

## Post-Treatment Care

Acupuncture needling of shortened muscles can be followed by:

• Post-isometric stretch techniques (Muscle energy).

• Muscle stretching with pre-stretch surface cooling using fluorimethane or ice. Only the skin, not the muscle, should be cooled.

The practitioner should encourage the patient to exercise and to use heat to reduce post-treatment soreness.

## Patients Refractory to Treatment

When patients who have myofascial pain do not respond to the these protocols, the practitioner should reassess the patient, looking for perpetuating factors. The most common factor is ligamentous insufficiency. Gait and foot disorders, medical problems and nutritional problems are common perpetuating factors, as well.

If a patient does not respond to milder treatment techniques, the practitioner can use a bleeding needle or a cataract scalpel at muscle triggers. This results in even larger local bleeding and hemodynamic effects.

# Sprains & Strains

Sprain and strains should be treated as early as possible to prevent the development of complications.

## Acute Stage

The following are the most important aspects in the treatment of sprains/strains.

### Minimizing Bleeding

Treatment of acute injury should be directed toward the prevention of bleeding and edema. Most injuries involve rupture of small blood vessels and arresting hemorrhage is the primary concern. The extravasation of blood will produce far more disability than the loss of a few fibers of muscle, tendon, or ligament (Garrick and Ebb *ibid*). Microscopic capillary bleeding in deep neck muscles has been shown to persist up to 5 days after motor vehicle collision injuries (Aldman 1987).

The majority of sprains and strains are of the mild or moderate variety, and therefore, by definition, the injured structure generally retains anatomic continuity and ability to function. The accompanying bleeding however, may distort normal anatomical relationships, resulting in pain and loss of motion. Bleeding and inflammation are essential for proper healing. However, it is best to prevent the blood from seeping into unaffected tissues causing unnecessary inflammation. Also inflammatory responses are often excessive and may be out of proportion to severity of the injury.

COMPRESSION. Compression is the most effective means of stopping hemorrhage. But to be effective, compression must be selective. Compression must be directed toward, and be in contact with, the hemorrhaging site. For example, tissues injured around the SI joint are deep to the bony surfaces and lay in a depression under the PSIS's, where a pressure wrap or tape may be applied. If a pad which allows for contact with the tape above the bony and other soft tissues is not used, the compressive force will probably only redistribute the swelling to areas where it will do more harm. Therefore, to effectively transfer compression to the tissues deeper to the PSIS's, a thick padding is needed over the desired area. This also is important in sprained ankles were a U shaped pad should be used.

CRYOTHERAPY. Cold application is helpful, but not as important as immediate compression. The efficacy of cold therapy has been studied on ankle sprains, showing an average of 15 days reduction in the time of recovery (Knight et al. 1980). Cryotherapy has several effects, including reduction of cell metabolism and oxygen consumption which can prevent secondary hypoxic injuries in uninjured tissues (Knight 1978). Cold also has an analgesic effect by acting as a counter irritant, and decreasing inflammatory responses (Cailliet 1991). Cold therapy has been criticized as it can cause edema, especially in the acute phase (Leduc et al. 1979).

Cold packs or ice should be combined with compression. Crushed ice or frozen gel capable of contouring around the anatomy is applied for a minimum of 20 minutes, repeating every two to four hours. Icing of the spine to treat deep seated lesions is ineffective, and in facet sprains may be detrimental by causing muscle cooling and spasm. In sprains of the SI joint, ice is helpful often but should be applied over the SI only, avoiding the lumbar muscles. Icing is helpful in interspinous ligamentous injuries, costotransverse and costosternal sprains, hyperextension/flexion injuries (whiplash) in the neck, tendinitis (both acute and chronic) and in the early stage of muscular strain. Cryotherapy is especially helpful in peripheral joint sprains and musculotendinous injuries.

The application of heat in acute injuries has been shown to be detrimental in the early stages (Hohl 1975). Heat is helpful in the chronic stage.

ELEVATION. Elevation, or at least avoidance of weight bearing, is the third element in the initial treatment of an acute injury. Painful movements should be avoided, but other movements should be encouraged in order to avoid the development of weak-

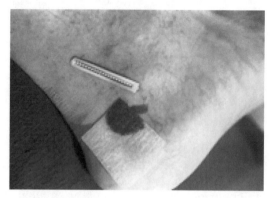

*Figure 2-1:* Bleeding congested vessels around the ankle.

ness from disuse.

**THERAPEUTIC EXERCISE.** Passive movement toward the direct or indirect direction (limited or non-painful) should be within the allowable joint play and range, and should be started as soon as possible.

**CROSS FIBER MASSAGE.** Cross fiber massage can be used gently for a minute or two, and may help prevent adhesions.

**BLOOD LETTING AND ACUPUNCTURE.** Blood letting (an OM technique) of visibly congested blood vessels in the area is helpful to reduce local pressure and encourages circulation—often leading to immediate reduction of pain and throbbing sensations (Figure 2-1). The Sinews channel is activated and supeficial local needles are inserted to surround the area. The appropriate Connecting channel is used often.

**MEDICINAL HERBS.** Medicinal herbs are prescribed according to the stage of the injury (page 297).

**SURGERY.** Although surgery may be necessary at times, several studies have shown that, at least at the knee joint, non-operative management of medial collateral ligament ruptures have as good an outcome as surgery.

## Subacute Stage

The subacute stage starts about 36-48 hours post injury, approximately when edema has stabilized. The practitioner is advised to treat swelling as quickly after the injury as possible, because edema becomes harder to manage once established. When patients present at the office a day or two post injury the treatment principles remain the same, first arresting all swelling, then eliminating edema and then restoring function.

- *Electrogalvanic Stimulation.* Once swelling is stabilized, the addition of high-intensity electrogalvanic or interferential stimulation with the muscle in the shortened position can help eliminate swelling.

- *Blood Letting and Acupuncture.* Blood letting of surrounding, visibly congested (dark colored) blood vessels, is effective in eliminating the swelling. The Sinews and Connecting channels are activated.

- *Topical Herbal Soaks.* Topical herbal soaks and plasters with or without massage are effective and should be used.

- *Contrast Therapy.* Contrast therapy (alternating hot and cold baths) should start at this time, first soaking the affected area in warm water (100 $^0$ F.) for about 4 minutes, followed by one minute of a cold icy water bath.

  Heat can increase blood flow, reduce pain and muscle spasm and relax joints. Encouraging active movement during the heat treatment is very important, as this will facilitate lymphatic, and other fluids, movement and drainage.

- *Exercise Therapy.* Exercise therapy within the nonpainful range is started, both actively and passively. Passive motion should be applied first in the indirect direction (i.e. toward the nonrestricted barrier) and initiated within the allowable joint-play and range. These measures may prevent the formation of troublesome adhesions. Direct movement into the restricted barriers is carried out as tolerated.

Patients usually respond to pain with guarding and avoidance of painful movements. Consequently, the resulting prolonged disuse leads to muscle weakness. Furthermore, because movements become uncomfortable, the muscles responsible for that action become less active, and the joint loses the stability afforded by these muscles, therefore increasing the likelihood of a recurrent injury. Strengthening exercises at the subacute phase should not be started too soon (especially if a tendon is involved), before the tissue has a chance to form a scar. They are started about 2-3 weeks after the injury. Light isometric muscle contractions are safe usually, and will not aggravate the condition (unless a tendon is involved) and should be gauged appropriately. The patient is taught particular exercises and instructed to perform about 5 repetitions hourly while awake. Vigorous activity should only be resumed after normal function has been restored. Otherwise, immature fibrous healing may rupture and maintain the disability. Also, the body will try to compensate for the dysfunction and establish abnormal patterns that may place unfamiliar stresses on numerous muscles and joints, causing a cascading increase in symptoms that may be much more difficult to deal with than those directly resulting from the original injury.

## Chronic Phase

The same treatment approach can be used in the chronic phase with more aggressive techniques. However, in tendinitis or muscular strains excessive strain from exercise can be detrimental. Often muscle length must be restored first.

## Stabilization & Exercise

Management of activity is part of the OM treatment approach of acute injuries, as well. Stabilization and restriction of movement with simultaneous exercise was described early in the Yang Dynasty in the medical book *Secret Formula of God for Management of Trauma and Fracture:*

> Sprains and fractures of the hands and feet are treated by topical application of ointment wrapped with cloth, and with intermittent exercise. The applicable exercises should be individualized, and the patient must neither overexercise nor underexercise.

For injuries to soft tissues, in order to promote Qi and Blood circulation, prevent stasis and adhesion, and promote healing, the practitioner must balance the need for immobility, stabilization, and mobility. In the acute and middle stages, movement must be soft and fluid to avoid aggravating the condition. In the late and chronic stages, the patient also can use strengthening exercises. Commonly-used, especially in acute disorders, are exercises that use Tai Chi and Qi Gong techniques. More specific muscle strengthening, stretching, and coordination training is used in middle and chronic stages.

## Herbal Management

In the early and middle stages of acute soft tissue injury, the main treatment principle is to activate the Blood and clear Heat. This facilitates elimination of Blood stasis and swelling, and it stops bleeding and pain.

A guiding oral and topical herbal formula for early stage sprain strain is:

Radix Angelicae Sinensis (Dang Gui)
Radix Rehmanniae (Sheng Di Huang)
Radix Paeoniae Alba (Bai Shao)
Radix Paeoniae Rubra (Qi Shao)
Rhizoma Ligustici Wallichii (Chuan Xiang)
Gummi Olibanum (Ru Xiang)
Resina Myrrhae (Mo Yao)
Herba Lycopodii (Shen Jin Cao)
Frctus Liquidambaris (Lu Lu Tong)

Semen Plantaginis (Che Qian Zi)
Flos Loncerae (Jin Yin Hua)
Flos Chrysanthemi (Ju Hua)
Rizoma Paridis (Zao Xiu)

If swelling is prominent:

Radix Bupleuri (Chai Hu)
Flos Carthami (Hong Hua)
Radix Paeonae Rubra (Chi Shao)
Semen Persicae (Tao Ren)
Sanguis Draconis (Xue Jie)
Radix Glycyrrhiza (Gan Cao)
Suama Manitis (Chuan Shan Jie)
Semen Trichonsanthes (Gua Lou Ren)
Radix et Rhizoma Rhei (Da Huang)
Resina Myrrhae (Mo Yao)
Gummi Olibanum (Ru Xiang)
Spina Gleditsiae (Zao Jiao Ci)

In the late stage of acute soft tissue injury and in chronic soft tissue dysfunction, the main pathology is disharmony of the Sinews and channels, which manifests as pain and fatigability of the affected tissues.

Treatment consists mainly of:
• Nourishing the Blood.

• Reharmonizing the collaterals.
• Warming the channels to stop pain.

A guiding oral and topical formula for late-stage with stiffness and pain is:

Radix Angelica Sinensis (Dang Gui)
Radix Peaoniae Rubra (Chi Shao)
Caulis Spatholobi (Ji Xue Teng)
Radix Salviae Miltiorrhizae (Dan Shen)
Ramulus Mori Albae (Sang Zhi)
Flos Carthami (Hong Hua)
Rhizoma Ligustici Wallichii (Chuan Xiong)
Radix Gentianae Macrophyllae (Qin Jiu)
Radix Clematidis (Wei Ling Xian)
Rhizoma Curcumae Longae (Jiang Huang)
Rhizoma seu Radix Notopterygii (Qiang Huo)

The practitioner uses OM individual diagnosis and techniques, alternating formulas accordingly.

Table 6-1 on page 299 summarizes the basic treatment principles used in the treatment of injuries. Table 6-2 on page 300 summarizes commonly used formulas for external application in all stages. Table 6-3 on page 301 summarizes commonly used formulas for oral intake in all stages.

*Table 6-1.* INJURY: BASIC TREATMENT PRINCIPLES

| TREATMENT PRINCIPLES | • Activate Blood<br>• Dissolve Stasis<br>• Eliminate Swelling<br>• Regulate Qi to Stop Pain |
|---|---|
| COMMON FORMULAS | • Three Colors Herbal ointment (Sanshe Gao)<br>• Dissolving Blood Stasis plaster (Huaxue Zhi Gao)<br>• Stopping Pain ointment (Zhitong Gao)<br>• Regulate Qi to Stop Pain Plaster (Liqi Zhitong Gao) |
| LOCAL HEAT/REDNESS | If the injury has local heat and redness, in order to<br>• Dissolve Blood Stasis<br>• Clear Heat<br>• Eliminate Toxin<br>• Reduce Swelling<br>• Stop Bleeding<br>Use<br>• Activating Blood ointment (Huoxue Gao)<br>• Clearing Ying ointment (Qing Ying Gao)<br>• Four-Yellow paste (Sihuang Gao)<br>• Gold-yellow paste (Jinhuang Gao) |
| MINOR INJURIES | For minor injuries, in order to<br>• Relax Sinews<br>• Activate the Blood<br>Use<br>• Thousand Flower oil (Wanhua Yao)<br>• Fr. Foeniculi oil (Xue Xiang oil) |

*Table 6-2.* **External Applications: Acute Injuries Late Stage, Certain Chronic Stages**

**External Herbal Applications**
**Acute Injuries Late Stage, And Certain Chronic Stages**

| Late Stage, Certain Chronic Stages | Pain Prolonged, Tissues Impaired Functionally |
|---|---|
| Treatment Principles | • Activate the Blood<br>• Stop Bleeding<br>• Dispel Stasis<br>• Stop Pain |
| Common Formulas | • Thousands of Responses ointment (Wan Fu Zi Gao)<br>• Pearl ointment (Zhen Zhu Gao)<br>• Transforming channels plaster (Huajian Gao) |
| Chronic Stages | Skin Over Lesion Cold, Somewhat White<br>Muscles and Tendons Hardened, Swollen, Spasmodic |
| Treatment Principles | • Warm the channels<br>• Stop Pain<br>• Facilitate Joint Movement |
| Possible Formulas | • Herbal hydrotherapy<br>• (Ba Xian Shao Yao Tang, Hai Tong Pi Tang)<br>• Topical spirits<br>• Huoxue Jiu (activate Blood spirit) |
| Chronic Pain with Wind-Damp Bi (rheumatism) | |
| Treatment Principles | • Warm the channels<br>• Eliminate Wind-Damp<br>• Stop Pain |
| Possible Formulas | • External application of steamed herbs<br>• Teng Yao, Tang Feng Shan<br>• Plaster<br>  — Dog skin plaster (Goupi Gao)<br>  — Transform channels plaster (Juajian Gao)<br>• Oils/Spirits |

*Table 6-3.* **INTERNAL HERBAL MEDICATION: ACUTE SOFT TISSUE INJURIES**

| **INTERNAL HERBAL APPLICATIONS: ACUTE SOFT TISSUE INJURIES** | |
|---|---|
| Pathologic Processes | • Blockage of Qi<br>• Blockage of Blood circulation<br>• Bleeding<br>• Severe pain due to stasis and ecchymosis |
| Treatment Principles | • Activate the Blood<br>• Dissolve Stasis<br>• Stop bleeding<br>• Regulate Qi! |
| Injury with Bi Syndrome (Wind-Damp/rheumatism), also: | • Eliminate Wind-Wet<br>• Harmonize the Collaterals |
| Weak Muscles/Tendons | • Supplement Spleen, Liver and Kidney with above principles |
| Early Stage      Treatment Principle<br>Common Formula | • Dissolve Stasis, Stop Pain, Stop Bleeding<br><br>• Stop Pain powder (Zhi Tong San), Yunnan White Powder (Yunnan Baiyao) |
| Middle Stage<br>  Treatment Principle<br><br><br><br>Common Formulas | Swelling and Pain Reduced Gradually and Noticeably<br>• Relax the Sinews<br>• Activate the Blood<br>• Reduce swelling<br>• Relaxing Tendon pill (Shu Jin Wan)<br>• Relaxing Sinew and Activating Blood Tea (Shu Jin Huo Xue Teng)<br>• Supplementing Sinew pill (Bu Jin Wan) |
| Late Stage,<br>Chronic Stage<br><br><br>Treatment Principles<br><br><br><br><br>Common Formulas | Often accompanied by Wind-Damp, manifest as local swelling, fatigue, muscle contractions, loss of normal function, pain (may be aggravated by weather changes).<br>• Nourish the Blood<br>• Harmonize the Collaterals<br>• Disperse Wind<br>• Stop Pain<br><br>• All-Inclusive Great Tonifying Tea (Shi Quan Da Bu Tang)<br>• Minor Invigorate the Collaterals Special Pill (Xiao Luo Luo Dan)<br>• Fantastically Effective Pill to Invigorate the Collaterals (Huo Luo Xiao Ling Dun)<br>• Major Invigorate the Collaterals Special Pill (Da Huo Luo Dan)<br>• Remove Painful Obstruction Tea (Juan Bi Tong) |
| Elderly/Weak      Treatment Principles<br><br>Common Formulas | • Supplement Liver and Kidney<br>• Eliminate Wind<br><br>• Bushen Zengjin Tong (Tonify Kidney Strengthen Sinews Tea)<br>• Bushen Huoxue Tong (Tonify Kidney Invigorate Blood Tea)<br>• Major Invigorate the Collaterals Special Pill (Da Hou Luo Dan) |

# Chapter 7: *The Neck and Head*

The cervical spine can perform a wide range of movements that are necessary for normal function and visual accommodation. Highly mobile due to the facets arrangement—oblique at angles of 45° (anterosuperior to posteroinferior) at the C2-3 joint tapering down to 10° at C7-T1—this part of the spine regularly takes part in intricate motions that strain the neck's musculoskeletal structures. The head alone requires complex movements for balance and rotation. One consequence of the cervical spine's flexibility is that the structure can become unstable easily. Degenerative changes, and associated pain, occur frequently.

The incidence of neck pain in the uninjured or pre-injured general population has been estimated to be about 7% (Deans et al. 1987). In a more recent report Bland (1989) reports that about 12% of women and 9% of men have neck pain at any given time. Hardin and Halla (1995) report that at one time or another neck pain may affect one-third of the adult population. In 10-15% of affected patients it can persist for 6 months or longer. Following car accidents, about 30% of car occupants suffer neck pain; many remain symptomatic for a prolonged period (Orthopade 1994). Head, neck and shoulder pain also can arise from tension, stress and other emotions (Johansson and Rubenowitz 1994; Pierti-Taleb at al. 1994).

Acupuncture (with attention to the neck) is a valuable tool for treatment of acute or chronic neck, shoulder and arm pain (Petrie and Langley 1983; Loy 1983; Laitenen 1975; Marcus and Gracer 1994; Gunn 1977). It is helpful during narcotic detoxification in chronic pain patients (Kroening and Aleson. 1985), and for treatment of headaches (Jensen et al. 1979; Hansen and Hansen 1983; Loh et al 1984; Vincent 1990).

## Anatomy & Biomechanics

The cervical spine has two functional segments: the typical vertebrae (C3-C7) and the atypical vertebrae (C0-C2), (Figure 7-1).

### The Typical Segments (C3-C7)

The typical cervical spine segments are the C3-C7 vertebrae. (The inferior facets of C2 have typical orientation, as well.) Described as a universal joint, a typical vertebra has a body, two laminae, two pedicles, two vertebral arches and a spinous process. Each of the C3-C6 vertebrae has a foramen for the vertebral artery. Each C3-C7 transverse process has an anterior tubercle and a posterior tubercle that serve as attachments for the scalene muscles anteriorly, and for the longus capitis and longissimus cervicis muscles posteriorly. The cervical nerve roots run under the transverse processes, through a trough in front of the facets.

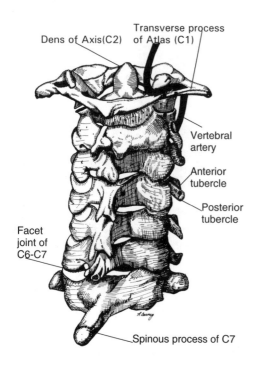

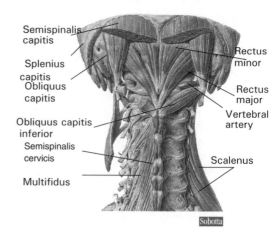

*Figure 7-2:*   Neck muscles.

brae is believed to function as guides for motion.

*Figure 7-1:*   Cervical spine (With permission Dorman and Ravin 1991).

## The Atypical Segments (C0-C1-C2)

The *atypical* segments of the cervical spine are the occipitoatloid joint (occipital bone and atlas) at C0-C1, and the atlantoaxoid joint (atlas and axis) at C1-C2.

On the typical cervical vertebrae, the zygoapophyseal (facet) joints face backward and upward at an angle of about 34° from the horizontal. These joints allow for flexion, extension, translation and sidebending, with coupled ipsilateral (type II) rotation. The greatest range of motion (ROM), about 17°, is at C5-6.

Adjacent vertebrae are linked by a disc, posterior and anterior longitudinal ligaments, facet joints, ligamenta nuchae, ligamenta flava, and the interspinous and intertransverse ligaments. From a reductionist viewpoint, the anterior column of the lower cervical vertebrae is believed to function as shock absorbers, and the posterior column of the lower cervical verte-

### The Occipitoatloid Joint (C0-C1)

The head-to-neck junction at C0-C1 is called the occipitoatlantoid or occipitoatloid joint. Articulation at this junction is of a modified-spherical type. Primary movement, which takes place in the transverse axis through a gliding motion of the upper surface of the joint, occurs posteriorly on flexion and anteriorly on extension.

On the average, motion across the transverse axis (about 24°) is limited by the bony and soft tissues that surround this joint. Sidebending takes place around the sagittal axis (z-axis) and measures about 5°. Occurrence of coupled sidebending and rotation at this joint is minor, but loss of these movements can be significant clinically. The total range of flexion and extension is 15% (Kapandji 1994).

The principal component of the occipitoatloid joint is the atlas (C1), a solid ring of bone that does not have a body and that articulates with the axis and the odontoid (dens) process. Other components of C1 are:

- Two oval-shaped, lateral pillars that run obliquely, anteriorly and medially and that bear the bi-concave articular surfaces (facets).

- An arch that, anteriorly, provides a small, cartilaginous, oval-shaped articular facet for the odontoid.

The rotator muscles of the head are attached to the transverse processes of the atlas. Since the atlas has no vertebral body, its facet joints (zygoapophyseal) are the only weight-bearing compression members at the joint.

### The Atlantoaxoid Joint (C1-C2)

C2 (axis) also called the odontoid (dens) vertebra, is a solid ring of bone from which the odontoid process rises vertically and to which the rotator muscles of the head are attached. The facets of the C2, which are located at the anterior aspect, articulate with the atlas. The splenius cervicis muscle attaches at the transverse process of axis. The nerve roots of the first and second spinal nerves lie superiorly and posteriorly to the articulating lateral masses of C1 and C2 (Bogduk and Twomey 1991).

ATLANTOAXOID JOINT MOTION. Motion at the C1-C2 joint is primarily rotation to the right and left. Other motions are slight flexion, extension, translation and sidebending. Motions occur in four articular vectors:

- Flexion and Extension.
  At this level are about 10°.

- Rotation.
  The total rotational range, about 50°, accounts for about 50% of rotation in the cervical spine.

- Sidebending.

Sidebending, 10° on the average, is possible only with coupled rotation. On sidebending, C1 rotates to the contralateral side while C2 rotates to the ipsilateral side of the bending (Kapanji 1974).[1]

### The Uncovertebral Joints

The uncovertebral joints are pseudojoints which do not contain articular cartilage and synovial fluid. They are thought to add lateral stability to the anterior column. The uncovertebral joints are a common cause of neuroforaminal narrowing due to degenerative arthritis.

## Innervation

The anterior aspect of the cervical spine is innervated by the anterior primary rami and its branches—the sinovertebral nerves. The posterior aspects are innervated by the posterior primary rami. The nerve roots run horizontally and laterally exiting at the intervertebral foramen. The roots contain both motor and sensory branches that are formed by the convergence of rootlets from the dorsal (sensory) and ventral (motor) aspects of the spinal cord. Outside the intervertebral foramen the roots again divide into dorsal and ventral branches and are joined by the cervical sympathetic chain.

## Cervical Spine Flexion

Cervical spine flexion takes place in two phases: first occurring at the C0-C1 and then at the C2-C7 joints.

Restriction of flexion in the C0-C1 and C1-C2 joints is produced by the:

- Nuchal ligament.

- Posterior longitudinal ligament.

---

1. Description of the range of motions at this joint vary considerably between authors.

- Longitudinal fasciculus of the cruciform ligament.

- Tectorial membrane.

- Posterior muscles.

Flexion of the head and neck depends on the anterior muscles of the neck. Table 7-1 summarizes innervation of the head and neck flexor muscles.

## Extension

In the cervical spine, the posterior muscles of the neck (Table 7-2), (Figure 7-2) perform the extension function. Extension is limited by bony limitation, anterior muscles, alar ligaments, and the anterior longitudinal ligament. Most of flexion-extension at the lower cervical spine takes place at the C3-C6 joints (especially C5-C6), (Kapanji *ibid*).

## Sidebending

The sidebender muscles of the head and neck achieve their action by mostly unilateral contraction of cervical muscles (Table 7-3 on page 307).

The total range of movement for the entire cervical spine in sidebending is approximately 45°; from C0 to C3 the ROM measures about 8°. When the neck is in extension, usually no sidebending of significance occurs, due to mechanical restrictions and the alar ligaments. Sidebending is greatest when the neck is in slight flexion. Coupled sidebending and rotation occurs, and is greatest, at C2-C3 and decreases at the lower cervical segments (Kapandji *ibid*).

## Rotation

Because most neck muscles are capable of contributing to neck rotation, the rotator muscles function as a complex system of combined muscle actions (Table 7-4 on page 308).

*Table 7-1.* FLEXOR MUSCLES OF THE HEAD AND NECK

| MUSCLE(S) | INNERVATION |
| --- | --- |
| Rectus capitis anterior | C1-C2 |
| Longus capitis cervicis | C1-C3 |
| Infra and Supra-Hyoid muscles | Facial nerve Inferior alveolar nerve |
| Sternocleidomastoid | C2, Accessory |
| Anterior, Medius, Posterior Scalene muscles | C3-C8 |
| Obliquus capitis superior | V1 |

Table 7-2. EXTENSOR MUSCLES OF THE HEAD AND NECK

| MUSCLE | INNERVATION |
| --- | --- |
| Splenius cervicis | C6-C8 |
| Splenius capitis | C4-C6 |
| Semispinalis cervices | C1-C8 |
| Semispinalis capitis | C1-C8 |
| Levator scapulae | C3-C4 |
| Intertransversarii | C1-C8 |
| Longissimus capitis | C6-C8 |
| Trapezius | C3-C4, Accessory |
| Sternocleidomastoid | C2, Accessory |

Table 7-3. SIDEBENDING MUSCLES OF THE HEAD AND NECK

| MUSCLE(S) | TO (SIDE) | INNERVATION |
| --- | --- | --- |
| Trapezius | Either | C3-C4, Accessory |
| Sternocleidomastoid | Opposite | C2, Accessory |
| Longissimus capitis | Same | C6-C8 |
| Longissimus cervicis | Same | C6-C8 |
| Splenius capitis | Same | C4-C6 |
| Splenius cervicis | Same | C4-C6 |
| Obliquus capitis inferior | Same | C1 |
| Levator scapulae | — | C3-C4 |
| Iliocostalis cervicis | — | C6-C8 |
| Rotatores brevis | — | C1-C8 |
| Rotatores longi | — | C1-C8 |
| Longus colli | — | C2-C6 |
| Scalenes | — | C3-C8 |
| Multifidus | — | C1-C8 |

*Table 7-4.* ROTATOR MUSCLES OF THE HEAD AND NECK

| MUSCLE(S) | TO (SIDE) | INNERVATION |
| --- | --- | --- |
| Sternocleidomastoid | Opposite | C2, Accessory |
| Trapezius | Opposite | C3-C4, Accessory |
| Splenius capitis | Same | C4-C6 |
| Splenius cervicis | Same | C4-C6 |
| Semispinalis capitis | Same | C1-C8 |
| Semispinalis cervices | Same | C1-C8 |
| Longissimus capitis | Same | C6-C8 |
| Longissimus cervicis | Same | C6-C8 |
| Obliquus capitis inferior | Same | C1 |
| Scalene | Opposite | C3-C8 |
| Rotatores brevis | Same | C1-C8 |
| Rotatores longi | Same | C1-C8 |
| Intertransversarii | — | C1-C8 |

# Imaging

Radiological studies play an important part in the evaluation of acute cervical trauma. No attempt is made within these pages to address the acute situation. Radiographs can give the clinician information about the bones themselves, but more often, subtle changes of position and asymmetries afford clues to altered tensile strength and the elasticity of restraining ligaments and fascia. A clearer observation of these somatic dysfunctions can be obtained with movements. Imaging studies are static. An approximation to the changes with movement is arrived at by obtaining X-rays in neutral positions and in the extremes of movement. Somatic dysfunctions are more troublesome and also are enhanced in appearance in the standing, weight-bearing position; therefore, it is a general principle in Orthopaedic Medicine to obtain films upright, whenever possible.

## Upper Cervical Spine

The occiput, atlas, and axis function as a unit and should be studied radiologically as a unit. At least three views should be obtained, including:

1. The anterior view of the upper cervical spine.

2. Lateral view (usually taken with that of the lower part of the neck).

3. Open-mouth or odontoid view.

   Additional views include (Jackson 1958).

4. Open-mouth view with left-headed rotation.

5. Open-mouth views of the odontoid with right-and-left-head rotation.

6. Lateral views of the neck in flexion.

7. Lateral views of the neck in extension.

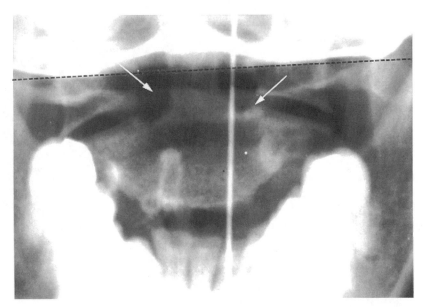

*Figure 7-3:* Normal open-mouth view of odontoid. The closed arrows point to the equal sulci. Note the base of the occiput (dotted line) is nearly horizontal. The white line is a vertical marker.

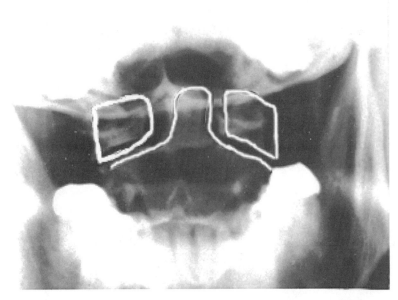

*Figure 7-4:* Open-mouth view of the odontoid and atlas. Note the unequal sulci and asymmetry of the lateral masses of the atlas. The two images are essentially the same and represent slight differences in radiographic technique.

Careful scrutiny of the several odontoid views may show asymmetry of its position. The recess or sulcus between the odontoid and the lateral mass of the atlas is best seen in the open-mouth view. The restraining ligaments are the apical and two alar ligaments. Alignment will be abnormal in the presence of asymmetrical tension from an injury. On rotation to the side of the intact alar ligament, movement is normal. On rotation to the side of the weakened alar ligament, subluxation is enhanced. Despite technical inconveniences, there is an advantage in obtaining these films upright (Figure 7-3 and Figure 7-4).

In the anterior-posterior (AP) view, slight head tilting often is visible. It usually signifies somatic dysfunction below the second cervical vertebra (Figure 7-5).

Many practitioners in the osteopathic and chiropractic professions have maintained that the position of the atlas is particularly important, not only for cervical dynamics, but also in regulating the whole spine.

In whiplash injuries the transverse ligament of the atlas may be attenuated. This can be demonstrated in lateral views taken in flexion and extension. The atlas will be seen to separate a little from the odontoid in flexion.

*Magnetic Resonance Imagery & Computed Tomography of the Upper Cervical Spine*

Transaxial imaging with magnetic resonance imagery (MRI) or computed tomograpy (CT) is best for evaluating acute trauma of the upper neck: CT is best for imaging bony structures and MRI shows soft-tissue abnormalities better, particularly those of the neuroaxis. Acutely injured patients can be managed in the supine position obviating the need for

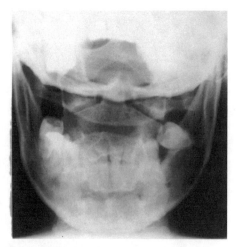

*Figure 7-5:* Anterior-posterior view of the upper cervical spine with the head tilt and asymmetric atlanto axial points. The head tilt is an essential change and is not an artifact in patient positioning.

moving them, so that the risk of aggravating neuroaxis injuries is assessed first.

Evaluation of chronic neck pain with MRI and CT is being used more in the quest for disc disease. Somatic dysfunction often is visible as a bonus in these images (Penning, Wilmick 1987; Dvorák 1987; Epstein 1988). When vertebral rotation is seen in static films, it probably represents a disparity in the tension of the soft tissues and not a chance position. The occipital condyles, the atlas, and the axis may not seem to be imaged equally or symmetrically. This should not be dismissed merely as positional. Patients without soft-tissue problems are able to lie straight in the gantay. Recognition of asymmetry therefore is meaningful (Mazzara 1989; Penning 1978; Clark 1987). Whenever possible, a space-oriented analysis, taken together with the clinical findings, gives a first approximation to a positional diagnosis.

**The Lower Cervical Spine**

In the lower cervical spine, attention to the images also can be divided between observations of the bones themselves and

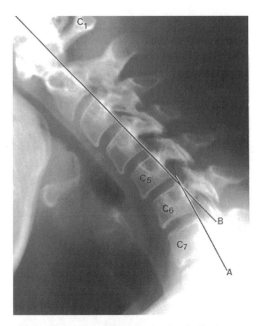

*Figure 7-6:* Lateral cervical spine in flexion. Lines A and B show the site of maximum stress at the C5-6 level. Note the normal and equal fanning of the spinous processes.

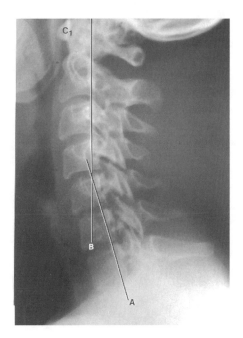

*Figure 7-7:* Lateral view of cervical spine. The lines indicate the site of normal stress. The site of intersection of lines A and B is the location of the greatest stress. Normal is at the middle of C5. Line A is drawn parallel with the posterior edge of C7 and line B is parallel with the posterior aspect of C2.

positional observations that reflect ligament and facial tension asymmetries. In the presence of long-standing dysfunction, soft-tissue abnormalities can affect the bony appearance secondarily. The presence of osteophytes is an example of this. A partial tear of a ligament attached to zygoapophyseal (facet) joint or vertebral body can lift the periosteum slightly, and, when the bone reforms under the rent, an osteophyte is formed.

Curves of the spine reflect tensions in soft tissues. Likewise, asymmetry in bony positioning with rotation should be noted. Unfolding of the spine should occur evenly with bending in any direction. The smoothness of the movement of bending is an important clinical observation. Its radiological counterpart should not be neglected (Foreman 1988). Because the study of somatic dysfunction is a dynamic one, abnormalities on imaging may bring the observer to the point of recognizing their presence but not necessarily defining them. This, however, is a first approximation. In the lateral film, the normal cervical spine has a lordotic curve. An evaluation of the region of the greatest stress can be estimated by drawing lines along the posterior surfaces of C6 and C7. Their point of intersection indicates the apex of the stress of the lordotic curve (Jackson 1977), usually falling between C3 and C5 (Figure 7-7- Figure 7-6).

Ligamentous or soft-tissue injuries (somatic dysfunction) can cause straightening of the cervical spine and loss of the natural lordosis. The site of maximal straightening may represent the major locus of the abnormality. Two considerations should be kept in mind. On the one hand, attenuated ligaments between vertebrae might allow increased movement between them. On the other hand, the reactive inflammation from the injury may bring on protective, reactive muscle contraction, so that the segment may be seen to move less. Imaging the bones, therefore, cannot replace a careful clinical assessment (Figure 7-9—Figure 7-10).

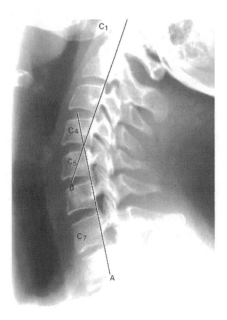

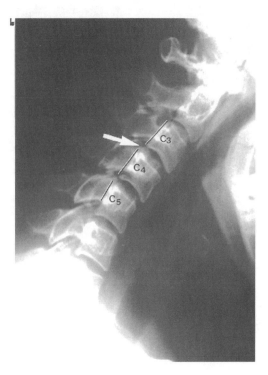

*Figure 7-8:* The lateral cervical spine in extension. Lines A and B demonstrate the greatest stress at C4-5. Note the normal and equal approximation of the spinous processes.

*Figure 7-10:* Lateral view of cervical spine with anterior subluxation in flexion of C3 on C4. The arrow points to the site of the anterior displacement.

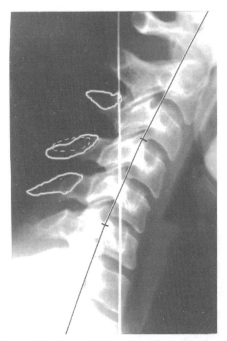

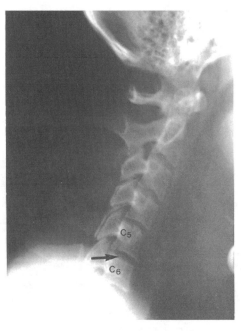

*Figure 7-9:* Lateral View of cervical spine with unequal fanning and the "flat spot" at the site of somatic joint dysfunction in flexion. (The vertical white line is a true vertical marker).

*Figure 7-11:* Lateral view of the neck with closed arrow pointing to the one narrow disc space at C5-6.

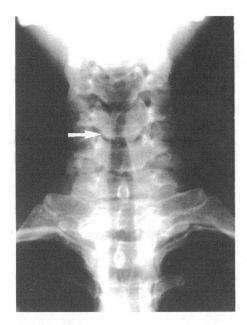

*Figure 7-12:* Anterior-posterior view of lower cervical spine with the arrow pointing to the asymmetric uncovertebral joint. The zygoapophyseal joints in this view are not clearly visible.

Evaluation of the height of the discs is best made on the lateral view. The normal disc tapers from the front backwards. The height is two to three times greater anteriorly. This contributes to the lordosis normally present. The height of the discs increases progressively by a small amount between the second and seventh spaces. Abnormal proximity of the vertebrae is an indirect sign of intervertebral disc attenuation. Although these abnormalities also are discernible on AP views, their assessment is more precise on the lateral ones (Figure 7-11).

Evidence that the degenerative process is primarily of a ligamentous nature comes in part from the development of osteophytes early in this process. Degenerating discs also may have visible gaseous vacuolation.

The synovial uncovertebral joints of Luschka are subject to this same degenerative process. Osteophytes growing from these joints are responsible for the bony spurs that encroach occasionally on the intervertebral foramina and that are notoriously responsible for episodes of true radiculopathy.

The uncovertebral joints are essential in the gliding intervertebral movements of the vertebrae in side bending and rotation (Penning and Wilmick 1987; Kapandji *ibid*). In the AP view, their alignment can be visualized and any asymmetry noted. A persistent asymmetry in several views indicates somatic dysfunction at the level concerned (Figure 7-12—Figure 7-13).

The zygoapophyseal joints are important structural elements of the vertebral column. Not surprisingly, trauma to the spine usually involves the capsules of these joints. In the case of the neck, the context usually is that of a whiplash injury. Osteophytes are a manifestation of healed injuries at these sites. The narrowing of the joint space also is a manifestation of injury at these sites but is somewhat hard to assess radiologically (because the static view of any particular

Just as the smooth, fan-like movement of the vertebrae depends on normal function of the intervertebral discs, so is the dysfunction of the discs responsible for uneven unfolding with bending.

In particular, a posteriorly or posterolaterally displaced fragment of an annulus can block extension at that level when trapped between the posterior margins of the vertebrae. It also can block flexion when trapped between the vertebra and the posterior longitudinal ligament. Pain, of course, is an important accompaniment of the latter situation.

Listhesis of the vertebrae always indicates ligament attenuation and usually is noted in flexion or extension. In forward spondylolisthesis of a vertebra on the one below, the major attenuation is to the posterior restraining structures, and vice versa. It is likely that the zygoapophyseal capsular ligaments also are injured and all restraining structures are affected to some extent.

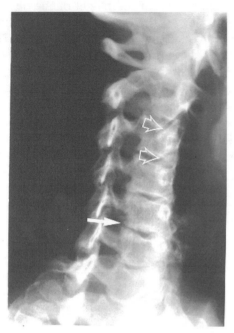

*Figure 7-13:* Oblique x-ray of the cervical spine. The closed arrows point to the bony "spurs" arising from the uncovertebral joints that are encroaching on the neural canal of C-5- 6. The open arrows point to the zygoapophyseal joints that are also visible in the projection.

dysfunction by viewing flexion and extension lateral films and then this level is scrutinized on an AP film, a subtle abnormality of alignment might be identified. All spinal movements include coupled side bending and rotation; hence an approximation to the nature of the somatic dysfunction might be attempted by viewing the films as a set.

Interestingly, a search for asymmetry of the bones when viewing MRI and CT scans can yield information even if the images were taken for other purposes. Isolated vertebral rotation almost always represents somatic joint dysfunction and is not merely positional. The vertebrae concerned will not be sliced symmetrically. One transverse process is likely to be demonstrated better than the other, and the vertebral body may appear rectangular rather than square. In the transverse images and in the presence of somatic joint dysfunction, the zygoapophyseal and uncovertebral joints are visualized unequally in any individual slice.

film may not be tangential to the joint space (Figure 7-14).

The extent of zygoapophyseal joint dysfunction can be evaluated in part in lateral and oblique extension views. In extension the joints are closed. With backward slippage, the spinous processes of the vertebrae approximate and may abut; thus, further extension may provoke slight subluxation of the zygoapophyseal joint. These movements encroach on the vertebral foramina. In the presence of osteophytes, this encroachment can be critical to the traversing nerve roots.

In normal spines, the anteroposterior diameter of the vertebral canal is about the same as the anteroposterior diameter of the vertebral body at each level. The normal ratio is equal or greater then 1.0: 0.8; a lesser ratio is considered abnormal.

If one particular level of the cervical spine is identified as the site of somatic

## Cervical Spondylosis

Ligament and fascia attenuation leading to and associated with degeneration of the intervertebral joints, the zygoapophyseal joints, and the uncovertebral joints, with their radiological manifestations, sometimes are labeled together as cervical spondylosis. The radiological inventory of abnormalities includes:

**1.** Disc space narrowing.

**2.** Osteophyte formation anteriorly and posteriorly at the disc level.

**3.** Osteophyte formation at the uncovertebral joints of Luschka.

**4.** Bone spurs anteriorly at the zygoapophyseal joints.

It is suggested here that these are indirect manifestations of ligament and fascial attenuation.

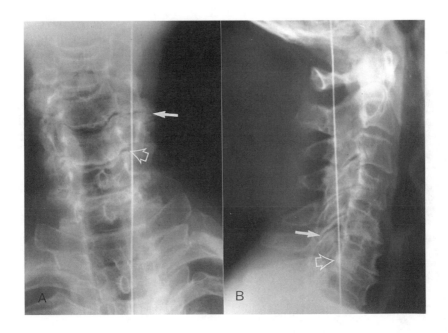

*Figure 7-14:* A and B x-ray changes of degenerative intervertebral joint disease of the lower cervical spine. Note the osteophytes from the joints of Luschka (open arrow) and zygoapophyseal joints (closed arrow).The neck list is structural.

Severe narrowing of the spinal canal can damage the cord—cervical spondylotic myelopathy. Posterior vertebral spurs usually make an important contribution to this disease. It is only through radiographic studies that this can be assessed accurately. The CT study is best for imaging bony abnormalities, but MRI gives more accurate information about the spinal canal and neuroaxis attenuation.

Because the differential diagnosis of cervical spondylotic myelopathy includes single and multiple disc herniation, MRI often is most helpful. When evaluating cervical spondylosis, it is important to remember that the degree of neurological deficit rarely coincides with the area of greatest degenerative change demonstrated on X-ray.

## Other Processes

The cervical spine, like other bones in the body, may be afflicted with other disease processes—primary and secondary neoplasms, infections, missed or unidentified fractures, metabolic bone diseases, and collagen vascular disease, all have radiological manifestations, which are not the subject of this text.

## Soft-Tissue Imaging of the Front of the Neck

While inspecting the lateral view of the spine, the retropharyngeal space should be noted for focal swelling, particularly after a recent injury. Although rare, it can be an important finding for ligament hematoma, as well as for occult fracture. When suspected, MRI or CT studies may be called for.

The lateral view also demonstrates the soft tissue behind the nasopharynx. Although the thickness of this area varies, a number of nasopharyngral disorders can be detected (Miles 1988).

The larynx and trachea air shadows should be noted. These subtle air lucencies are frequently distorted by asymmetrical contraction of the anterior neck muscles. This is particularly true when there is a dis-

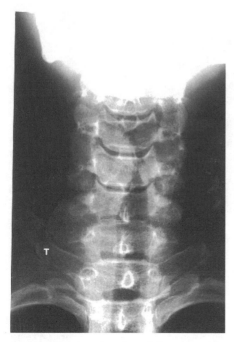

*Figure 7-15:* Anterior view of the neck with tracheal distortion by muscle spasm of the omohyoid anteriorly. Note the perfect bony anterior-posterior alignment, but the tracheal alignment is not symmetrical.

parity between the position of the chin and the neck, suggesting abnormal tension in the omohyoid and sternothyroid muscles that often are involved first in extension injuries of the neck (Figure 7-15).

# OM Disorders

Treatment of soft tissue injury in the neck was described as early as (100 B.C.). The classic book *Canon of Spiritual Pivot* states:

> For difficulty in neck flexion and extension.... treat the foot Taiyang channel.... In difficulties of rotation.... treat the hand Taiyang channel.

In *Golden Mirror for Original Medicine, Orthopedic Outline* traumatic neck

pain is categorized as *drop, hit* and *fall.* Symptoms and signs are characterized as extended neck with loss of flexion, flexed neck with loss of extension and loosening of tendons or ligaments resulting in dislocation, stiffness and rigidity of the soft tissues. *Compilation of Traumatology* states that "stiff neck" may be caused by sprain or by misuse of pillows.

## Modern Classifications

In general, modern classifications distinguish between exogenous and endogenous causes. Exogenous and Independent causes are Wind, Cold, Damp, sprains and contusions.

### Wind & Cold Exposure

Pathogenic factors can cause a stiff neck and lead to stagnation of Qi and Blood which block the Channels and Collaterals leading to Painful Obstructive Disorders (Bi). When symptoms of neck stiffness, headache and temperature aversion are elicited by exposure to windy and cold weather, a more superficial stiff neck syndrome is present. This syndrome has a rapid onset but usually is self-limiting at 2-3 days. If symptoms are prolonged, complicating factors should be sought.

### Strain & Contusion

Strains can present as a painful stiff neck and palpation reveals muscle spasm, painful Ashi (trigger) and channel points.

Contusion results in a localized, slightly swollen and tender focus. Associated collateral (nerve) damage may cause symptoms of tingling and numbness.

### Internal/Endogenous Causes

Internal classifications or cervical syndromes usually are applied to chronic, painful neck disorders. Often the Liver and Kidney Organs and the Urinary Bladder, and Small Intestine channels are involved. The Yang Linking (Wei), Yin Motility (Qiao), and Governing (Du) Extra channels are implicated often, as well.

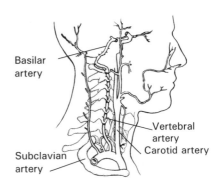

*Figure 7-16:* Vascular structures.

### Phlegm & Dampness

Phlegm and fluid accumulation (often secondary to Organ dysfunction) may rise to the neck region, obstructing the channels and collaterals.

### Stagnation of Qi & Blood

Any chronic or acute affliction can result in stagnation of Qi and Blood and development of pain and distention. Qi stagnation (distention pain) is associated often with ligamentous laxity, pain that is alleviated by movement and that increases with emotional and physical tension. Blood stagnation is associated often with a history of trauma and sharp pains.

# Biomedical Disorders

Pain in the neck, head, shoulder and arm regions can be due to a variety of disorders that should be ruled out. Table 7-5 on page 318 summarizes some of these. Because innervation of the craniocervical joints differs from innervation of joints in other regions of the body, a variety of clinical problems can result. The most notable of these problems is "cervical balance disorders" (Neuhuber and Bankoul 1994), which occur due to the thick-calibre neck muscle afferents that project directly to the external cuneate nucleus and to the vestibular nuclear complex. This projection, which is most prominent in segments C2 and C3, is scant or absent in the more caudal segments.

When considering the sources of cervical pain, the practitioner must review and consider nonorthopedic conditions that can evoke upper body pain. The practitio-

ner must be careful and remain alert to the potential effects of manipulation and related techniques that can have serious consequences.

## Vascular Disorders

The likelihood of vascular disorders is an important element in the diagnosis of the cervical spine. Potential of vascular compromise is inherent in certain mechanical therapies and other treatments of the neck. The differential diagnoses of vascular conditions include:

- Sudden arterial occlusions (as in coronary artery disease with angina).
- Thoracic outlet syndrome.
- Arteritis.
- Intermittent claudication (periodic insufficiency of blood supply, unlikely in the upper body).
- Raynaud's disease/phenomenon (upper extremity pain that is secondary to vasospasm).
- Basilar syndrome (a condition that affects the posterior cerebral and vertebral arteries), (Figure 7-16).

Table 7-6 lists predisposing factors in vascular compromise (Rivett 1994; Kunnasmaa 1994).

*Table 7-5.* **SOURCES OF UPPER BODY PAIN**

**NECK, HEAD, SCAPULA, ARM, HANDS**

Nonorthopedic

Vascular Conditions
- sudden arterial occlusions
- basilar syndrome
- intermittent claudication
- Raynaud's disease/phenomenon

Other Nonorthopedic Conditions
- rheumatoid arthritis
- secondary malignancy
- herpetic and trigeminal neuralgias
- neuroma
- neurofibromas
- amyotrophy
- muscular wasting such as in amyotrophic lateral sclerosis (Lou Gherig's disease)
- calcification of the ligamenta flava
- axial osteomalacia (softening of the bones)
- abdominal and chest diseases

**Orthopedic**

Musculoskeletal Cervical Lesions
- ligaments
- tendons
- muscles
- joints
- intervertebral discs

Trauma such as fracture

Vertebral and soft tissue dysfunction in cervical spine referred from more distal spine

*Table 7-6.* **FACTORS IN VASCULAR COMPROMISE**

| PREDISPOSING FACTORS | OTHER FACTORS |
|---|---|
| • hypertension | • diabetes |
| • fibromuscular dysplasia | • neoplasm |
| • oral contraceptive use | • arteritis |
| • arteriopathy | • multiple sclerosis |
| • cervical spondylosis | • aneurysm |
| • arteriosclerosis | • bony congenital abnormalities |
| • congenital asymmetry of the posterior circulation | • neurofibromatosis |
| • history of previous neck trauma | • steroid treatment |
| • cardiovascular disease | |
| • osteoarthrosis | |
| • segmental hypermobility | |
| • smoking | |

*Symptoms*

Pathology of the basilar artery and the vertebral artery (VA) can cause cervical pain, vertigo and tinnitus. The vessel affected most often in cervical vascular disorders is the anterior spinal artery. Neurological symptoms frequently are accompanied by acute pain that radiates segmentally. Rotation with extension to one side has been shown to obstruct the vertebral arteries on the stretched side (Gerlach 1984; Weintraub and Khoury 1995). However others saw no change in vascular flow (Weingar and Bischoff 1992), (for more detail see manipulation chapter 7).

Cervical vascular compromise can result in symptoms of anxiety, nystagmus (involuntary eye movements) and dizziness. Osteophytosis and arterial wall disease are thought to be the most common causes of CVA complications due to manipulation. (This assertion has been challenged, because most of these complications, from manipulation, are seen in patients between 30-50 years of age, and not in older patients as thought previously), (Grant 1988).

**SUBARACHNOID HEMATOMA.** Subarachnoid hematoma should always be suspected, especially if the patient has a sudden onset of severe headache.

**IDIOPATHIC SPONTANEOUS SPINAL EPIDURAL HEMATOMA.** Idiopathic spontaneous spinal epidural hematoma is rare. However, if a patient has a sudden onset of acute cervical pain, and especially if the patient is taking anticoagulation medication, the practitioner should consider this possibility. Usually the first symptom is severe neck pain, followed by radiating segmental pain.

**EXTRACRANIAL VERTEBRAL ARTERY DISSECTION.** Sturzenegger (1994) reports that, in patients who have extracranial vertebral artery dissection, the clinical features of headache and neck pain are always located on the side of the dissected vertebral artery. Some patients have head and posterior neck pain. Others have posterior neck pain only, no change in a chronic pre-existing headache, or no pain at all.

Pain starts suddenly, and is sharp in quality, severe in intensity, and different from any previous headache. Following acute onset, the pain is monophasic, with gradual remission of a persistent headache lasting one to three weeks. Most patients experience a delay between the onset of head or posterior neck pain and the onset of neurologic dysfunction. About 50% of patients report that this delay is less than one day; about 50% report the delay to be 1-21 days. Although this distinct type of pain is nonspecific as an isolated symptom, it should raise suspicion of an underlying vertebral artery dissection. Early confirmation of this diagnosis, and subsequent anticoagulation if dissection does not extend intracranially, may help prevent vertebrobasilar ischemic deficits.

**ANGINA PECTORIS.** Angina pectoris often manifests as tingling or pain in the face, neck, abdomen or chest. Occasionally it may manifest as facial or neck pain alone. If the patient has a risk factor for cardiovascular disease (such as hypertension, diabetes, smoking, family history, obesity or hyperlipidemia), and if the patient experiences these symptoms on exertion, heart disease should be considered. OM treatment for angina pectoris is similar to treatment for other vascular compromise conditions.

**TEMPORAL ARTERITIS.** Temporal arteritis can result in an intense temporal area headache, extremely tender scalp, and no pulsation of the temporal arteries. The erythrocyte sedimentation rate can be extremely elevated, generally over 100.

> **WARNING:** Temporal arteritis is a medical emergency. A delay in treatment can result in blindness.

### Intermittent Claudication

Intermittent claudication caused by ischemia secondary to arteriosclerotic plaque progression can cause the patient to complain of pain in the extremities on exertion (uncommon in the upper extremities). If neck movements do not provoke the extremity pain, this condition should be considered as a possible source.

## Examination for Vascular Compromise

The reliability of tests for vascular compromise is questionable. However, the practitioner should perform them, because a positive sign can be significant. (These tests should be performed for medicolegal reasons, as well).

Before considering cervical manual therapy, to assess the possibility of vascular compromise the practitioner should perform a provocation test such as the cervical Quadrant Test (over-pressure to the extended, rotated and sidebent neck) or Barrét's test.

The practitioner asks the patient to:

1. Stand with eyes closed and arms in front, with palms upheld horizontally.

2. Rotate his head to one side, hold it there for one minute, and then rotate it to the other side.

Any movement of the patient's stretched arms away from the parallel starting position, implies vascular compromise. No cervical manipulation should be performed.

**TREATMENT OF VASCULAR COMPROMISE.** If vascular compromise is present, a combination of OM and modern medicine—but not manipulation of the neck—can be used. If osteophytosis is present, surgery may be indicated. Arterial wall disease can be treated with a combination of OM (blood activation, stasis transformation, phlegm dispersion, opening of portals, and hardness softening, none of which are in the scope of this text) in conjunction with modern medical intervention.

## Headache

Headache, a common symptom of cervical dysfunction, can be due to mechanical, muscular, ligamentous and/or neurological lesions. Pain may or may not be felt at the neck and head and may be related to movement. The pain may be unilateral or bilateral and it may be felt over the occiput, the forehead, temples and the eye. Treatment directed to the cervical spine is often effective in treatment of headaches.

Bogduk (1992) has shown that, neuroanatomically, cervicogenic headache is transmitted by convergence in the trigeminocervical nucleus between nociceptive afferents from the field of the trigeminal nerve and the receptive fields of the first three cervical nerves.

## Acute, New Headache

An acute, new headache can be serious. The practitioner should consider conditions such as an impending CVA (cerebral vascular accident), subarachnoid hemorrhage, infections, malignant hypertension, arteritis, poisoning, intracranial tumor, and trauma.

## Chronic, Recurrent Headaches

Chronic, recurrent headaches are often due to musculoskeletal conditions such as ligamentous lesions, vertebral dysfunctions of the upper cervical spine, and myofascial syndromes.

**EARLY MORNING HEADACHE.** Early morning headaches are common with joint dysfunctions and ligamentous insufficiency, often seen in elderly patients. The pain usually improves after several hours of movement (posain).

**POSTERIOR NECK MUSCLE HARDNESS.** In studies of the "hardness" of trapezius and posterior paraspinal muscles in patients who had headaches, Sakai et al. (1995) found that hardness of these muscles in women was significantly greater than that of men, and that this correlated in patients of both sexes with the existence of headaches. Trapezius muscles were significantly harder than paraspinal posterior neck muscles measured at C5. Muscle hardness did not show a significant correlation with advancing age, blood pressure or subjective feeling of stiffness in the shoulder.

Sakai et al. noted a significant correlation between muscle hardness (by objective measurement) and stiffness scores evaluated manually through palpation. In patients who had tension-type headache (n = 60), the hardness of the trapezius muscles was significantly greater than that of normal subjects. There was no significant difference in muscle hardness between episodic tension-type headache and chronic tension-type headache.

MIGRAINE HEADACHE. Migraine headaches are believed to have a vascular origin—in the prodromal phase (before headache begins), intracranial blood vessels constrict, and characteristic visual and/or sensory disturbances occur. In the second phase the blood vessels dilate, which results in acute unilateral headache. Migraine headaches can be precipitated by cervical spine mechanical dysfunctions.

PHYSICAL MEDICINE TREATMENTS OF MIGRAINE AND OTHER HEADACHES. Many forms of physical medicine have been used in the treatment of migraine and other headaches. Most have been shown to be effective in shortening the duration and decreasing the intensity of the pain. However, most do not appear to reduce the frequency of the attacks. A high percentage of patients who have migraine headaches report neck symptoms in the premonitory phase, both during the headache phase and after (Blau and MacGregor 1994). Cyriax reported that migraine headaches sometimes can be aborted by strong traction on the neck (Cyriax 1982). Parker, Tupling and Pryor (1978) have compared chiropractic manipulation to manipulation by a medical practitioner or physiotherapist and to simple cervical mobilization. Although the study found no difference in frequency of recurrence, duration or disability, the chiropractic patients reported greater reduction in the pain associated with the attacks.

In treatment of chronic tension-type headaches, Boline et al. (1995) have compared the use of manipulation to use of amitriptyline (antidepressant) and found that, at the end of treatment (4-6 weeks), amitriptyline was slightly more effective but was associated with more side effects. Four weeks after cessation of treatment, however, patients who received spinal manipulative therapy experienced a sustained therapeutic benefit. By contrast, patients who received amitriptyline therapy reverted to baseline values. The toggle recoil technique (a type of manipulation) also has been shown to be effective (Whittingham, Ellis and Molyneux 1994).

ACUPUNCTURE. Acupuncture can be beneficial in tension and other types of headaches (Jensen et al. 1979; Vincent 1990; Loh et al. 1984; Hansen and Hansen 1985). Markelova et al. (1984) have shown that in migraine headache acupuncture responders the therapeutic effect is achieved by normalization of serotonin levels and not by analgesic effects from increased endorphin production.

## Other Nonorthopedic Conditions

Other nonorthopedic conditions that can evoke upper body pain include rheumatoid arthritis, malignancy, herpetic and trigeminal neuralgias, neuroma, neurofibromas, amyotrophy (muscular wasting such as in amyotrophic lateral sclerosis, also called Lou Gherig's disease), calcification of the ligamenta flava, and axial osteomalacia (softening of the bones), (Ombergt, Bisschop, ter Veer, Van de Velde 1995).

### Cervical Capsular Pattern

Cervical capsular pattern of movement limitation, which is equal limitation in both rotations, can be found in fractures, rheumatoid arthritis, ankylosis spondylitis, myelomas, secondary neoplasm and osteoarthrosis (Cyriax *ibid*).

## Paresthesia

Paresthesia (numbness and tingling) requires consideration of conditions such as diabetes, peripheral neuritis, nerve entrapment, transitory ischemic attack (TIA), strokes, and pernicious anemia.

## Scapular & Shoulder Pain

Scapular or shoulder pain can be felt in pleurisy and in conditions that irritate the diaphragm, such as ectopic pregnancy, gall bladder disease, and in inferior myocardial infarction.

## Neuralgic Amyotropy

This uncommon disorder can be seen more frequently in the cervical spine than at other spinal levels. The onset can be sudden, with central or bilateral severe neck pain that later radiates to both upper limbs. After a while the pain remains in one arm only. Movement is possible and paresthesia uncommon.The pain may be aggravated by coughing or deep breathing (Brown *ibid*).

## Herpetic Neuralgia

Herpetic neuralgia can present as pain before cutaneous lesions are visible.

## Trigeminal Neuralgia

Trigeminal neuralgia presents as severe paroxysmal (sudden bouts of second-long lacerating) facial pain in the distribution of the trigeminal nerve. This can be aggravated by cold air, shaving, chewing and other movements, but it is unaffected by cervical movements. Other symptoms of trigeminal neuralgia include muscle spasms, flushing of the face, lacrimation,

and increased salivation (Brown *ibid*). Neuralgias can be treated by OM methods. Treatment details are not in the scope of this text.

## Mononeuritis

Mononeuritis should be considered especially in patients with a history of trauma or viral infections. Symptoms are:

- *Long thoracic nerve.* Discomfort mostly over the scapular and upper arm area, with limitation of active arm elevation and a positive scapula-winging test.

- *Spinal accessory nerve.* Ache and weakness similar to long thoracic nerve neuritis except that resisted approximation of scapula is weak due to trapezius muscle weakness. There is no scapular winging.

- *Suprascapular nerve.* Constant pain in the scapular area and upper arm, movements of neck and scapula are normal, there is weakness of supraspinatus and infraspinatus muscles, (Ombergt, Bisschop, ter Veer, Van de Velde 1995).

## Neurofibromatosis

Neurofibromatosis (von Recklinghausen's disease) is a congenital, autosomal dominant condition that appears mostly in late childhood. Neurofibromas are tumors of nervous tissue that may appear on the skin or in the optic and acoustic nerves. Other manifestations include multiple, pedunculated soft tissue fleshy tumors, and café-au-lait-pigmented macules (café-colored plaque or patches). This condition is associated with pain that is confined to radicular patterns. A neurofibroma (Schwannoma) may also present as a single tumor without other associated symptoms. Symptoms often start in the periphery and progress proximally. Generally, the pain increases over time. Often, weakness occurs in muscles that are outside of a single myotomal pattern (Cyriax *ibid*).

## Infection

Infections that can affect the spine include osteomyelitis (often seen in younger patients), brucellosis (especially in farm workers), and tuberculosis (especially in immigrants, and in immunologically-weak populations). Gonococcal, staphylococcal, syphilitic, and viral infections should be kept in mind (Brown *ibid*).

## Organ Disorders

Diseases of the gall bladder, pancreas, spleen, or apex of the heart, any irritation of the diaphragm, and/or ectopic pregnancy frequently refer pain to the scapular and shoulder regions. However, scapular/shoulder pain is unlikely to be the only presenting symptom.[2]

## Rheumatoid Arthritis & Related Diseases

Rheumatoid arthritis (RA) usually shows migratory pains in joints and muscles, with signs of inflammation such as red, hot, swollen, tender and large joints. RA, ankylosing spondylitis,[3] psoriasis[4] and Reiter's disease[5] are unlikely to present with primary cervical involvement (Ombergt, Bisschop, ter Veer, Van de Velde 1995).

Inflammatory conditions, especially rheumatoid arthritis, can affect the transverse ligament, permitting the odontoid process of the axis to sublux. Other conditions such as Reiter's disease (mostly lower spine), psoriasis, and inflammatory bowel disorders also can lead to arthropathy.

For mild-to-moderate cases of these disease states, OM techniques can be effective. In severe cases the treatment

---

2. For treatment, see the author's book *Acute Abdominal Syndromes*. Blue Poppy Press.

3. A progressive disease in which the joint and/or its surrounding tissue become fixed; usually seen in young adults; four times more common in the white population than in the black population.

4. A dermatological and arthritic disorder.

5. A triad of arthritis with fever, conjunctivitis and urethritis.

plan should incorporate modern Western medicine. (A treatment plan for severe cases is not within the scope of this text.)

## Metabolic Destructive Processes

Metabolic destructive processes such as osteoporosis[6] and osteomalacia should be suspected in elderly, kyphotic patients or in patients in whom minor injuries cause severe, localized pain. (This is not as common in the cervical spine as in other parts of the spine).

Two forms of metabolic destructive processes are *Paget's* disease and *ochronosis*. Paget's disease (osteitis deformans), a chronic inflammatory disease of the bone by which the bones thicken and distort, is seen in 3% of adults over 40 years. It is twice as common in males as in females. Of patients who have Paget's disease, 90% are asymptomatic.

Ochronosis is a rare condition marked by dark pigmentation of cartilage, ligaments, fibrous tissue, skin and urine. Twice as common in males as in females, this condition is seen in mid-life and in patients with hyperparathyroidism (Brown *ibid*).

## Primary Neoplastic Disease

Neoplastic disease can cause pain and weakness associated with cervical radiculopathy. The examination of cervical range of motion (ROM) can show gross limitation in all directions. Often muscle spasms with an empty end feel are palpable, especially if the malignant deposits are in the lower four cervical vertebrae. Resisted movements also are painful, but more weakness is evident than is found typically in cervical disc disease (Cyriax *ibid*).

---

6. Four times more common in women—especially postmenopausal women—than in men.

*Metastatic Disease*

Early metastatic disease can be difficult to detect, because the physical signs can be subtle, and radiographs can be negative for abnormality at this stage. Deposits in the upper cervical spine and the upper thoracic vertebrae are difficult to detect because often nerve sequelae are absent. The most common sources of metastasis in the spine are prostate, breast, lung, kidney, thyroid and colon cancers (Ombregt, Bisschop, ter Veer and Van de Velde 1995).

Warning signs are:

- Pain that awakens the patient at night and that is unrelieved by rest.

- Expanding or rapidly-increasing pain.

- (Any) pain in an elderly patient.

- Constitutional symptoms such as weight loss, fever, excessive sweating and fatigue.

- Muscular spasm that increases with side-bending away from the painful side.

- History of cancer.

- Major neurological signs without significant root pain.

- Involvement of several roots.

- Severe bone tenderness when percussed.

Other malignancies such as esophageal cancers frequently refer pain to the neck and upper extremities.

Treatment should incorporate OM and modern Western medicine.

*Benign Tumors*

Primary benign tumors in the cervical spine occur more often in children than adults. The most common are: giant cell tumors, aneurysmal bone cyst, osteoblastoma haemangioma, osteochondroma, osteoid osteoma and eosinophilic granuloma (Brown 1995).

*Depression & Anxiety Disorders*

Depression and anxiety disorders are common contributing factors in neck pain. Patients who have been diagnosed with fibromyalgia syndromes score much higher on anxiety and depression scales. Although fibromyalgia is not thought to be a psychogenic disease (Schuessler G, Konermann 1993), these patients are helped by treatment for depression. Pain tends to be variable and is associated with fatigue, sleep disorders, head and other aches, and inability to cope with stress.

# Musculoskeletal Sources

Musculoskeletal sources of neck pain respond often to treatments described in this text.

## Ligamentous Pain

Ligamentous lesions, a common cause of pain in the upper body and extremities, can be a source of headaches, as well. Often, neck pain that comes from degenerated ligaments (which cannot be seen on radiographs) is attributed to osteophytes and degenerative disc disease, which can be seen on radiographs. By their very presence, the osteophytes and degenerative disc disease can mislead the practitioner. If the practitioner treats for degenerated ligaments, the symptoms often improve despite the fact that follow-up X-ray does not change. Osteophytes, which form to stabilize lax joints, can have beneficial effects.

### Upper Cervical Ligaments

Upper cervical ligaments are a common source of headaches (Figure 7-17).

**ALAR LIGAMENTS.** The alar (wing-shaped maxillary) ligaments, which are made up almost entirely of collagenous fibers (Saldinger, Dvorák, Rahn and Perren 1990), can be stretched only about 6-8% of their resting length without causing irreversible damage. They can rupture at 200 N (Dvorák, Schmeider and Rahn 1988).

The primary role of the alar ligaments is to limit axial rotation in the upper cervical spine (CO-C1,C1-C2.).

- The taut occipital segment of the alar ligament induces forced rotation of the axis toward the same side as sidebending (non-neutral coupled motion at C1-C2, and neutral coupled motion at CO-C1).

- Flexion in the upper neck is limited chiefly by the nuchal and posterior longitudinal ligaments and their extensions, the tectorial membrane, and the cruciform and alar ligaments.

The alar ligaments are susceptible to injury in rear-end motor vehicle crashes (Dvorák, Schmeider and Rahn 1988).

**CRUCIFORM LIGAMENTS.** The cruciform ligament has two components. The lateral component, called the transverse ligament of the atlas, assures physiologic rotation of the C1-C2 joint and protects the spinal cord. The second component is a longitudinal element between the anterior border of the foramen magnum and the posterior aspect of the vertebral body of the axis. When trauma occurs, these ligaments can rupture, primarily at the osteoligamentous interface (Dvorák, Panjabi, Grber, Wichmann 1987).

**LIGAMENTUM FLAVUM.** The ligamentum flavum at the upper cervical level connects the posterior arch of the atlas and the arch of the axis.

**LIGAMENTUM NUCHAE.** The ligamentum nuchae attaches to the external occipital protuberance and joins with the interspinous ligaments and supraspinous ligaments. The ligament retains elastic energy during flexion, the release of which assists in bringing the head back to neutral. Below C7 the ligament is detached from the inter-

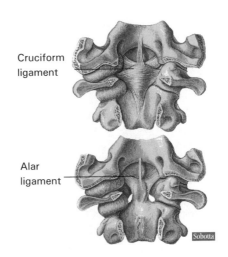

*Figure 7-17:* Upper cervical ligaments, CO-C1 joints.

spinous ligaments and supraspinous ligaments.

**POSTERIOR ATLANTO-OCCIPITAL MEMBRANE.** The Posterior atlanto-occipital membrane joins the posterior border of the foramen magnum with the posterior arch of the atlas.

**TECTORIAL MEMBRANE.** The tectorial membrane joins below with the anterior aspect of the posterior longitudinal ligament at the axis and above to the base of the occiput in front of the foramen magnum (Figure 7-18).

*Symptoms*

Lesions of the upper cervical ligaments and the bony attachments of the myofascial tissues often are associated with headaches and upper cervical pain (Figure 7-19). Provocative injections of paravertebral musculature, ligaments and facet joints reveals referred pain patterns. Provocative injections of the lateral atlantoaxial joint results in consistent referral patterns, whereas provocative injections of the atlanto-occipital joint produces

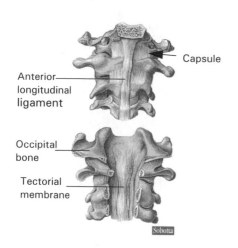

*Figure 7-18:* Ligaments and membrane of cervical spine.

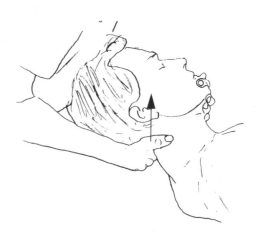

*Figure 7-20:* Aspinall's transverse ligament test. The practitioner holds the head in flexion and than applies an anteriorly directed force to the posterior aspect of the atlas. The test is positive if upon upward translation the patient feels a lump in the throat as the atlas moves toward the esophagus.

referral patterns that vary significantly. (Dreyfuss, Michaelsen and Fletcher 1994).

Instability of the upper ligaments can be dangerous and when suspected should be evaluated by motion x-ray. The joints should not be manipulated.

### Examination

Examination of the upper cervical ligaments can include a combination of passive examinations, palpation, Aspinall's Transverse Ligament Test (Figure 7-20),

the Sharp-Purser Test (Figure 7-21) and motion radiographs.

### Treatment

Treatment depends on the specific condition. Injection must be done with radiological control and may be very helpful.

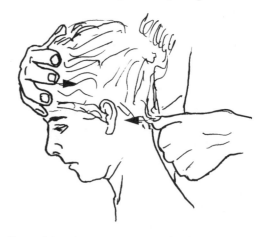

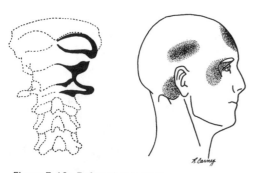

*Figure 7-19:* Referred pain from upper cervical soft tissues. (Reprinted with permission Dorman and Ravin 1991).

*Figure 7-21:* Sharp-Purser test. The head is pushed posteriorly gently against the practioner's thumb which is on the spinous process of the axis. The test is positive if a sense of gliding movement or a sound is heard as the atlas and the skull subluxate forward and backward.

*Ligaments: Middle & Lower Cervical Spine*

The middle (Figure 7-22) and lower cervical ligamentous structures (Figure 7-23, Figure 7-24) often evoke referred pain in the upper extremities.

**POSTERIOR/ANTERIOR LONGITUDINAL LIGAMENTS.** The posterior longitudinal ligament originates from the tectorial membrane and passes downwards along the posterior aspect of the vertebral body. The anterior longitudinal ligament runs from the anterior tubercle of the atlas and passes downwards along the anterior aspect of the vertebral body. The posterior and anterior longitudinal ligaments protect and support the intervertebral discs. The posterior ligament also protects the dura mater from the intervertebral discs. In the cervical spine (in contrast to the lumbar spine), the posterior ligament spans the full width of the vertebrae. The longitudinal ligaments are innervated both intrinsically and extrinsically (Willard *ibid*).

**INTERTRANSVERSE LIGAMENTS.** The intertransverse ligaments connect the transverse processes at each level.

**LIGAMENTUM FLAVUM.** The ligamentum flavum lies between the vertebral arches at each level. The ligament contains much elastic tissue which stores and releases elastic energy.

Symptoms

The ligaments of the middle and lower cervical spine can lead to local pain and referred symptoms in the shoulder, periscapular regions and arms. According to Ongley, the ligaments at the C7 transverse process can refer pain in three patterns (Figure 7-24),

- The anterior aspect of the transverse process refers anteriorly down the front of the chest.

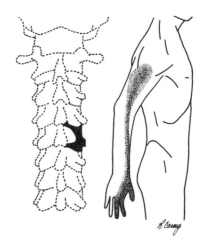

*Figure 7-22:* Referred pain from C5 sclerotome and soft tissue bony attachments. (With permission Dorman and Ravin 1991).

- A lesion proximal to the posterior tip refers to the medial scapula posteriorly.
- The tip refers pain to the shoulder (Dorman and Ravin 1991).

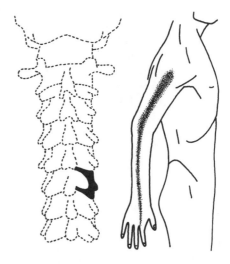

*Figure 7-23:* Referred pain from C6 sclerotome and soft tissue bony attachments. (With permission Dorman and Ravin 1991).

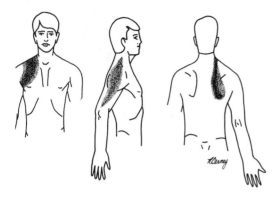

*Figure 7-24:* Referred pain from myofascial attachments to C7 transverse processes (With permission Dorman and Ravin 1991).

*Examination*

Examination can include evaluation of joint play, passive tests of the neck, palpation and motion radiographs.

*Treatment*

Treatment of the ligaments can be a combination of periosteal needling, acupuncture (especially basal tonification), cross fiber massage, electrostimulation, prolotherapy, manipulation, exercise and herbal medicine. In OM-style manipulations, often the practitioner (sometimes with the help of an assistant) attempts to increase pressure on these ligaments using traction, digit pressure with high-velocity thrust.

## Pain: Cervical Facet Joints

The facet joints and their ligamentous structures can refer pain. Fukui, Ohseto, Shiotani, Ohno, Karasawa, Naganuma and Yuda (1996) showed that with provocation under fluoroscopic control the main distribution of referred pain was as follows:

- Pain in the *occipital* region was referred from C2/3.

- Pain in the *upper posterolateral* cervical region was referred from C0/1, C1/2, and C2/3.

- Pain in the *upper posterior* cervical region was referred from C2/3, C3/4.

- Pain in the *middle posterior* cervical region was referred from C3/4, C4/5.

- Pain in the *lower posterior* cervical region was referred from C4/5, C5/6.

- Pain in the *suprascapular* region was referred from C4/5, C5/6.

- Pain in the *superior angle of the scapula* was referred from C6/7.

- Pain in *mid-scapular region* from C7/Th1.

## Cervical Spine Instability

Cervical rotational instability can be congenital or acquired, and can be due to congenital or degenerative changes in the dens of the axis. Trauma can lead to ligamentous rupture, often of the transverse ligament of the atlas, which can rupture at approximately 350 N force (Dvorák and Dvorák 1990). The resulting instability can be mild or severe.

*Unstable Degenerative Spondylolisthesis*

Unstable degenerative spondylolisthesis of the cervical spine is rare (Deburge et al. 1995). Usually the slips occur at the C3-on-C4 or C4-on-C5 levels, immediately above a stiff, lower-cervical spine (Figure 7-25). The two clinical patterns are neck pain alone and neck pain with neurological involvement that causes cervicobrachial pain or myelopathy. The diagnosis can be made by flexion and extension X-rays.

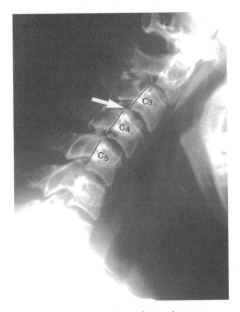

*Figure 7-25:* Lateral view of anterior subluxation in flexion of C3 on C4.

**SYMPTOMS.** Symptoms and signs of instability are:

* Paresthesia and neurological signs of the upper limbs.

* Bilateral symptoms, simultaneous or alternating, in both limbs.

* Symptoms crossing the midline.

* Chronic and persistent pain.

* Symptoms relieved by immobilization.

**TREATMENT.** Treatment depends on the severity of the instability. Surgery may be required.

In patients who have a recent soft tissue injury to the cervical spine and minimal or no neurologic deficits, a temporary improvement in symptoms following manual treatment may indicate instability. In such cases, *further manual treatment is contraindicated* until instability is ruled out.

### Ligament Examinations

Ligamentous disorders can cause pain that is evoked by stretching (or exerting pressure) on the abnormal ligaments.

Ligaments are difficult to palpate because, with the exception of the supraspinous ligament, they must be felt through many layers of tissues. Evaluation of most cervical ligaments requires a combination of passive motion examination and palpation. To palpate the deeper ligaments, with the patient sitting, the practitioner:

1. Sidebends the patient's neck and rotates it gently from side to side until maximum relaxation is achieved.

2. Applies pressure slowly and progressively.

3. (When resisting muscle tension begins) releases the pressure until relaxation returns.

4. Resumes palpation.

Using this technique, often it is possible to get a sense of the bone and ligaments without creating muscle guarding that hinders the examination.

### Treatment of Ligamentous Lesions

Treatment of ligamentous sprains and mild instability is achieved by correcting all vertebral dysfunctions (which can cause unnecessary ligament strain), compression, ice and by strengthening and balancing the affected muscles. If ligamentous insufficiency is moderate, periosteal acupuncture or prolotherapy may be needed.

### Forward Head Posture

Although often not symptomatic, non-optimal postures may result in abnormal stresses and accommodation in the musculoskeletal system. When head posture is "optimal" (Figure 7-26), the apex of the lordotic cervical curve usually is at C4-5, and the head's center of gravity is at a point

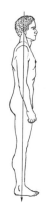

*Figure 7-26:* Optimal posture.

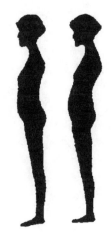

*Figure 7-27:* Adaptation to forward head posture.

just anterior to the cervical spine and just superior to the temporomandibular joint.

When the head is held forward, this changes: the lower cervical segments flex and (for the head to remain looking forward) the apex of the cervical lordosis shifts upward. This may result in increased compression forces on the lower cervical segments, which can lead to pathology of the lower segments (Figure 7-27).

### Cause of Forward Head Posture

According to Shaw (1992), forward movement of the head results from any joint dysfunction that affects the parallel plane of the eyes and ears, and from occlusion of the mandible in its horizontal plane. These new planes are maintained at the expense of normal function almost anywhere in the musculoskeletal system. This posture can result in significant effects on the entire musculoskeletal system. Such posture also can be secondary to any dysfunction as far down as the feet. The Alexander Technique recognizes this concept, and awareness and correction of head posture often is sufficient for correcting the entire body posture.

### Appearance of Forward Head Posture

Forward head posture is commonly associated with either a general increase in thoracic kyphosis or with "dowager's hump," i.e., an increased, localized kyphosis at the cervicothoracic area. However, especially if the patient is standing, in order to maintain the body's center of gravity the upper thoracic spine might extend (losing its usual kyphosis) and may appear to flatten.

### Development of Forward Head Posture

Although forward head posture is most obvious in mature patients, usually the condition begins early in life when posture becomes habitual. Since gravity tends to exert a force on the head and neck that makes them shift forward, and because the head can weigh as much as 15 pounds, poor posture during many daily activities such as working at computers and/or reading, and even postural laziness and emotional disturbances such as poor self-esteem and depression, can perpetuate this tendency.

## Effects of Forward Head Posture

Forward head posture may result in many joints being maintained at their extreme range. This can result in reduced motion and, therefore, regenerative activities at the joint, probably leading to degenerative changes in the joint complex. Abnormal resting joint positions may also lead to some ligaments being stretched continually resulting in loss of their tensile strength and hypersensitivity. This unbalanced posture alters weight-bearing, causing muscle compensations with shortening in some groups, and causing the muscle's antagonistic group to be inhibited and stretched (Janda *ibid*).

**FATIGUE AND SHORTENING.** One adaptation seen clinically is that the suboccipital muscles, levator scapulae, and upper fibers of trapezius and sternocleidomastoid fatigue and shorten as they work harder to maintain the head upright. The upper flexors then can become inhibited, stretched and weak.

**MUSCLE HYPERACTIVITY.** Another clinical presentation is hyperactivity of the upper flexor muscles and of the sternocleidomastoid and scalene muscles, which accentuates forward head posture. This hyperactivity can stretch and facilitate the suboccipital neck extensors and the levator scapulae, which often develop trigger points at their attachments to the scapula.

## Protraction of Shoulder Girdle

According to Shaw (*ibid*), the shoulder girdle (scapula) is the positional foundation of the head and neck. The shoulder girdle can protract, elevate, and internally rotate, causing a round-shouldered appearance. This dysfunction shortens the upper fibers of the trapezius and levator scapulae, elevating the scapula and leading to increased thoracic convexity and abduction. The result is a shortening of muscle such as the teres major and, reciprocally, inhibition of the lower fibers of the trapezius and rhomboids. The extension by the head on the atlas (for maintaining the visual plane) causes the suprahyoid and infrahyoid muscles to stretch and pull the mandible. This can give rise to temporomandibular joint disorders. Other types of compensation are possible, as well.

## Symptoms

Because forward head posture can affect such a variety of structures, symptoms can vary greatly. Headaches and myofascial pain are common, and temporomandibular joint disorders are seen (Ayub, Glasheen-Wray, Kraus 1984). Because the thoracic spine can compensate by either decreasing or increasing its kyphosis (depending on how the lumbar spine and lower extremities compensate for the load), (*ibid*), many patients develop low back pain, as well.

## Examination

Examination is by observation: forward head posture is evident in simple visual examination.

## Treatment

The best treatment approach is global, addressing joint dysfunctions, pelvic obliquities, foot mechanics, and myofascial adaptations. Postural training often is helpful, however, changes in tissues and general habits can take a long time. Postural training may not work in patients who have significant physiological tissue alterations.

**CHIN POSITION.** Often, postural awareness and alteration can be achieved by teaching the patient to pay attention to the position of their chin and shoulder girdle. One method for affecting this condition is frequent tucking-in of the chin, while elongating the spine through visualization.

**MUSCLE SHORTENING AND INHIBITION.** For patients who have shortening of the suboccipital muscles and inhibition of the flexor muscles, exercises to stretch the suboccipitals and strengthen the flexors tend to be helpful. Because this type of patient often has increased thoracic kyphosis, it may be necessary to first stretch the pectoral muscles and strengthen the rhomboids. The patient may need to keep the scapula retracted. If the flexor muscles are shortened clinically and the suboccipital and levator scapula develop trigger points, the practitioner should needle them and stretch the flexors.

## Myofascial & Contractile Unit Pain

Cervical muscles have an exceptionally high innervation ratio and are capable of very rapid and subtle movements. They are vulnerable and develop lesions often. Myofascial pain can occur as a primary condition or secondarily to underlying problems such as degenerative joint disease (DJD) or ligament insufficiency. Using magnetic resonance imaging (MRI) studies of patients who had chronic head and neck pain, Hallgren, Greenman and Rechtien (1994) found that, in patients who had substantial motion restrictions, related muscles had high-signal intensity, indicating replacement of tissue by "dead" suboccipital skeletal muscle with fatty tissue. The reduction in proprioceptive afferent activity in affected muscles may cause increased facilitation of neural activity that the patient perceives as pain.

In biopsies of ventral neck muscles (sternocleidomastoid, omohyoid, and longus colli) and dorsal neck muscles (rectus capitis posterior major, obliquus capitis inferior, splenius capitis, and trapezius) of patients who had cervical dysfunction of different etiologies, Uhlig, Weber, Grob and Muntener (1995) found signs of muscle fiber transformation in all muscles. Regardless of the type of disorder, fibers had an increased relative amount of type-IIC fibers.[7] In the ventral muscles and the obliquus capitis inferior, transformation occurrence correlated strongly with the duration of symptoms: In the ventral muscles, the vast majority of transformations occurred in patients who had a shorter history of symptoms, whereas the reverse occurred for the obliquus capitis inferior. For the other dorsal muscles, transformation events did not correlate with duration of symptoms.

### Affected Muscles

In myofascial syndromes of the neck, the most commonly affected muscles are the trapezius, multifidi, splenius and sternocleidomastoid. The levator scapulae, trapezius, and scalenes are commonly involved in neck, shoulder and upper extremity pain. The upper semispinalis, splenius rectus capitis and obliques can cause symptoms that refer pain to the suboccipital, temporal and supraorbital areas of the head (Kuchera and Kuchera ibid). Often, stretching of the affected contractile units produces pain and reveals shortening of the muscles. Resisted-movement examinations may or may not elicit pain. Frequently, when tendinous lesions are involved, strong resisted movements are painful.

### Evaluation

The practitioner should evaluate these muscles for tissue texture, shortening and hyperactive motor, trigger and/or acupuncture points.

DEEPER MUSCLE GROUPS. In mild or less severe conditions and injuries of the cervical spine, the deeper intrinsic muscle groups (multifidus, intertransverse and interspinous) may be the only involved muscles. They can be examined using motion techniques and/or palpation. To find a hyperactive trigger, exploration with a needle (thin gauge, #36) may be

---

7.  Transitional or intermediate fibers, identified by the pH lability of their myofibrillar ATPase.

necessary. For thin patients, since the deeper muscles are transverse and oblique, sometimes it is possible to palpate hard, tight bands using a vertically directed stroke.

**ENTIRE MUSCLE.** Involvement of an entire muscle in a cervical dysfunction is uncommon. Usually only isolated groups of fibers within the muscle are tight, stringy and tender. If entire groups of muscles are in spasm and cause immobilization of the cervical spine, a more severe lesion such as disc herniation or fracture should be suspected (Cyriax *ibid*).

**TIGHT MUSCLE BANDS.** Examination of a tight muscle band includes palpation of the tight muscle's and bony attachment to evaluate the possibility of tendinosis.

### Shoulder Girdle

The shoulder girdle is innervated by C4 and C5 and the myotome is of C5 and C6. Lesions at these levels can cause muscle dysfunctions of the rotator cuff. (Since these lesions are secondary manifestations, treatment always should be directed primarily to the source.)

### Treatment

Treatment is directed to the primary lesion and can include manipulation, acupuncture, dry needling, massage, countertension-positioning, scraping, stretching, post-isometric stretching, muscle energy, exercise, and/or oral and topical medications.

## Myofascial Syndromes

Myofascial syndromes in the neck and shoulder regions are common. These areas often are stressed in this computer-and-car age. Many people hold tension in these regions, possibly resulting in development of hemodynamic changes and chronic myofascial pain. Often myofascial pain is

secondary to joint dysfunctions and ligamentous disorders.

### Muscles of The Posterior Neck

The posterior cervical muscles lie in four layers:

| LAYER | IS FORMED BY THE |
|---|---|
| 1 (outer) | trapezius |
| 2 | splenius capitis and cervicis |
| 3 | semispinalis capitis, levator scapulae |
| 4 (deepest) | multifidi, rotators, small suboccipitals |

Table 7-7 on page 338 summarizes the muscles of the posterior neck, by layer.

### Layer 1 (Outer):

**TRAPEZIUS.** The most superficial of the posterior cervical muscles, the trapezius is shaped like a large coat hanger that has a connecting inferior triangle. The muscle fibers, which extend in a multitude of directions, can function independently (Figure 7-29).

**ATTACHMENTS.**

The upper fibers:

- Attach superiorly to the medial third of the superior nuchal line of the occiput.

- Connect at midline to the ligamenta nuchae and the spinous processes of the C1-C4 vertebrae.

- Meet inferiorly, laterally and forward, where they attach to the lateral third of the clavicle.

Acting unilaterally, the upper fibers elevate the shoulder, and sidebend the head and neck.

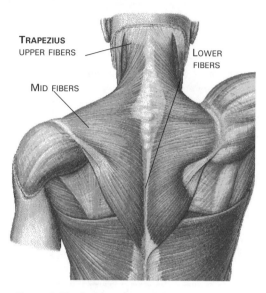

*Figure 7-29:* First layer muscles.

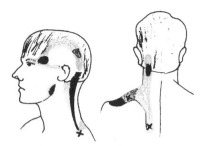

*Figure 7-30:* Referred pain from trapezius muscle triggers. (After Travell and Simons).

The lower fibers:

• Attach medially to the spinous processes and interspinous ligaments of the T4-T12 vertebrae.

• Ascend laterally.

• Converge at the tubercle, at the medial end of the spine of the scapula, just lateral to the lower attachment on the levator scapulae muscle.

The lower fibers retract the scapula and rotate the glenoid fossa upward. They also assist in flexion and abduction of the arm. The trapezius is innervated by the accessory nerves and the C3-C4 nerves.

The middle fibers:

• Attach medially to the spinous processes and interspinous ligaments of the C6-T3 vertebrae.

• Attach laterally to the acromion process and superior lip of the spine of the scapula.

These muscle fibers adduct the scapula and assist in arm abduction.

**SYMPTOMS.** Symptoms vary, depending on the fibers involved. Typically symptoms are felt across the shoulder, neck and head. Dysfunction of the trapezius in association with the levator scapulae or splenius cervicis can cause an acute stiff neck (Travell, Simons 1983), (Figure 7-30).

**EXAMINATION.** Examination often reveals pain at full rotation and contralateral side-bending. In this type of lesion, full flexion is rarely painful. Rotation to the same side produces pain only if other muscles are involved, as well.

**TREATMENT.** Acupuncture needling—especially using the Gall Bladder Sinews channels, Large intestine Sinews channels, Small Intestine Sinew channels and Yang

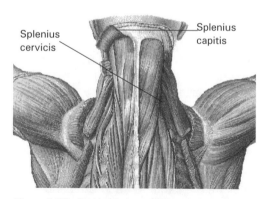

*Figure 7-28:* Second layer muscles.

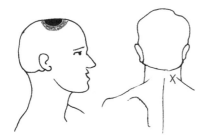

*Figure 7-31:* Referred pain from splenius capitis muscle trigger (After Travell and Simons).

Linking (Wei) channel—countertension-positioning, and/or stretching usually are effective treatment methods.

## Layer 2

**SPLENIUS CAPITIS AND CERVICIS.** The second-layer muscles extend and rotate the neck to the same side (Figure 7-28).

**ATTACHMENTS.** The splenius capitis and cervicis attach as follows:

• The splenius capitis and cervicis attach inferiorly to the spinous processes of the lower cervical and upper thoracic vertebrae.

• The cervicis attach superiorly to the transverse processes of the upper cervical vertebra.

• The capitis attaches to the mastoid process of the skull.
  Innervation of both come from branches of the dorsal primary divisions of the C2-C4 spinal nerves.

**SYMPTOMS.** Symptoms due to lesions in the splenius capitis and cervicis muscles can present as neck, cranium and eye pain. During examination, rotation of the neck is limited by pain, with some restriction of flexion. Eye pain with blurred vision also may be elicited (Travell, Simons *ibis*) (Figure 7-31).

**EXAMINATION.** Examination begins with palpation for tissue texture. The practitioner

should also assess cervical rotation and flexion.

**TREATMENT.** Treatment consists of needling of the myofascial trigger points, with needling of the bony attachments, and acupuncture, especially the Urinary Bladder Sinews and Gall Bladder Sinews channels, Yang Motility (Qiao) and Yang Linking (Wei) channels. Stretching may be needed in chronic cases. Countertension-positioning is effective.

## Layer 3

**SEMISPINALIS CAPITIS AND CERVICIS AND LEVATOR SCAPULAE.** The third-layer semispinalis capitis and cervicis muscles are the primary extenders and rotators of the neck (Figure 7-32, Figure 7-33). They are innervated by spinal nerves C1-C8.

**ATTACHMENTS.** The third-layer semispinalis capitis and cervicis attach inferiorly to the transverse processes of the T1 through T7 vertebrae.

The semispinalis capitis:

• Also attaches below to the transverse processes of C3-C6.

• Attaches to the occiput between the superior and inferior nuchal lines.
  The cervicis attach superiorly to the spinous processes of C2-C5.

The levator scapulae (Figure 7-32) attaches to the transverse processes of the four cervical vertebrae above, and to the superior angle of the scapula below.

**SYMPTOMS.** Symptoms that result from triggers in these muscles often cause pain over the back of the neck and head (Figure 7-34). Pain from the levator scapulae concentrate at the angle of the neck and along the vertebral border of the scapula (Figure 7-35).

**EXAMINATION.** Examination of the neck's range of movement may show restricted

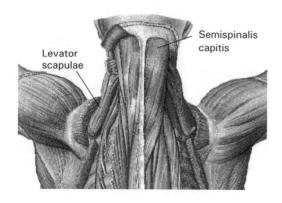

Figure 7-32: Third layer muscles.

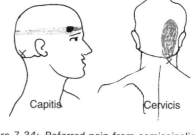

Figure 7-34: Referred pain from semispinalis capitis and cervicis muscle triggers (After Travell and Simons).

flexion, and possibly rotation, secondary to tight extensor muscles. Neck extension, however, is restricted only slightly. On palpation, the muscles are tender.

Tightness of the levator scapulae results primarily in restriction of neck rotation.

**TREATMENT.** Layer 3 of the cervical spine muscle may not benefit from massage and soft tissue mobilization techniques in the way the more superficial layers benefit. Needling is more effective. Countertension-positioning is effective, as well. The practitioner can use muscle energy to address vertebral dysfunctions. Chronic dysfunctions may require stretching techniques to prevent exacerbation. Acupuncture using the Urinary Bladder and Small Intestines Sinews channels and Main channels is often effective.

*Layer 4*

**MULTIFIDI, DEEP ROTATORS, SUBOCCIPITAL TRIANGLE.** The fourth layer of muscles of the posterior cervical spine is synergistic primarily with the third-layer muscles (Figure 7-36),

- The multifidi are synergistic with the semispinalis capitis in extension of the neck.

- The deep rotators are synergistic with the semispinalis cervicis in rotation (Travell and Simons *ibid*).

They are innervated by spinal nerves C1-C8.

Spasm in the multifidi and deep rotators muscles can cause and maintain non-

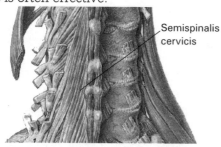

Figure 7-33: Third layer muscles.

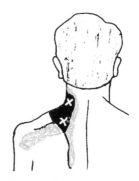

Figure 7-35: Referred pain from levator scapulae muscle triggers. (After Travell and Simons).

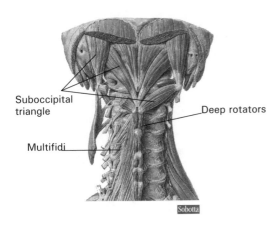

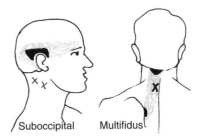

*Figure 7-37:* Referred pain from suboccipital and multifidus muscle triggers (After Travell and Simons).

*Figure 7-36:* Fourth layer muscles.

neutral vertebral dysfunction in the neck.

**ATTACHMENTS.** The suboccipital triangle muscles connect the occiput with the first and second cervical vertebrae. This triangle consists of the inferior oblique, superior oblique and rectus capitis posterior muscles.

- The inferior oblique extends horizontally and laterally from the spine of the axis to the transverse processes of the atlas.
- The superior oblique extends from the transverse processes of the atlas to the occipital bone.
- The rectus capitis posterior major extends upward and backward from the spine of the axis to the occipital bone.
- The less significant rectus capitis posterior minor lies deep and medially to the triangle of muscles, and extends from the spine of the atlas to the occipital bone.

**SYMPTOMS.** Lesions in these muscles are a common cause of headache in the occipital region or referred to the forehead, temples or jaw (Travell and Simons 1983), (Figure 7-37).

**EXAMINATION.** Examination consists of palpating for tissue texture, and assessing cervical rotations, OA and C1-C2 functions. For the multifidi and deep rotators muscles, joint play and coupled sidebending and rotation are assessed.

**TREATMENT.** Layer 4 of the cervical spine muscles may not benefit from massage and soft tissue mobilization techniques in the way the more superficial layers benefit. Dry needling is more effective for these muscle groups. Countertension-positioning and postisometric relaxation (muscle energy) are effective, as well. The practitioner can use muscle energy to address vertebral dysfunctions which are often seen. Chronic disorders may require stretching techniques to prevent exacerbation. Acupuncture to the Yang Linking (Wei), Urinary Bladder and Gall Bladder channels is often effective.

To relieve headaches due to somatic dysfunction and facilitated suboccipital muscles, the practitioner treats the occipital atlas (OA) and C1-C2 vertebral dysfunctions. Muscle energy, countertension-positioning, dry needling and massage are very effective.

Table 7-7 on page 338 summarizes the muscles and myofascial syndromes of the ventral neck region.

*Table 7-7.* **Posterior Neck Muscles**

| Layer, Formed by | Innervated by | Description |
|---|---|---|
| **I (OUTER)**<br>Trapezius | Accessory Nerves<br>C3-C4 Nerves | FUNCTIONS<br>• Fibers extend multiple directions, can function independently<br>• Upper fibers elevate shoulder; sidebend head and neck<br>• Middle fibers adduct scapula; assist in arm abduction<br>• Lower fibers retract scapula; rotate glenoid fossa upward; assist in arm flexion and abduction<br>SYMPTOMS<br>• Vary, depending on fibers involved<br>• Typically felt across shoulder, neck, head<br>• Dysfunction in association with levator scapulae or splenius cervicis can cause acute stiff neck<br>• Often pain felt at full rotation & contralateral sidebending<br>• Full flexion rarely painful<br>• Rotation to same side painful only if other muscles involved<br>TREATMENT<br>• Dry needling<br>• Acupuncture — especially using the Gall Bladder sinew channel, Large Intestines sinew channel, Small Intestines sinew channel and Yang Linking/Wei Vessel<br>• Countertension-positioning<br>• Stretching<br>• Massage<br>• Scraping |
| 2 Layer<br>Splenius Capitis<br>Cervicis | Branches of Dorsal Primary Divisions of Spinal Nerves C2-C4 | FUNCTION<br>• Extend and rotate neck to same side<br>SYMPTOMS<br>• Pain in neck, cranium, eye (w/ blurred vision)<br>• Neck rotation limited by pain<br>• Some flexion restriction<br>TREATMENT<br>• Dry needling of myofascial trigger points<br>• Needling of bony attachments<br>• Acupuncture, especially the Urinary Bladder sinew channel, Gall Bladder sinew channel, Yang Motility/Qiao and Linking/Wei Vessels<br>• (Chronic dysfunctions) stretching<br>• Manipulation<br>• Muscle energy<br>• Massage<br>• Counterstrain-positioning |

*Table 7-7.* **POSTERIOR NECK MUSCLES (CONTINUED)**

| LAYER, FORMED BY | INNERVATED BY | DESCRIPTION |
|---|---|---|
| 3 Layer<br>Semispinalis Capitis<br>**Levator S**capulae | Spinal Nerves<br>C1-C8 | FUNCTION<br>• Primary neck extenders and rotators<br>SYMPTOMS<br>• Pain over back of neck, head and scapula<br>• ROM<br>  — restricted flexion (possibly rotation) secondary to tight extensor muscles<br>  — neck extension restricted only slightly<br>  — restricted rotation with levator scapulae tension<br>TREATMENT<br>• Dry needling<br>• Acupuncture using the UB and SI sinew channels and Main channels<br>• Muscle energy to address vertebral dysfunction<br>• (Chronic dysfunctions) stretching techniques (to prevent exacerbation)<br>• Counterstrain-positioning<br>• Massage |
| 4 Layer<br>Multifidi<br>Rotators<br>Small Suboccipitals | Spinal Nerves<br>C1-C8 | FUNCTIONS<br>• (Primarily synergistic with third-layer muscles)<br>• Multifidi synergistic w/semispinalis capitis in neck extension<br>• Deep rotators synergistic with semispinalis cervicis in rotation<br>SYMPTOMS<br>• Spasm can cause/maintain non-neutral vertebral neck dysfunction<br>TREATMENT<br>• Same as for other neck muscles<br>• For headache due to OA and C1- C2 somatic dysfunction, muscle energy, dry needling, and counterstrain-positioning<br>• Acupuncture to the Yang Linking/Wei and Urinary Bladder Main channel |

*Myofascial Syndromes: Muscles of the Anterior Neck.*

The anterior neck muscles, the scalenes and the sternocleidomastoid are accessory muscles that often are involved in neck, head and arm pain. Table 7-8 on page 342 is a summary description of these muscles.

*Scalenes*

Each side of the neck has three scalenes, which originate from the anterior transverse processes of the C3-C7. The main function of the scalenesis is to suspend the thoracic outlet (more accurately, "inlet") and to maintain it level. During inspiration the scalenes raise the first rib and (indirectly) the lower ribs (Basmajian and De Luca 1983). The scalenes also stabilize the cervical spine against lateral movement. They are innervated by the anterior division of spinal nerves C2-C7 (Table 7-8 on page 342).

**ATTACHMENTS.** The scalenes attachments are:

- The first two scalenes insert into the upper surfaces of the first rib.

- The posterior scalene inserts into the second rib.

**SYMPTOMS.** Symptoms of scalene lesions can be primarily myofascial, or they can be secondary with sensory and motor nerve involvement such as in neurovascular entrapment (thoracic outlet syndrome). Referred pain from the scalenes is commonly the source of shoulder and upper arm pain syndromes (Long 1956), (Figure 7-38). Pain on the radial side of the hand indicates a referred myofascial source. Pain on the ulnar side with puffiness of the hand suggests brachial plexus or subclavian vein entrapment (Travell and Simons *ibid*). Abnormally attached or enlarged scalenes can cause thoracic outlet symptoms (Liu, Tahmoush, Roos and Schwartz-

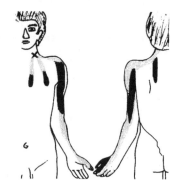

*Figure 7-38:* Referred pain from scalene muscle triggers (After Travell and Simons).

man 1995).

**EXAMINATION.** Examination often reveals a shortened, tender scalene muscle.

Travell and Simons describe a Scalene Provocation Test in which the patient rotates the head toward the painful side, and then pulls the chin down into the hollow above the clavicle actively by flexing his head.

If the lesion is in the scalenes, this movement elicits local neck pain. Lesions in the scalenes are often accompanied by psoas muscle lesions, which manifests as slouched posture with a flexed head.

**TREATMENT.** The scalenes usually respond well to muscle energy, post-isometrics, countertension-positional release, and at times to massage and dry needling. Acupuncture to the Stomach and Liver Sinews channels and Main channels, and Yin Motility (Qiao) are often effective.

*The Sternocleidomastoid Muscle (SCM)*

The SCM (Table 7-8 on page 342), which runs down the neck obliquely, is accentuated when the head is rotated to the opposite side.

**ATTACHMENTS.** This muscle consists of two divisions, sternal and clavicular, that blend to form common attachments at the

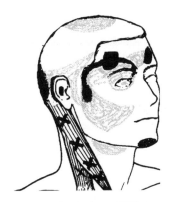

*Figure 7-39:* Referred pain from SCM muscular triggers (After Travell and Simons).

lateral surface of the mastoid process and the lateral half of the superior nuchal line of the occipital bone.

- The sternal division attaches below, at the anterior surface of the manubrium of the sternum.

- The clavicular division attaches inferiorly to the superior border of the anterior medial third of the clavicle.

The SCM is supplied by cranial nerve XI.

**SYMPTOMS.** The most common symptom seen with a trigger point in the SCM is tension headache. Travell (*ibid*) reports postural dizziness and imbalance. Neck pain is rare, although extreme neck rotation, extension and (at times) flexion can intensify the pain.

**EXAMINATION.** Examination often reveals a tender muscle. Neck movements usually are full, but extension or flexion may be reduced slightly. Rotation to the opposite side may be reduced, as well. Sidebending toward the pain combined with rotation to the other side is seen with muscle spasm—"blackbird's sign".

**TREATMENT.** Treatment consists of massage, countertension-positional release and dry needling. Acupuncture to the Stomach, Large Intestine and Liver Sinews and Main channels, and Yin Motility (Qiao) channel are often effective.

*Myofascial Pain & Insomnia/Depression/ Fibromyalgia*

If myofascial pain syndrome is accompanied by insomnia or depression, or if the patient has fibromyalgia, the practitioner should consider including antidepressants, amino acids, melatonin, St. John's wort, Kava, vitamins, calcium, magnesium and Chinese herbal medication (see appendix A).

## Facet Syndromes

Facet irritation is a common cause of neck, head and shoulder pain. The "facet syndrome" however is controversial.

Zygoapophyseal (facet) joint strains often lead to irritation of the scalene muscles and cause pain in the hand, arm, shoulder, periscapular area and chest. A thoracic outlet compression with brachial plexus pain may be seen. These joint strains are more common in C3-C5 (Bogduk et al. *ibid*).

Another common cause of neck pain is thought to be internal derangement of a "meniscoid" in the facet joints. These structures may be formed by intra-articular inclusions. Mercer and Bogduk's (1993) showed three types of intra-articular inclusion in the cervical spine:

- Fat pads occur regularly in the atlanto-occipital joints but rarely in the zygoapophyseal joints.

- Capsular rims occur occasionally at all levels.

- Fibroadipose meniscoids occurred regularly in the atlantoaxial and facet joints.

Mercer and Bogduk posit that the function of fibroadipose meniscoids is to protect the articular cartilages in gliding joints that subluxate during normal movement. These structures may act as a nidus for intra-articular fibrosis, and meniscus entrapment may be a mechanism for torticollis.

Patients who have internal derangements almost always suffer also from liga-

*Table 7-8.* ANTERIOR NECK MUSCLES

| Muscle | Innervated by | Description |
|---|---|---|
| SCALENES<br>(3 on each side) | Anterior Division of Spinal Nerves C2-C7 | FUNCTIONS<br>• Suspend thoracic outlet<br>• Maintain thoracic outlet level<br>• (During inspiration) raise first rib, (indirectly) lower ribs<br>• Stabilize cervical spine against lateral movement<br>**SYMPTOMS**<br>• Primary myofascial or secondary sensory with motor nerve involvement<br>• Referred pain from scalenes (common source of shoulder and upper arm pain syndromes)<br>• Pain on radial side of hand (indicates referred myofascial source)<br>• Pain on ulnar side with hand puffiness (suggests brachial plexus or subclavian vein entrapment)<br>• (Often) shortened, tender scalene muscle<br>• (Often) accompanied by psoas muscle dysfunction manifest as slouched posture with flexed head<br>• Travell and Simons Scalene Provocation Test elicits pain in scalenes<br>TREATMENT<br>• Muscle energy<br>• Post-isometric techniques<br>• Countertension-positioning<br>• Dry needling |
| STERNOCLEIDOMASTOID | Cranial Nerve | FUNCTIONS<br>• Rotation to opposite side<br>• Bilateral action flexes neck<br>SYMPTOMS<br>• (often) tender muscle<br>• neck movements usually full, but possible slight reduction in extension/flexion<br>• possible reduced rotation to opposite side<br>TREATMENT<br>• massage<br>• countertension-positioning<br>• dry needling |

mentous laxity, muscular deconditioning and other spinal functional disorders, all of which should be treated.

**NON-FACET JOINT PAIN.** Bogduk and Aprill (1993) have demonstrated that, of patients who had post-traumatic neck pain, only 23% had facet joint pain alone (Barnsley et al. found 54% 1995):

• 41% had a combination of disc and facet lesions.

• 20% had a disc lesion alone.

• 17% had neither.

## Treatment

Treatment of facet disorders can include manual therapy (muscle energy or manipulation); acupuncture to involved muscles, and to the joint capsule if it is hypermobile, and stabilization exercises. Prolotherapy is required often.

## Fracture

An acute fracture of a vertebral body leads to limitation of movements in all directions (especially extension), (Cyriax *ibid*). Treatment might include surgery and should include acupuncture and herbal medicine, both oral and topical to hasten the recovery time.

## Treatment

In the early stages, herbal treatment is directed at activating the Blood, transforming Stasis, clearing Heat from the Blood, subduing swelling and alleviating pain.

In the middle stage, the aim of herbal treatment is to aid union of bone, muscles and ligaments.

Late-stage treatment consists of activating the collateral systems (energy, Blood, and neural circulation) and relaxing of joints and soft tissues.

## Disc Disorders

The cervical intervertebral discs are relatively thicker, posteriorly broader and anteriorly higher than those of the thoracic spine. This increased thickness is thought to have developed in response to excessive strains on discs, due to extensive cervical motions. The nucleus of the cervical intervetebral disc is located somewhat anteriorly, allowing for a forward and backward gliding motion.

## Cervical Disc Nuclear Displacement

According to Cyriax, although cervical disc nuclear displacement is rare, it can be the source of nerve root impingement. For this type of lesion, the usual course is spontaneous resolution within four months.

## Symptoms

Patients with lateral cervical disc protrusions display (Lunsford et al. 1980):

- Neck pain in 80%.
- Radicular pain 77%.
- Shoulder pain 35%.
- Interscapular pain 8%.
- Headache 13%.
- Numbness in one arm 53%.
- Numbness bilaterally 5%.
- Weakness in one arm 36%.
- Weakness bilaterally 1%.
- Single myotomal deficits in 50%.
- Multiple myotome deficits in 25%.
- Normal reflexes in 35-47%.
- Abnormal reflexes in 50-64%.

Patients with acute cervical disc protrusion will often lean the head toward the side of the root being compressed in order to push the nucleus to other side.

## Examination

Examination can reveal a "partial articular pattern"—i.e. some movements being limited and painful while others are not:

- Movements that engage the blocked joint or increase nerve compression increase the pain.
- Active or passive rotation toward the painful side nearly always elicits pain, although many patients posture the neck toward the painful side.

— Foraminal Compression Test is positive and increases symptoms (Figure 7-40).

— A Distraction Test may relieve symptoms (Figure 7-40).

— In lower cervical root compression of C5-C7, the Limb Tension Test can be positive and painful (Figure 7-41).

— Resisted movements usually are painless.

— Pain can be segmental or extrasegmental, depending on the extent of the disc protrusion and ligamentous or muscular involvement.

— Cervical disc pain usually is unilateral and is felt in the neck, and in the scapula, arms and hands.

— With disc lesions, segmental cervical motions are restricted, usually at the level of the disc. Often additional segments are affected, as well.

— Usually, also at the level of the disc, motion to one side is restricted, with a painful, hard end feel, and a springy end feel on the contralateral side.

*Treatment*

Treatment consists of traction, indirect techniques, and distal acupuncture. If thrust manipulation is used, it always should be directed to the nonpainful direction and should be performed with the cervical spine in traction. Hypomobility evident in the secondarily-involved segments can be treated in both directions. Treatment with chiropractic manipulative therapy, longitudinal cervical traction and interferential therapy has been reported to be effective (Brouillette and Gurske 1994; Beneliyahu 1994).

*Nerve Root Impingement*

According to Cyriax cervical discs that impinge on a single nerve root usually

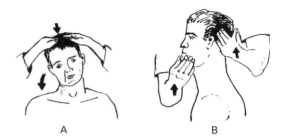

*Figure 7-40:* A: Foraminal compression test is positive if it increases symptoms, B: Distraction test is positive if it decreases symptoms.

refer pain in a single dermatomal distribution (Figure 7-42). This is due to the anatomy of the cervical spine, which restricts the disc to compression of the nerve root immediately inferior to the disc (e.g., the disc at the 5th joint affects the 6th cervical root). Lunsford et al. (1980) however, found that 50% of disc herniation cases will have a single myotome deficit and 25% will have multiple myotome deficits. Normal reflex can be found in 35%-47% of cases.

The highest incidence of nerve root impingement occurs in people aged 35-60. In younger patients who exhibit nerve root signs, a neuroma should be suspected. In older patients, the intervertebral discs usually are drier, making rupture or protru-

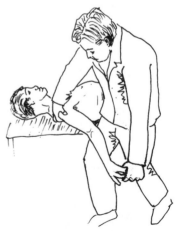

*Figure 7-41:* Limb tension test. Test is positive if arm and wrist extension increases the pain.

sion less likely, and significant osteophytosis or metastasis should be considered (Cyriax *ibid*).

**SYMPTOMS.** The symptoms of cervical nerve root impingement include:

- Scapular pain caused by pressure on the dura mater.
- Dermatomally-distributed pain due to pressure on the dural sleeve of the nerve root.
- Weakness in the associated myotome.
- Tingling secondary to involvement of parenchyma (functional aspect of cell) (Cyriax *ibid*).

Table 7-9 summarizes examples of segmental muscular weakness that occurs as a result of cervical disc lesions.

**EXAMINATION.** Orthopedic and neurological examinations should be performed. The sensory examination should focus on radicular or segmental deficits, and espe-

cially on perception of pain. Hypoesthesia (lessened sensibility to touch) and paresthesia (tingling and numbness) are also seen in pseudoradicular syndromes.

**TREATMENT.** The approach depends on the severity of nerve root compression. Treatment can vary, from techniques such as those described in this text to surgical intervention. Root pain usually resolves regardless of treatment in about 6 months. If pain persists or worsens one suspects a more serious condition such as malignancy (Cyriax *ibid*).

### Segmental Muscular Weakness Due To Cervical Disc Lesions

Nerve root impingement produces the articular signs of passive movement limitations (often the only symptom in the initial stages), increasing pain in the arm or paresthesia in the hand on neck movement, and segmental muscular weakness.

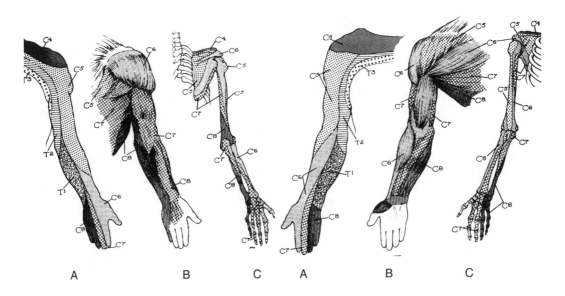

*Figure 7-42:* Segmental innervation: A—Dermatome, B—Myotome, C—Sclerotome (Reproduced with permission, Inman VT. Referred pain from skeletal structures J Nerv Ment Dis 99:660, 1944).

*Table 7-9.* SEGMENTAL MUSCULAR WEAKNESS DUE TO CERVICAL DISC LESIONS

| LOCATION OF LESION | WEAKNESS |
|---|---|
| C8 | ulnar deviation at the wrist<br>thumb adduction and extension |
| C7 | wrist flexion<br>elbow extension<br>arm adduction |
| C6 | wrist extension |
| C5-C6 | elbow flexion |
| C5 | shoulder abduction and rotation |
| Mostly C4, also C2, C3 | shoulder shrug |
| C3 | neck sidebending |
| C1, C2 | neck flexion |
| C1 | neck rotation |
| **THE DEEP TENDON REFLEXES** | |
| C5-C6 | biceps reflex reduced<br>brachioradialis reflex reduced |
| C7-C8 | triceps reflex reduced |
| Cranial nerve V | jaw bite reflex reduced |

**FIRST AND SECOND CERVICAL ROOTS.** The first and second cervical roots are affected rarely, since the uppermost cervical joints do not have discs. Pain and paresthesia of the vertex of the skull (innervated by C1) and in the temple, forehead and eyes (innervated by C2) often are attributed wrongly to upper nerve root lesions. These symptoms are likely to be due to mechanical, ligamentous and musculotendinous lesions of the upper cervical spine. However, an osteophyte that impinges on the second cervical nerve root can produce these symptoms and should be considered a possible source in the elderly patient.

**THIRD CERVICAL ROOT.** Compression of the third cervical root gives rise to unilateral pain in the neck and paresthesia and numbness in the lower ear, the cheek and the temporal areas. Rarely paresthesia and numbness in one cheek and the chin are the only symptoms.

**FOURTH CERVICAL ROOT.** Fourth cervical root lesions are uncommon. However, this type of lesion can produce pain and paresthesia of the mid-neck and shoulder, including the deltoid.

**FIFTH CERVICAL ROOT.** If a lesion affects the fifth cervical root, pain may be felt in the arm, forearm or scapular regions but *does not extend to the thumb*. Paresthesia from this source can extend to the thumb. Weakness of the deltoid and bicep muscles and a sluggish biceps reflex may be seen, as may a weak brachioradialis reflex.

**SIXTH CERVICAL ROOT.** Sixth cervical root lesion pain propagates down the arm and forearm to the radial side of the hand. Paresthesia and cutaneous analgesia are felt in the *thumb* and *index* finger. Weakness of the biceps, brachialis, supinator brevis and extensor carpi radialis muscles can result from a lesion at this cervical level. The biceps reflex may be reduced or absent (sometimes this is the only positive finding during examination).

**SEVENTH CERVICAL ROOT.** The seventh cervical nerve root is affected most frequently. According to Cyriax, 90% of disc lesions that result in a nerve root palsy of the cervical spine occur at this level. Pain is felt from the scapular area, down the back of the arm, to the outer forearm and to the fingertips. Paresthesia is felt in the index, *middle and ring fingers*. Weakness of the triceps, and sometimes of the radial flexors and wrist extensors, may be observed. The deep tendon reflex of the triceps may be affected. Frequently, cutaneous analgesia is detected at the dorsum of the middle and index fingers.

**EIGHTH CERVICAL ROOT.** Pain of the eighth cervical root involves the lower scapular area, the back or inner side of the arm, and the inner forearm. The patient reports paresthesia in the *middle, ring and little fingers*. Weakness is evident in the extensor and adductor muscles of the thumb, and in the extensors of the fingers. Cutaneous analgesia may be felt at the little finger.

*Spinal Cord*

If the spinal cord is affected, the practitioner may see signs such as uncoordinated lower limbs, spastic gait and/or a positive Babinski sign (backward flexion of the great toe, elicited by stroking of lateral aspect of sole of foot). Many pathological reflexes may be found (Babinski, clonus and hyperreflexia) and they are often grouped under the name "long tract signs".

**McKenzie System**

The McKenzie system is helpful in the evaluation and treatment of disc derangements. Loading strategies that include static postures and dynamic movements are assessed. The patient is first asked to perform a single movement for each loading strategy examined. The practitioner assesses the range and quality of movement and not symptoms. Then, the patient is instructed to perform repeated movements in each of the planes—repetitive movements are necessary to accurately assess each movement plane. A single movement or moment's positioning may give a false impression. At the end of each movement series, symptoms, especially peripheralization, are noted. If necessary, over pressure by the practitioner can be added at the end range of each movement. Static postures, at end range, are evaluated by asking the patient to hold each position for some time. Static loading tests are used generally when dynamic tests do not reveal a clear result (McKenzie and Jacobes *ibid*).

In the cervical spine the practitioner evaluates:

1. Full passive flexion sitting (Figure 7-43).

2. Retraction sitting (retraction results in flexion in the upper and extension in the lower cervical spine).

3. Protrusion (protrusion results in extension of the upper, and flexion in the lower cervical spine). Retraction-then-protrusion sitting (Figure 7-44).

4. Retraction supine (Figure 7-45).

5. Full passive extension (Figure 7-46).

6. Retraction-then-extension supine (Figure 7-47).

7. Retracted sidebending sitting (Figure 7-48).

8. Retraction rotation (Figure 7-49).

Movements and postures that result in reduced symptoms and centralization are used for treatment. The appropriate therapeutic movement may change and reevaluation should be performed frequently.

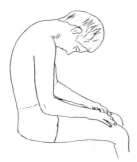

*Figure 7-43:* Passive flexion.

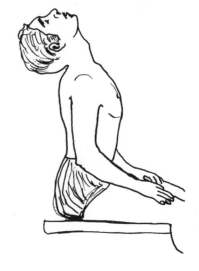

*Figure 7-46:* Passive extension.

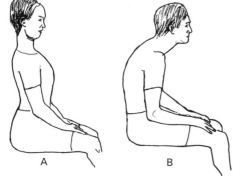

A                    B

*Figure 7-44:* Retraction — A; protrusion —B.

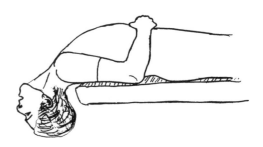

*Figure 7-47:* Retraction-extension supine.

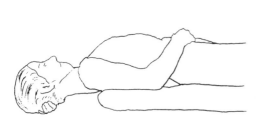

*Figure 7-45:* Retraction supine.

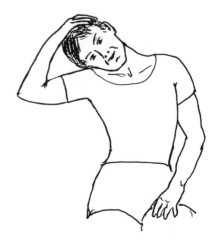

*Figure 7-48:* Retraction-sidebending.

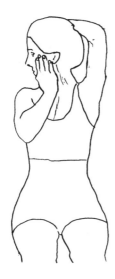

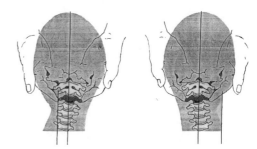

*Figure 7-50:* Assessment of typical cervical joint function. Test is positive if translation to one side is reduced and the end feel is altered as compared to the other side. (With permission Mitchell 1995).

*Figure 7-49:* Retraction rotation.

## Vertebral Dysfunction

In the cervical spine, vertebral dysfunctions are categorized as applying to the *typical vertebrae* (C3-C7) or *atypical vertebrae* (CO-C1 and C1-C2).

The cervical spine is unique in that no neutral group dysfunction is possible. Although a small amount of rotation and sidebending occurs in the opposite direction in the CO-C1 articulation, this is the only cervical vertebra capable of this type of motion, and therefore no group (neutral) dysfunction is possible (Greenman *ibid*).

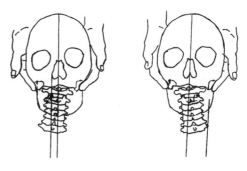

*Figure 7-51:* Assessment of OA junction. Test is positive if translation to one side is reduced and the end feel is altered as compared to the other side. (With permission Mitchell 1995).

*Examination*

Examination for cervical vertebral restrictions is best performed with the patient supine. The practitioner:

*Restrictions*

CO-C1 restrictions mostly affect flexion and extension, limiting posterior gliding of CO on C1 with flexion, anterior gliding with extension, and to a lesser but important extent, sidebending. C1-C2 restrictions largely involve rotational movements. In the typical (C3-C7) segments, both flexion restrictions (ERS) and extension restrictions (FRS) are common.

1. Translates the head from side to side— both in extension and flexion—for the typical segments— and notes the end feel and range (Figure 7-50).

2. Adds anterior and posterior glide for assessing the OA junction. Notes end feel and range (Figure 7-51).

3. Performs rotation (with the neck in full flexion) to assess C1-2 function. Notes end feel and range (Figure 7-52).

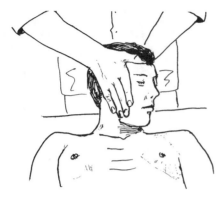

*Figure 7-52:* Assessment of C1-C2 rotation. Test is positive if rotation to one side is reduced and the end feel is altered as compared to the other side.

## Treatment

Vertebral dysfunctions in the neck respond well to thrust manipulation, muscle energy techniques and needling. For dysfunction in the typical segments, both muscle energy and needling can be used, with the neck positioned at a restricted barrier.

**FLEXION RESTRICTION (ERS).** For ERS dysfunction, the neck is flexed, sidebent and rotated away from the dysfunctional side (the side to which the vertebra is rotated when the spine is flexed; the side to which the segment resists sidebending), until the feather edge of these motions are engaged. The joint must remain loose-packed. The practitioner:

Needles superficially over the contracted deep rotatory muscle. Activates the appropriate dorsal Sinews, and Main channels.

or:

Resists the patient's effort of sidebending or extension (Muscle Energy).

**EXTENSION RESTRICTION (FRS).** For FRS dysfunctions, the neck is extended, sidebent and rotated toward the dysfunctional side.[8] The practitioner:

Needles superficial points over the contracted scalenus and longus colli muscles anteriorly. Activates the appropriate ventral Sinews, and Main channels.

or:

For muscle energy, resists the patient's effort at sidebending or flexion.

**C0-C1 AND C1-C2 DYSFUNCTION.** C0-C1 and C1-C2 dysfunctions are best treated with muscle energy, although needling of the suboccipital muscles with the neck engaging the barrier may be helpful, as well.

## Multiple Lesions

Neck Pain with arm pain indicates that the arm pain can be either local or referred. The practitioner should consider a distal cause, as well. As with all pain syndromes, the practitioner should rule out nonmusculoskeletal sources first.

The possibility of more than one lesion should be suspected always until proven otherwise. For example, a patient who has neck and hand numbness may have both a cervical problem and carpal tunnel syndrome. In patients with arm pain and/or numbness the following are considered:

- Thalamic ischemia (especially in older patients or history of cardiovascular disease—often with associated symptoms around the face and mouth.

- Disc disorders.

- Radiculopathy.

- Cervical spondylotic myelopathy (in older patients).

- Spinal stenosis or space occupying lesions (stenosis in older and space occu-

---

8. The side to which the TrPs is rotated toward when the neck is in extension; or away from the side to which the segment is rotated (positioned); or toward the side to which the segment resists sidebending with the spine in extension.

pying lesions in both young and old patients).

- Joint dysfunctions.

- Myofascial/ligamentous pain syndromes.

- Thoracic outlet syndrome (especially if traumatic history).

- Pancoast's tumors (especially in smokers or with Horner's syndrome).

- Shoulder, elbow or wrist disorders.

- Cardiac ischemia.

- Neuropathies.

- Amyotrophic lateral sclerosis.

- Spinal cord myelopathy.

If a patient has two culprit abnormalities, it is recommended to treat the proximal lesion before the more distal one. In such cases, the practitioner should manage spinal involvement first, because the two entities may have a mechanical, neurological or vascular relationship. In tennis elbow for example, cervical manipulation was shown to produce significant improvement in pressure pain threshold, pain-free grip strength, neurodynamics and pain scores relative to placebo (Vicenzino, Collins, and Wright 1996).

## Osteoarthritis

Osteophytes of the cervical spine are predominately asymptomatic unless they compress nerves, ligaments or arteries (Figure 7-53). Generally they should not be considered significant. However, they suggest a degenerative process and, therefore, other possible pathology.

Electromyographic analysis of neck muscle fatigue, in patients who have osteoarthritis of the cervical spine, shows a higher fatigue of the anterior and posterior neck muscles. Rehabilitation programs should consider these muscular changes to obtain optimal outcomes. (Gogia and Sab-

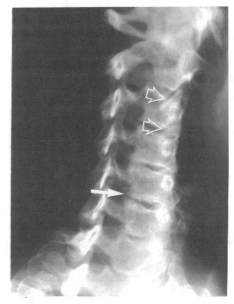

*Figure 7-53:* Oblique x-ray showing arthritis with bony spurs (closed arrow) encroaching on the neural canal of C5-6. The open arrows point to the facet joints.

bahi 1994). Often symptoms are due to ligamentous laxity.

## Thoracic Outlet Syndrome

Thoracic outlet syndrome (TOS) describes a variety of conditions that affect compression of the brachial plexus, resulting in neuropathy.[9] This syndrome can lead to vascular compromise and may be associated with an anomalous cervical rib (McCarthy, Yao, and Schafer et al. 1989). Often either cervical spine involvement or first rib dysfunction is present, as well.

Traumatic history has been found in 86% of 668 patients undergoing surgery for TOS (Sanders and Pearce 1989). The mechanisms are probably due to the development of swelling and adhesions in the fascia or fibrous bends of the anterior and/or middle scalenes (Cailliet 1988).

---

9. "Thoracic inlet" is a more accurate term, since the nerves enter at this location and exit further down.

*Symptoms*

Thoracic outlet syndrome can cause a variety of symptoms, often presenting with nocturnal symptoms of paresthesia in the arms or hands, possibly bilaterally. This sensation, which may awaken the patient at night, is a phenomenon of release of pressure on the brachial plexus nerve trunk. Normal daytime activity causes compression of the brachial nerve from the weight of the arms or contracted myofascial structures, and leads to mechanical pressure on the brachial plexus. During sleep the tension is relaxed and this causes onset of paresthesia.

In patients with thoracic outlet syndrome that did not respond to conservative therapy for over 7-12 months, Liu, Tahmoush, Roos and Schwartzman (1995) found a compressive brachial plexopathy from abnormally-attached or enlarged scalene muscles that affected the upper trunk of the brachial plexus. In some patients, at least one fibrous band compressed the lower trunk of the brachial plexus, as well. The patients had pain and sensory changes in a brachial plexus distribution, aggravation of pain with use of the affected extremity, pain on palpation over the brachial plexus, no intrinsic hand muscle atrophy, and normal nerve conduction studies. Electromyography (EMG) showed mild chronic neuropathic changes in some patients.

Liu et al. concluded that neurogenic thoracic outlet syndrome can occur from cervical band and scalene muscle anomalies without intrinsic hand muscle atrophy from abnormalities such as the presence of cervical ribs or enlarged C7 transverse processes and can occur with or without abnormalities of EMG readings.

*Examination*

No simple (fool-proof) examination for thoracic outlet syndrome exists. Tests designed to obliterate radial pulses are not specific for TOS. The practitioner can:

1. Ask the seated patient to abduct his arms to 90°. Externally rotate his hands so that they face the ceiling, keeping the shoulders retracted. Then open and close his hands rapidly for 3 minutes. The exam is positive if symptoms and fatigue are produced on the symptomatic side while the asymptomatic side remains unchanged.

2. Ask the patient to carry a 5-lb weight in each hand for 3 minutes. The examination is positive if symptoms are reproduced on the symptomatic side.

3. Ask the patient to rest the patient's arm on the patient's head for several minutes. If paresthesia occurs after several minutes, the patient is likely to be suffering from thoracic outlet syndrome.

4. Order an X-ray, which is needed to diagnose a cervical rib dysfunction.

*Treatment*

Treatment is directed to the underlying condition and may present a clinical challenge. Treatment may consist of manual therapy, acupuncture and dry needling. In some cases (Cyriax *ibid*), simple, frequent shoulder shrugging is all that is required to alleviate symptoms. Local heparin injection may be tried in patients that do not respond (Ellis personal communication). If symptoms are severe and are unresponsive to less invasive treatment, surgical intervention might be necessary.

## Acute Torticollis

Acute torticollis is common in middle aged patients, and is less common in younger and older patients. In children, torticollis may be congenital due to a non painful contracture of the sternocleidomastoid muscle. If not, congenital torticollis in children may represent a serious condition of infectious, neurological, or neoplastic origin (Ombergt, Bisschop, ter Veer and Van de Velde 1995).

## Symptoms

Symptoms and signs of acute torticollis are:

- Most often the patient awakens in the morning with a stiffness ("kink') and antalgic posture of the neck.

- Weight-bearing or any attempt to rotate the neck is painful.

- The pain usually is unilateral and may extend to the shoulder and periscapular regions.

- Occasionally the pain extends to the arm or is felt bilaterally.

- Similar symptoms may arise suddenly doing some movement or a trivial incident (Mcnair 1986).

- If due to a disc lesion the neck is held often in pure sidebending (without rotation component) away from the painful side.

## Examination

Inspection and examination for torticollis follows the usual pattern in the cervical spine:

- Extension dysfunction will present usually with a flexed, rotated and sidebent segment, usually toward the painful side.

- Flexion dysfunction will present usually with extended rotated and sidebent segment toward the painful side.

- Resisted movements often are painful and weak (due to pain).
  Often arm movements are painful as well, especially ipsilateral arm elevation.

- Pure sidebending posture away from pain occurs often with disc lesions.

TREATMENT. Treatment of torticollis follows the usual techniques presented in the text.

## Whiplash Injury

The term *whiplash injury* was used first by Crowe in 1928 to describe neck injuries that are due to automobile rear-end collisions. Whiplash is a nonspecific term that neither conveys the character of the injury nor indicates a diagnosis. It refers to cervical hyperextension-flexion injury, also called acceleration/deceleration syndrome. Another current term for injuries due to low-speed, rear-end collision is LoSRC.

Automobile accident injuries are common, and their clinical importance tends to be underestimated. Even mild and moderate whiplash can cause tears of muscles, tendons, ligaments and joint capsules. The threshold (for male subjects) seems to be at 5 m.p.h. for mild cervical strain injury, which is caused by rapid compression-tension cycle directed through the musculoskeletal neck (McConnell et al 1993). In a review of 32 studies from 1980 to 1994, Nordhoff (1996) found that about 40% of automobile accident victims have long-term, persistent symptoms. The upper neck, the weakest part of the spine, is most vulnerable to this form of trauma (Tsuchisashi et al. 1981). Whiplash can occur due to other traumas such as sports injuries, as well.

Whiplash can cause injury to many structures, because the direction of collision is variable, and the seat belt provides a pivot line that tends to lead to torsional strains. While the use of seat belts prevents serious injuries and saves lives, their use does increase the risk of sprain/strains in the neck and low back (Orsay et al. 1990). Because the cervical system is linked mechanically to the rest of the spine, concomitant brain, spinal cord, facet and peripheral nerve injuries are probable, and common (Ward *ibid*). The most commonly involved tissues probably are the cervical ligaments and muscles. In severe trauma, the anterior longitudinal ligament can rupture, which causes the upper facets to move downward on the lower facets, markedly relaxing the ligamentum flavum. This sliding of the vertebrae can damage the spinal cord and can even cause death (Cyriax *ibid*). Traumatic syrinx, a pathological, tube-shaped cavity in the brain or spinal cord, also has been noted on MRIs secondary to traumatic cord injury (Brown 1995).

## Mechanisms of Injury

For diagnosis and treatment of whiplash injury, determining the direction and mode of an injury may be important.

**REAR-END COLLISION.** During a rear-end collision (Figure 7-54), the trunk accelerates forward, leaving the head relatively behind resulting in hyper-extension injury. Even low-velocity rear end collisions can cause significant injuries to muscles, ligaments, discs, and even vertebral body fractures (Dunn and Blazar 1987). Low speed rear-end collisions can cause more symptoms than higher speed front-end collisions (Hyde1992):

- The 8-15 pounds of the head whips backward into hyperextension.

  The excessive extension probably is due, in part, to the unopposed movement of the neck that occurs because ventral muscles that usually protect against hyperextension do not have time to react. Hyperextension leads to stretch injury of the anterior structures such as the anterior longitudinal ligament, anterior disc herniation, joint infringement into the intervetebral foramen, fracture of the cervical vertebrae, and compression injury of the facet structures posteriorly.

- Usually flexion follows, limited by the seat belt and by the chin hitting the chest.

  As the head hits the head rest and the soft tissues are stretched, the head is whipped forward. Release of elastic energy from the head rest, recoil of the car seat and soft tissues and a stretch reflex (reflex contraction) in the ventral (flexors) muscles are contributing

factors. The head whips forward, because of the preset cervical flexors tension, and their reactive forceful contraction (reactive to forceful stretch). Also, the timing of flexor muscle recoil appears to have an additive affect with the recoil effects of the seats, therefore the head thrusts forward violently. Hyperflexion results in posterior soft tissues injury (Dorman 1997).

**FORWARD COLLISION.** Forward collision (often called deceleration injury), (Figure 7-55), causes cervical hyperflexion, which can be followed by hyperextension. The hyperflexion leads to trauma of the posterior cervical ligaments, most often at C5-C6 (Jackson 1958), subluxation and sprain of the facets, capsular tears, and posterior disc herniation.

## Pathology

Little direct information is available on the pathological processes of *non-fatal* whiplash injuries. MacNab reports damage to the longus colli muscles and widespread soft tissue contusion in the neck, including anterior longitudinal ligament tears, sympathetic nerve involvement, and bruising of the esophagus (MacNab 1964, 1973).

**LONG-TERM DEGENERATIVE CHANGES.** Long-term X-ray follow-up on whiplash injuries shows an increased rate of degenerative changes in patients who originally had normal X-ray findings. Typically these changes are confined to one or two segments at the C5-6-7 level, as compared to the non-traumatic, diffuse degeneration pattern seen in the elderly. Pre-existing degenerative disease does not seem to contribute significantly to prolonged symptoms in cases of whiplash injuries (Meenen, Katzer, Dihlmann, Held, Fyfe and Jungbluth 1994). However, other studies find a high correlation between pre-existing cervical spondylosis and persistence of pain after whiplash injury (Miles et al. 1988).

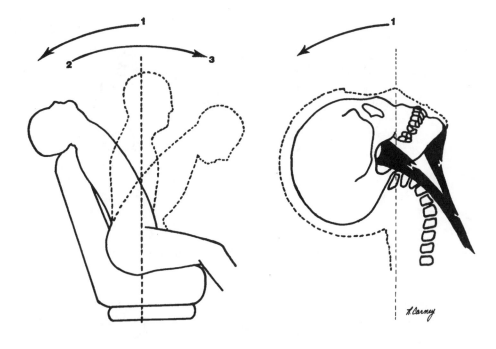

*Figure 7-54:* In rear-end collisions whiplash injuries damage the anterior ligaments and soft tissues

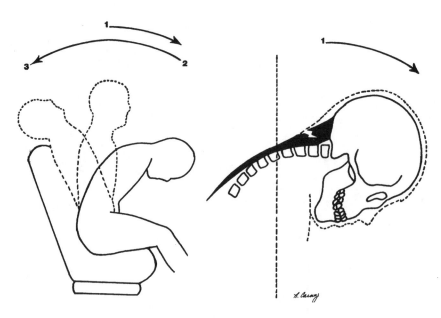

*Figure 7-55:* Injury to posterior tissues from forward collisions (With permission Dorman and Ravin 1991).

**DISC LESIONS.** Whiplash also might result in fatal disc lesions. Hinz (1968) demonstrated that, in 41 cases of fatal whiplash, the most common lesion was a disc rupture, usually at the C3-C4 level. Postmortems also show common isolated avulsions of the annular fibers from the rim of the cervical vertebral body, with annular ruptures extending into the central disc, usually at C5-C7 (Jónsson 1991; Eliyahu 1989).

**FACET LESIONS.** In a diagnostic block study of patients who had chronic neck pain following whiplash injury, Barnsley et al. (1995) reported that the prevalence of cervical facet joint pain occurred in 54% of patients. Barnsley concluded that cervical facet joint pain was the most common source of chronic neck pain following whiplash.

**TYPE OF IMPACT.** In rear-end collisions, replica studies of *hyperextension* injury show that the greatest deformation (about 57%) occurs in the longus colli. The scalenus anterior muscle was deformed in 21% and was more common than deformations in

the sternocleidomastoid, longus capitis and scalene posterior muscles (Deng and Goldsmith 1987).

MacNab (1971) has implicated (in hyperextension injuries) the sympathetic plexus, anterior longitudinal ligaments with separation of cervical discs, trapezius, splenius capitis, semispinalis capitis, scaleni, longissimus capitis, rectus capitis, rhomboid, inferior and superior oblique capitis, and longus capitis.

*Hyperflexion* neck injuries produce primarily ligamentous-disc injuries (Yoganandan et al. 1989). A replica study showed that the splenius cervicis and splenius capitis muscles bear the greatest deformation, about 50%, (Deng and Goldsmith 1987). If the neck is flexed at the time of impact, the T-1 to T-4 areas will bear the greatest stress (Pintar et al. 1989).

*Rotational* spinal soft tissue injuries affect primarily the ligaments and zygoapophyseal (facet) joints complex (Yoganandan et al *ibid*).

*Side collisions* result in sidebending injury. Side collisions tend to affect the middle-to-upper neck regions more than other crashes. A replica side collision study showed the longus capitis bearing the majority (57%) of deforming forces (sidebending in the cervical spine is always coupled with rotation).

## Diagnostic Limitations

When whiplash occurs, diagnosis is complicated by the fact that currently available imaging techniques are deficient in visualizing the cervical soft tissues. Ultrasound, which is being explored as a diagnostic tool, may be valuable for documenting swelling in soft tissues. Woltring et al. (1994) suggest that helical axis may provide objective assessment of joint pathology and dysfunction. This would help significantly in assessing whiplash injuries and settling litigation issues. Currently, in many cases the patient's complaints are dismissed because "objective" evidence is lacking and ulterior motives such as litigation are suspected. The evidence that litigating prolongs recovery from automobile accidents is unconvincing (Mendelson 1982, 1984).

### POOR CORRELATION WITH MRI FINDINGS. In studies in which patients were examined clinically and by MRI, Pettersson et al. (1994) reported that 26 of 39 cases of whiplash neck injury showed changes on the MRI. Twenty-five of those cases showed disc lesions, of which ten were identified as disc herniations and one was identified as a muscle lesion. The correlation between the MRI findings and the clinical symptoms and signs was poor.

## Initial Findings after Injury

In studies of the relationship between accident mechanisms and initial findings after whiplash injury, Sturzenegger et al. (1994) found that the passenger's position in the car, use of a seat belt, and the presence of a head restraint showed no significant correlation with findings. Rotated or inclined head position at the moment of impact was associated with a higher frequency of multiple symptoms, with more severe symptoms, and signs of musculoligamental-cervical strain and neural involvement, particularly radicular damage. Unprepared occupants had a higher frequency of multiple symptoms and more severe headache. Rear-end collision was associated with a higher frequency of multiple symptoms, especially of cranial nerve or brainstem dysfunction. Sturzenegger et al. concluded that three features of accident mechanisms were associated with more severe symptoms:

- An unprepared occupant.
- Rear-end collision, with or without subsequent frontal impact.
- Rotated or inclined head position at the moment of impact.

## Important Considerations

Because whiplash can cause a variety of symptoms that can manifest at different times, the practitioner must stay alert for possible long-term complications.

### DELAY IN SYMPTOMS. Pain due to whiplash usually begins several hours, days, or even weeks (typical of ligamentous pain) after the accident (Hirsch, Hirsch and Hiramoto 1988). Unless the practitioner obtains a thorough history for trauma, this delayed onset of symptoms can cause the practitioner to miss the precipitating mechanism of injury. In a study of 5,000 patients, 25% showed significantly-prolonged onset of symptoms that were secondary to whiplash injury. In more severe injuries, the pain usually was immediate. In the delayed group, the most frequently reported symptom was headache (Balla and Karnaghan 1987). Upper-extremity radiating symptoms may not appear until several months after injury (Bugduk *ibid*).

### HEADACHE FOLLOWING WHIPLASH. Headache following whiplash injury has been reported to occur in 48-80% of patients (Norris and Watts 1983). In a study of the prevalence of third occipital nerve head-

ache among whiplash patients, Lord et al. found that a third occipital nerve block was effective in patients whom the diagnosis was positive. These patients were significantly more likely to be tender over the C2-3 facet joint (Lord, Barnsley, Wallis, Bogduk and 1994).

**PROGRESSION OF SYMPTOMS.** Following whiplash injury, the victim typically complains of a wide variety of symptoms. Immediately after the injury, the only complaints usually are of shock and anxiety without pain, probably due to stress analgesia. Later, general aching, mild neck pain, occipital pain, headache, limitation of cervical movement, and perhaps blurred vision, tinnitus and dyspahagia are seen. Often these symptoms intensify with time. Unless treated properly, they can last for years. Most patients who require medical attention and then recover, do so within the first two years (Gargan and Bannister 1990).

Injuries of the upper cervical spine develop earlier. Often they are accompanied by sympathetic/cranial/central involvement such as headache, tinnitus, diaphoresis, dizziness, altered sensorium and blurred vision. This may be due to the sympathetic afferents from the cranial vessels, which pass their sensory information through the upper cervical roots (Lambert and Bogduk et al. 1991), or from brain or spinal cord injury. These symptoms were described first in 1926 as the Barré-Lieou syndrome, in which a series of symptoms including headache, vertigo, tinnitus and ocular problems were associated with post-traumatic disc prolapse at the C 3-4 level.

Other symptoms reported at various stages of whiplash include anxiety, fatigue, irritability, insomnia and flashbacks (Dalal and Harrison 1993). Dysphagia or discomfort on swallowing may be seen in up to 30% of patients (Norris and Watt 1983). Usually this is due to injury of ventral soft tissues. Low back pain may be seen in 57-71% of patients (Foreman and Croft 1988).

**IMPAIRMENT OF ATTENTION.** In their evaluation of attention and memory function of patients two years following a whiplash injury, Stefano and Radavov (1995) found no memory impairment in symptomatic patients. However, symptomatic and matched asymptomatic individuals had differing levels of attention. In tasks that required divided attention, symptomatic patients had difficulties that could not be explained as having occurred due to use of medicines that might affect ability to perform divided-attention tasks.

**POST-CONCUSSION SYNDROME.** Head injuries from mild traumas (and whiplash) can lead to chronic symptoms or "post concussion syndrome" in as many as 50% of patients (Alves et al. 1986). Symptoms often include cognitive, behavioral and pain complaints (Alves and Jenttner 1986).

**DELAYED RECOVERY.** In their study of the predictive relationship between psychosocial factors and the course of recovery in patients who have whiplash injury, Radanov et al. (1994) found that patients who remained symptomatic at one year had:

- Significantly higher ratings of initial neck pain and headache.

- A greater variety of subjective complaints.

- Higher scores on the "nervousness" scale from the personality inventory.

- Worse well-being scores.

- Poorer performance with regard to focussed attention.

The study's regression analysis revealed that the initial variables that correlated significantly with poor recovery at one year were higher age, complaint of sleep disturbances, and higher intensity of initial neck pain and headache.

*Treatment of Whiplash Injury*

Treatment for acute whiplash can consist of compression, icing and bracing of the neck as soon as possible.[10] Microscopic capillary bleeding in deep neck muscles has been shown to persist up to 2-5 days after motor vehicle collision injuries (Aldman 1987). Bracing for a prolonged period has been shown to cause muscle atrophy, joint contracture, and prolonged rehabilitation (Ruskin 1984). Treatment can include indirect techniques to relax muscles, acupuncture, and herbs for pain control. Bracing and cervical collars can be used in:

- Severe neck pain (in patients who have severe spasm, suspected fracture, and ligamentous instability).
- Temporarily during activities that aggravate pain.
- During sleep.

Thrust manipulation is rarely used to restore function and free entrapped tissues. When mild signs of disc involvement (such as partial articular pattern and joint dysfunction) are present without radicular signs, direct and/or indirect cervical manipulation often is helpful. However, the practitioner must be sure of the diagnosis and the technique, because serious instability may exist. Acupuncture can be used early for its analgesic effect and resulting improved mobility.

> **WARNING:** Thrust manipulation in a patient with instability can have catastrophic consequences

**NOTE:** The appropriateness of nonsteroidal anti-inflammatory agents (NSAIDs) use is debatable, because they inhibit inflammation and therefore interfere with healing of wounded tissues. If NSAIDs are used, they should be combined with OM hemostatic herbs. Use of these herbs will help keep to a minimum the microbleeding that occurs due to the antiplatelet action of NSAIDs. This will prevent inflammation in areas that will not benefit from inflammation. NSAID use should probably be limited to the first several days.

**TREATMENT OF FACET JOINT INJURY.** Injury to the cervical facet joints is thought to be a common problem following whiplash injury. Barnsley et al. (1994) report that, following whiplash injury, injection of betamethasone into the facets is not effective. This study indicates that, when the facets are involved, the pain probably is due to mechanical dysfunctions, not just inflammation.

Thermal ablation of the nerve that supplies a symptomatic facet can result in complete relief of symptoms, in chronic patients (Bogduk 1997).

**TREATMENT OF CHRONIC-STAGE WHIPLASH.** To treat chronic-stage whiplash, the practitioner should address all mechanical and myofascial/ligamentous components globally. Rehabilitation should involve (Fitz-Ritson 1995) exercises that address coordination of eye-head-neck-arm movements, coordination of the entire vertebral column, and returning the "phasic" component of the musculature to functional levels.

Acupuncture can have a 71% to 91% positive clinical response (Su and Su 1988). Acupuncture has been used successfully in combination with manual medicine techniques, as well (Pearson 1990).

---

10. Some researchers say that the neck should not be kept immobile. The author prefers only early bracing, but finds that immobilizing the neck during sleep periods is helpful at later stages.

# General Treatments: Neck & Head Pain

The following techniques are rewarding often in the treatment of musculoskeletal disorders of the neck region.

# Acute Pain

In acute cases, the practitioner emphasizes distal points and the Sinews channel, limiting local deep needling to a maximum retention of ½-minute and to a few trigger, acupuncture or motor points. If needles are left for a longer duration, the needling depth should be superficial and electricity may be added. The practitioner:

1. Needles the distal points, either on channels that have been demonstrated to have dysfunctions or for motions that increase pain (see tables below).

2. Asks the patient to mobilize the neck gently.

3. Reevaluates for mechanical dysfunctions and adds specific needles to address these.

## Point Combination

When the patient is prone, a useful point combination is to needle ear points and upright tendons (needle subcutaneously),[11] (Figure 7-56), with the addition of wrist points and Beside Three Miles (see chapter 5). This protocol can be used in most cases of acute cervical pain. Moxa,

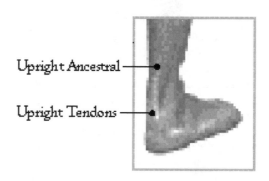

*Figure 7-56:* Correct Tendons

heat or electrical stimulation to points on the Sinews channels are important, as well.

## Local Points

Local points can be very helpful when treating acute neck pain. The practitioner:

1. Positions the neck such that the painful movement is just engaged.

2. Needles superficially over the affected muscles.
   If needed quickly inserts a needle into the muscle body.
   IF NEEDED.

3. Needles the tip of the fifth cervical transverse process and facets.

4. Taps periosteal junctions when appropriate (Figure 7-57).[12]

## Herbal Therapy

A guiding oral analgesic formula for acute neck pain with or without neuralgia and headache is:

Radix Aconiti Agrestis (Cao Wu and Chuan Wu)
Eupolyphagae Seu Opisthoplatiae (Tu Bie Chong)
Lumbricus (Di Long)
Semen Sojae (Dan Dou Chi)
Moschus Moschiferi (She Xiang)

---

11. Two Tong-style points located in the achilles tendon.

12. Clinical judgment must be used as to the benefit of a more aggressive needling.

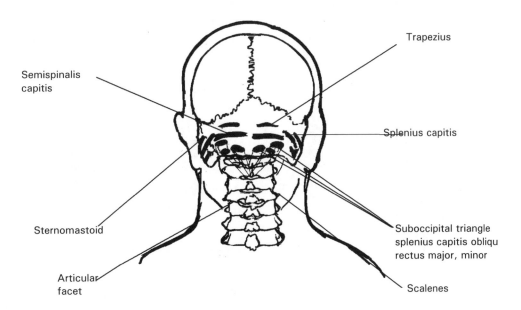

Trapezius

Semispinalis
capitis

Splenius capitis

Sternomastoid

Suboccipital triangle
splenius capitis obliqu
rectus major, minor

Articular
facet

Scalenes

*Figure 7-57:*Important bony attachments to dry needling in neck and head pain
(After Gunn 1989).

A guiding oral formula for acute stiff neck from climatic, sleep (morning kink), and mechanical pain is:

Rhizoma seu Radix Notopterygium (Qiang Hou)

Semen Coix (Yi Yi Ren)

Radix Lederouriella (Fang Feng)

Clematis (Wei Ling Xian)

Rhizoma Ligusticum (Chuan Xiang)

Radix Salvia (Dan Shen)

Rhizoma Curcumae (Jiang Huang)

Radix Pueraria (Ge Gen)

Radix Glycyrrhizae (Gan Cao)

A guiding topical formula for acute neck pain from myofascial source with or without headache is:

Fructus Gardenia (Jee Jee)

Angelica Sinensis (Dang Gui)

Radix Pseudoginseng (San Qi)

Rhizoma Corydalis (Yan Hu Sou)

Flos Carthami (Hong Hua)

Rhizoma Drynariae (Gu Sui Bu)

Myrrha (Mo Yao)

Gummi Olibanum (Ru Xiang)

Eupolyphaga seu Opisthoplatiae (Tu Bie Chong)

Radix Gentianae Macrophyllae (Qin Jiao)

Herba Lycopi (Ze Lan)

Fructus Liquidambaris (Lu Lu Tong)

Cortex Acamthopanacis radicis (Wu Jia Pi)

## Chronic Neck Pain

For chronic cases, local needling is more effective. Electroacupuncture can be used. The practitioner applies the anode pole of a stimulator locally in a local-distal combination, starting with mild stimulation and, if needed, using the more vigorous techniques described in the section on contractile unit dysfunction (chapter 6). Extra and Sinews channels, as well as channel-draining therapies are effective. The Main channels are used according to the patient's general condition.

CAUTION: The practitioner must remind the patient, especially when more vigorous techniques are used, that this treatment is long-term, and that before the pain resolves, healing pain might increase temporarily.

To treat chronic pain, the practitioner:

**1.** Gently needles specifically over all facilitated (spasm) muscles.

(if needed) Needles into the muscle belly.

**2.** Gently needles the tendinous insertions, following the direction of the fibers without penetrating the tendons.

**3.** Uses channel draining and Extra channel techniques.

**4.** Considers two factors:

• Significant Inflammation.
If significant inflammation (pain) is present, the practitioner starts with a monopolar stimulation connecting the anode (+) at the local site and the cathode (-) at the ear or distal channel points, keeping the needle in for five to fifteen minutes, stimulating at 100-200 Hz. This reduces nervous excitation and edema in the area around the anode (+)

• Significant Degenerative Changes or Ligamentous Insufficiency.
If the patient has either significant degenerative changes or ligament insufficiency, stronger stimulation might be necessary at the articular pillars, and facets of the applicable segment.

**5.** Starts at the local site of injury, usually at the ligamentous and tendinous structures, where proliferation of tissue is desired.

**6.** Needles the periosteum. Applies the anode (+) pole of a monopolar stimulator locally for one hour using 100-200 Hz. (Some patients respond better to (-) pole stimulation.

**NOTE:** (If the procedure is too painful for the patient) administers 200 mg. of Yanhusuoyisu Pian[13] (tetrahydropalmini sulfate) 15 minutes prior to start of treatment.

Any time a patient is to be left lying on the table with needles inserted (acupunc-

13. Currently not available in US.

ture point treatment without active patient movement), the practitioner positions the patient such that muscle guarding is at a minimum. Pillows or other devices may be needed to help the patient achieve maximum relaxation.

CAUTION: Treatment of these muscles by dry needling means a delicate balance between injury and therapy. A slow technique and close attention to the needle feel is the only way to know when stimulation is sufficient and when it is injurious.

## Herbal Therapy

A guiding oral formula for chronic neck pain from mechanical or myofascial source with or without headache is:

Rhizoma Corydalis (Yan Hu Suo), (Vinegar extracted)

Rhizoma Ligusticum (Chuan Xiong)

Radix Gentianae Macrophyllae (Qin Jiao)

Rhizoma Curcumae (Jiang Huang)

Semen Coix (Yi Yi Ren)

Caulis Milletii (Ji Xue Teng)

Radix Puerariae (Ge Gen)

Eupolyphagae Seu Opisthoplatiae (Tu Bie Chong)

Lumbricus (Di Long)

Semen Sojae (Dan Dou Chi)

Tortoise Plastrom Glue (Gui Ban Jiao)

Fructus Lycii (Gou Qi)

Herba Asari (Xi Xin)

Another guiding formula for chronic neck pain from mechanical and myofascial source (with/out headache) in a patient with more symptoms of fatigue and chill is:

Radix Angelica Sinensis (Dang Gui)

Rhizoma Corydalis (Yan Hu Suo)

Flos Carthami (Hong Hua)

Rhizoma Drynariae (Gu Sui Bu)

Resina Myrrhae (Mo Yao)

Gummi Olibanum (Ru Xiang)

Eupolyphaga seu Opisthoplatiae (Tu Bie Chong)

Herba Lycopi (Ze Lan)

Fructus Liquidambaris (Lu Lu Tong)

Aconiti Agestis (Cao Wu and Chuan Wu) plus (ethanol extracted)

Ramulus Cinnamomi (Gui Zhi)

Radix Gentianae Macrophyllae (Qin Jiao)

Cortex Acamthopanacis radicis (Wu Jia Pi)

A guiding oral formula for neck, arm and head pain from cervical spondylopathy is:

Radix Angelica Sinensis (Dang Gui)

Radix Salviae (Dan Shen)

Ramulus Mori (Sang Zhi)

Fructus Hordeum Vulgare (Mai Ya)

Radix Rehmanniae (Sheng Di Huang)

Herba Pyrolae (Lu Xian Cao)

Rhizoma Drynariae (Gu Sui Bu)

Herba Cistanchis (Rou Cong Rong)

Pollen Typhae (Pu Huang)

Caulis Millettiae (Ji Xue Teng)

Periostracum Cicadae (Chan Tui)

A guiding oral formula for non-specific headache is:

Gypsum Fibrosum (Shi Gao)

Radix Curcumae (Yu Jin)

Radix Paeoniae Alba (Bai Shao)

Flos Chrysanthemi (Ju Hua)

Bombyx Mori (Jiang Can)

Fructus Vitalizes (Man King Zi)

Semen Zizyphi Spinosae (Suan Zao Ren)

Caulis Polygoni Multiflori (Ye Jiao Teng)

Os Draconis (Long Gu)

Fructus Gardenia (Zhi Zi)

Flos Carthami (Hong Hua)

Herba Dendrobii (Shi Hu)

Rhizoma et Radix Ligustici (Gao Ben)

Rhizoma Ligusticum (Chuan Xiong)

## Scraping

Scraping is helpful often in patients with myofascial tightness. The patient's affected region is scraped until a mild hematoma (bruise) is created. The procedure is repeated once a week until the symptoms improve and/or the area no longer reacts by busing (Figure 7-58).

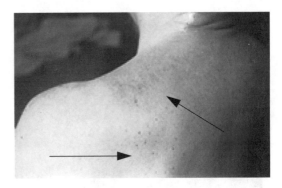

*Figure 7-58:*Hematoma as result of scraping.

## Channel Therapy

**SINEWS CHANNELS.** Sinews channels are used frequently during the acute phase of a cervical sprain. There are several ways to activate the Sinews channels.

- Tap the Well and first four points of the channel quickly with a burning incense stick.
- Needle the well points; electrical stimulation can then be used between the well point and local lesion or termination points.
- Needle the termination points on the head or trunk.
  SI-18 for the Yang-Leg Sinew channels.
  GB-13 for the Yang-Arm Sinew channels.
- Treat local points (Ashi, triggers) at painful areas with superficial techniques.

**CONNECTING CHANNELS.** Commonly used Connecting channels are: the Lung/Large Intestine, Small Intestine/Heart, Pericardium/Triple Warmer, Urinary Bladder/Kidney and Gall Bladder/Liver. The practitioner tonifies or sedates the appropriate Source point on the affected channel and the contralateral Connecting point on it's paired channel. Dark and visible superficial blood vessels are bled and the Connecting channel which passes through the region is activated. The connecting channels are used any time there is swelling and circulatory involvement.

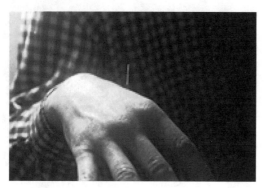

*Figure 7-59:  Laozhen.*

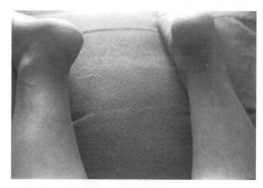

*Figure 7-60:*Correct Tendons

**YANG LINKING (WEI) CHANNEL.** The Yang Linking (Wei) channel, which combines aspects of the Small Intestine, Triple Warmer, Urinary Bladder, Gall Bladder, and Governing channel are used on patients who have:

- Cervical pain from degenerative processes.
- Headache that radiates from the base of the head (GB20) to the forehead or behind the ipsilateral eye.
- Any lateral (parietal) headache.
- Laterally radiating pain such as cervical radiculopathy.

The Master point for the Yang Linking (Wei) channel is TW-5, the Coupled point is GB-41, the Activation point is UB-63 and the Accumulating (Xi) point is GB-35.

**YANG MOTILITY (QIAO) CHANNEL.** The Yang Motility (Qiao) channel is used often for cervical stiffness, muscular weakness, and/or pain in the lateral and central aspects of the neck and shoulder. The channel also can be used for post-concussion visual disturbances.

The Master point of the Yang Motility (Qiao) is UB-62, the Coupled point is SI-3, the Activation point is UB-62, and the Accumulating (Xi) point is UB-59.

**GOVERNING (DU) CHANNEL.** The Governing (Du) channel is used often in disorders of the head, neck and back, especially mid-line pain. A sense as though one cannot hold the head up often is associated with the Governing (Du) channel.

The Master point of the Governing (Du) channel is SI-3, the Coupled point is UB-62, the Activation point is GV-1.

*Stiff Neck*

For treatment of stiff neck (especially if treated early), the point Laozhen (stiff neck), (Figure 7-59) can be helpful. It can be treated contralaterally to the direction to which the neck is turned (if right rotation is difficult, or left sided pain, treat the right side) or by choosing the side in which the point is more tender. The needle should be twirled continuously while the patient performs side-to-side neck rotation for five minutes.

*Posterior Neck Pain, Occipital Head Pain*

For posterior neck pain and or occipital head pain, the Correct Tendons points can be used (Figure 7-60), leaving the needles in place for one hour (or longer) while the patient mobilizes the neck. The needle must penetrate, go through the achilles tendon, and touch bone.

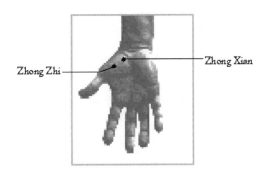

Zhong Zhi — Zhong Xian

*Figure 7-61:*Double Child/Immortal

## Neck & Periscapular Pain

Double Child/Immortal (Figure 7-61) are especial useful in neck and periscapular pain. Ipsilateral SI-6 can be added. The shoulder girdle and neck are mobilized.

## Multi-Channel Disorders

If more than one channel is involved, through and through acupoint stimulation can be used, e.g., if both Tai Yang and Shao Yang are involved, the practitioner needles TW-5 through to SI-6. The eight Extra channels are appropriate, as well.

## Marrow/bone Disorders

For disorders involving the bones, joints and or brain, K-3, UB-11 and GB-39 can be used. The Kidney Divergent channel should be used, as well.

## Sprain Strain

For sprain/strain of the neck, SI-3 UB-62 and SI-6 can be used as the major points.

## Cervical Soft Tissue Disorders

For disorders of the ligaments, tendons and fascia, GB-34 and Liv-8 can be used. The Liver Divergent channel should be used, as well.

For muscle, especially weakness, St-36, SP-2, 3, CV-6 (moxa), Yang Motility (Qiao) or Yin Motility (Qiao) treatments can be used.

## Timing of Symptoms

The practitioner uses: UB-62 if symptoms increase during the day and K-6 if symptoms increase at night.

## Recurrent Dysfunction

For a weak, deficient patient who has recurrent joint dysfunctions, the practitioner uses: Alarm (Mu) points connected with Back Shu (Transporting points) of the weak Organs followed by; Lu-7 (sedate), LI-4, 11 (sedate), St-36 (tonify or moxa), Sp-6 (tonify).

or

SI-3 and UB- 62 (with ion cord).

or

Moxa ST-36, CV-4 and GB-39.

## Wandering Pain (Bi)

For pain that constantly moves and changes, the practitioner needles in the valleys between the muscles and adds: GB-20, UB-17, Liv-3, SP-3, GV-16, LI-4 and GV-14.

## Common Points & Combinations

The common points and combinations listed in Table 7-10 on page 366 are useful in treatment of headache. The common points and combinations listed in Table 7-11 on page 367 through Table 7-14 on page 368 are useful in treatment of neck pain.

*Table 7-10.* **POINTS: TREATING HEADACHE**

| SYMPTOM | POINTS |
|---------|--------|
| Frontal | GV-23; LI-4, 7; ST-36, 44 and Yinteng through to UB-2, Sp-4, 9 |
| Parietal | GV-21, 20<br>UB-64,65 |
| Posterior parietal | Liv-3; SP-6 |
| Occipital | Taiyang; ST-7; 8 TW- 5<br>GB-38; UB-10, 64 |
| Temporal | TW-1-5; GB-1, 14, 38, 41; LU-7; ST-43<br>or<br>Beside Three Miles |
| Vertex or Deficient | K-1; UB-65<br>or<br>Liv-2,3 |
| Occipital radiating to forehead or eye | GB-41, 35, 20; TW-5; UB-63 |
| Migraine | TW-6; GB-37, 20, 4<br>or<br>Taiyang ST-8; TW-5, GB-7, 38, 41<br>H-8<br>or<br>UB-64 and 65<br>or<br>Beside Three Miles |

*Table 7-11.* **POINTS: TREATING MOVEMENT RESTRICTIONS AND ROTATION**

| Symptom | Points |
|---------|--------|
| Resistance to cervical rotation | GB-21 |
| Sudden neck muscle spasm with limitation of neck rotation | UB-10 |
| Acute shoulder pain with resistance to cervical rotation | ST-38 |
| Sudden neck muscle spasm with limitation of neck rotation | UB-37,10; SI-3; GB-21 |

*Table 7-12.* **POINTS: TREATING CERVICAL EXTENSION AND/OR FLEXION**

| Symptom | Points |
|---------|--------|
| Resistance to cervical extension and/or flexion | UB-11 |
| Resistance to cervical extension and/or flexion Also good for neck pain and headache | UB-64; UB-65 |
| Increased symptoms and signs with extension and/or flexion movement | UB-64; UB-11 |
| Relieves pain and stiffness in the head and back of the neck, especially painful extension | UB-64, 11 CV-24 |

*Table 7-13.* **POINTS: TREATING GENERAL CERVICAL STIFFNESS**

| Symptom | Points |
|---------|--------|
| Stiff neck | TW-16; SI-3 |
| Stiff neck | CV-24; GV-16; SI-3 |
| Stiff neck | Laozhen and Ashi (tender) points, SI-3; GB-3 |
| Stiff neck | CV-24; SI-3; GV-16 |
| Stiff neck | UB--64, 37, 11, 10; GB-21; TW-16; SI-3 |
| Stiff neck with superficial syndrome | UB--65, 10 |

*Table 7-14.* POINTS: TREATING NECK AND SHOULDER PAIN

| Symptom | Points |
|---|---|
| Severe neck and shoulder pain, especially in levator scapula reference pattern | UB-62; SI-3 |
| Severe neck and shoulder pain | SI-6; UB-10 |
| Neck and shoulder pain | TW-14 |
| Neck pain that radiates into the back and shoulder | TW-10 |
| Levator scapula muscle reference pattern; neck and periscapular | SI-1 (moxa); SI-3 1/2; Double san |
| Immobile, severely painful neck | SI-1, 2, 3, 5; UB-2, 60; GB-12; H-3 |
| Pain due to supraspinous and interspinous ligaments | GV-26; SI-3 |
| Pain of lateral part of vertebra, radiating periscapularly | SI-3, 6 |
| Neck pain radiating to the upper border of scapula | TW-5; GB-39 |
| Pain and spasm of SCM muscle | LI-4; LU-7; K-6 |
| Medial pain, occipital pain, disc pain | Upright Tendons |

## Cervical: Fascia Restrictions

Fascial layers in the neck and shoulder often become restricted. Unless treated, they can remain restricted permanently. The practitioner:

1. Identifies restricted fascial areas in the patient's neck and shoulder.

2. Determines the direction of maximum fascial restriction.

3. (In the restricted direction) repeatedly threads one 1.5-inch needle subcutaneously in a fan shape.

   (For needle technique, see "Wrist and Ankle Acupuncture," chapter 5). No rotation or retention of the needle is necessary).

4. Uses massage and other manual therapies.

## Cervical: Ligamentous Insufficiency

Periosteal acupuncture can be helpful for mild instability. More significant instabilities often require prolotherapy.

Treatment for mild cervical instability always begins at the spinal segments that show motion loss. Often treatment to these segments takes the strain off of the ligaments at the hypermobile joint that is compensating for the motion loss, thereby allowing healing. If further stabilization is needed, the practitioner:

1. Identifies the affected segment

   (Because this treatment may be painful) gives the patient 200 mg. of Yanhusuoyisu Pian (tetrahydropalmini sulfate) and waits 15 minutes before beginning the treatment.[1]

2. Keeps the patient's head flexed maximally and rotated slightly.

3. Uses a lateral approach to needle the articular pillars, facets, and transverse and spinous processes.

   The practitioner pecks at the periosteum, using one needle repeatedly at all locations. (It is possible to treat both sides simultaneously by using a posterior approach. However, this tends to be more painful, and the patient's reactions can cause greater difficulty in controlling the needle and in sensing where the needle tip is located), (Figure 7-62).

4. Identifies the locations that best reproduce the target symptoms.

---

1. Currently not available in the US.

**5.** Leaves the needles in place for one hour (only if sites are close to bone, not muscular tissue).

The practitioner connects a monopolar electrical stimulator with the anode (+) locally and (-) cathode distally, and applies them throughout the hour (some patients do better with the (-) pole locally).

**6.** Tells the patient to expect healing pain for several days following treatment.

The patient must understand that this process increases local inflammation and (usually) pain, and that the inflammation is required in order to rebuild tissues.

CAUTION: For the needling to be effective, the patient must not take anti-inflammatory agents such as aspirin, ibuprofen and naproxen for several months.

Ligamentous stabilization is needed only occasionally. Usually other treatments are effective. A practitioner who is in a referral practice might encounter a disproportionate number of patients who need ligamentous stabilization.[2]

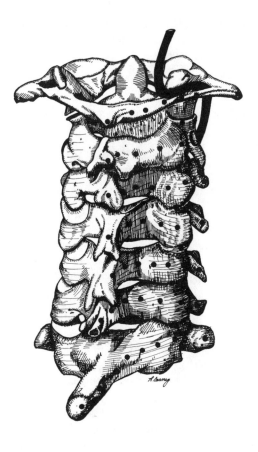

*Figure 7-62:* Important sites used in needling and prolotherapy (With permission Dorman and Ravin 1991).

### Needling for Motion Restriction

To treat motion restriction in the cervical spine, the practitioner positions the spine so it engages the restricted barrier and needles superficially over the shortened muscle that is maintaining the dysfunction. If needed the muscle belly may be needled.

During needling, the practitioner might find abnormal loci that can be responsible for maintaining the muscle tightness (joint dysfunction). These loci, which feel hard, fibrous and sensitive, might need more vigorous treatment.

**FLEXION RESTRICTION.** For flexion restriction (non-neutral dysfunctions[3]), the practitioner needles over the intrinsic (deep cervical) muscle. For example, in flexion restrictions the segment is extended, rotated and sidebent to one side, restricting flexion, rotation and sidebending to the other side (called ERS dysfunction). The practitioner:

---

2. The author has treated many patients successfully using the above method. However, a significant number of patients who are treated with periosteal acupuncture might be resistant and might still need referral to prolotherapy.

3. In the cervical spine (C2-C7) sidebending is coupled with rotation to the same side (non-neutral movement).

1. Positions the patient's neck in flexion until sensing movement of the first (upper) segment.

2. Sidebends the neck, rotates the head away from the dysfunctional side, until sensing the first barrier to motion at this level.

3. Needles over the intrinsic muscle that overlies the dysfunction.

   (If needed) needles the muscle belly.

4. (As the barrier increases) re-positions the spinal segment at the new barriers and needles again.

5. Needles any other active points.

6. Needles the appropriate channels that serve the joint.

**EXTENSION RESTRICTIONS.** For extension restriction (non-neutral dysfunctions), the practitioner needles over the ventral muscles. For example, in extension restriction the segment is flexed, rotated and sidebent to one side, restricting extension, rotation and sidebending to the other side (called FRS dysfunction). The practitioner:

1. Positions the patient neck in extension, keeping the patient's chin somewhat tucked, until the practitioner feels movement of the first segment.

2. Sidebends the neck and rotates the head to the dysfunctional side, until he senses the first barrier to motion at this level.

3. Needles superficially over the ventral muscles that overlie the dysfunction.

4. (As the barrier increases) re-positions the spine into the new barrier, and needles again.

5. Needles any other active points.

6. Needles the appropriate ventral channel that supplies the joint.

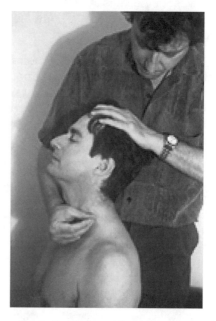

*Figure 7-63:* Needling position for treatment of extension restriction.

7. (If necessary), needles the facets and deeper tissues (Figure 7-63).

   These techniques treat mechanical dysfunctions, myofascial patterning and the channels simultaneously.

# Muscle Energy (Manipulation Without Thrust)

For treatment of joint dysfunctions in the cervical spine, muscle energy is the preferred manual therapy technique because it is effective, less traumatic to the patient, and less risky than thrust techniques. (Occasionally, however, thrust techniques succeed where muscle energy fails). Although some manual therapy techniques used in OM use contract/relax methods to achieve a therapeutic affect, specific muscle energy techniques described in this section are of western osteopathic origin.

For this type of manipulation, the practitioner positions the patient such that the restricted barrier is engaged. The joint must remain loose-packed. The patient tries to move against the practitioner's resistance while the practitioner keeps the joint fixed at the pathological barrier.

### Dysfunctions of Occipitoatloid Joint

*Restriction of Flexion at CO-C1*

For treatment of restrictions of flexion at C0-C1, the patient is supine.

The practitioner:

1. Holds the patient's head with one hand at the base of the head and the other on the chin such that he can resist flexion.

2. Translates the patient's head toward the floor, to the feather edge of the barrier.

3. Sidebends the patient's head to the feather edge of the barrier.

4. Rotates the patient's head to the opposite side, again to the feather edge of that barrier.

   The joint must remain loose-packed.

5. Asks the patient to extend his head gently, against the practitioner's resistance. (After 6 seconds) asks the patient to relax.

6. Repeats the process with the new barrier engaged.

Usually the technique is repeated 3-5 times during a session (Figure 7-64). In patients with recurrent dysfunctions the Gall Bladder, Triple Warmer or other appropriate channels are treated at the same time.

*Restriction Of Extension At CO-C1*

For restrictions of extension at C0-C1, the technique is reversed. The patient is supine. The practitioner:

1. Holds the patient's head with one hand on the chin and the other one at the base of the head.

2. Translates the patient's head toward the ceiling, to the feather edge of that barrier.

3. Slightly extends to edge of the barrier.

4. Sidebends the patient's head to the feather edge of the barrier.

5. Rotates the patient's head to the opposite side, again to the feather edge of that barrier.

6. The joint must remain loose-packed.

7. Asks the patient to extend or sidebend his head gently, against the practitioner's resistance. (After 6 seconds) asks the patient to relax.

8. Repeats the process with the new barrier engaged (Figure 7-65).

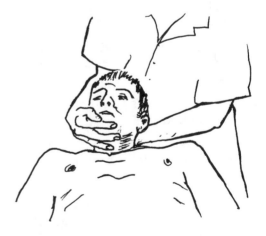

*Figure 7-64:*Muscle energy technique for flexion and right rotation restriction at CO-C1 — ES(rt) R(lt).

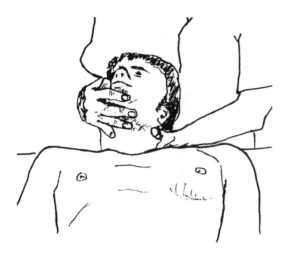

*Figure 7-65:* Muscle energy technique for extension and right rotation restriction at CO-C1 — FS(rt) R(lt).

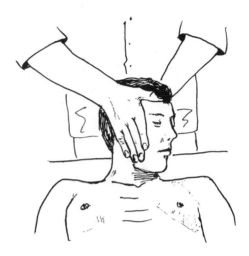

*Figure 7-66:* Muscle energy technique for rotation restriction to the left at C1-C2.

Usually the technique is repeated 3-5 times during a session. In patients with recurrent dysfunctions the Gall Bladder, Triple Warmer and other appropriate Main channels are treated at the same time.

**Dysfunctions of Atlantoaxoid Joint**

For treatment of C1-C2 dysfunctions, the patient is supine. The practitioner:

1. Holds the patient's head on both sides while keeping the patient's chin gently tucked in.

2. Flexes the patient's neck until sensing tissue tension at C2.

3. Rotates the patient's head to the feather edge of the restricted barrier.
   The joint must remain loose-packed.

4. Asks the patient to rotate the patient's head gently to the opposite side, against the practitioner's resistance.

5. (After 6 seconds) asks the patient to relax.

6. Repeats the process with the new barriers engaged.

Usually the technique is repeated 3-5 times during a session. In patients with recurrent dysfunctions the Gall Bladder, Tripple Warmer and other appropriate channels are treated at the same time (Figure 7-66).

**Typical Vertebrae**

*Extension Restrictions (FRS Dysfunction)*

For treatment of FRS Dysfunction of the typical vertebrae, the patient is supine. The practitioner:

1. Monitors the segment firmly with his fingers.

2. Extends the patient's neck while the patient's chin remains somewhat tucked, until the feather edge of movement at the segment is felt first.

3. Sidebends and rotates the patient's neck to the side of dysfunction (away from the side toward which the segment is rotated, or, toward the side that resists sidebending when the spine is in

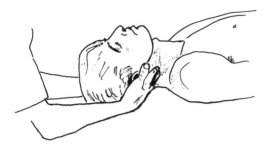

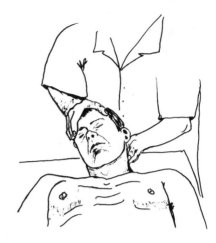

*Figure 7-67:* Muscle energy technique for extension restriction to the right — FRS (lt).

*Figure 7-68:* Muscle energy technique for flexion restriction to right — ERS (lt).

extension), until the first sign of that barrier is engaged.

The joint must remain loose-packed.

**4.** Resists the patient's attempt at sidebending.

**5.** (After 6 seconds) asks the patient to relax.

**6.** Repeats the process with the new barriers engaged.

Usually the technique is repeated 3-5 times during a session. In patients with recurrent dysfunctions the Stomach, Kidney, and other appropriate Main channels are treated at the same time (Figure 7-67).

### Flexion Restrictions (ERS Dysfunctions)

For treatment of ERS dysfunction of the typical vertebrae, the patient is supine. The practitioner:

**1.** Helps the patient keep a somewhat-tucked chin.

**2.** Flexes the spine until first sensing motion at the upper dysfunctional segment.

**3.** Sidebends the patient's neck and rotates it away from the dysfunctional side (the side to which the vertebra is rotated

when the spine is flexed, or the side to which the segment resists sidebending) until the barrier is engaged.

The joint must remain loose-packed.

**4.** Resists the patient's effort at neck sidebending.

**5.** (After 6 seconds) asks the patient to relax.

**6.** Repeats the process with the new barriers engaged.

Usually the technique is repeated 3-5 times during a session. In patients with recurrent dysfunctions the Urinary Bladder and other appropriate Main channels are treated at the same time (Figure 7-68).

# Thrust Manipulation

The dangers of thrust manipulation have been exaggerated greatly. The inherent risk of thrust manipulation and non-thrust procedures in which the head and neck are rotated, (especially if extended at the same time) must however, be kept in mind.

Weintraub and Khoury (1995), have documented by magnetic resonance angiographic analysis, and others (Ombergt, Bisschop, ter Veer and Van de Velde 1995) by other techniques, that neck and head positions of rotation and hyperextension can result in abnormalities of perfusion at the atlantoaxial and atlantooccipital junction and in the distal vertebral artery.

- Rotation slightly decreases blood flow in the ipsilateral vertebral artery, and significantly decreases blood flow in the contralateral artery.

- Sidebending slightly decreases flow in the ipsilateral artery and has no effect on blood flow in the contralateral artery.

- Pure flexion or extension do not effect blood flow at all.

  — However flexion combined with rotation significantly reduces flow bilaterally and flexion combined with sidebending and contralateral rotation slightly decreases flow in the contralateral artery, while complete cessation of flow is seen in the ipsilateral artery.

- Patients with degenerative joint disease are at increased risk.

A 1993 estimate states that one in 17,000 manipulations results in *mild* complications, most commonly a *transient* disturbance of consciousness or radicular signs (Dvorák, Baumgartner and Antinnes 1993). More serious complications have been reported. Kunnasmaa (1993) recently reviewed all European journal reports and found 139 cases of cerebrovascular accidents (CVA). Kunnasmaa reported 31 deaths and 29 severe residual neurological deficits following cervical manipulation.

Considering that at least several million manipulations are performed each year, and that so few reports of complications are published, the procedure can be regarded as safe when performed appropriately. Estimates for CVA range from one-per-million to three-per-million manipulations (Middleeditch 199; Carey 1993).

In comparison, nonsteroidal anti-inflationary (NSAIDs) medications result in 20,000 *deaths* and cost $200,000,000 for treatment of side effects in the US., alone. It is estimated that 8% of the world adult population is prescribed an NSAID for a variety of conditions (Simon 1997).

Manipulation can be performed in the pain-free direction, as determined by provocation tests. When the practitioner has mastered this technique, he uses motion restriction, rather than pain, as a guide. Slack is taken up in the spinal segments adjacent to the dysfunctional joint. Localization of movements should be painless. The thrust must be sufficient to gap and move the restricted joint in the desired direction, or to stimulate the antagonist muscle to release the joint (via reciprocal inhibition). This is achieved by a quick thrust of low amplitude (distance).

Contraindications to thrust manipulation are:

- Evidence of upper motor neuron lesion (cord signs and symptoms).

- Spinal cord compression.

- Adherent dura.

- Basilar ischemia.

- Blood clotting disorders.

- Drop attacks.

- Catalepsy.

- Infection and active inflammation, including ankylosing spodylitis.

Relative contraindications to thrust manipulation are:

- Anticoagulant therapy.

- Rheumatoid arthritis or other destructive lesions.

- Weakness and pain associated with pain on contralateral sidebending (often a sign of a tumor).

- Instability of the spine (can be caused by rheumatoid arthritis, by trauma or congenital).

- Disc protrusions and radial tears that pass from the annulus into the nucleus.

*Table 7-15.* SAMPLE CONSIDERATIONS FOR THRUST MANIPULATION

| PRESENTATION | CONSIDERATION |
|---|---|
| Articular Signs | If the patient has articular signs, limitation of movement in some directions, no clear root signs, and at least three directions of free movement, manipulation therapy can be tried |
| Acute Facet Sprain | If the patient has an acute facet sprain with hemarthrosis, thrust techniques often are painful and unhelpful |
| Nervousness or Muscle Guarding | If the patient is nervous or has severe muscle guarding, the practitioner applies acupuncture, massage and indirect techniques first |
| Root Signs | In the presence of root signs, thrust manipulation often fails—especially if a nucleus protrusion has occurred—and even might aggravate symptoms. In these cases, the practitioner applies traction first |

• Hyper-sensitivity.

Thrust manipulation should follow the findings of the examination, as described in the examples in Table 7-15 on page 375.

If dysfunction is found in one or two segments, or if multiple dysfunctions are found in different sides of the neck, they should be treated with specific techniques applied to the dysfunctional segment. If multiple segments are dysfunctional unilaterally, or if (in chronic cases) restriction due to adhesions is suspected, the practitioner can use a less specific technique such as Cyriax's or OM techniques.

Adhesions are diagnosed by assessing the end feel, which usually is abrupt and without a bony feel to it, and in which spasm is absent. For adhesions, use more strength, for multiple site dysfunctions on the same side, use less strength. If mild disc lesions are suspected, thrust manipulation should be performed only with traction. When treating the neck, start at the bottom and work up, except for extension restrictions, which should be treated from superior to inferior.

## Joint Crack

In 1995 Reggars and Pollard reported that in 50 patients, a relationship between the side of head rotation and the side of joint crack during "diversified" rotatory manipulation of the cervical spine was found. When they analyzed the "joint crack"

sound by wave analysis of digital audio tape recordings, 94% exhibited cracking on the ipsilateral side to head rotation; one subject exhibited joint cracking on the contralateral side only; and two subjects exhibited bilateral joint crack sounds. Statistically, the rate of exclusively ipsilateral joint cracking in subjects who had a history of neck trauma was significantly lower. The joint crack sound is thought to result from joint space enlargement. The fluid within the joint may transform from a liquid to a gases state (like opening a champagne bottle) resulting in the popping sound.

## Thrust Techniques

Thrust techniques can be designed by either:

• Assessing which cervical movements are painful, and then manipulating away from the pain.

• Assessing motion restrictions and correcting them (rotational and sidebending thrust).

MANIPULATING AWAY FROM THE PAIN. Both Cyriax and OM manipulation use the first technique, which is simple and easy to learn. The text describes a variation that allows for somewhat more specificity.

The advantages of this system are its simplicity and relative safety. The disadvantage is the possibility of missing a

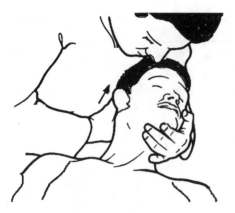

*Figure 7-69:* Thrust with traction technique for upper cervical spine

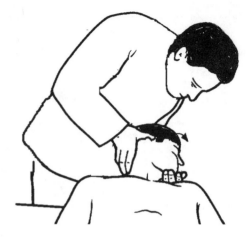

*Figure 7-70:* Rotation thrust.

hypomobile segment that requires treatment. Also, manipulation often is applied to segments that are only reactive to a hypomobile segment, and that often are hypermobile. Although techniques directed specifically to hypomobility and restricted motions are more difficult to learn, they often can be more effective and comfortable.

Each maneuver should be followed by reexamination.

### Occipitoatloid (OA) Joints

For lesions of the occipitoatloid (OA) joints, a simple traction thrust often is sufficient. The patient is supine, head at midrange. The practitioner sits at the head of the table. The practitioner:

1. Positions the patient in a way such that restricted components are engaged (if a rotation, extension or flexion component is present).

2. Pulls the patient's neck slightly, localizing other planes as needed until all of the slack is taken up.

3. Quickly pulls the patient's head toward him (during exhalation, with the patient relaxed), (Figure 7-69).

### Atlantoaxoid Joint (C1-C2)

Atlantoaxoid lesions usually are rotation restrictions. Manipulation here is by pure rotation, with the head in neutral position. The patient is supine, head resting on a small pillow. The practitioner sits at the head of the table. The practitioner:

1. Holds the patient's occiput with one hand and the patient's chin with the other.

2. Asks the patient to inhale, then to exhale.

   Performs a quick, short increase of rotation in the restricted direction or away from pain (during exhalation, with the patient relaxed), (Figure 7-70).

### Typical Cervical Spine

In lesions of C2-C6, where non-neutral mechanics occur, restrictions of movement usually are in flexion, extension, rotation and sidebending. There is little difference in manipulation treatment of restricted rotation and sidebending, except in degree. The main principle in manipulation at these levels is to first secure facet locking by sidebending and rotation to the opposite side.

ROTATIONAL THRUST AND SIDEBENDING THRUST FOR MOTION RESTRICTIONS AND PAINFUL DIRECTION. This section focuses on two basic manipulations: releasing rotation and sidebending. Lesions of the upper cervical spine generally respond better to rotational thrust; lesions of the lower cervical spine respond better to sidebending thrusts. Often traction can be added.

Before performing the rotational thrust or sidebending thrust, the practitioner identifies the painful segment by assessing segmental provocation tests and finding the planes of painful movements or identifying segmental restrictions.

ROTATIONAL THRUST. The rotational thrust is best for dysfunctions of the upper cervical spine. The patient is supine. The practitioner sits at the head of the table. The practitioner:

1. Supports the patient's head with his index finger in contact with the nonpainful side of the facet joint to be treated.

2. Lifts the patient's head slightly, until the applicable joint is engaged.

3. Lets the patient's head slide slightly down into extension.

4. Rotates the patient's head away from the painful side, until he can feel the affected joint engage (with one hand on the patient's chin and the other at the affected level).

5. Adjusts all planes of motion minimally (mostly by first using lateral translation/sidebending to the opposite direction of rotation), taking up all slack and localizing the thrust to the joint.

CAUTION: The barriers just before the area of manipulation should have a slight springiness. If the barrier is painful, or if guarding and/or radicular signs (arm or scapular pain, pins and needles) are present, the practitioner should try to re-localize the maneuver. If signs continue to be present after re-localizing, the practitioner should stop the maneuver.

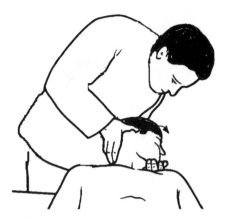

*Figure 7-71:* Rotation thrust.

6. Makes a short, quick rotation of the patient's head, (to perform the correction) using the hand that is holding the chin and assisted by the index finger at the dysfunctional level.

The practitioner also can use the index finger, with a rotary, pushing maneuver over the articular pillars (Figure 7-71).

The same procedure can be performed to correct motion restrictions. The practitioner engages the restricted barriers in a similar manner, except that sidebending and rotation is to the same side (e.g., with ERS (right) the neck is flexed, left sidebent and left rotated).

SIDEBENDING THRUST. The sidebending thrust technique works best for dysfunctions of the middle to lower cervical segments. The patient is supine. The practitioner sits at the head of the table. The practitioner:

1. Supports the patient's head with one hand.

2. Places his other hand and index finger at the apex of the patient's articular pillar, opposite painful side.

3. Lifts the patient's head slightly.

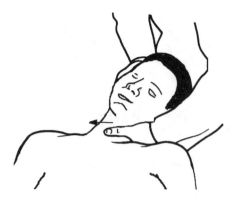

*Figure 7-72:* Side thrust — mid cervical spine.

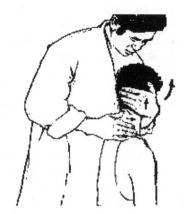

*Figure 7-73:* OM Tui-Na manipulation under traction. Note both short and long levers are used.

**4.** Sidebends the patient's neck over the fulcrum provided by the index finger, away from the painful side.

**5.** Rotates the patient's head toward the painful side, until movement of the dysfunctional segment is first sensed.

**6.** Localizes the motions carefully in order to achieve maximum comfort for the patient.

**7.** (To perform the correction) gives a quick and short thrust of the fulcrum hand toward the eye of the painful side.

This maneuver also can be performed with the addition of slight traction (Figure 7-72).

**EXTENSION RESTRICTION OR FRS DYSFUNCTION.** The sidebending thrust can be used to correct facet loss of extension (FRS dysfunction). Since extension restriction might be due to inability of the facet to close, the practitioner:

**1.** Places his fulcrum hand just above the dysfunctional segment.

**2.** Directs the thrust downward toward T1, with the neck in extension.

(e.g., for FRS (left), the neck is extended, right sidebent and slightly rotated left).

In the lower cervical and upper thoracic spine, extension, sidebending and rotation to the opposite side are necessary to localize the manipulation and protect the neck.

*Manipulation With Traction*

Intervertebral disc lesions respond best to manipulations under traction, a method also used widely in Chinese medicine (Figure 7-73). In some studies, traction has been shown to increase vertebral artery occlusions. In other studies it did not (Tatlow, Brown and Issingtone 1963; Thiel, Wallace, Donat and Yong-Hing). Cyriax, who reported no serious complications associated with his manipulation traction techniques, describes a series of maneuvers that the practitioner performs sequentially, reassessing between each maneuver. These techniques include the straight pull, rotation with traction, side flexion during traction, and anteroposteroir glid. One other technique is lateral gliding which is done without traction.

**THE STRAIGHT PULL.** According to Cyriax, the straight pull (which is both therapeutic and diagnostic) should be the first maneuver performed on every patient. For this

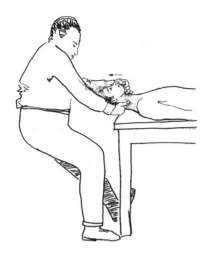

*Figure 7-74:*The straight pull.

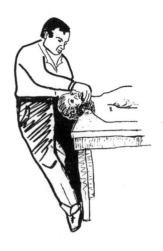

*Figure 7-75:*Rotation with traction technique.

technique, the patient is supine and his shoulder is level with the end of the table. The practitioner is at the head of the table. An assistant or a strap holds the patient in place during the traction maneuver. The practitioner:

1. Places the patient's head in neutral position (midline without flexion, extension or rotation).

2. Holds the patient's occiput with one hand and places his other hand under the patient's chin.

3. Applies a straight pull for 2-3 seconds.

The first pull is mild, followed by pulls of increasing strength, until the joint play is restored (Figure 7-74).

**ROTATION WITH TRACTION.** This technique, which is needed only rarely, is useful for treating patients for whom other techniques have failed. It may work by rupturing adhesions or freeing trapped tissues. The patient is supine; his shoulder is level with the end of the table. The practitioner is at the head of the table. An assistant or a strap holds the patient in place during the traction maneuver. The practitioner:

1. Leans backward, pulling until his own arms are extended, and holds for two seconds.

2. Rotates the patient's head away from the painful side (maintaining traction).

3. Releases traction while maintaining extension (when tissue resistance is first felt).

4. Repeats step three until all slack is taken up at the joint.

5. Delivers a quick, short, rotation thrust with the hand that is holding the patient's jaw (if the end feel is not hard) (Figure 7-75).

**SIDE FLEXION DURING TRACTION.** This technique is needed only on rare occasions, when side flexion is still painful after other techniques have failed. The patient is supine. An assistant is positioned such that he can prevent the patient from slipping sideways and from sliding up the table. The practitioner:

1. Braces one of his legs against the side of the table on which sidebending is required.

2. Positions his other leg in front of the braced leg.

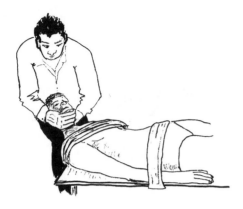

*Figure 7-76:*Sideflexion with traction technique.

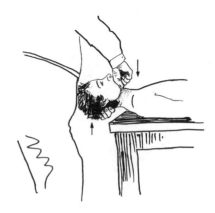

*Figure 7-77:*Anteroposterior glide with traction.

**3.** Leans back to apply traction, and swings his own front leg backward, pulling the patient's neck into side flexion (keeping his own arms partly flexed).

**4.** Makes a quick thrust by drawing his own elbows together, toward his body (When all slack is taken up), (Figure 7-76).

**ANTEROPOSTERIOR GLIDE WITH TRACTION.** This technique is indicated when the range of extension has not improved with rotation and/or lateral flexion techniques. The patient lies supine with his head over the edge of the table. An assistant holds the feet or the patient is strapped down to the table. The practitioner:

**1.** Stands at the back of the patient's head.

**2.** Supports the patient's head under the occiput with one hand, and the other hand is put at the patient's chin.

**3.** Places his feet against the legs of the table and leans backward.

**4.** (After having taken up the slack) glides the head anteriorly and posteriorly as far as it would go.

**5.** A sudden thrust is then added (Figure 7-77).

**LATERAL GLIDE.** This technique is useful to get rid of post-manipulative soreness. It is useful also when soreness or pain shifts to the other side as a result of treatment. The patient lies supine with head over the edge of the table. An assistant holds the feet or the patient is strapped down to the table. The practitioner:

**1.** Stands at the patient's head with his feet apart.

**2.** Supports the patient's head on both sides of his head.

**3.** Moves his weight over to one leg and then to the other, therefore moving the patient's head from side to side (no sidebending of the neck should occur), (Figure 7-78).

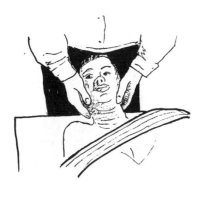
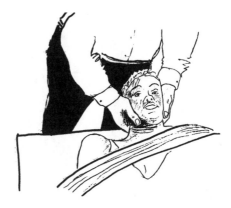

*Figure 7-78:*Lateral glide technique.

# Post Isometric Muscle Relaxation (Muscle Energy)

Post-isometric muscle relaxation (PIR) techniques are very useful for treatment of shortened muscles. They can be used to treat muscle tension and post-treatment stiffness. In general, the practitioner:

1. Positions the muscle at its first comfortable stretch barrier, and then releases it slightly.

2. Asks the patient to push against the practitioner's resistance. The practitioner does not allow any motion to occur.

3. Holds the position for 5 seconds before releasing.

4. Stretches the muscle to its new barrier, and then releases the muscle slightly.

5. Repeats steps 2 and 3 three-to-four times, until the muscle is lengthened sufficiently.

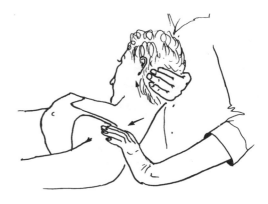

*Figure 7-79:* Levator scapulae PIR.

Postural muscles that often become shortened and require treatment are the levator scapulae, trapezius, scalenes, multifidi, rotatores and the sternocleidomastoid (Figure 7-79 through Figure 7-83).

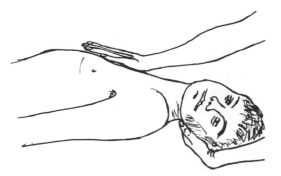

*Figure 7-81:*Sternocleidomastoid PIR (against gravity).

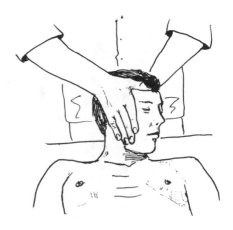

*Figure 7-82:*Mulitidi and rotatores PIR (left).

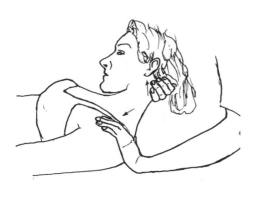

*Figure 7-80:*Upper trapezius PIR.

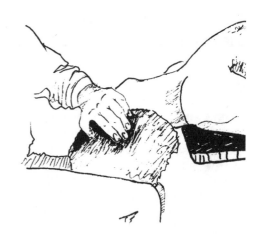

*Figure 7-83:*Scalene PIR.

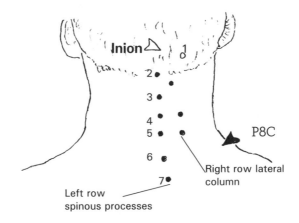

*Figure 7-84:*Posterior cervical Jones points (After Jones, Kusunosa and Goering 1995).

# Countertension-positional Release

Countertension-positional release is an effective technique for treatment of facilitated muscles. It is particularly helpful during the acute stages when the patient may be guarding his neck. This section presents examples for muscles that frequently are involved in cervical injuries.

With vertebral dysfunctions, tenderness at the "Jones Points", which are labeled by vertebra and as anterior (A) or posterior (P), develops often. These points then define the treatment position. Countertension-positional release can be used also for any shorted muscle (without having a tender Jones point), as well.

## Posterior Cervical Vertebrae Dysfunctions

Posterior cervical dysfunctions are named, in the countertension-positional release system, in patients who may find forward bending painful and in whom an extremely tender point is present on the dorsal aspect of the neck (Figure 7-84).

**POINT P1C** is found in two locations:

- P1C (inion) point, located on the medial side of the posterocervical muscle mass, where it is attached to the occiput about 3 cm below the posterior occipital ridge.

- P1C-1, on the occiput, lateral to the main posterocervical muscle mass, about 3.5 cm from midline between the muscle mass and the mastoid.

**FIRST CERVICAL VERTEBRA (STRAINED RECTUS CAPITIS MAJOR, MINOR MUSCLE, AND RECTUS CAPITIS POSTERIOR MINOR).** This treatment works for both Point P1C and Point P1C (inion), rectus capitis major and minor muscle strains, and rectus capitis posterior minor. The patient is supine. The practitioner is at the head of the table and:

1. Holds the patient's head by putting one hand on the occiput and the other hand on the forehead.

2. Pulls the patient's occiput up and pushes the forehead down, flexing the head markedly while keeping the chin tucked.

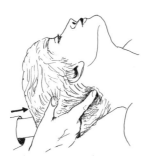

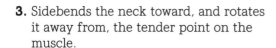

*Figure 7-85:* Counter tension technique for posterior C1.

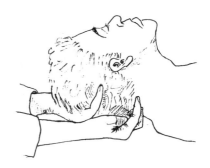

*Figure 7-86:* Countertension technique for posterior C2.

**3.** Sidebends the neck toward, and rotates it away from, the tender point on the muscle.

**4.** Fine tunes these movements until the point is no longer tender.

**5.** Holds this position for 90 seconds.

**6.** Slowly returns the patient's neck to neutral position (Figure 7-85).

**SECOND CERVICAL VERTEBRA (STRAINED OBLIQUUS CAPITIS SUPERIOR).** The obliquus capitis superior Point (P2C) is tender in dysfunction of the second cervical vertebra. P2C is found in two locations:

• On the lateral side of the muscle mass just below the occiput, and 1.5cm from the midline.

• On the upper surface of the spinous process of the second vertebra.

For treatment, the patient is supine. The practitioner is at the head of the table. The practitioner:

**1.** Holds the patient's head, placing one hand on the occiput, the other hand either on top of the head or on one (either) side.

**2.** Flexes the lower cervical spine by lifting his hand under the occiput and pressing on top of the head. This extends the upper cervical spine and shortens the muscle.

**3.** Adds slight sidebending and rotation away from the tender point.

**4.** Fine tunes these positions until the point is no longer tender.

**5.** Holds this position for 90 seconds.

**6.** Slowly returns the neck to neutral position (Figure 7-86).

**THIRD CERVICAL VERTEBRA (STRAINED ROTATORS, MULTIFIDUS, INTERSPINALIS).** Points for the rotator, multifidus and interspinalis muscles, which lie on the inferior surface of the spinous processes of C2-C7, reflect dysfunction of the vertebrae below. Point P3C is located at the inferior surface of the spinous process of the second vertebra. For treatment, the patient is supine. The practitioner stands at the head of the table. The practitioner:

**1.** Holds the patient's head with one hand on top and the other on the side of the tender point.

**2.** Sidebends the patient's head, and rotates it away from the tender point.

**3.** Extends the neck to approximately $45^0$.

**4.** Applies pressure to the top of the head caudally.

**5.** Fine tunes the position until the tender point is relieved.

**6.** Holds the position for 90 seconds.

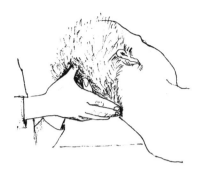

*Figure 7-87:* Countertension technique for posterior C3.

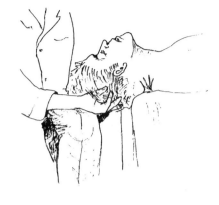

*Figure 7-88:* Countertension technique for posterior C4.

**7.** Slowly returns the patient's head to neutral position (Figure 7-87).

**FOURTH CERVICAL VERTEBRA.** Point P4C is located on the spinous process of the third vertebra. For treatment, the patient is supine. The practitioner stands at the head of the table. The practitioner:

**1.** Holds the patient's head and monitors a tender point laterally to the P4C point on the muscle mass.

**2.** Rotates the patient's neck and sidebends it away from (but sometimes toward) the tender point, while adding extension and slight compression force on the occiput.

**3.** Fine tunes these positions until the tenderness is reduced.

**4.** Holds the position for 90 seconds.

**5.** Slowly returns the patient's neck to neutral position (Figure 7-88).

**REMAINING CERVICAL/UPPER THORACIC VERTEBRAE.** The rest of the lower cervical and upper thoracic vertebrae are treated in the same manner. The lower the dysfunction is in the cervical spine, the more extension the practitioner must introduce. No compression force is needed for dysfunctions of the lower vertebrae (Figure 7-89).

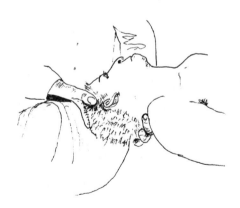

*Figure 7-89:* Countertension technique for posterior lower cervicals.

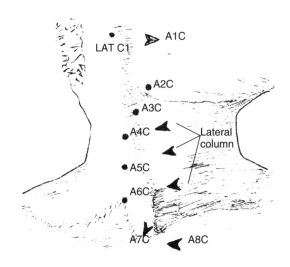

*Figure 7-90:*   Anterior cervical Jones points (After Jones, Kusunosa and Goering 1995).

### *Dysfunctions: Anterior Cervical Vertebrae*

Anterior cervical dysfunctions are found in patients for whom backward bending may be painful and for whom an extremely tender point is present on the ventral aspect of the neck. Counterten-sion-positioning can be used to treat these dysfunctions (Figure 7-90).

**A1C (FIRST) CERVICAL DYSFUNCTION (STRAINED ANTERIOR RECTUS CAPITIS, AND DIGASTRIC STRAINS).** The first cervical joint (A1C) is located at the posterior surface of the ascending ramus of the mandible, approximately 1 cm superior to the man-dibular angle just under the ear. Another point for the first cervical joint (A1C rare), is found on the inner table of the mandible 2 cm anterior to the angle of the mandible.

- A1C is tender with strained anterior rec-tus capitis.

- A1C (rare) is tender with digastric strains.

For treatment, the patient is supine. The practitioner is at the head of the table. The practitioner:

1. Supports the patient's occiput with one hand, and rotates the patient's head markedly, away from the tender point.

2. Places the fingers of his other hand on the patient's occiput and on the tender point.

3. Adds slight neck flexion, extension, or sidebending away from the tender point until tenderness is reduced.

4. Holds this position for 90 seconds.

5. Slowly returns the patient's head to neutral position (Figure 7-91).

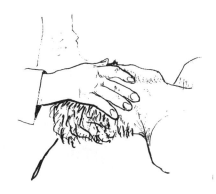

*Figure 7-91:* Countertension technique for anterior C1.

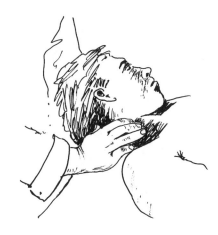

*Figure 7-92:* Countertension technique for anterior C2.

**THIRD CERVICAL TROUGH SIXTH (A2C-A6C) DYSFUNCTIONS (LONGUS COLLI STRAIN, SCALENUS ANTERIOR AND LONGUS).** With minor variations, this treatment can be used for dysfunctions of the third cervical A1C and longus colli strain.

Jones points (A3C-A5C) are tender with Anterior Fourth-Through-Sixth Cervical Vertebrae dysfunction and scalenus anterior and longus colli strains. Jones Points A3C-A6C are located at the tips of the transverse processes of the affected joint.

For treatment, the patient is supine. The practitioner is at the head of the table. The practitioner:

1. Holds the patient's head, with one hand on the occiput and the other hand monitors the tender points.

2. Flexes the patient's neck markedly and sidebends it slightly toward the tender point.

3. Rotates the patient's neck to the other side.

4. Holds for 90 seconds.

5. Returns the patient's head to neutral position (Figure 7-92).

**A7C DYSFUNCTION OF THE SEVENTH CERVICAL JOINT (STRAIN OF SCM ATTACHMENT).** Point A7C is located at the posterior superior surface of the clavicle, 3 cm lateral to the medial end. The patient is supine. The practitioner is at the head of the table. The practitioner:

1. Finds A7C by pushing inferiorly on the superior edge of the clavicle.

2. Holds the back of the patient's neck (not the head) with one hand, and monitors the tender point with the other hand.

3. Flexes the lower neck markedly.

4. Rotates the lower neck slightly, away from the tender point.

5. Sidebends the lower neck markedly, toward the tender point.

6. Fine tunes the movements until the tenderness is reduced markedly.

7. Holds this position for 90 seconds.

8. (Slowly) Returns the patient's neck to neutral position (Figure 7-93).

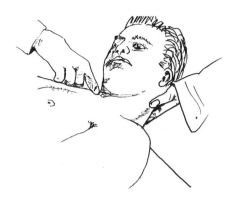

*Figure 7-93:* Countertension technique for C7.

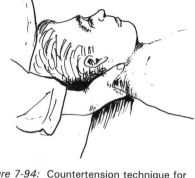

*Figure 7-94:* Countertension technique for lateral C1.

**A8C DYSFUNCTION OF EIGHTH CERVICAL JOINT (STRAINED STERNOHYOID OR OMOHYOID).** The A8C Point is located at the medial end of the clavicle. Tenderness at this point is uncommon and is treated like A2C-A6C.

**LATERAL FIRST CERVICAL JOINT DYSFUNCTION.** This technique is for treating lateral first cervical (rectus capitis lateralis) joint dysfunction in which the transverse process of the first cervical vertebra is approximated to the mastoid process on the involved side. Tenderness might be found when palpating the position of the TrPs of the first cervical vertebra in either side, by pinching the tips of the mastoid processes between index fingers and the thumbs of both hands and permitting the fingertips to move down and more deeply medial, to feel the TrPs of the vertebra just below. The patient is supine. The practitioner:

1. Holds the base of the patient's head on both sides.

2. Sidebends the patient's neck toward the dysfunctional side.

3. Supports the patient's head by leaning it on his head.

4. Monitors until tenderness is reduced markedly or the position of the TrPs is restored (Figure 7-94).

**ANTERIOR LATERAL COLUMNS.** These points are found in the throat area on the anterior surface of the lateral columns. The patient is supine. The practitioner is at the head of the table. The practitioner:

1. Flexes the neck markedly.

2. Rotates the head away from the tender point.

3. Sidebends the neck slightly toward the tender point.

4. Holds for this position for a short time.

5. (Slowly) Returns the patient's neck to neutral position (Figure 7-95).

**WARNING:** Prolonged pressure over the internal carotid artery and its plexuses of nerves (from the above position) can cause a loss of consciousness.

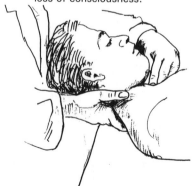

*Figure 7-95:* Countertension technique for anterior lateral columns.

# Chapter 8: *The Thorax*

Diagnosis of pain in the thoracic areas is complicated by referred pain from chest and abdominal organs and from numerous structures that make up the rib cage.

## Anatomy

The thoracic spine comprises one of the primary curves of the spine and exhibits a mild kyphosis (posterior convexity). The thoracic spine consists of twelve heart-shaped vertebrae that have vertically oriented facets, with a 60° inclination around the horizontal axis, and a 20° inclination around the vertical axis (White and Panjabi, 1978).

The remainder of the boney thorax consists of 24 ribs, costocartilages and the sternum. A thoracic vertebra has ten separate articulations, any one of which can become dysfunctional (Figure 8-1).

LIGAMENTS. Stability in the thoracic spine is maintained by the costovertebral, costotransverse and sternal articulations. The costovertebral and transverse articulations are stabilized by the strong ligamentum capitus costae radiatum, costotransverse ligament, and ligament of the tuberculi costae (Figure 8-1).

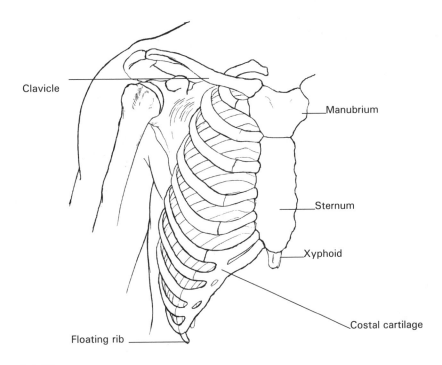

Clavicle

Manubrium

Sternum

Xyphoid

Costal cartilage

Floating rib

*Figure 8-1:* Rib cage.

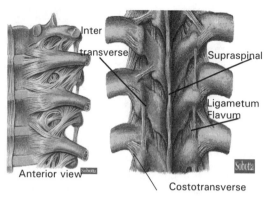

*Figure 8-1:* Ligaments

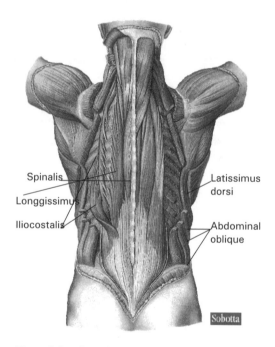

*Figure 8-2:* Superficial and Intermediate Muscles.

**THORACIC SPINAL CORD.** The thoracic spinal cord supplies sympathetic innervation to the arms and to 50% of the legs, and the heart, lung, mucous membranes of the head and neck, GI tract, kidneys, adrenals and gonads.

Table 8-1 on page 391 summarizes mus-

cles of the thoracic spine (Figure 8-2).

# Imaging

The upper thoracic vertebra are difficult to visualize on routine imaging of the thoracic spine. The lower eight vertebra are some what easier to identify on plain films and their size and shape can easily be evaluated. In the lower thoracic spine the disc space heights are consistent with little variation between the highest most visualized and those near the lumbar spine. The disc space height of the lower thoracic discs can be evaluated on both the anterior-posterior and the lateral films. The vertebral bodies in the thoracic spine also are most square radiographically with some slight trapezoidal shape to the middle vertebral (T3-6) that creates the kyphosis of the spine in this region. The shapes of the discs and the vertebral bodies are nicely seen on CT's and MRI's of these parts.

## Imaging Considerations

Although thoracic herniated discs are very rare they do occur, but at most they represent no more than 2% of all discs (Vallo 1982; Ombregt et al. *ibid*). They occasionally create some plain film findings such as disc space narrowing and a calcified disc, but these findings are notoriously unreliable and if these diagnoses are likely then an MRI or CT should be used liberally to aid in the diagnosis of these problems.

In general, with plain films the radiologist notes:

**1.** Any wedging of the vertebrae.

**2.** Do the disc spaces appear normal.

**3.** Is there any Schmorl's nodes.[1]

1. Herniation of the intervertebral disc into the vertebral body.

*Table 8-1.* **MUSCLES OF THE THORACIC SPINE**

| FUNCTION | MUSCLES |
|---|---|
| Flexion | Rectus abdominus, external and internal abdominal obliques (bilateral contraction) |
| Extension | Spinalis thoracis, iliocostalis thoracis (bilateral), semispinalis thoracis (bilateral), longissimus thoracis (bilateral), multifidus (bilateral), rotators (bilateral) and interspinales |
| Rotation and Sidebending | Iliocostalis (to same side), longissimus thorcsis (to same side), internal abdominal oblique (to same side), semispinalis thoracis (to opposite side), multifidus (to opposite side), rotators (to opposite side), external abdominal obliques (to opposite side) and transverses abdominus (to opposite side) |

**4.** Is the ring epiphysis, if present, normal.

**5.** Is there a "bamboo" spine, indicative of ankylosing spondylitis.

**6.** Is there any scoliosis or excessive kyphosis.

**7.** Any malposition of trachea, lung or heart.

**8.** Normal symmetry of the ribs.

**9.** Any osteophytes or bony cysts.

**10.** Facet arthropathy or other degenerative disease.

## OM Disorders

Disorders affecting the thoracic areas are often associated with Liver and Gall Bladder dysfunctions, which may arise due to depression and emotional stresses.

External, Independent or Miscellaneous factors are often related to symptoms of the upper back. Excessive Dampness can transform to Phlegm and obstruct the free flow of Qi and Blood. Over indulgence in greasy and spicy foods leads to accumulation of Heat in the Stomach channel and Collaterals which further obstructs the Qi and Blood. Chest pain can develop resulting in cardiovascular symptoms. Sprains and traumas are a common cause of symptoms, as well.

## Biomedical Disorders

Many conditions that affect the cervical spine also affect the thoracic spine. Symptoms felt in the thoracic area can arise from a wide variety of sources, including:

- Metabolic.
- Visceral.
- Infectious.
- Cancerous.
- Musculoskeletal from, spine, ribs, costal articulations, ligaments and myofascial sources.

When the source of symptoms is musculoskeletal, movement of the affected structure elicits pain. This however, is true also for many visceral disorders. When a deep breath or a cough, produces pain, a non-musculoskeletal source must be considered. Chest pain also is due to joint dysfunctions, but also can be visceral in origin.

### Non-Musculoskeletal Disorders

Non-musculoskeletal origins must be kept in mind as these are frequently encountered in this area. The quality of pain is of little help as pain from visceral and musculoskeletal origin is the same. Pain arising from visceral origin often leads to pain that is affected by posture, breathing and other physical activity. Consequently, a careful history and physical should always be done (Ombregt, Bisschop, ter Veer and Van de Velde 1995).

*Ankylosing Spondylitis*

Ankylosing spondylitis is an inflammatory condition that produces pain that comes and goes for years, unrelated to activity. Pain often is worst in the morning.

*Nerves*

Herpes zoster, a common cause of thoracic pain, can be felt before the vesicles appear, usually three to four days, but infrequently up to 2 weeks prior to the vesicular phase. Occasionally, especially in patients with history of herpes, the vesicles never show up. Post-herpetic neuralgia can continue for a long time after the vesicles have healed.

    *Neuritis* of the long thoracic, supraspacular or spinal accessory nerves results in constant pain on the affected side, usually lasting about three weeks.

    *Neuromas* may initially be symptomatic only at the posterior thorax. Later, if confined to one side of the spine, neuromas can painfully limit sidebending away from the painful side. A spreading patch of skin numbness may forewarn the development of a neuroma (Cyriax *ibid*).

*Heart & Vascular Disorders*

Conditions such as myocardial infarction, insufficiency, endocarditis and pericarditis may refer pain to the thorax. The myocardium is developed from the first, second, and third thoracic embryonic segments. Heart pain can be felt in these dermatomes. Pain may spread from the thorax to the neck, jaw and upper limbs, most often to the left arm (20 times more common than right). Retrosternal, parasternal, and epigastric pains are common. Pain may be confined to any of the above areas alone, as well.

    Vascular conditions such as aneurysm (local abnormal dilatation of blood vessel), pulmonary embolism (a mass of undissolved matter in the blood), and venous thrombosis (blood clot occlusion), also can refer pain to the thorax. Hematoma due to intra-aortic injection can elicit left-sided lower thoracic pain (Ombregt, Bisschop, ter Veer and Van de Velde 1995).

*Neoplastic Disorders*

Primary neoplasms in thoracic spine are rare. Metastases does occur however (often in the ribs) from lung, breast, prostate, kidney and thyroid cancers. Horner's syndrome may be seen (Ombregt, Bisschop, ter Veer and Van de Velde 1995).

*Pulmonary Disorders*

Pneumothorax, pneumonia/pleurisy, infarction and prolonged coughing all can result in pain at the thoracic areas.

*Esophageal Disorders*

Esophageal spasm, reflux/esophagitis and rupture can result in thoracic pain.

*Abdominal Disorders*

Disorders of the gall bladder, liver, bile ducts, diaphragm, kidney, ureters, pancreas, stomach, duodenum, and ectopic pregnancy should be considered.

    Many conditions that affect the cervical spine also affect the thoracic spine. The reader is referred to that section in the text.

## Musculoskeletal Disorders

The most common cause of musculoskeletal pain in the thoracic area is a lesion in the lower cervical or thoracic joints and ligaments. Because there is considerable dermatomal overlap within an individual, and variation between people, pain patterns serve only to guide the practitioner to the sources of pain (Cyriax *ibid*).

## Pain of Cervical Origin

Disc lesions at the third and fourth cervical roots radiate to the base of the neck and upper thoracic areas. From the fifth and sixth roots pain radiates to the interscapular areas. The seventh root refers pain to the midthoracic area, often most intensely to the lower angle of the scapula. Cervical sclerotomes and myotomes also refer to the upper thorax. The lower cervical joints, C4-C7, refer pain to the upper thoracic areas, often around the scapulae (Cyriax *ibid*).

## Pain From Thoracic Structures

Thoracic joints are a common cause of pain. Internal derangement gives rise to pain felt in the center of the spine, or to one side of the posterior thorax. The upper thoracic, T1-T4 levels, are the stiffest part of the spine, and pain due to these levels usually is felt locally. Lesions in the midthoracic (T5-T7) facet joints, are commonly felt in the center of the spine, or in one side of the posterior thorax. T8-T10 refer pain commonly to the sides and anteriorly. Rib articular problems also are common at these levels. Lesions in the lower thoracic spine (T11-L1), result in pain referral to the lumbar, iliac crest areas, and occasionally to the testes (Cyriax *ibid*).

## T4 Syndrome

McGuckin (1986) has described the T4 syndrome, which is characterized by tenderness and stiffness at T3-T5, and by vague, nonsegmental pain and paresthesia in the hands, arms and posterior neck, and vague head pains.

## Disc Lesions

Disc lesions are more common in the lower thoracic spine, starting at T9, and are most common at T11-12. In primary posterolateral disc herniations, pain is felt unilaterally and anteriorly. Occasionally, a thoracic disc initiates sternal pain which may be confused with heart disease. With first and second thoracic disc lesions (rare), the ache is felt at the lower scapular areas, radiating to the ulnar side of the palm or to inner arm (Cyriax *ibid*).

## Myofascial Disorders

Sprains of the *latissimus dorsi* and *pectoralis major* can refer pain diffusely (not well localized) to the thorax, shoulder, arm and elbow. The latissimus dorsi can also refer pain to the lower back. The *intercostal muscles* (Cyriax *ibid*) can get slightly torn when a rib breaks. Pain is well-localized at the site of the lesion. The muscles often are sprained from injuries, including whiplash injury. Other communally affected muscles are the *serratus anterior*, *serratus posterior inferior*, *iliocostalis*, *multifidus* and *rhomboids* (Travell *ibid*).

## Ligaments

The characteristics of ligamentous pain in the thoracic regions are the same as in other spinal areas. The most common symptoms are pain and low tolerance to sitting and physical work, with posain and nulliness.

## Bone Fractures

According to Cyriax, a wedge fracture usually gives symptoms for no more than three months. Often for the first week there is girdle pain. Commonly ligamentous pain supervenes and may last indefinitely (Cyriax *ibid*).

## Vertebral Dysfunctions.

Vertebral dysfunctions in the thoracic spine are of the neutral and non-neutral variety. Flexion restrictions (ERS) and extension restrictions (FRS) can be seen. Findings are similar to those of the lumbar spine (see chapter 9), except that here the ribs may be affected, as well.

## Ribs

The ribs, costovertebral and costosternal joints are common areas of dysfunction, pathology and pain. Fractures are common, resulting in local pain lasting up to 6 weeks. "Spontaneous" rib fractures have been reported (Fam et al 1983) and may be due to severe coughing, RA, osteoporosis and cancers. Pain from the costovertebral joints usually is felt locally, about 3-4 cm from midline.

Dysfunction of the costovertebral joints can refer pain posteriorly to the chest wall, or anteriorly to the chest— often mimicking visceral pain, which must be ruled out. If the joint is responsible, pain usually is provoked by deep breathing and pressure on the affected rib.

COSTOCHONDRITIS. *Costochondritis*, a common cause of pain, usually is felt locally but can radiate widely along with local tenderness. The tenderness tends to involve multiple sites. The 2nd to 5th cartilages are affected most frequently (Calabro et al. 1880). Structural rib dysfunction often is the cause of costochondritis (Greenman *ibid*). Treatment directed at the rib joints results often in immediate improvement. Dysfunctions of the upper three ribs are a frequent cause of rib pain. The strong ligaments at these sites can become strained.

STRUCTURAL RIB DYSFUNCTIONS. Structural rib dysfunctions may be divided into anterior, posterior or superior subluxations. Ribs may develop torsion and compression syndromes, as well (Greenman *ibid*). Rib subluxations have been reported with chest pain syndromes (Heinz and Zavala 1977).

The "slipped rib syndrome" is thought to be traumatic in nature, often involving the lower (non-true) ribs, as these are structurally the weakest areas of the chest. Pain from subluxed ribs commonly affect the abdominal areas (upper quadrant or epigastric), and may be confused with pain of abdominal origin—the patient may react to the pain with vomiting and nausea. Pain may be also felt below the lower margins of the ribs and back. The mobility of the anterior costal cartilage increases (Bonica 1990).

To assess for rib subluxations the posterior and anterior rib angles are checked. Normally these should be smooth. With a rib subluxation both the anterior and posterior rib angles are found either too posterior or anterior. If one rib is found to be anterior and the other posterior a "compression syndrome" is suspected. Rib torsions usually are secondary to vertebral dysfunctions (Greenman *ibid*).

# Treatment

Treatments of disorders affecting the thoracic areas depend on the diagnosis and follow the general rules. Needling thoracic spine structures is commonly needed to prevent relapses of mechanical dysfunctions, replace overactive nociceptors with fibrous tissue, and reset muscle and fascia length and tone. In chronic patients, in whom relapses are frequent, joint stabilization may be needed. Periosteal acupuncture or prolotherapy often are necessary.

### Superficial Fascia: Needling

After identifying fascial restrictions by assessing tissue drag and skin movement over the thoracic areas, the patient is placed such that the affected tissues are maximally stretched. The practitioner then inserts a 1-1/2 inch needle subcutaneously (see hand and wrist acupuncture for detail), directing the needle toward the restricted direction.

*Muscle Shortening & Hyperactivity*

After locating all shortened, or electrically and mechanically (tender) hyperactive muscles, the affected muscles are treated with needling. If the patient is extremely sensitive, insert the needle gently without needle rotation. When a needling sensation is obtained (referred sensation, ache, twitch), the needle is withdrawn. Then all the muscle attachments are treated by periosteal acupuncture.

*Instability*

As this procedure may be painful, a pre medication with 200mg of Yanhusuoyisu Pian (tetrahydropalmini sulfate),[2] may be useful. With the patient supine, or in the lateral recumbent position, and spine flexed (to open the facets), one needles all ligamentous periosteal junctions, including the interspinal, flava (between vertebral arches), and intertransverse ligaments. First the practitioner identifies the edge of the vertebral bodies and leaves a needle there as a marker. The same is done at one of the transverse processes, and at several rib angles. These needles are used as guides for needle depths, and then all of the above structures are treated. The needle is pointed inferiorly to minimize the danger of penetrating the cord. Only one side is needled at a time, in case an accidental pneumothorax occurs (punctured lung, air in the pleural cavity), so that the patient still has one fully-functional side. The needle should penetrate the facets. When correctly needling a facet joint the needle-feel is as though a tough capsule is being penetrated, first, and then the needle loses resistance as the joint is penetrated. When the needle is directed superiorly and laterally, great care must be used as it may bend and take its own course and penetrate the cord. The patient should understand that aggravation and healing pain can be expected after the treatment.

---

2. Currently not available in US.

## Acupuncture

Many of the points used for the cervical spine can be used to treat the thoracic spine (especially upper). Needling local Ashi (tender) points, moxa, compresses, cupping, scraping and electrical stimulation often are used, as well. The Liver, Gall Bladder, Pericardium and Yin Linking (Wei) channels are especially important. Table 8-2 on page 396 summarizes important points and point combinations for treatment of the thoracic areas.

## Herbal Therapy

As disorders of the thoracic area often are associated with the Liver and Gall Bladder channels, the herb Radix Bupleurum (Chai Hu) is added to the formulas, as a messenger herb to bring the formula to the mid-back and costal regions. A guiding formula for midthoracic, chest, and rib pain from myofascial and mechanical sources is:

Radix Bupleurum (Chai Hu)

Cyprus (Xiang Fu)

Rhizoma Ligusticum (Chuan Xiong)

Radix Peony Alba (Bai Shao)

Radix Angelica Chinensis (Dang Gui)

Semen Persica (Tao Ren)

Pericarpium Citri Reticulatae (Chen Pi)

Herba Leonurus (Yi Mu Cao)

Fructus Aurantii (Zhi Qiao)

Radix Curcumae (Yu Jin)

Radix Corydalis (Yan Hu Suo)

Semen Citri Reticulatae (Ju He)

Radix Puerarae (Ge Gen)

Fructus Meliae Toosendan (Chuan Lian Zi)

Herba Taraxaci Mongolici Cum Radice (Pu Gong Ying)

Semen Coicis (Yi Yi Ren)

Radix Glycyrrhizae (Gan Cao)

*Table 8-2.* IMPORTANT POINTS AND POINT COMBINATIONS FOR THE THORACIC AREAS

| POINTS | USES |
|---|---|
| SI-11and SI-6 | Pain and weakness in the arm and shoulder regions<br>Pain in the chest and lateral costal regions<br>Pain and or neuralgia and numbness in the scapular and the posteromedial aspect (SI channel) of the arm and elbow<br>Levator scapula, infraspinatus, supraspinatus and upper posterior trapezius lesions |
| LI-15 | Upper back and shoulder pain especially due to muscle channel dysfunctions<br>Spasm of the upper anterior trapezius, scalenus anterior, and the deltoid muscles |
| St-44 | Anterior chest pain<br>Rib dysfunctions |
| P-6 | Anterior chest and rib pain and dysfunctions<br>Fourth through twelfth rib pain<br>Pain in the ventral aspect of the arm and forearm |
| Lu-8-9-10 | Anterior chest and rib pain<br>Dysfunctions of the upper two ribs and clavicle<br>Lesions in the scalenus muscles |
| Lu-5 | Upper chest, rib, and neck pain with inability to raise the arm |
| H-8-7 | Anterior chest and rib pain<br>Dysfunctions of the second third and fourth ribs<br>Lateral costal pain |
| TW-5 | Lateral trunk pain. |
| GB-21 | Upper back, neck, shoulder and arm pain<br>Trapezius lesions |
| GB-39 | Acute upper back and neck pain and tightness |
| Team of Four Horses 88.17-18-19 | Lower and/or upper back pain<br>Rib dysfunctions, costal pain and flank pain in a weak patient (for unilateral pain needle contralaterally) |
| SI-14 and GB-21 | Local pain, numbness and weakness in upper thoracic and shoulder regions |
| St-36, St-32, Sp-10, GB-30, GB-31and GB-34 | Musculoskeletal pain in the upper and lateral back, chest and upper limbs. |
| Two + yellow (a combination of three points) 88.12, 88.14 and Passing Heaven 88.03 | Upper back pain with degenerative disc and joint disease<br>Spinal deformity |
| Lu-7 -> Lu-8 and subcutaneous needling along superior border of the clavicle<br>Or in the direction of skin drag restriction | Upper chest, neck, and arm pain from scalene muscle lesions |

## Manipulation

Manipulation of the thoracic spine often is rewarding. However, relapse of symptoms is common, and stabilization of affected joints by periosteal acupuncture, exercise, or prolotherapy often is necessary.

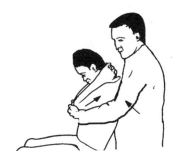

*Figure 8-3:* Thrust technique for bilateral joint dysfunction.

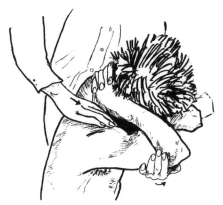

*Figure 8-4:* Thrust technique for rotation dysfunction.

Manipulation techniques of the thoracic spine can be divided roughly by the level manipulated. The upper segments (C7-T3) are stiff and require more skill, the middle (T3-T10) and lower (T8-L1) segments are relatively easy to manipulate. Manipulation can be performed in the supine, prone, and sitting positions. They can also be performed under traction.

Contraindicated to manipulation are listed on page 374.

### Manipulation, Upper Thoracic Spine.

Manipulation for bilateral flexion/extension dysfunctions can be performed with the patient seated and with his hands clasped behind his neck, and elbows approximated in front (putting the neck in flexion, which helps localize the treatment to the upper thorax). The practitioner stands behind and:

1. Holds the patient's elbows and leans the patient against his own chest (a towel can be used to increase the fulcrum against the chest).

2. (During patient exhalation). takes up all the slack.

3. (Then with an upward scooping motion, and simultaneous forward and upward) thrusts with his chest (Figure 8-3).

**A VARIATION FOR ROTATION DYSFUNCTIONS.** The patient is positioned as above, but this time the patient is not holding his elbows

together (results in less neck flexion). The practitioner stands at the patient's non-painful side and holds the under-arm of the patient, on the opposite side, with the thumb (or heel of hand) of the practitioner's other hand on the spinous process below the dysfunctional segment. (When treating the upper thoracic joints side-bending the neck first and rotating it to opposite side is desirable as it locks the facets and protects the cervical spine). The practitioner:

1. Rotates the spine by pulling the patient's arm—taking up all the slack.

2. Flexes or extends as needed for localization (or away from pain).

3. (During exhalation when the patient is relaxed) thrusts primarily with the thumb toward the spinous process (Figure 8-4).

For extension restriction, the thrust is delivered in an inferior direction from the upper aspect of the joint.

**ROTATION UNDER TRACTION.** For rotational dysfunction at C7-T2, the cervical rotation with traction technique may be effective when other techniques fail. These however, are seldom needed.

*Manipulation of Mid-thoracic Spine*

Manipulation of midthoracic levels can be achieved in the supine or prone positions.

**SUPINE TECHNIQUES (T4-T10).** These techniques vary depending on which level is treated and on whether flexion, extension or neutral thrust is appropriate. The direction of treatment can be achieved by patient placement, or by the position of the fulcrum hand, and the angle of thrust. Described here is a method of patient positioning, in flexion, extension, or neutral. A position is chosen away from painful movements or directly into the restricted barriers.

**SUPINE MANIPULATION IN NEUTRAL.** Patient is supine close to the edge of table and with his head supported by a pillow. The practitioner stands at the side of the table and:

1. Crosses the patient's arms, having him hold his opposite shoulder with the arm opposite the practitioner uppermost.

2. Rolls the patient toward him and places his fulcrum hand under the dysfunctional segment.

3. Rolls the patient on his back and localizes the fulcrum by slightly leaning over the patient and sidebending the spine into the joint barriers (this must be comfortable both to the patient and the practitioner).

4. Asks the patient to relax and exhale, takes up all the slack, then thrusts in a

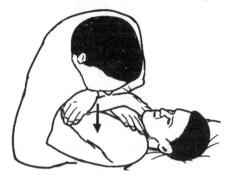

*Figure 8-5:* Supine technique in neutral.

downward direction with his chest (Figure 8-5).

**SUPINE MANIPULATION IN EXTENSION.** Patient is supine close to the edge of table and head without a pillow. The practitioner stands at the side of the patient and:

1. Interlocks the patient's hands behind his neck with elbows together as close to the chin as possible (this puts the spine in extension).

2. Holds the patient's elbows and rolls the patient toward him. Places his fulcrum hand under the dysfunctional segment (may use a ball to increase the fulcrum).

3. Rolls the patient on his back, slightly leaning over the patient's elbows.

4. Moves the elbows superiorly to increase extension and sidebends the spine, as needed (engaging the joint barriers).

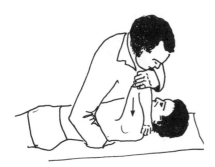

Figure 8-6: Supine technique in extension.

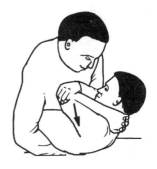

Figure 8-7: Supine technique in flexion.

**5.** Takes up all the slack and thrusts downward through the elbows.

**SUPINE MANIPULATION IN FLEXION.** Patient is supine, close to the edge of the table and with his head supported by a pillow. Patient's hands are interlocked behind the neck and elbows are held together. The practitioner:

**1.** Holds the patient's elbows and rolls him toward himself. Places his fulcrum hand under the dysfunctional segment.

**2.** Holds the patient's elbows, which should point inferiorly (brings spine into flexion).

**3.** Localizes, by leaning slightly over the patient and sidebending the spine into the joint barriers.

**4.** Takes up all slack and thrusts downward using the arms, hands and chest.(Figure 8-7).

*Manipulations Prone Position (T4 -T12)*

These techniques are easy to learn and are used widely by OM, Cyriax and other systems. They can be designed to treat the spine in extension, flexion, and rotation (although the thrust is into extension).

To treat *flexion dysfunctions*, the front of the table is lowered, positioning the patient in flexion. For greater accuracy the practitioner thrusts slightly below the dysfunctional segment. For *extension restrictions*, the practitioner puts a pillow under the patient's chest, and for greater accuracy thrusts directly above the segment. For *neutral dysfunctions*, the patient lies flat on the table, and the practitioner thrusts just above the segment with one hand, and below the segment with the other hand. For primarily rotation dysfunctions, a crossed-hand technique is used to increase rotation.

Only the last, i.e., rotation technique, is shown here as the other techniques are very similar except that the position of the pisiform is on both sides of the spine and at the same level, or at the center between two spinous processes.

**PRONE ROTATION TECHNIQUE.** Patient is prone, head turned to the comfortable direction. Practitioner at the nonpainful side of the patient. The practitioner:

**1.** Leans over the patient, with his extended wrists crossed so that the pisiform is in contact with two vertebra. One hand on the dysfunctional transverse process, and the other (the side closer to him) on the transverse process of the vertebra below.

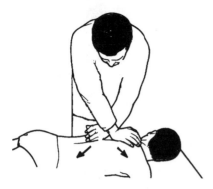

*Figure 8-8:*  Prone rotary technique.

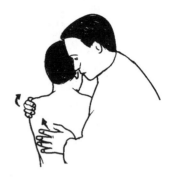

*Figure 8-9:*  Thrust technique for rotation dysfunction of low to upper spine.

**2.** Takes up the slack by leaning over the patient, while asking the patient to exhale (one may also sidebend the patient engaging this plane).

**3.** Applies a short quick thrust by leaning over the patient (Figure 8-8).

*Lower Thoracic Spine (T8-l1)*

For dysfunctions of the lower thoracic spine the lumbar roll techniques can be used (see lumbar chapter 9).

A technique for the lower thoracic rotational dysfunctions can be done with the patient seated.

**SEATED TECHNIQUE.** Patient is seated with his hands crossed over, holding his shoulders. The practitioner stands behind the patient, with the pisiform of one hand placed at the level to be manipulated, the other hand reaching in front of the patient, grasping either the patient's opposite shoulder or opposite arm and:

**1.** Introduces rotation with sidebending to the same or opposite sides, as needed.

**2.** Introduces flexion or extension, or keeps the spine in neutral, as needed.

**3.** Engages the joint in all three planes, and takes up all the slack.

**4.** During exhalation, a rotary thrust is carried out against the transverse process with a combination of the practitioners hands and body. (one may also emphasize sidebending during the thrust) (Figure 8-9).

Modifications of all of the above techniques can be applied for dysfunctional ribs. The fulcrum is placed more laterally at the rib angles, or at the costotransverse joint. Manipulation of the ribs can be achieved also by a thrust on the anterior angles.

**Muscle Energy**

Muscle energy techniques for the thoracic spine are principally the same as used in the lumbar and cervical spine with a few modifications. When treating the upper thoracic spine, from C7 to T5, the patient's head and neck are used to localize the movements to the barriers (similar to techniques of the cervical spine), (Greenman *ibid*).

*Upper-Thoracic Spine*

**EXTENSION RESTRICTIONS (FRS).** When treating extension restrictions (FRS dysfunctions) it is better to, either passively or actively, tuck the patient's chin.

Patient seated and practitioner on the side or behind the patient. The practitioner then:

1. Places his monitoring hand over the dysfunctional segment, thumb over the spinous process (touching it and the neighboring spine firmly), and fingers over the articular pillar. His other hand is used to control the head and neck movements.

2. Extends the patient's spine from below by asking the patient to push his belly forward, until the feather edge of motion is felt with the monitoring hand, at the lower portion of the dysfunctional segment.

3. Extends the patient's neck from above while keeping the chin tucked.

4. Sidebends and rotates the patient's neck toward the dysfunctional side, by translating the patient, and rotating his head until the feather edge of movement is sensed with the monitoring fingers.

5. Resists active flexion or sidebending of the patient's head for 3-5 seconds.

6. Repeats steps 4-6 three to four times.

7. Rechecks (Figure 8-10).

Bourdillon describes a technique that can be used in patients where no cervical extension is tolerated. Here the patient holds his shoulder with his opposite hand. Then the practitioner pulls the elbow upwards to introduce extension. Sidebending and rotation at the level is introduced with the monitoring hand below, and by control of the patient's elbow from above. The localization is by translation rather than simple sidebending and extension. After all three barriers are engaged, the

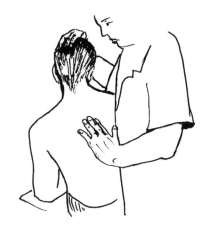

*Figure 8-10:* Muscle energy technique for extension, right sidebending and rotation restriction at upper thoracic spine — FRS (lt).

patient's effort of pushing his elbow down and forward is resisted by the practitioner.

**FLEXION RESTRICTIONS (ERS).** Patient and practitioner positions are the same as above. The practitioner:

1. Flexes the spine from below, by having the patient slump until he first senses motion over the lower aspect of the spinous process below the dysfunctional segment.

2. Flexes from above by moving the head and neck forward until the feather edge of movement is felt at the upper adjoining spinal process.

3. Sidebends and rotates the spine away from the dysfunctional side by translating the patient and rotating the head until he first feels movement at the dysfunctional segment with the monitoring fingers.

4. Resists active extension or sidebending of the patient's head for 3-5 seconds.

5. Repeats steps 4-6 three to four times.

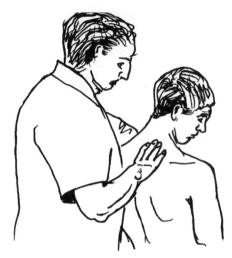

*Figure 8-11:*  Muscle energy technique for flexion, right sidebending and rotation restriction at upper thoracic spine — ERS(rt).

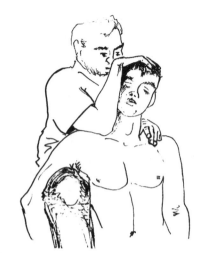

*Figure 8-12:*  Muscle energy technique for neutral restriction of left sidebending and right rotation — NS(rt).

**6.** Rechecks (Figure 8-11).

**NEUTRAL GROUP DYSFUNCTIONS.** Patient and practitioner positions are the same as above, except the practitioner's thumb monitors the muscles, over the apex of the convexity of the dysfunctional group. The spine remains in neutral, no flexion or extension is introduced. The practitioner:

**1.** Sidebends the spine toward the convexity of the group by a pressure over the shoulder with the monitoring hand, and by side bending the head toward the same shoulder.

**2.** Rotates the head to the opposite side of sidebending, until motion is first sensed with the monitoring hand.

**3.** Resists the patient's active movement of his head against the practitioner's hand, for 3-5 seconds.

**4.** Repeats steps 2-4 three to four times.

**5.** Rechecks (Figure 8-12).

## Lower Thoracic Spine

Techniques for the lower thoracic spine are similar to the techniques used in the lumbar spine (see chapter 9). Alternatively, the patient can be treated sitting, and localization done by using the patient's shoulders and spine, instead of the head and neck (Figure 8-13 through Figure 8-15).

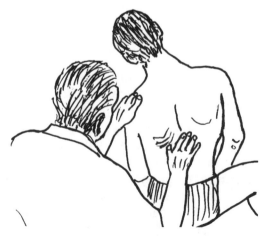

*Figure 8-13:*  Muscle energy technique for FRS(rt) at lower thoracic spine.

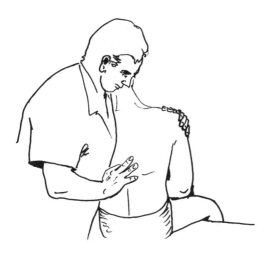

*Figure 8-14:* Muscle energy technique for ERS(rt) at the lower thoracic spine.

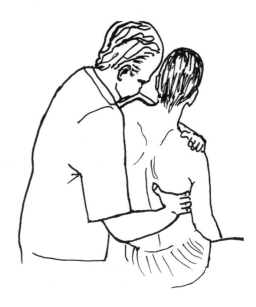

*Figure 8-15:* Muscle energy technique for neutral dysfunction at lower thoracic spine.

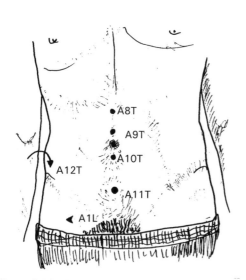

Figure 8-16:  Anterior lower thoracic Jones
points (After Jones, Kusunose and Goering 1995).

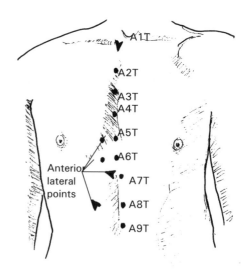

Figure 8-17:  Anterior upper thoracic Jones
points (After Jones, Kusunose and Goering 1995).

nothyroid and internal intercostal muscle
spasm.

For treatment of A1T the patient is
seated in front of the practitioner with his
hands on top of his head (this fixes the
force to the upper thorax). He then leans
back against the practitioner (a pillow can
be used between the patient and practitioner for comfort). The practitioner:

1. Places his arms around and under the
   patient's axila locking them in front.

2. Instructs the patient to slump forward
   and adds pressure with his chest.

3. Fine tunes with rotation until
   tenderness at the point is minimal.

4. Holds for 90 seconds and slowly
   releases (Figure 8-19).

**A2T-A4T.** Treatment of the third through
sixth joints uses similar techniques except
for increasing the amount of flexion.

Treatment of the third and fourth levels is achieved by pulling the patient's
arms and shoulders backward into extension (Figure 8-18).

## Countertension Postional Release

For countertension techniques the thoracic spine is divided into anterior, posterior, and rib dysfunctions. Here only
techniques for anterior and posterior dysfunctions are described.

### Anterior Dysfunctions

Several Jones points are located over the
manubrium, sternum, and xyphoid process labeled A1T-A6T. These points are
tender with anterior dysfunctions of the
first through the sixth thoracic joints (Figure 8-17 and Figure 8-16).

**A1T (STERNOTHYROID AND INTERNAL INTER-
COSTAL MUSCLES).** The first point, A1T is
located at the suprasternal notch. Tenderness at A1T is tested by applying anteriorly directed pressure onto the notch. The
point is tender with lesions of the first and
second thoracic vertebra and whith   ster-

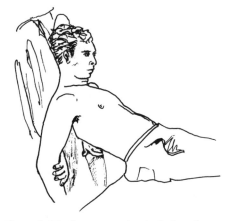

*Figure 8-18:* Countertension technique for anterior T3 and T4.

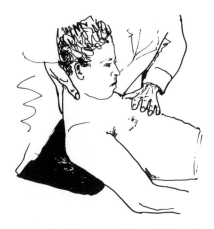

*Figure 8-21:* Countertension technique for anterior T5-T7.

**A5T** THROUGH **A7T**. For the fifth through seventh thoracic joints considerable amount of flexion is needed, which is achieved by having the patient lean against the practitioner's thigh (Figure 8-20). Or by having the patient lie supine and just far enough off the table that the practitioner can apply strong force by pushing against the upper thoracic with the side of his femur and hip (Figure 8-21). This technique is especially helpful for the seventh and eighth (A8T) levels with ten-

derness around the xyphoid junction.

**AT5** THROUGH **AT9** JOINTS ANTERIOR LATERAL DYSFUNCTIONS (DIAPHRAGORATIC CRURA AND TRANSVERSES THORACIC MUSCLES). For the fifth through the ninth thoracic areas and for the diaphragoratic crura and transverses thoracic muscles, the Jones points are located on the costal cartilages close to the side of the sternum for T5 and T6, and off an inch or more to the side of the xyphoid process on the medial, inferior surfaces of the costal cartilage for T7 and T8.

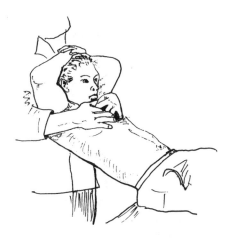

*Figure 8-19:* Countertension technique for anterior T1-T2.

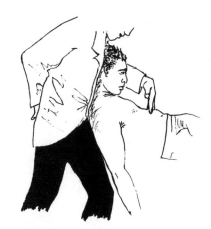

*Figure 8-20:* Countertension technique for anterior T5 -T7 (Second option).

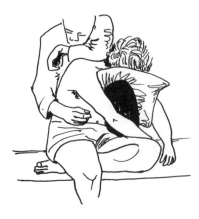

*Figure 8-22:*  Countertension technique for anterior lateral T5-T8

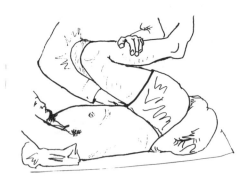

*Figure 8-23:*  Countertension technique for anterior T9-L1

For treatment the patient is seated in front of the practitioner with his legs and feet resting on the table, to the side of the practitioner's leg, which is also placed on the table opposite to the tender point. The patient leans over toward the practitioner's thigh, and rests his arm over a pillow which is placed over the practitioner's thigh. The practitioner:

1. Places his hands over the tender point.

2. Sidebends the patient's body toward the tender point somewhat, by translating the trunk to the opposite side.

3. Rotates the patient's trunk by placing the patient's arm on the involved side, across the front of his body, away from the tender point.

4. (When tenderness at the point is minimal) holds the position for 90 seconds and then slowly returns the patient to neutral (Figure 8-22).

**A9T-AL1. (DIAPHRAGORATIC CRURA, TRANSVERSES THORACIC AND PSOAS MUSCLES).** These points are tender often in patients with low back pain. Tender points, except for the A12T are located near the midline deep in the abdomen. A9T is about one cm above the umbilicus, A11T is about two inches below the umbilicus. The point

A12T is found on the inner table of the ala of the ilium, in the midaxillary line. A1L is included here because it is treated in the same way.

For treatment the patient lies supine with a pillow under his chest and pelvis. The practitioner:

1. Flexes the patient's knees to induce flexion at the spine.

2. Sidebends the spine (about 20°) by pulling the patient's knees toward the tender side slightly.

3. Fine tunes and holds the position for 90 seconds.

4. Returns the patient to neutral by slowly returning the legs and removing the pillow from under the hips (Figure 8-23).

*Posterior Dyfunctions.*

The Jones points for the posterior thorax are located in three lines. One is located in the interspinal areas, on the sides of the spinous processes. The second line is located paraspinally, and the third over the rib angles (Figure 8-24).

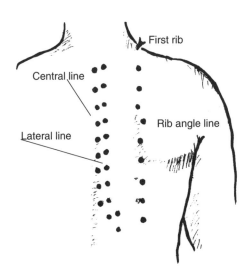

Figure 8-24: Posterior thoracic Jones points
(After Jones, Kusunose and Goering 1995).

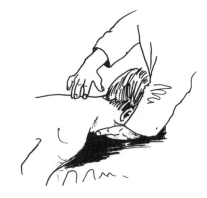

*Figure 8-25:* Countertension technique for posterior T1-T3.

The upper thoracic Jones points become most tender on the sides of the spinous processes with joint dysfunction. The lower thoracic points become tender usually paravertebrally, or just lateral to the spinous process. At the thoracolumbar junction, the most sensitive points are found on the posterior tips of the transverse processes. Sometimes, the most tender points are found on the spinous process. Tenderness is best palpated with the patient supine.

When treating the posterior thorax, the closer the sensitive point is to midline, the more extension is needed. The further the tender point is from midline, the more sidebending away from the tender point is needed.

**P1T THROUGH P3T (INTERSPINALES, MULTIFIDUS AND ROTATOR MUSCLES).** P1T and P3T are used to treat the lower posterocervical and upper posterior first through third thoracic joints and interspinales, multifidus and rotator muscles. P1T through P3T Jones points are located on the sides of spinous processes of T1 through T3.

For treatment the patient is prone with arms along the sides of his body. One of the practitioner's hands is placed under

the patient's chin, while the other monitors the tender point. The practitioner:

1. Slowly extends the patient's head and neck to the level of involvement.

2. Sidebends and rotates the head slightly, usually away from the sensitive point, until tenderness at the point is at a minimum.

3. Holds for 90 seconds and slowly returns the patient to neutral (Figure 8-25).

**P4T-P6T (INTERSPINALES, MULTIFIDUS AND ROTATOR MUSCLES.)** P4T-P6T are used to treat the   fourth, through sixth posterior thoracic tender points and joints. Jones points P4T through P6T are located on the sides of the spinous processes of T3-T6. Treatment at these levels is essentially the same as the upper 2 thoracic joints, except that the arms are now extended above the head.

For treatment the patient is prone with arms along the sides of his head. One of the practitioner's hands is placed under the patient's chin, while the other monitors the tender point. The practitioner:

1. Slowly extends the patient's head and neck to the level of involvement.

2. Sidebends and rotates the head slightly, usually away form the sensitive point,

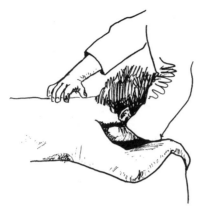

*Figure 8-26:*  Countertension technique for posterior T4-T6.

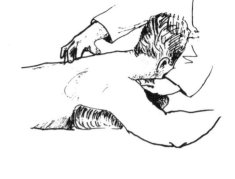

*Figure 8-27:*  Countertension technique for posterior T7-T9.

until tenderness at the point is at a minimum.

**3.** Holds for 90 seconds and slowly returns the patient to neutral (Figure 8-26).

### P6T-P9T (Multifidus, Rotators And Levator Costorum Muscles).

Treatment at these levels is essentially the same as the upper T4-T6 thoracic joints, except that now a pillow is used to extend the upper thoracic spine. The practitioner may need to stretch the neck farther to get the action down to the necessary level.

For treatment the patient is prone with arms along the sides of his head. One of the practitioner's hands is placed under the patient's chin, while the other monitors the tender point. The practitioner:

**1.** Slowly extends the patient's head and neck to the level of involvement.

**2.** Sidebends and rotates the head slightly, usually away form the sensitive point, until tenderness at the point is at a minimum.

**3.** Holds for 90 seconds and slowly returns the patient to neutral (Figure 8-27).

### P10-11-12T and P1L (Multifidus, Rotators And Quadratus Lumborum Muscle).

P10-11-12T are used to treat mid and lower thoracic dysfunctions, with tender points in the midline, or near the spinous processes; and for multifidus, rotators and quadratus lumborum muscle spasms. P10-11-12T usually are found laterally to the spinous processes, or on the tips of the transverse processes. These points however, may be found more centrally and then treated with more extension and less sidebending.

For treatment the patient is prone, propped up with a pillow under the chest, or if available, by raising the head of the treatment table. The practitioner stands on the opposite side of the tender point and with one hand over the point and the other hand under the ASIS, at the side of the tender point. The practitioner:

**1.** Pulls the ASIS up and toward the tender point, creating rotation of approximately 30-45°. Sometimes it may be necessary to add sidebending away from the tender point by translating the legs.

**2.** Fine tunes until the point tenderness is at a minimum, and holds the position for 90 seconds.

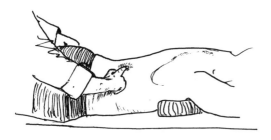

*Figure 8-28:* Countertension technique for posterior thoracic T10-L1.

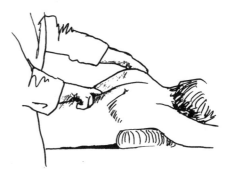

*Figure 8-29:* Countertension technique for posterior thoracic with marked deviation of spinous processes.

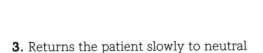

**3.** Returns the patient slowly to neutral (Figure 8-28).

**POSTERIOR THORACIC WITH MARKED DEVIATION OF SPINOUS PROCESSES**. These points tend to be tender in the lower thoracic spine but can become tender anywhere along the thoracic spine.

For treatment the patient is prone with a pillow under his chest. The patient's arm, on the involved side, lies along the side of the head, while the other arm hangs off the table.

The practitioner stands on the opposite side of the tender points and grasps the patient's arm on the involved side, near the axilla, without undue pulling of sensitive skin. The other hand monitors the tender point.

The practitioner:

**1.** Pulls the arm toward himself, and superiorly, creating mostly sidebending with a mild rotation and extension, until tenderness at the point is at a minimum.

**2.** Holds for 90 seconds and slowly returns the patient to neutral (Figure 8-29).

# Chapter 9: *The Low Back*

Low back pain is the most common cause of musculoskeletal disability, and apparently has been so for thousands of years; the classic *Simple Questions* (200 B.C.) devoted an entire chapter (chapter 41) to low back pain. In modern times some 60-80% of people will suffer a disabling episode of back pain once in their life. After excluding traditional orthopedic, medical and neurological conditions, 83% of back pains are said to be idiopathic (Kraus 1988). Holbrook et al. (1984) found that at any one time 17% of the US population is having back pain. The cost of low back pain on the economy from medical treatment, legal proceedings and work loss is enormous (Snook 1987). Most of individuals who have acute low back pain recover within 6 weeks, whether they are treated or not (Bann and Wood 1975). It is the 5-15% that do not recover which account for the majority of the cost (Webster and Snook 1990).

## Anatomy & Biomechanics

The usual lumbar spine has five vertebrae. The wide part of the vertebral body is situated anteriorly, and the dorsal arch posteriorly. There is a disc between adjacent bodies. The vertebral body is thicker in front (anteriorly) and wider transversely. Together with the discs, which are also thicker anteriorly, they give the lumbar spine its lordotic curve. L5 is much thicker anteriorly, as is the disc at this level, accounting for the angular lumbosacral junction. In some people L5 is fused with the sacrum—called sacralization. The nucleus pulposus in the lumbar spine is located centrally within the disc. This allows for rocker-like movement.

The posterior arch, which is united with a thick pedicle to the vertebral body, is composed of a thick and broad spinous process and two transverse processes (TrPs). The arches of L1 through L3 originate from the juncture of the pedicles and laminae, and are horizontal. The TrPs of the lower two vertebrae arise from the pedicles and posterior portion of the body, and are inclined posteriorly (Bogduk *ibid*).

The articular facets, in the upper lumbar region, are oriented in a vertical sagittal (vertical and anteroposterior) plane that permits flexion and extension, but which resists sidebending when the spine is in a neutral position (the lumbar lordosis is maintained but is not excessive). However, a very small amount of rotation and sidebending is present throughout the lumbar spine and increases when there is slight flexion. Flexion/extension and rotation are greatest at L5-S1. Sidebending is greatest at L3-4 (White and Panjabi 1978). The orientation of the lumbar facets do not permit compression and are not designed for weight bearing (Figure 9-1), (Brown 1995).

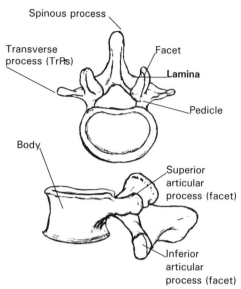

*Figure 9-1:* Lumbar vertebra.

*Table 9-1.* **APPROXIMATE LOADS AT L3 IN A 70KG INDIVIDUAL**

| ACTIVITY | APPROXIMATE LOAD (KG/CM2) |
|---|---|
| Lying Supine | 30 |
| Sitting | 100 |
| Coughing; Jumping | 110 |
| Laughing; Bending Forward to 20% | 120 |
| Hyperextending Actively while Supine | 150 |
| Doing Sit-Ups | 180 |
| Lifting a 20kg load with Straight Back | 210 |
| Lifting a 20kg load with Back Forward Bent | 340 |

The anterior portion of the functional units of the spine (vertebral bodies and the discs) are considered to be weight bearing, shock absorbing structures. The discs in the lumbar spine account for about 30% of the column length. Approximate pressure loads at L3 in a 70 kg individual have been measured (Nachemson and Elfstrom 1970) and summarized in Table 9-1.

The posterior portion of the functional units are triangular structures composed of two vertebral arches, two TrPs, a central posterior spinous process, and paired articular facets. The posterior portion is believed to be non-weight bearing, and the facets within them regulate motion available in the lower spine. Muscles and ligaments, which attach to the TrPs and spinous processes, act as tension members and contribute to lumbar mobility and stability. Abnormal disc function, ligamentous weakening and excessive lordosis may weaken the integrity of the lumbar spine and shift weight bearing to the posterior portions of the vertebral unit, which are not as suitable to carry this load.

## Lumbar Spine: Movement

Movement in the lumbar spine is produced by the coordinated action of nerves, muscles and levers. Elastic energy stored in the fascia and ligaments also provides momentum (spring) to movement. Agonistic muscles (prime movers, muscle that are contracting) initiate and carry out movement, whereas antagonist muscles often control and modify it (Lindh 1980). Spinal movements are always a combination of the actions of several segments, and side-bending is coupled with rotation and translation. During active gait, the spine responds (mostly passively) to the primary propellants—the lower extremity and pelvic systems.

### Flexion

Flexion in the lumbar spine consists of rotation, coupled with translation, of one vertebra on it's adjoining inferior vertebra, and usually involves the simultaneous movement of the lumbar spine and pelvis in one plane. The superior vertebra glides anteriorly, compressing the disc anteriorly. The posterior aspect of the disc is unloaded and therefore widens. During forward bending the nucleus pulposus moves backward and the axis of rotation is thought to moved with it (Kapandji 1974).

The effects of flexion on forces exerted by the lumbar back muscles was studied by Macintosh, Bogduk and Pearcy (1993). In flexion, the lever arm length decreases slightly (produced by the spine), which results in up to 18% decrease of the maximum extensor magnitude exerted across the lumbar spine. Compression loads are not significantly different from those generated in the upright subject. However, there are major changes in shear forces, in particular a reversal from a net anterior to a net posterior shear force at the L5/S1 segment. Flexion causes substantial elongation of the back muscles, which results in reduction of their maximum active tension. However, when the increase in passive tension is considered, it appears that the compression forces and tension exerted by the back muscles (in full flexion) are not significantly different from those produced in the upright posture (Basmajian and Nyberg 1993).

Flexion is limited by the geometry of tissues; ligamenta flava, the facet (zygoapophyseal) joint capsules, the interspinous ligaments and, except for the lower vertebrae, the supraspinous ligament. The annulus of the disc also limits forward flexion (Bogdug *ibid*).

During flexion the erector spinae muscles elongate and help to decelerate forward flexion by eccentric contraction. At the end of flexion the erector spinae muscles are inactive (based on EMG). Heavy lifting or unguarded movement with the spine flexed, may strain structures stressed by flexion, or which help restore the body to the upright posture. During heavy lifting, the pelvis often rotates first with the ligaments of the lumbar spine bearing the brunt of the stress. At 45° (based on EMG) the muscles of the back become active (Bogduk 1980). The quadri-

ceps femoris, iliotibial, and glutiel muscles assist in flexion and may be strained.

Cailleit (1981) has designated the movement during flexion the "Lumbo Pelvic Rhythm." Initially the lumbar portion flattens. As flexion continues, a gradual reversal of the lumbar curve occurs, most prominently at the lower portion of the spine. With back pain, guarding often does not allow for normal pelvic rhythm.

### Extension

Extension is achieved through a combination of pelvic and extensor muscle shortening and support through the thoracolumbar fascia and latissimus dorsi (Bogduk 1980). The pelvis rotates backward, and then the spine extends. The body of the superior vertebra rotates and translates posteriorly, compressing the posterior portion of the disc. The nucleus is pushed anteriorly. Extension is limited both by tissue and bony geometry of the vertebral arch and by tension which develops in the soft tissues anteriorly.

The sacrospinalis (erector spinae) muscle is ensheathed by the thick lumbar part of the thoracolumbar fascia, which is attached medially to the lumbar vertebrae, and which becomes continuous laterally with the aponeurosis and fascia of the latissimus dorsi and anterior abdominal muscles (Bogduk and Twomey *ibid*). These form a tube around the spine adding protection and stability when the fascia tightens and expands due to the broadening of the extensor muscles during extension.

Bogduk, Macintosh and Pearcy (1992) showed that in the upright position the thoracic fibers of the lumbar erector spinae contribute 50% of the total extensor movement exerted on L4 and L5. The multifidus contributes some 20%, and the remaining extensor tension is exerted by the lumbar fibers of the erector spinae. At upper lumbar levels, the thoracic fibers of the lumbar erector spinae contribute between 70% and 86% of the total extensor tension.

In the upright posture, the lumbar back muscles exert a net posterior shear force on segments L1-L4, but exert an anterior shear force on L5. Collectively, all the back muscles exert large compression forces on all segments.

Loss of extension has been shown to correlate with low back pain more closely than flexion (Troup 1987).

### Sidebending/Rotation

Sidebending to any extent (even though slight) in the lumbar spine is coupled always with translation and rotation. During sidebending the upper vertebra tilts ipsilaterally, compressing the disc on the same side. The nucleus is displaced contralaterally.

When the lordotic curve is intact, sidebending is coupled with rotation to the opposite side (neutral or type I motion). According to Fryett if the facets are engaged during flexion or extension, sidebending will be coupled with rotation to the same side (non-neutral type II motion). With non-neutral or Type II lumbar mechanics the spine is less stable, and injury is more likely to occur (Greenman *ibid*). During rotation the back and abdominal muscles are active on both sides of the spine.

Sidebending is limited by the geometry of both bony and soft tissues. The ipsilateral facet closes and the contralateral facet opens, and soft tissues are stretched (Kapandji *ibid*).

Restrictions in sidebending and rotation have been shown to correlate with the degree of low back pain (Mellin 1986).

### Muscle Torque

The maximal single fascicle of axial torque generated by the lumbar back muscles was studied by Mactintosh et al. (1993). Torque was measured in the longissimus thoracis, iliocostalis lumborum and the lumbar mul-

tifidus in subjects during standing, both in the upright position and in full flexion.

- The above muscles in upright subjects exerted no more than 2 N/m of axial torque.

- The collective torque of all muscles acting on a single segment did not exceed 5 N.

- All torques were considerably reduced in full flexion.

From these measurements the lumbar back muscles appear to exert very little torque on the lumbar spine, and contribute about only 5% of the total torque involved in trunk rotation. According to Macintosh none of the lumbar back muscles should be considered as rotators. The abdominal oblique muscles appear to be the principal rotators of the trunk (Macintosh, Pearcy and Bogduk 1993).

## The Pelvic Girdle

The pelvis is a three-part bony ring with two sacroiliac (SI) joints posteriorly and the pubic symphysis anteriorly. The role of the sacroiliac joint in musculoskeletal pain has been controversial. Older literature stated that the SI joints are functionally fused and therefore no dysfunction could occur. (This error was probably due to early anatomical studies that were done on very old subjects with pathological joints.) It is now well established that the SI joints are true synovial (diarthrodial) joints with an articular capsule, joint space, and cartilage in which movement does occur. A recent controlled study of low back pain has shown that 30% of patients had pain related to the SI joints. In these patients tears of the ventral capsule were documented (Schwarzer, Aprill and Bogduk 1995).

Several rotational axes in the SI joint, and translation or gliding motions have been described in the literature (Kapandji 1974; Colachis et al. 1963; Egund 1978;

Lavignolle et al. 1983; Vleeming et al. 1992).

In the osteopathic literature specific motions and dysfunctions of the sacroiliac are described well, as are techniques to restore normal position and function (Greenman 1989).

The pelvis and sacroiliac joints are key pivots in which there is interaction between the downward gravitational force of the trunk and the upward reaction forces from the ground. The pelvis must withstand great forces in various directions. Pelvic motions are essential for increasing functional rotation of the spine. The joints are rich in mechanoreceptors which probably function as proprioceptors amidst these forces.

No primary muscle movers are responsible for SI motions. The two muscles that contribute to sacral movement are the piriformis (the only muscle that crosses the sacrum), and the aponeurosis of the erector spinae, which attach to the posterior surface of the sacrum. The abdominal, latissimus dorsi (through the thoracolumbar fascia), perineum, quadratus lumborum, iliopsoas, gluteus maximus, gluteus medius, pelvic diaphragm and other lower extremity muscles all contribute indirectly to sacroiliac motions via their connections to the pelvis.

The SI joints are described by Vleeming as compression joints which rely for stability on forces adducting the ilia onto the sacrum—which he calls force closure. The sacrum has also been described by Grant as being suspended in the ilia by the interosseous, posterior SI, sacrotuberous and spinous ligaments—and therefore vulnerable to shear. Stability of the joint is achieved primarily by these ligaments. Vleeming also has evidence that self-bracing against shear is provided by interaction of the rough surfaces of the joint with ligaments, muscles and fascial forces on the joint. In the sitting position it has been suggested that the force closure contributed by the muscles is reduced (Snijders, Vleeming and Stoeckart 1992), which may lead to increased instability in the seated patient and may explain the increased pain often seen after prolonged sitting.

Depending on posture, several muscles can either increase the loads on the sacrum, or contribute to self-bracing. These are the gluteus maximus, erector spinae, quadratus lumborum, abdominal (oblique and rectus), latissimus dorsi and psoas. The gluteus maximus and piriformis muscles are thought to increase friction forces and self-bracing. Weakness of the above muscles is thought to cause mechanical pelvic dysfunction (Snijders, Vleeming and Stoeckart *ibid*).

According to Snijders, Vleeming and Stoeckart (1992) the biceps femoris, piriformis, coccygeus and gluteus maximus muscles and the deep layer of the lumbodorsal fascia can influence the ligamental tension that regulates SI joint stability. The lumbodorsal caudad fascial fibers extend to the contralateral side, and function synergistically with the contralateral gluteus maximus muscle.

In forward bending, for example, the transverse and oblique abdominal muscles, and gluteus maximus muscle in particular, are important in providing stability by increasing force closure of the ilia onto the sacrum. Tightness of the biceps femoris or gluteus maximus will restrict sacral flexion (nutation) whereas weakness will allow increased flexion (nutation) of the sacrum (Vleeming 1989). This can increase and add to the gravitational forces from the upper body pushing down on the sacral base (the Z-axis, sagittal plane when subject is standing).

Tightness or weakness of the piriformis can effect either sacral torsional or sidebending movements, and will influence the tone of the sacrospinous ligament, as they both share a common attachment at the anterior sacrum. Both movement and sacrospinous ligament tone are necessary in normal mechanics and stability.

Structural and functional integrity are important physiologically for normal pelvic and spinal function. This integrity is essential for the storage of elastic energy. Dysfunction of this integrity increases

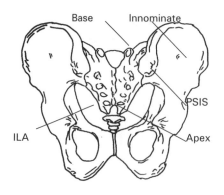

*Figure 9-2:* Sacrum and innominates.

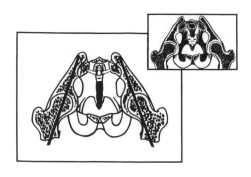

*Figure 9-3:* Suspended sacrum (Reprinted with permission Dorman and Ravin 1991).

oxygen consumption during normal walking. Correcting the dysfunction and the accompanying ligamentous laxity remedies this excess oxygen consumption (Dorman 1995).

Even in normal people, the two SI joints are never symmetrical. However, when there is joint dysfunction or pathology, one usually can detect loss of motion and functional asymmetry. The pelvis is also important in the osteopathic respiratory and circulatory models because of the relationship of the pelvis to the urogenital diaphragm, and in the osteopathic craniosacral system (Kuchera *ibid*).

The sacrum is most frequently formed by 5 (can be 2-6) fused vertebrae and ossified intervertebral discs in a triangular shape. Situated with its base (the wider aspect) superior, its first vertebra has a prominent, oval upper surface with a significant, forward slope. Attached to it is a thick disc that unites the sacrum to L5. The inclination of the superior surface of S1, results in L5 tendency to slide inferiorly and anteriorly—often resulting in spondylolysis.

The sacrum is suspended between the ilia (Figure 9-3) with its base (superior aspect) anterior to its apex (the inferior end), like the platform of a suspension bridge. Therefore, the narrow apex is positioned posteroinferiorly. The apex articu-

lates with the coccyx. The two bony edges inferior and lateral to the apex, just lateral and inferior to the fifth vertebra and sacral cornu, are the sacrum's inferior lateral angles (ILA). The ILAs are important landmarks for sacral function and position assessment. Developmentally the ILAs are the TrPs of S5 (Mitchell *ibid*). The sacrum is viewed as part of the spinal vertebral (trunk) axis in the osteopathic literature (Figure 9-2).

*The Innominates*

The innominates (hip bones) are each formed of the fused ilium, ischium and pubis, and in the osteopathic literature are functionally viewed as part of the lower extremities. The femur is connected to the innominate anteriorly via the hip joint. It is also anterior to the innominate's axis of rotation, believed to be at S2. Therefore, viewed from the side, any rotation at the innominate influences the apparent leg length (Greenman *ibid*).

*The Symphysis Pubis*

The symphysis pubis is an amphiarthrosis (an intermediate joint between diarthrosis and synarthrosis in which the articular bony surfaces are connected by an elastic cartilaginous substance) with strong superior and inferior ligaments and a thinner posterior ligament. Movement of the pubis occurs during the normal walking cycle and has been described as rotation of one pubic bone on the other around a transverse axis. Vertical movement (shear) has been described as abnormal for the symphysis pubis during walking (Kapandji 1978). However, others consider this motion normal, especially during prolonged one-legged standing, and self-correcting when weight is put on the other leg (Dihlmann 1980).

Dysfunction and laxity of the symphysis pubis is common during pregnancy under the influence of the hormone relaxin. It has been suggested that use of a sacral belt in the last months of pregnancy prevents such dysfunctions (Vleeming 1994). The abdominal and leg adductor muscles can both influence pubic joint function and maintain dysfunctions—often due to abnormal nervous input from dysfunction at T11-L2 (Mitchell *ibid*).

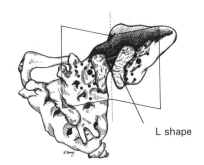

*Figure 9-4:*   L-shaped SI joint surface (with permission Dorman and Ravin 1991).

*The Sacroiliac Joint*

The SI joint is derived embryologically from a number of segments. An L-shaped joint (Figure 9-4), its upper and lower limbs have different orientations. The upper is broader posteriorly and the lower broader anteriorly. With its irregular articular surfaces, the joint has a convex/concave relationship between the sacrum and the ilia. It is relatively flat compared to other, more stable joints. This bony configuration is thought to provide some stability as the sacrum wedges in the ilia and leads to an interlocking (wedging in) at S2 (Greenman *ibid*). Therefore, the sacrum has been described as a keystone of an arch. However, since its base is anterior to the lumbar spine, and certainly when one is weight-bearing on one foot as in walking, it cannot function as a true architectural keystone, which is stable by compression alone. The sacrum is most likely stable by compression from bones and from tension

of soft tissues (therefore it has been compared to a platform of a suspension bridge). Additional forces are needed to achieve what a tie-beam (or more accurately, a come-along) does. This is accomplished by tension elements and possibly force closure from soft tissues on the ilia, and from ligaments that cross the joint. According to Greenman, in about 10-15% of individuals the opposing joint surfaces are quite flat, and the function of bony compression is lacking, leaving the soft tissues completely responsible for joint stability, and therefore more vulnerable to shear forces.

*Ligaments*

The body weight is thought to be transmitted from the sacrum to the innominates chiefly by the sacroiliac ligaments, which are thick and strong posteriorly and thinner anteriorly (although through tensegrity other tension and compression elements are involved as well). The sacrum is suspended from the iliac portion of the innominate by these ligaments.

ILIOLUMBAR LIGAMENTS. The iliolumbar ligaments are attached to the anterior surface of the ilia and to the TrPs of the lower lumbar vertebrae. The lower fibers extend anteriorly and join the anterior SI ligaments. Superiorly they join the TrPs of L4 and L5. This superior band passes from the TrPs of L5 to the posterior surface of the medial part of the iliac crest where the quadratus lumborum also originates, in part. The iliolumbar ligaments were thought to be formed during adolescence from the quadratus lumborum muscle; however, newer information shows the ligament to be present in babies, as well (Willard *ibid*).

The iliolumbar and the lumbodorsal fasciae are important restraining and stabilizing structures in all lumbosacral movements. The iliolumbar ligaments function as guy wires and give lateral stability to the lumbosacral column.

Sprain of the iliolumbar ligament is common, often due to torsional injuries or an unleveled sacral base. Often it is the first ligament that causes back pain, as it may be affected by both spinal and innominate sprains (Kutchera and Kutchera *ibid*). The quadratus lumborum is frequently involved as well. Pain from the iliolumbar ligaments is felt in L1-4 sclerotomes (Dorman *ibid*), (Figure 9-5).

**LUMBOSACRAL LIGAMENTS.** The lumbosacral ligaments are a common cause of low back pain in the midline. Pain (posain) from the lumbosacral and interspinous ligaments is provoked by prolonged standing, sitting or lying. Often the pain spreads symmetrically across the low back and is aggravated by prolonged sitting and flexion to full range. Rotation often is normal At times extension is painful, as fibers may be squeezed between the spines (Dorman *ibid*), (Figure 9-5).

**POSTERIOR (DORSAL) SI LIGAMENTS.** The posterior (dorsal) SI ligaments can be divided into three layers (Kapandji *ibid*; Dorman *ibid*):

- The most posterior ligaments span the sacral crest vertically and attach to the ilium. The superficial long ligament fibers are more vertical and blend with the sacrotuberous ligament, which is continuous with the tendon of the long head of the biceps femoris.

- The intermediate layer overlies most of the posterior aspect of the SI joints and runs from the posterior arches of the sacrum to the medial side of the ilium.

The short fibers of the posterior SI ligaments are oriented transversely and are intertwined. Therefore, when pulled upon they tighten (like a rope), approximating the two ilia. They form the major support for the sacrum. These ligaments are an important part of the force closure mechanism of the ilium on the sacrum. When gravitational forces from the trunk push on the sacrum, the dorsal SI ligaments pull the ilia closer to the sacrum.

- The deep layer of interosseous ligaments attaches laterally to the medial aspect of the PSIS and to the anterior foramina of S1 and S2. They are strong and form the principal union between the two bones (Figure 9-5).

**SACROSPINOUS LIGAMENT.** The sacrospinous ligament runs under the sacrotuberous ligament. It attaches medially by its broad base to the sacrotuberous ligament and to the anterior surface of the sacrum. Laterally it attaches to the spine of the ischium (Figure 9-5).

**SACROTUBEROUS LIGAMENT.** The sacrotuberous ligament is attached superiorly by a wide flat base to the posterior, superior and inferior iliac spines. Then the ligament runs inferiorly to the lower sacrum and is attached to the ischial tuberosity. This ligament is connected with the posterior SI ligaments at the PSIS. The lower fibers of the gluteus maximus are attached to the sacrotuberous ligament, as well. Below, it is, in part, connected to the tendon of the biceps muscle which directly affects its tension (Vleeming *ibid*), (Figure 9-5).

The sacrotuberous and sacrospinous ligaments function to oppose upward rotation of the sacral apex (bottom of sacrum) under the downward force of the spine on

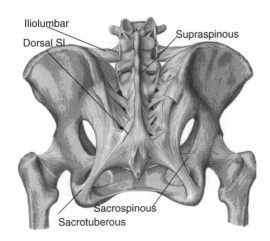

*Figure 9-5:* Lumbopelvic ligaments.

the anteriorly positioned sacral base (top of the sacrum), (Figure 9-2).

## Motion In The Pelvis

Motions of the pelvic ring have been studied, although much disagreement is found among researchers. Analysis of walking shows that counter-rotations of the two innominates is an important part of normal walking. This movement can occur only if the pubic symphysis can rotate around a transverse axis. The sacrum rotates toward, and sidebends away from, the side on which the innominate rotates posteriorly. This type of movement is called anterior torsion (Mitchell 1948). Other movements occur as well. Any restriction in these motions renders the walking cycle abnormal, and can affect function and lead to pain in the back and legs. Dorman also hypothesizes that, during walking, the SI joint must lock and unlock on alternating sides, allowing for maximal efficiency of the pelvic "differential-like mechanism".

When the patient is standing on the right leg, the left innominate is pushed posteriorly by the weight of the trunk, pushing the SI joint caudad (inferiorly) while the supporting leg pushes the hip superiorly. The hanging leg (left in this example) will pull and rotate the left

innominate anteriorly. (These motions are used to evaluate the SI joint with the Gillet's-Stork Test), (Figure 9-6), (Brown 1995)

### Osteopathic Pelvic Motions

Movements of the sacrum between the innominates are described as sacroiliac motions. These are all physiological movements that can become restricted or exaggerated (Greenman *ibid*; Mitchell *ibid*; Bourdillon, Day and Brookhout 1992).

**NUTATION.** Nutation is movement of the sacral base anteriorly and inferiorly (down the L shaped track of the joint) between the innominates. It involves a rotation of the sacrum about a transverse axis and translation of the sacrum caudally (inferiorly) within the joint. Sacral nutation is a normal, coupled movement to extension of the lumbar spine. Bilateral restrictions are rare; unilateral restrictions are common.

**COUNTERNUTATION.** Counternutation (posterior nutation) occurs when the base moves posteriorly and superiorly on the innominate bones in the same axis as nutation. The sacral base becomes prominent posteriorly, and the ILAs less so. Counternutation is a normal reaction to extreme lumber flexion. Restrictions can occur both unilaterally and bilaterally.

**NUTATIONAL DYSFUNCTIONS.** Nutational Dysfunctions are probably maintained due to SI ligamentous insufficiency and lack of muscle stabilization on the joint.

**SHEARS.** Sacral shears (downward movements) have been described in the literature as non-physiological. However, they are part of the normal sacral movement during nutation and counternutation. True dysfunctional shears probably represent ligament insufficiency.

**SACRAL TORSIONS.** Anterior (forward) torsion is a normal movement around a theo-

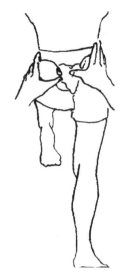

*Figure 9-6:* Gillet's Stork Test.

# Imaging

The lumbar spine and pelvis frequently are imaged together. Many of the considerations regarding the radiological studies have been touched on elsewhere in this text. This section covers only the topics of interest to the orthopedic practitioner that usually are not dealt with in standard radiology texts. Apart from setting out to seek and exclude neoplastic and bony disease proper, the images mostly are used to obtain *indirect* information about supporting tissues; therefore, a search is made for asymmetry and for disordered relationships between the visible parts. This quest is marred by three factors:

1. Large variations exist between individuals. (Although some congenital abnormalities of bony formation, such as spina bifida, have weak correlations with instability and back pain, their presence is by no means an indication of the cause of trouble), (Figure 9-7).

2. Asymmetries between the two sides also are frequent. (They also bear a moderated relationship to the development of strains in the restraining soft tissues. Their presence is not in itself diagnostic.)

3. Alignment of the subject in the X-ray beam affects the projection of the images on the film. The problem of correct placement of the patient arises here.

retical oblique axis accompanying the counterrotation of the two innominates and the lateral shifts of the spine in normal walking. During walking, the lumbar sidebending muscles on the swing leg side contract at mid-stride elevating the hip so as to allow the swing leg to pass. The piriformis muscle on the non-swing side contracts and stabilizes the sacrum, creating an axis by which the sacrum rotates. This probably creates an oblique axis between the lower and the opposite upper sacroiliac region. The sacrum rotates toward the side of the oblique axis (Mitchell 1993).

*Posterior (backward) torsions* occur during lumbar non-neutral mechanics that result in co-contraction of lumbar side benders and hip external rotator muscles. This induces a backward torsional movement of the sacral base on an oblique axis. Backward torsional movements are thought to be a normal physiological motion in response to non-neutral lumbar movements.

Backward torsion dysfunctions are maintained by the lumbar sidebenders, principally quadratus lumborum and piriformis on the same side (Mitchell personal communication).

The alignment of the endoskeleton within the overall dimensions of the torso—in this case, the low back, low abdomen, and buttocks—is altered *internally* in disorders of the musculoskeletal system. Should the midpoint of the torso represent the point of reference or should pairs of bony landmarks be the defining factors? This problem of malalignment of the endoskeleton, or part of it, versus the "sausage" of the torso is dealt with elsewhere in this text. The problem of interpreting asymmetry in images needs to be recognized. The recognition of imperfections in

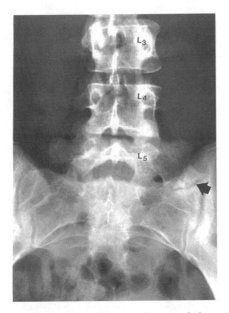

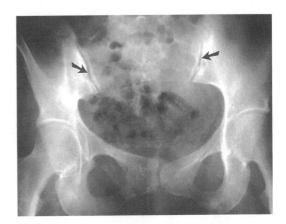

*Figure 9-8:* A pelvis with alar asymmetry and sacroiliac joint osteoarthritic changes (closed arrows). Note the asymmetry of S-1 joint, the ilial rotation, and the symphysis pubis. These are changes of a pelvis in asymlocation.

*Figure 9-7:* The pelvis showing sacral alar and transverse process of L5 asymmetry and the presence of a pseudoarthrosis (closed arrow) between these two structures on the left. The L4-5 relationship is near normal, but there is right rotation and right side bending of L3 on L4.

alignment radiologically can supplement clinical observations in the assessment of strains in the ligament and fascial supporting tissues and help identify somatic dysfunctions. (A number of lines can be drawn on the films as visual aids.)

## Plain Films of the Pelvis

Anteroposterior and lateral standing films are recommended (Denslow et al. 1983). The patient should stand on a level floor. Leaning sideways can affect the level of the femoral heads if the feet are not parallel. To eliminate this artifact, the patient should stand as straight as possible, and the heels should be placed under the femoralheads. A close approximation to this can be achieved by drawing parallel lines on the floor 6 inches apart and asking the patient to align the medial aspects of the feet to the outside of these markings. The

Bucky should be upright and aligned accurately in all planes. Horizontal and vertical lines thus will be parallel to the edge of the film. A spirit level or plumb line should be used to check these alignments. Visualizing the pelvis as a symmetrical inverted triangle helps in viewing the films (Figure 9-9), (Kapndji *ibid*). Lines drawn across the femoral heads are expected to be horizontal (Beal 1987; Kraus 1949) as well as a line drawn across the iliac crests. A third line, which should be horizontal, is drawn across the sacral base. The radiographic landmark recommended is to the small indentation just lateral to the facet joints or the sacral sulcus. (These lines usually are easily identifiable and are far enough apart to assess their inclination to the horizontal.) This landmark is not always clearly discernible, however, and asymmetries in its structure are not always associated with overall asymmetry in the position of the sacrum. An alternative landmark using the inferior aspects of the sacroiliac joints has been recommended. Because this landmark is subject to more variation, difference in height of these points offers a weaker clue to important dysfunction.

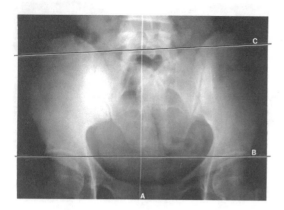

*Figure 9-9:* Pelvis with visual aids. Line A is a true vertical line. Line B shows that the legs are of equal length. Line C, which is on the sacral base, slopes down on the right, and demonstrates a sacral tilt. This is radiographic evidence of sacral asymlocation. Note the midline position of L5 and the symphysis pubis but the asymmetry of the sacrum and the iliac bones.

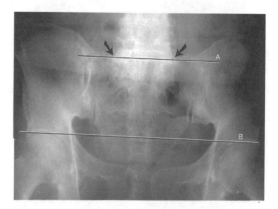

*Figure 9-10:* This is a pelvis with sacral tilt, but the slope to the left is created by unequal leg lengths. The line across the sacral base (A) is parallel with the line across the femoral heads (B) but not level with the horizon. The closed arrows point to the sacral notches, which are a good location to establish the sacral base.

Instances are found when leg-length discrepancy is present, and, although these several lines are not horizontal, they are parallel (Figure 9-10), (Kappler 1983). Leg-length discrepancy is usual, but it has been found that the recommendation for heel elevation is best made on clinical grounds (Greenman *ibid*). When the lines marking the sacral base and the femoral heads are not parallel, sacral torsion or dysfunction is indicated (Figure 9-8 through Figure 9-11).

**3.** An effect produced by the lines of projection when the image was recorded.

When the entire pelvis is turned in one direction by 5-10°, a striking change in the image is created.

## Sacroiliac Joints

The sacroiliac joints are notoriously asymmetrical (Fryette 1954; Solonen 1957). Radiographic asymmetry may be caused by:

**1.** A natural or congenital structural asymmetry.

**2.** Asymmetric projection from an acquired dysfunction, such as sacral asymlocation.

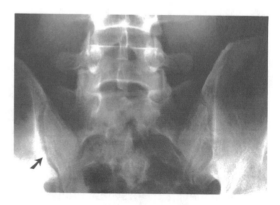

*Figure 9-11:* Close-up of a pelvis with sacral asymlocation. Note the unilateral osteitis condensans ilii (closed arrow).

*Osteitis Condensans Ilii*

Increased density of the iliac bone in proximity to the sacroiliac joints goes by the name osteitis condensans ilii. The phenomenon is attributed to increased stress in the iliac bone from increased stress at the sacroiliac joints and is more commonly seen in women (Figure 9-11), (Kricum 1988). When an increased density involves the whole of one iliac bone, the condition is termed *generalized osteitis condensans alii* and does not have this significance (Figure 9-12).

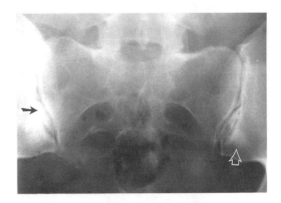

*Figure 9-12:* Close-up of sacrum with generalized osteitis condensans ilii on the right (closed arrow) and localized osteitis on the left (open arrow). Asymmetric osteitis condensans ilii is a common finding with sacral asymlocation. The "bull's eye" effect is created by a gas shadow over the left S-1 joint.

*Local Manifestations of Arthritis at the Sacroiliac Joint*

In young persons a small site of bone loss can be seen at the lower end of the sacroiliac joint on the sacral side. This is an early radiographic pointer to acute joint dysfunction or strain and may precede more obvious osteoarthritic changes, such as formation of osteophytes (Figure 9-14 and Figure 9-13).

The sacroiliac joint space is hard to evaluate on X-ray. The lucency represents subsynovial cartilage and normally varies between 2mm and 5mm. When identified and seen to be reduced, the loss represents disease, either degenerative or inflammatory process.

**Lateral Film of Pelvis**

Lateral films of the pelvis are notoriously difficult to evaluate, but some useful information can be gleaned. A line drawn along the anterior surface of the sacral base creates an angle with the horizontal. This is called *Ferguson's angle*. This angle is large in cases in which the sacrum tends toward the horizontal. There is an increased lordosis, as well. In this situation, increased stress occurs at the lumbosacral zygoapophyseal joints (Figure 9-15). The position of the coccyx should be noted in the lateral film (Figure 9-16).

**Magnetic Resonance Imagery & Computed Tomography of the Pelvis**

Ordinarily, the patient will lie supine for MRI and CT scans. In some instances, the patient is unable to lie flat comfortably. This alone might be responsible for asymmetry of the bony structures in the image; but in cases in which the posteriorsuperior iliac spines and apex of the sacrum make contact with the plinth, asymmetry in appearance of bony landmarks probably indicates an acquired distortion of the pelvic ring, such as an ilial upshear or sacral asymlocation (Figure 9-17 and Figure 9-18). (An asymmetry in the width of the sacroiliac joint itself also depends on the three factors listed), (Resnik 1985).

Because of the large amount of three dimensional information acquired with computer-assisted imaging, these modalities have the prospect of providing detailed information on acquired malalignment and other dysfunctions. The precise classification of this information and its integration into clinical nomenclature represents an exciting challenge.

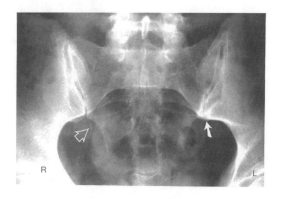

*Figure 9-13:* Pelvis demonstrating degenerative joint disease of the sacroiliac joint. Left sacroiliac joint with prominent osteophytes inferiorly (closed arrow) and loss of space. The open arrow points to right S-1 joint, which shows unequal loss of joint space. The open arrow points to a small vascular calcification.

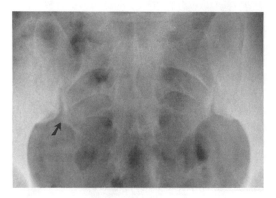

*Figure 9-14:* Anterior-posterior view of the pelvis and sacrum with the arrow pointing to the site of the demineralization at the inferior margin of the right sacroiliac joint. This is an early sign of degenerative joint disease.

When the pelvic ring is distorted, as in sacral asymlocation, it is common to observe one ilium rotated anteriorly. This is analogous to the movement in the rear differential of a car. In these cases, it is observed that when the patient lies flat, the anterior-superior iliac spines in the gantry before taking an image (with the help of a spirit level in these cases) may produce asymmetry of the posterior elements of the pelvic ring on the images. During walking, the pelvic ring moves with every step. In cases in which it does not return to symmetry on lying down, there is an appearance of leg-length discrepancy. This can be corrected by the Wilson/Barstow maneuver in those cases in which the asymmetric position is not stuck (Mitchell 1979; Don Tingny 1985). It is not known if there is any difference in the appearance of the images in these cases (versus those of pain from a stuck asymlocation). It would be surprising if there were.

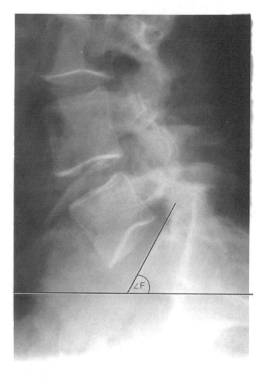

*Figure 9-15:* Lateral lumbar spine at the lumbosacral junction. Ferguson's angle (F) is demonstrated and is abnormal, that is greater than 45°.

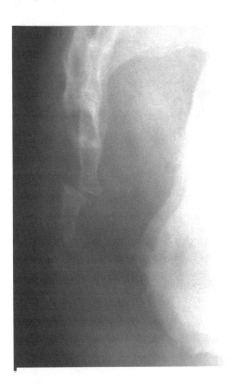

Figure 9-16: Lateral view of sacrum with dislocated coccyx.

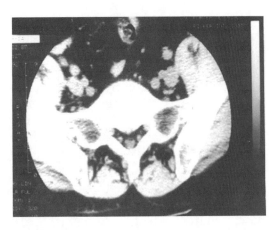

Figure 9-18: CT scan of the pelvis. Note the asymmetries. This is interpreted as a "sacral torsion" and not because of patient positioning on the scanning table.

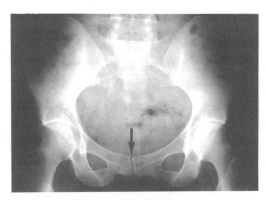

Figure 9-19: Right symphysis pubis (arrow) is high. Note the other changes of pelvic dysfunction, and the side-bending of L5.

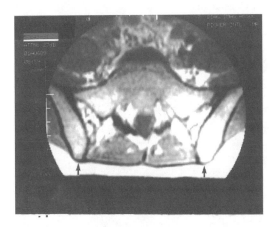

Figure 9-17: MRI scan of normal sacrum and ilii. Note the symmetry of the ilii and that the sacral ala are parallel with the base of the film. The closed arrows point to the PSIS.

## The Symphysis Pubis

Anatomic asymmetry in this fibrocartilaginous joint often is visualized radiologically, particularly in ilial up-slip and down-slip, as defined by osteopathic medicine (Figure 9-19).

Acute shears at this site, labeled *pubitis*, can cause widening of the joint space. Chronic pubitis can be manifested by loss of joint space and osteophyte formation Figure 9-20).

## Imaging Considerations in the Lumbar Spine

The lumbar spine is normal in 10% of X-rays (Ford 1966). Degenerative changes of apophyseal joints or disc space narrowing at one or more levels is seen in 50% of the X-rays taken in a survey of an apparently normal population. Abnormal flexion and extension views or altered motility can be demonstrated in 25% of samples of otherwise healthy persons. Abnormal facet joints and an abnormal number of vertebrae occur in 10% of all cases. The clinical importance of the situation depends on the situation (Frymoyer 1986; Nachemson 1975; Scavone 1981).

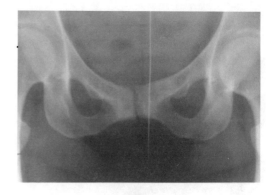

*Figure 9-20:* Acute pubitis. There is considerable adjacent bony sclerosis and loss of symphysis pubis joint space.

### Congenital Abnormalities

The identification of congenital abnormalities in the lumbar spine is important because some abnormalities will influence the treatment and others will explain the patient's symptoms. An attempt to identify the number of lumbar vertebrae might be hampered by transitional abnormalities. Spina bifida occulta of the vertebrae occurs in 20% of spines (Boone 1985). If prolotherapy of the lumbar spine is contemplated, the presence of this congenital defect might change the approach to the interspinous ligaments. In the presence of spina bifida, the possibility of an arachnoid cyst at these levels should be kept in mind. A transverse process of L5 may form a joint with ipsilateral sacral ala, creating an unstable situation with a pseudoarthrosis that may be a source of pain (Figure 9-7), (Jonsson 1989). The iliolumbar ligament also traverses this space and may become inflamed sympathetically. Injecting the pseudoarthrosis with a small amount of local anesthetic and steroid can be helpful.

### Zygoapophyseal Joints

It would seem logical that the orientation of the zygapophyseal joints at the lumbosacral junction *should be* the same on both sides. Asymmetry in the orientation will create an area of stress in the supporting fascial and ligament tissues. It, therefore, is not surprising to find that when these joints are asymmetric in their orientation, osteoarthritic or degenerative changes are common (Fryette *ibid*). If the lumbosacral apophyseal joints are mainly coronal in their orientation (that is, thoracic-like), they allow more rotation and side bending than the typical sagittal-lumbar-type zygoapophyseal joints. The orientation easily can be seen on MRI and CT scans but can also be determined from an AP lumbar X-ray (Van Schaik 1985).

### Visual Aids

Many geometric lines and angles have been drawn as diagnostic aids on films. Two angles are described below:

**1.** On the plane lateral film on the lumbosacral junction, a line is drawn along the anterior surface of the sacral base, creating an angle with the horizontal. This, as stated previously, is defined as *Ferguson's angle*. This angle is large when the sacrum tends toward the horizontal and there is an increased lordosis. In this situation increased stress occurs at the lumbosacral zygoapophyseal joints.

2. The lumbosacral angle is measured by drawing a line through the L5-S1 disc space and a second line through the T12-L1 disc space. The angle between them defines the pelvic tilt in degrees and also is a comment on the lumbar lordosis. Several exercise programs have been developed in an attempt to alter this angle, some leading to claims of clinical benefit (Gracovetsky 1989).

*Soft-Tissue Observation*

The psoas muscles are the major flexors of the lower trunk and thighs. They also stabilize the lumbar spine in side bending. By and large they are not palpable, so observations on them are indirect. Trunk list and somatic dysfunction in the lumbar and thoracolumbar spine are maintained by psoas contraction. On plain AP X-rays, the psoas shadow usually can be made out. If then shadows representing the muscle are asymmetric, spasm can be suspected. The *bulging* of one psoas compared to the other can result in a slight increase in density of the muscles and manifest as a *whitening*. This is often associated with a type 1 lumbar scoliosis to the side of the muscle spasm. Changes in the appearance of the muscle with trunk list also are visible on CT and MRI images, sometimes giving a clue to muscle spasm. These imaging modalities allow the radiologist to measure the cross section of the muscle and compare the sides. In scoliosis the muscle on the concave side lies further from the midline and its cross section is rounder. This is the equivalent of bulging and whitening seen on plain film (Mayer 1989; Gordon 1984; Tracy 1989).

On plain films it often is possible to identify renal shadows. When these shadows are abnormally low in standing films the term *ptosis* can be applied. In modern practice, the concept of disease from renal ptosis is obsolete to the point of taboo. Nonetheless, there are instances that seem to indicate that (in some cases) low back pain can arise from this uncertain entity, presumably by traction on the perirenal fascia, thus provoking psoas spasm. this problem may be connected with flexion injuries occurring over a seatbelt (Barral 1989).

The bones on the plain films should be screened for abnormalities that might represent metabolic or other bone disease, such as primary or secondary bony neoplasms. The soft tissues should be screened for extraneous information (such as calcification of the abdominal aorta, the presence of lower abdominal masses, kidney stones, gallstones, faecoliths, and the like).

# A New Understanding of the Human Pelvis[1]

## Prelude

Advances in human acumen peak when East meets West. Concepts, ideas, and science stagnate in the dogma of stable societies. The paradigm shift was defined for modern philosophy by Thomas Kuhn (1962). It has, however, been a distinction of our civilization, Western civilization, that after each cycle of decay it has arisen, like a phoenix, five times, with each resurgence rising to higher levels of achievement, always following an Eastern challenge (Ouigley and Carroll 1966) and contrasting with the doom of the other twenty-four civilizations recorded in available history (Spengler and Oswald 1932). It

---

1. This section is written by Thomas Dorman MD.

is fitting, therefore, to place the account which follows in a book which challenges West with East, a book which raises fundamental questions about what we are doing with health care in the West. Our scientific paradigm hails from Descartes. The reductionist analysis of the body/machine is based on its component parts. This paradigm contrasts with the holistic one which marked the Middle Ages and was represented diacritically by the famous Jewish Arabist philosopher and healer, Maimonides (ben Maimon 1075).

All work is built on contemporary foundations. Extraordinarily, this is true of major religions (Baigent et al. 1991). Contrariwise, new concepts are said to arrive, seemingly immaculately formed, in the minds of inventors during sleep (O'Neill, Prodigal genius). Whether discoveries are planted in these selected minds by intuition, preternatural influences or merely through the unconscious grinding of the gears of logic remains an enigma. Pondering upon this is best left to the intimate thoughts of the reader.

## Locomotion & Oscillation

Foreword advancement of any organism, in its own medium, be it flight, swimming or walking, is by a process of cyclic movements. This usually involves more than one organ, whereby energy is restored into the system rhythmically through oscillation. The momentum, the flywheel effect, is achieved either through the recoil of elastic tissues or the oscillation of a weight like pendulum. The trunk of the bounding cat, the tail of the hopping kangaroo, the limbs of a galloping camel all represent these mechanisms. It was believed until recently that in the case of human walking (in contrast to running) no energy is stored and released (McNeil 1988). Whether the development of mechanical clocks took its cues from nature is unknown. Be that as it may, the mechanism of a pendulum is one where kinetic and antigravitational potential energy alternate. The clockwork mech-

anism allows the escapement of the stored (mainspring) energy to be released regularly, rhythmically, efficiently through the use of a pendulum. It was the invention of Christiaan Huygens (1629-1695), a Dutch watchmaker, who was first able to store elastic energy in a spring liberating reliable time-keeping mechanisms for the first time from what we now call long-case clocks. In the spring-driven escapement we have an analogy to the second oscillating mechanisms in locomotion of organisms including that of our own.

## Human Walking

Amongst mammals only Homo sapiens is an erect organism. Even the species which are closest to humans, as judged by comparative anatomy, the apes, are essentially quadruped creatures, which, like the domestic dog, can rise on their hind legs temporarily. In walking, humans swing their arms. These short pendulums store and release antigravitational energy and contribute to the overall efficiency of the locomotor mechanism, which, in reality, is the whole of our body. Note that the arms swing to and aft alternately on the two sides, thereby creating torque through the upper girdle, and in brisk walking note how the upper girdle rotates alternately with each step versus the pelvis. This torque represents storage and release of elastic energy in the fascial layers of the trunk, particularly the paraspinal ligaments. The lower limbs also serve as pendulums. An easy way to appreciate their role as pendulums is to watch an individual walking on a treadmill. In this situation the body is stationary against the surrounding room and it is easy to see how each leg rises and falls alternately with the other and how the advancement of the trunk of the walking person is not continuous but oscillates depending on the phase in the cycle of movement of the legs. As the swing-leg accelerates, the trunk slows, relatively, and with planting that leg decelerates while the trunk speeds up. The trunk accelerates and decelerates with each leg swing cycle. This phenomenon is repeated, of course, when the other leg takes over the pendular-swing function. It is self-evident that the legs have the additional function of stance, and it is also self-evident that these functions alternate between the sides and within the cycle. How is the energy of momentum, the kinetic energy, transferred from the leg (pendulum) to the trunk? It is evident that they are attached by the pelvis. Before answering how the forces are transferred, let us look at the example of the dynamic passive walker. This is a mechano-like assemblage in which the equivalent of a human torso is mounted on "thighs" through a horizontal transverse axle representing 'hips'. The knees are similarly represented (with extension blocks) and the feet are rockers. This mechanical contraption can imitate human forward walking down a slope angled at 3°, once it is started, without additional energetic input. The kinetic pendular energy of each leg is sufficient on planting, to transfer sufficient momentum to the torso to lift the second leg off the ground and bring it into swing. This device demonstrates, therefore, that walking is a dynamic-passive attribute of the balance and linkage geometry of the upright human (McGeer 1990). Experientially we know, of course, that taking a stroll on the level is an "exercise" consuming little effort. We see then that walking can be achieved through kinetic pendular mechanisms with little energy. The transfer of forces is simply through the mechanical linkages. Clearly, this applies to the human frame likewise and the pelvis is the relevant linkage.

Each of us will have had the experience of trying to walk without swinging the trunk or arms and have found it somewhat inconvenient. The swing of the arms and upper trunk is indeed not merely an atavistic neuronal release but a mechanical contribution through an oscillating mechanism. As a first approximation the efficiency is mechanical, dynamical and antigravitational. Additionally, however, in the living organism, we need to look at elastic energy as well. In the passive dynamic walker, there are no elastic components. On the other hand, the energy stored and released anti-gravitationally by the upper limbs (pendulums) is transferred into a torque of the trunk which in turn is applied through ligaments and fasciae which bind the lower lumbar vertebrae and sacrum to the ilia. The torque is transferred diffusely through the soft tissues. The mechanical loci of transfer are the (propeller-shaped) sacroiliac joints. It is through the *sacroiliac mechanism* that the flywheel effect of the rotation of the trunk with its attendant (upper limb) pendulums contributes to the momentum of walking.

### The Role of the Pelvis

It is becoming apparent that the construction of this mechanism is predicated on a unique role of the human pelvis. It has the task, so to speak, of combining stability in stance with mobility in swing. The mobility is not merely passive but has to allow the release of the stored elastic energy in the fasciae into the other moving parts. It is not surprising, therefore, when we find that the unique joints of the pelvis, the sacroiliac joints, are different anatomically and functionally from all other joints of the body. All other synovial joints are low friction devices. Contrariwise, the sacroiliac joint, though allowing (a small range of) movement, is a high friction device analogous to the clutch of a shift-stick automobile. It is in the unique anatomical characteristic that we also find the unique physiologic one—that is to say, the ability to maintain force closure on the stance side and unlock allowing the transfer of the elastic energy on the swing side.

An understanding of this relationship has developed in the last decade. The recognition of the unique characteristics of the sacroiliac joint, that of force closure, comes from the research of a group in Rotterdam (Vleeming, Steockart et al. 1990; Vleeming, Volkers et al. 1990). These researchers tested the friction coefficient of the surfaces of the sacroiliac joint by mechanical means and reviewed the macroscopic and microscopic anatomy of these surfaces. Measurements of the efficiency of walking, by way of assessing oxygen consumption while walking on a treadmill, were performed at Cal Poly State University in California, and it was found that arm swinging, the rise and fall of the trunk, leg swing, and rotation of the trunk each contribute to the efficiency of walking. This was evaluated through measuring the oxygen consumption of each of these components in itself and comparing the sum with the actual consumption of oxygen with normal walking (Dorman et al. 1993).

### Sacroiliac Joint Movement

There has existed in this century some erroneous teaching about the sacroiliac joints. A number of texts have stated categorically that no movement occurs at these joints (except in parturition). This chapter is not the place to contradict this fallacy. Suffice it to say that stereo photogranrratic studies (Egund et al. 1978; Lavingnolle et al. 1983) and actual radiologic cadaver imaging (Weisl 1955) have demonstrated movement at these joints. In life, movement has been demonstrated by placing Kirschner nails in the sacrum and ilium and watching the movement in walking individuals (Colachis et al. 1963). The range of movement and the axis of rotation, however, have been found to be extraordinarily variable amongst individuals, a finding which is not surprising in the face of the extraordinary variability in the anatomy of the joints themselves (Solonen 1957). Here there is an example where a reductionist analysis of movement, the analogy with moving mechanical devices, fails. The forces are transmitted through the soft tissues and attempts to analyze the mechanics in a manner analogous to that of moving parts and machinery has dissipated a lot of research energy with little yield. The *instantaneous access of rotation*

is a term used by engineers in attempts to define the mechanical relationship between irregularly moving surfaces predicated on the tension of the soft tissues. This writer has found this approach not useful from a biological and medical perspective.

### Pelvic Dysfunction

When a person stands on one leg he does not fall down. The vertical poise against gravity is predicated on balance as the upper part of the body is broader than the base (foot). Our ability to maintain balance in one legged stance is an achievement which physicists have graced with the term unstable equilibrium. We all know that in this situation minor sways of the body are countered by muscle action bringing the center of gravity back over the narrow base. It is the brain which senses the balance and commands the muscles. The second factor which allows us to remain in balance is the stability of the leg, the stable strut should, one would think, be made best of a pillar of bone. However, as we inspect the anatomy of our legs we find that the foot is mounted through the hinge of the ankle by the tibia, the femur is mounted on top of it through another hinge. The ball and socket of the hip is superseded by the last joint in this chain, the sacroiliac joint. The (floppy) spine is mounted on top. How is it then, that this loose jointed collection of bones serves as a pillar, and why all the joints? It is plain that the joints facilitate locomotion. The great architect was confronted, then, with the need for stability and mobility in the same structure. This article will concentrate on pelvic dysfunction, but first, a brief review of the other section of the pillar. The foot is planted and the leg hinges over the ankle as we walk over the stance foot. During this phase the knee is locked in (hyper) extension which converts the hinge to a solid leg as long as the force of gravity maintains the slight hyper-extending pressure. The quadriceps muscle guards this position; but in a normal knee stability is maintained passively by the ligaments.

In the case of the ball and socket (hip joint), as long as the femur is upright, the acetabulum has nowhere to go. Try standing on one leg, you will find that whether you allow your pelvis to sag (in the Trandelenberg position) or whether you hoist your body over your standing femur, the righting reflex maintains your center of gravity right over the leg, so that only slight muscular action is needed.

Stability at the sacroiliac joint is based on a more complex mechanism, which has recently been called *selfbracing* (Snijders, Vleeming and Stoeckart 1992). This is an excellent term, but is conceptually little different from the ex-center stability maintained through the knee. First let us review some anatomic details of the sacroiliac joint. This synovial joint, in contrast to the other synovial joints of the body, has a rough surface. This has been demonstrated both microscopically and macroscopically (Spengler and Oswald *ibid*). When the auricular surface is inspected frontally it has, as the name indicates, the approximate appearance of a pinna. As a simplified first approximation it is L shaped and opens backwards. The major stabilizing ligament of this joint, which incidentally is the thickest ligament in the human frame, is located at the elbow of the L. The collagenous fibers of this ligament are intertwined diagonally as they traverse the very short distance between the bones. The surfaces of the sacroiliac joints are not oriented in any of the primary body planes. As a first approximation one can see that the ilial surface faces medially, forward and superiorly. In adults the joint is not planar. The medial, superior and anterior facing applies to the upper (and larger) section of the joint. The inferior part is even more variable than the superior, but modally, usually faces medially, posteriorly and superiorly. It is helpful to think of the joint surface as similar to a propeller, or a corkscrew. The geometry of screws is best defined by the direction in which they

tighten (for instance clockwise tightening, the familiar direction). Tightening between sacrum and ilium in the case of the sacroiliac joint is not dissimilar. In contrast to a wood screw, the tightening of the sacroiliac joint is controlled by the main central ligament (which you might think of as a rope). As torque is applied the fibers are squeezed together and the rope tightens. As it is a very short rope the ilium and sacrum are forced together. The rough surfaces between them maintain stable approximation, hence the stability when weight is borne on one leg.

The direction of closure and tightening of the surfaces of the sacroiliac joint is based on its geometry. Closure is achieved as the superior end of the sacrum moves backward against the ilium. This has been defined as *counter nutation*. It is instinctual for us to think of rotation round an axis, but in fact the movement of most joints consists of a combination of rotation and gliding (Miller, Schultz and Andersson 1987). Engineers, in order to maintain their terminology of rotation, have coined the term *instantaneous axis of rotation* to define the minute fraction of the movement which has a theoretical axis at each degree of movement. This "point" moves with the glide, so they speak of a *moving instantaneous axis of rotation*. The interrelationship of these axes are a physicist's Ptolemaic calculus. To the clinician the action is in the ligaments. Here tightening through a twist is achieved and the bony surfaces are approximated. There is an extraordinary degree of variation in the detailed bony anatomy between individuals and even between the two sides. In any case the geometry of the joint goes through changes in each of us with aging. It is the function which remains the same during the walking phase of life. So in walking, through counter-nutation, with approximation of the bones and a variable glide of the auricular surfaces on each other, stability of the pillar is maintained during the stance phase. The pillar reverts to a flexible pendulum as the stride advances and the leg alternates into the swing phase; the knee unlocks, flexion occurs at the hip, and at the sacroiliac joint nutation occurs on that side; the sacroiliac ligament unwinds a little (incidentally restoring some elastic energy into the mechanism of locomotion) as the ilium moves slightly backward and medially on the sacrum.

The mechanism of locking at the sacroiliac joints alternates between the sides, locking on the stance side and unlocking on the swing side. Efficient walking is predicated on the mechanism being reliable. The fidelity consists of maintaining a stable strut in stance and unlocking on cue.

In the case of the movement of the peripheral joints, locking in stability, where it occurs is dependent on position and the forces surrounding the joint, but not dependent directly on the function of another joint. The sacroiliac joints are not so "lucky" because they share the sacrum. Even this versatile bone can move only in one direction at a time. Additionally, the ilia are united anteriorly at the syndesmosis of the symphysis. Herein lies the weakness of the human pelvis. In normal walking the sacroiliac joints lock and unlock on either side alternately, so that counternutation (locking) and nutation (unlocking) define the cyclic sequence; the phases being opposite on the two sides. As locking consists of a backward movement of the upper portion of the sacrum (Greenman 1990) versus the ilium, if locking were to occur simultaneously on both sides, there would be extreme counter nutation of the sacrum versus both ilia. Because of the angle of the sacroiliac joint in the coronal plane, the pelvic circumference would tend to enlarge. The ligaments will allow so much stretch that as the sacrum gets wedged, backward, between the two ilia, the ligaments are finally tightened. Due to the locking mechanism, discussed earlier, it is possible for the sacrum to become trapped in this position. The inferior surfaces of the sacroiliac joints are such that for entrapment at the lower level

of the pelvis to occur (as seen in the coronal plane) the inferior surface of the sacrum would need to move forward between the two ilia (this is also defined in the movement of counter nutation). As mentioned earlier, there is no distinct axis of rotation, so that this phenomenon, of self bracing, with entrapment of both sacroiliac joints (through counter nutation of the sacrum bilaterally) can occur in the upper portion of the pelvic ring, and at the level of the inferior portion of the sacroiliac joints, or at both simultaneously.

To make matters even more complicated entrapment can occur when the ilia are aligned symmetrically about each other, or when one is relatively more foreword than the other. The usual situation being an anterior right ilium in right handed individuals (LaCourse et al. 1990). Ligaments are elastic. When stretched, the abducting forces contained in the elasticity of the ligaments of the pelvic ring, particularly the posterior sacroiliac ligaments, tend to maintain the entrapment. The self bracing mechanism of the sacroiliac joint, through its propeller shape and rough surfaces, partakes in this entrapment. And so it is that if both legs play the role of being in the stance phase of locomotion simultaneously this phenomenon of pelvic entrapment can occur. Conceptually this is no more complicated than driving a wedge into a tight space. The terminological definition of the various possible positions of the three pelvic bones in relation to each other has exercised the profession of osteopathy for a hundred years, and it has been systematized only recently (Greenman 1989). It is estimated that the anterior rotation of the ilia, on one or both sides relative to the sacrum is common in a back pain population and is the root cause of most pelvic dysfunction, which in turn is responsible for many remote secondary soft tissue strains defined usually in osteopathic circles as local areas of somatic dysfunction. Manual correction, followed by self treatments of the anterior rotation and strengthening of the abdominal muscles relieves the problem in a large portion of the patients (DonTigny 1992). In most cases the first clinical observation is the loss of lordosis with pain in attempted extension at the lumbosacral level while standing. The usual range (for that patient) of rotation and side bending is also reduced, because the slack, usually present in the ligaments which would ordinarily allow these movements, is taken up by the abnormal (entrapped) position of the sacrum (Stevens 1992). The importance of the slack in the soft tissues was described first in the case of cross referred pain from dysfunction in the sacroiliac joints in pain from attempted straight leg raising (Mennell 1960). Pseudo-leg-length-discrepancy on lying supine is also usual, but can be found in individuals without pain as well. The presence of the asymmetry in normals, while it becomes more pronounced in patients with entrapment has been called asymlocation (Dorman 1991).

In the frontal plane the sacrum is seen to be wider at its cephalic end. This has led to the time honored impression that it functions like a *keystone* in an arch. Seemingly this observation is correct only when it is in *dysfunction*. It is, however, an observation of this practitioner that patients with pelvic dysfunction lose up to 2cm in height when their pelvis is dysfunctional. Some height is regained after successful manipulation. This (unpublished) observation supports the notion that the sacrum descends between the ilia with wedging, at least in some instances, with entrapment.

The human pelvis is mechanically unique. The phenomenon of entrapment through the maintained adducting forces of the elastic ligaments, which hold the three pelvic bones together, can last for long periods. When the sacrum is firmly entrapped this way the patient becomes dependent on an *external force* to unlock the dysfunction—manipulation. Sometimes the degree of entrapment is less severe and then certain maneuvers, which the patient can do himself, might suffice to restore optimal symmetry, or at least reduce the severity of the dysfunction.

This phenomenon of entrapment, of *somatic dysfunction*, is characteristic of but not confined to the human pelvis. Pelvic dysfunction is, however, usually present when the osteopath finds somatic dysfunction at any level of the axial skeleton. It is persistent or recurrent unless the pelvis is restored to normal. It is suggested here that the reason is the *unique quality of the human pelvis—entrapment*. The osteopaths' aphorism that pain is a liar is due to the fact that through the transfer of the tension in ligaments and fascia, the strain might be felt at a distant site.

Bipedality, by its inherent nature, necessitates alternating stance and swing phases of the legs. The transfer of weight from the central axial skeleton alternately to the legs is responsible for the inexorable mechanics of the human pelvis. These mechanics are quite different from those of all other creatures. The other bipedal animals, birds and dinosaurs, have different mechanics because they balance their tail and trunk like a see saw, in contrast to humans who balance the vertical torso over a point

We find, then, that a mechanical analysis of the function of ligaments affords us an understanding of the dynamical forces active in locomotion and explains both the function and dysfunction of the *unique* human pelvis. Future textbooks of medicine should contain a section on ligaments with a subsection on disordered mechanics after a suitable analysis of normal mechanics. The chapter headings regarding the management of dysfunction should include manipulation because when there is entrapment only manipulation can release it. The altered strength and elasticity of ligaments should be addressed. The available modalities of treatment include:

1. An adjustment in frequency of usage (rest and exercise).

2. Metabolic support systemically (nutrition).

**3.** Locally (prolotherapy [Ongley, Klein and Dorman 1987]).

Preventative measures should include advice about maintaining satisfactory alignment of mechanics. Perhaps ligament weakness can be attributed to a sedentary life style punctuated with acceleration deceleration forces on the axial skeleton. Does posture play a role? It is an unconfirmed observation that in primitive societies there is less back pain. It has been suggested that forces transferred via the hamstrings and the sacrotuberous ligament to the infero-lateral angle of the sacrum, tending to bring on nutation are present during squatting while maintaining lordosis of the lumbar spine (Martin 1975). These forces might serve pelvic alignment and training better than sitting in a chair. Is it possible that the epidemic of back pain in Western civilization is a side effect of comfortable furniture and the toilet seat?

### The Role of Prolotherapy

Hyperplasia of collagenous tissue can be achieved through stimulating inflammation. Indeed, it is the process of inflammation as originally defined by Eli Metchnikoff (1893) and subsequently studied by Cohnheim (1889) which has been known throughout the contemporary era of biological studies to be the source of organismal repair. It is this very inflammation which every surgeon (rightly) relies upon for wound repair in anticipation of suture removal. It has been known since the days of Hippocrates (Adams 1946) that the irritation of fibrous tissue can provoke hypertrophy and the term *sclerotherapy* was introduced by the osteopathic profession as early as 1937 (Gedney 1937) as an adaptation of the previously established techniques of healing used by herniologists before the advent of aseptic surgery. Scars were indeed produced by the marked irritant effect induced in these areas. With the recognition of the increasing epidemic

of ligamentous and fascial injuries in modern times, George Hackett (1958), an industrial surgeon from the Midwest, introduced a concept that the hypertrophy of ligamentous tissue might be achieved successfully without necessarily provoking scars and postulated that through fine tuning the amount of inflammation it might be possible to achieve that exact result. For this purpose he introduced the term prolotherapy and spent a number of years experimenting with several irritant solutions and observing the effect on experimental animals. Thereby, through a process of trial and error which by now was taken on in other English-speaking countries and in particular by M.J. Ongley in New Zealand, a number of substances were found to have the maximal therapeutic yield with minimal risk.

### Manipulation

The role of manual therapy has been subject to controversial argumentation to a large extent because of the mind set of establishment medicine introduced with the reorganization of medicine in 1910 (Flexner and Abraham 1910). Its undoubted usefulness has gained recognition through the force of the market place and was reported to constitute, in chiropractic hands alone, a four and a half billion dollar yearly industry in 1991 (Lawrence and Dana 1991). It is only in recent times that authoritative scientific writing has yielded a small place in the dejure scientific pantheon to what is defacto a common experience of most individuals who have suffered back pain and have been treated manually (Shekelle et al. 1992).

### Combined Management of Back Pain

In spite of some comments earlier in this chapter about the possible limitations of the reductionist approach, the use of diagnosis has remained central in orthopedic medicine. The cardinal characteristics of ligaments are clinical manifestations of dysfunction. These have been defined elsewhere (Dorman *ibid*). In abbreviated summary, one might state that persistent pain from maintenance of tension for long periods (posain) and a phenomenon on a false sensation of a numb-like feeling (nulliness) have been recognized. These terms have been used in the last half decade seemingly propitiously. Finally one should comment that ligaments lend themselves to imaging poorly and dysfunction does not have an imaging counterpart at all in these structures. Finally there are no laboratory tests for abnormal ligaments. The clinicians have, therefore, been thrown back on their bedside skills and a knowledge of anatomy, both waning in an age of the quick fix, the reductionist approach, and molecular biology. Its not surprising, therefore, that the remnant of practitioners waging these skills are found at the margins of the profession amongst foreign and older doctors who are a little less influenced by the whirlwind of political, academic and scientific correctness which are formatting received opinion and practice guidelines like a gel.

## Ongley's Technique

The combination of manipulation with ligament refurbishing, or prolotherapy, can be seen as the logical outcome of the discussion above. We owe, however, to the genius of that man the combination of manipulation with prolotherapy and a number of additional essential components creating what is now called the Ongley technique. It goes without saying that this approach is appropriate only in cases where the diagnosis of persistent somatic dysfunction in the pelvis is confirmed and where more significant disease has been excluded. Does the refurbishment of the posterior sacroiliac ligaments with prolotherapy work? The clinical effectiveness has been subject to two clinical trials (Ongley *ibid*; Klein, Eek, DeLong and Mooney

1993) and the mechanical changes in the alignment of the iliac bones versus each other, tending to symmetry with treatment has also been shown. Most recently it has also been found that the efficiency of walking, as judged by oxygen consumption improves after treatment (Dorman et al. 1995). This last observation ties the treatment by Ongley's technique into the new understanding of the role of the pelvis in locomotion.

## The Sliding Clutch Syndrome

In back pain clinics it seems there are a number of individuals who report episodic falling. The leg gives way when entering into stance irregularly and unexpectedly. This is an intrinsic injury (Mennell 1964). The patient's reaction is one of embarrassment and persistent dysfunction is never seen. It is, of course, important for the clinician to separate these episodes of falling from other causes of loss of function such as epilepsy, cardiac arrhythmias, and loose bodies in joints. In any case, it has been found by this writer that in a number of cases, who were treated with prolotherapy to the posterior sacroiliac joint ligaments, these episodes of falling cleared up. So, through serendipity, it was realized that the falling (dysfunction) was due to momentary slippage of the sacroiliac joint (clutch) as the subject entered into stance. This caused them to lose balance and fall. Not surprisingly, no defect of the central nervous system can ever be detected in these cases. The sobriquet given to this condition, the slipping clutch syndrome, is an attempt at an analysis of the cause as well as a shorthand description.

## In Summary

The tenets of this chapter are:

1. The human pelvis is unique in bipedal locomotion. Its function is that of a gearbox transferring forces for the enhanced efficiency of walking.

**2.** The efficiency of walking is predicated on the flywheel effect of the moving parts.

**3.** Antigravitational pendular limb movements contribute to the storage and release of energy.

**4.** Elastic recoil in ligaments and fasciae throughout the body contribute to the storage and release of energy.

**5.** The ligamentousfascial organ functions as a whole.

**6.** Dysfunction of the clockwork, or transducer-like role of the pelvis, is predicated on its unique delicate balance.

**7.** With persistent dysfunction, in addition to pain, there is inefficiency in walking.

**8.** Dysfunction at the sacroiliac joint can manifest itself by mechanical failure, the slipping clutch syndrome, and with pain.

**9.** An understanding of the mechanics and mechanical dysfunction explains the effectiveness of the two clinical tools.

**10.** The clinical tools for dealing with the problems (in addition to correct diagnosis) are manipulation and prolotherapy.

**11.** Tensegrity is the term used to convey the phenomenon of transferred forces through a structure constituted of tension and compression members, like the skeletal ligamentous system. An understanding of tensegrity is required, therefore, in management.

## OM Disorders

Back pain was described over 2,000 years ago in the medical writings of Dr. Chun Yu Yi. In the classic book *The Canon of Inter-*nal Medicine, he states that the back is the Fu of the Kidney. Dr. Chun relayed several etiologies for back pain such as traumatic injury and invasion of Wind-Cold and Wind-Heat, and he stated that back pain is related closely to the Zhong Fu (Organs) and channels. The classic book *General Treatise on the Causes and Symptoms of Diseases* divides back pain into five general categories:

**1.** Dysfunction of the Shao Yin system.

> The Kidney is part of the Shao Yin system, and its Yang Qi is weakened in October. This can result in back pain due to Kidney Yang Qi damage.

**2.** Wind Bi (painful obstruction), Wind-Cold invasion.

**3.** Overexertion weakening the Kidney Qi.

**4.** Trauma.

**5.** Sleeping in a wet, cold area.

In the Ysui dynasty, authors suggested that the Kidney system controls the back and legs, realizing that back pain and lower extremity pain may be related.

Injury, weakening and laxity of soft tissues have been described as causes of many chronic back conditions in OM. The chapter Exploration of Pathology in *Familiar Conversation* states:

> People in their fifties are in a state of deficiency. Their Liver Qi is deficient and therefore their sinews are rigid, their Kidneys are exhausted, impairing healing and regeneration of tissues, their Bone Marrow is empty, leading to weak bones.... Deficiency of the Governing and Girdle channels leads to looseness of sinews and spinal deterioration.

Back pain is generally divided into Internal and External causes. External and Independent causes are seen with sprains, Qi and Blood stasis, and/or Wind-Cold, Wind-Damp and Wind-Heat. External causes effect mostly the channels.

Internal causes generally are divided into; Kidney deficiencies (Yin, Yang or Essence), and Liver dysfunctions (Blood, Qi or Yin deficiency, and/or stasis). Some channel dysfunctions that result in back pain, especially of the Girdle (Dai) channel, Governing (Du) channel, Penetrating (Chong) and Yang and Yin linking (Wei) channels can be considered internal. Strains, that often result due to weakness, have an internal component, as well.

# Biomedical Disorders

Table 3-13 on page 631 (appendix B) summarizes some non-orthopedic biomedical causes of back pain.

## Ligamentous Disorders

Ligamentous disorders are extremely common causes of chronic low back pain. They are seen often in patients with recurring pain and spinal and sacroiliac joint instability. Pain is characterized by the so called "cocktail syndrome" where the patient has a difficult time standing still. Pain is worse in the morning and improves with movement. A numb like sensation (nulliness) is common. Table 3-2 on page 439 summarizes ligamentous pain from the lumbo-sacral areas. Figure 9-21 through Figure 4-23 on page 438 illustrate the pain patterns.

### Sacroiliac Ligaments

Pain from different areas of the SI ligaments can be referred to various regions of the pelvic area and leg. It usually skips the knee or other large joints. (Hachett, Hemwall, and Montgomery 1991).

Pain from the *upper portion* of the sacroiliac joint tends to refer to the outside of the buttock, the outer part of the thigh, and the lateral part of the upper calf over the upper portion of the fibula. Pain in L4

and L3 distributions is seen as well (Dorman and Ravin 1991).

Pain from the *lower part of the upper portion* of the SI ligaments refers in a sacrotuberous ligament distribution. Dorman posits that pain from the sacrotuberous ligament is the most common cause of *false sciatica*. Often pain is felt in wide distribution at the upper, outer buttock, with radiation to the posterolateral thigh and leg, sometimes reaching the sole of the foot. Pain from the *portion below* (of upper portion) refers a little more medially, to the posterolateral part of the buttock, and to the thigh and calf, a little more posteriorly than that which came from the upper ligamentous portion.

Pain that arises from the ligamentous attachments of the *middle portion* of the sacrum (aponeurosis over the multifidus muscle) approximately at the level of S3 spreads across the middle of the buttock in an inverted horseshoe shape distribution (Dorman and Ravin 1991). Pain from the sacrococcygeal ligament is felt down both thighs in S1-2 distribution. Unilateral back pain often originates from the posterior SI ligaments.

Pain from the *lowest portion* refers in the sacrospinous distribution. Pain from the sacrospinous ligament is felt over the upper, outer buttock, with a thin line radiating down the midline and into the fold of the buttock and, if severe, down the midline of the leg as far as the heel.

EFFECTS OF SACRAL MOVEMENTS. Usually sacral rotations are to the opposite side from L5 movements. During lumbar flexion the base of the sacrum extends (counternutation), and during lumbar extension the sacrum flexes (nutation). When a patient leans back, extending the spine, the sacral base moves anteriorly and the apex moves posteriorly and superiorly. This stretches the sacrospinous and tuberous ligaments, and it can provoke symptoms of these ligaments. Sidebending away from the affected side is painful, as well. In flexion the sacral base moves posteriorly (counternutation) and increases tension in

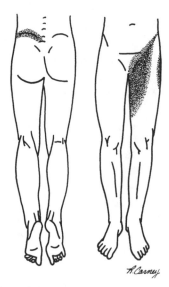

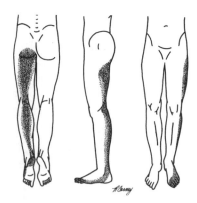

*Figure 9-23:* Referred pain from sacrotuberous ligament (With permission Dorman and Ravin 1991).

*Figure 9-21:* Referred pain from the iliolumbar ligament (with permission Dorman and Ravin 1991)

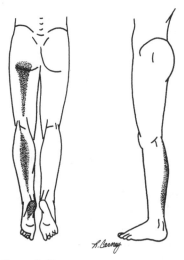

*Figure 9-22:* Referred pain from sacrospinous ligament (With permission Dorman and Ravin 1991).

cific radiographic control, can lead to pain of the buttock, thigh, and calf. The larger the volume injected the more distal the pain is referred. Facet irritation can limit the straight leg raise (SLR) and increase tension of the hamstrings and inhibit the local reflex arc. The level of the lumbar spine injected does not change the referral pattern significantly. The L3-4 facet refers a little more laterally. This evidence suggests that facet dysfunction cannot be differentiated from other sources of pain by the pattern or distribution of pain observed (Mooney and Robertson 1976), and is probably due to facet innervation which comes from 3 neural segments (Brown 1995).

The facet joints contain or develop menisci which can lead to internal derangement (Mercer and Bogduk 1993). The multifidus muscle attaches to the facet capsule and has the potential to move this meniscus. Pain from the posterior capsule, which is associated with spasms in the multifidus muscle—that cross the joint, and are innervated by the same nerves may be referred to the buttocks and may be indistinguishable from discogenic pain (Taylor and Twomey 1992). The multifidus muscle is a stabilizer of the facet joints as well as being an extensor of the spine. Lesions in the multifidus muscles may result in pain with similar distribution.

the lumbosacral ligaments (Dorman *ibid*). *These patterns should always be considered when a patient presents with "sciatica" like pain.*

### FACET DISORDERS

Mooney has shown that injection of the facets with hypertonic saline, under spe-

The relative contributions of the disc and facet joint in chronic low back pain has been studied by Schwarzer et al. (1994). The authors found that about 40% of patients had a probable discogenic source, and about 20% had a facet source. Less than 10% had a combination of both. They concluded that in patients with chronic low back pain, the combination of discogenic pain and facet joint pain is uncommon.

They also studied the clinical features of patients with pain stemming from the lumbar facets. They found that the response to facet joint injection was not associated with any single clinical feature or set of clinical features, and concluded that the facet joint is an important source of pain, but the existence of a "facet syndrome" must be questioned (Schwarzer, Aprill, Derby, Fortin, Kine and Bogduk 1994).

*Table 9-2.* **LIGAMENTOUS PAIN**

| LIGAMENT | GENERAL CHARACTERISTICS | FELT AT |
|---|---|---|
| **ILIOLUMBAR LIGAMENT** | Sprain is common<br>  — due to torsional injuries or an unleveled sacral base<br>Often the first ligament that causes back pain<br>  — quadratus lumborum is frequently involved as well | Pain felt in L1-4 sclerotomes<br>Pain provoked by trunk rotation to and sidebending away from ligament |
| **LUMBOSACRAL AND INTERSPINOUS LIGAMENTS** | Common cause of midline low back pain | From the ligamentous attachments to the middle portion of the sacrum (aponeuroses over the multifidus muscle) the pain:<br>  — spreads across the middle of the buttock in an inverted horseshoe shape distribution<br>Pain provoked by prolonged standing, sitting, lying or full flexion<br>Rotation often is normal.<br>At times extension is painful, as fibers may be squeezed between the spines |
| **DORSAL SI** | Very common cause of back and leg pain | Referred to various regions of the pelvic area and leg<br>It usually skips the knee or other large joints |
| **SACROSPINOUS LIGAMENT** | Commonly seen with hip-like pain | Felt over the upper, outer buttock<br>  — with a thin line radiating down the midline and into the fold of the buttock<br>  — if severe, down the midline of the leg as far as the heel |
| **SACROTUBEROUS LIGAMENT** | Commonly mistaken as sciatica | Similar to Sacrospinous<br>  — but in a wider distribution<br>  — may affect the heel only |
| **SACROCOCCYGEAL LIGAMENT** | Often with local semipros | Felt down both thighs in S1-2 distribution |

## Disc Disorders

Disc lesions in the lumbar spine can be divided generally into internal disc derangement, annular fissures and the more traditional disc excursions (for more information see chapter 3).

### The Mckenzie System

The McKenzie system is helpful in the evaluation and treatment of disc derangements. Loading strategies that include static postures and dynamic movements are assessed. The patient is first asked to perform a single movement for each loading strategy to be examined. The practitioner assess the range and quality of the movement and not symptoms. Then, the patient is instructed to perform repeated movements in each of the planes—repetitive movements are necessary to accurately assess each movement plane, a single movement or moment's positioning may give a false impression. At the end of each movement series symptoms, especially periferalization, are noted.

If necessary over pressure by the practitioner can be added at the end range of each movement. Static postures, at end range, are evaluated by asking the patient to hold each position for some time. Static loading tests generally are used when dynamic tests do not reveal a clear result (McKenzie and Jacobes 1996).

In the lumbar spine the practitioner evaluates: Flexion standing (Figure 9-25).

**6.** Extension standing (Figure 9-24).

**7.** Flexion supine (Figure 9-26).

**8.** Extension prone (Figure 9-27).

**9.** Extension with lateral shift prone (Figure 9-28).

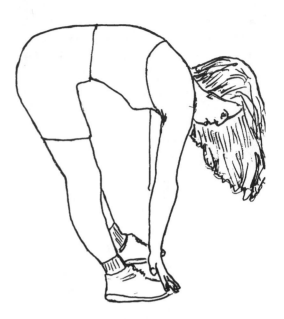

*Figure 9-25:* Standing flexion.

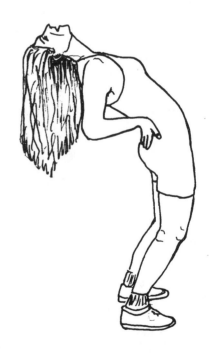

*Figure 9-24:* Standing extension.

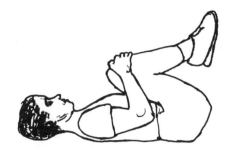

*Figure 9-26:* Supine flexion.

These fissures often are open and leak chemical inflammatory mediators into the CSF and around the nerve root. Such chemical irritants have been postulated to be the cause of a chemical rediculite that can simulate a disc protrusion-like pain (Brown *ibid*).

## Disc Protrusions

When significant disc material encroaches on the nerve root, radicular pain may ensue, followed by palsy (although MRI studies show nerve root compression in

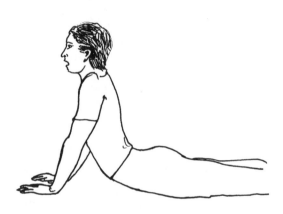

*Figure 9-27:* Extension prone.

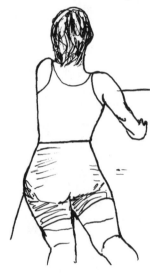

*Figure 9-28:* Extension with lateral shift prone.

Postures and movements that *centralize* and reduce the pain are used for treatment. Figure 9-29 shows a side-gliding technique for the treatment of lateral disc deviations.

## Annular Fissures

Annular fissures are characterized by chronic low back pain that may simulate SI joint and ligament like pain. This syndrome is considered to be very recalcitrant to conservative treatment.Usually the patient presents with a history of having failed therapy and stabilization training.

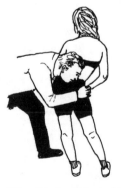

*Figure 9-29:* Side-glide treatment of lateral disc deviations.

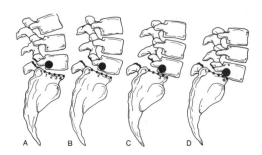

*Figure 9-30:* Spondylolisthesis, first through fourth grade (With permission Dorman and Ravin 1991).

normal, asymptomatic people, as well). Typically the patient experiences shooting pain in a dermatomal distribution. In posterolateral lesion the pain may be felt only in the leg, without back pain. This type of leg pain (sciatica) without back pain usually recovers by itself in 12-18 months. If pain spreads down the leg and at the same time increases in the back, this may be a danger sign of an expanding lesion. Serious lesions, such as a space occupying lesion or metastases should be excluded (Cyriax and Cyriax 1993).

Table 3-14 on page 633 summarizes symptoms related to the lumbar nerve roots. Table 3-15 on page 635 summarizes symptoms related to pressure on the sacral nerve roots. The dermatomes are illustrated in Figure 4-7 on page 81.

## Spondylolysis-Spondylolisthesis

Spondylolysis is a stress fracture and separation of one part of the vertebra, the pars interarticularis. The body pedicle and the superior articular pillar can slide anteriorly, while the spinous process, the laminae and the inferior articular pillar are held posteriorly. This, or a slip of the entire vertebra (due to facet or ligament pathology), can be seen at any age. It may be congenital, traumatic or degenerative. However, recent studies have shown the that the lytic defect develops principally during childhood and adolescence (Figure 9-30 through Figure 9-32).

*Spondylolisthesis* can be separated into several types, the most common of which is fatigue separation of the pars interarticularis. A congenital arrangement in which the facets are more horizontal (sagittally) may result in a slippage forward of one side of the vertebra. Degeneration of the facets and of other ligaments may account for the remaining types. Spondylolisthesis is found in about 5% of asymptomatic populations (Brown *ibid*).

Spondylolisthesis may or may not cause pain, and when it does it is often intermittent. It comes on after prolonged standing, is aggravated by activity, and usually is felt in the low back, but can radiate to the buttock, outer thighs and legs. Usually the pain is bilateral and often is relieved by lying or sitting. Squatting often is restful (Dorman *ibid*). (Squatting is thought by some to be the reason back pain is less common in countries in which toilet seats are not used).

Hamstring tightness, limited flexion and marked lordosis is common. The resulting excess lordosis may shift gravitational loads more to the posterior elements (less on vertebral bodies and discs, more on the facet joints), wearing them out. The nerve roots may rub over a bony ledge.

Inspection often reveals a step-like abnormality that may be seen on standing or during motion, and which may disappear in the prone position. If the step remains the same between standing and lying, it may be considered stable, and it is less likely to cause symptoms or to progress (Brown *ibid*).

In symptomatic patients, the interspinous ligaments over the segments are tender. Bilateral leg pain is common and is aggravated by standing and is alleviated by flexion. Spinal claudication syndrome should be considered (Paris *ibid*).

Just as ligament insufficiency is common with spondylolisthesis, so is recurrence of symptoms.

**IMAGING.** This lesion of the pars interarticularis can be identified on the AP and lat-

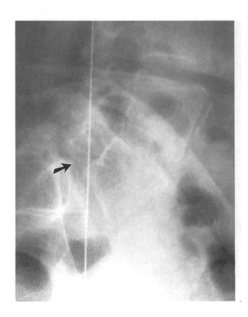

*Figure 9-31:* Lateral lumbar spine with degenerative spondylolisthesis. Note the arrow points to the area of anterior displacement of L5 on the sacrum.

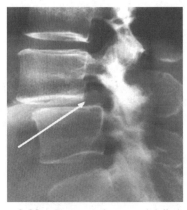

*Figure 9-32:* Degenerative spondylolisthesis at L4. Note the arrow points to the area of anterior displacement of L4 on L5.

eral X-ray. These views are relatively high in radiation and should be used sparingly and with forethought. The oblique image demonstrates the lesion and is identified as the "collar of the scotty dog" (Figure 9-33). In degenerative spondylolisthesis the degree of anterior displacement usually is not more than about a fourth of the lower vertebral body width (first or second degree).

### Treatment

Treatment with techniques described in this book may be of help in some cases, depending on severity. Moderate and severe cases may require prolotherapy or surgical fusion.

**MANUAL THERAPY.** Treatment is directed to decreasing lordosis, correcting vertebral dysfunctions, stabilizing the segment and correcting abnormal muscular patterning. Manual therapy can be done with the patient standing against a wall or lying supine and with the trunk flexed. Then, pressure applied ventrally several segments above the lesion will result in a posterior glide of the subluxed segment and will restore normal alignment. Another way is to press on the segment below. No thrust techniques should be attempted in the subluxed area, as instability is the rule.

**OTHER TREATMENTS.** Periosteal acupuncture, electric stimulation, and herbal application to the interspinous ligaments can be performed. In addition, needling of the facet joints, the intertransverse ligaments and the ligamenta flava could be attempted. All lumbopelvic, thoracic, leg and hip muscles should be assessed and treated. Often the hamstrings and quadratus lumborum are involved and should be treated. Post-isometric stretches and countertension release may be helpful.

Orthotics such as negative heels or heel lifts may be helpful, both to address an un-level sacral base and to decrease lordosis (Paris *ibid*). Bracing and corsets may be necessary during acute phases, but should be removed as soon as possible, as they weaken the supporting muscles of the back (Magora 1976). The use of a Levator[tm] has been advocated (Jungmann 1992) to aid in decreasing postural decompensation as measured by the pelvic index, reducing the lumbosacral angle and transferring postural stress off the posterior tissues (Kuchera and Kuchera 1993).

Exercises for spondylolisthesis should be designed to stabilize the lumbosacral region and to reduce lumbar lordosis. Exer-

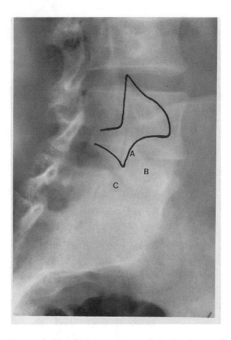

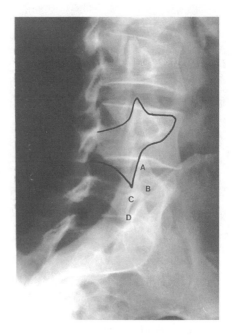

*Figure 9-33:* Oblique views of the lumbar spine with "collar on the dog," which is the area of no bone in the pars interarticularis (C). The normal dog is outlined on the vertebra above.

*Figure 9-34:* Oblique view of a normal lumbar spine with no "collar" on the dog. There is a line around the dog to demonstrate what a normal dog looks like. A, ear; B, eye; C, neck (no collar); D, legs.

cise should be only of flexion-type rather than flexion/extension. Pelvic narrow and coil exercises with the knees bent in the supine position are effective. Flattening the back against a wall while standing, and bringing the chest to the thigh while sitting in a chair (Kuchera and Kuchera *ibid*), and squatting can be beneficial.

The patient should be educated as to back mechanics and proper exercises, including proper lifting, sitting, bending, and standing. The patient should also be instructed to avoid high heels, as they increase lordosis.

## Spondylosis

Lumbar spondylosis (degenerative arthritis) is an almost universal condition that occurs with aging. Many people who have X-ray findings of spondylosis are pain free and only manifest stiffness. However, this gradual degenerative condition of all aspects of the functional unit can predispose one to somatic dysfunction and to myofascial pain, if the segment is unstable. When spodylosis is severe it may lead to narrowing of the spinal canal and intervertebral foramen. Compression of the cauda equine and nerve roots may result, and surgery may be needed.

Patients usually are over 50 years of age, and may have a history of spinal trauma. Pain usually is local and may radiate to the buttocks. Neuralgias or claudication may be seen in severe cases. Pain is aggravated by activity and by sitting. Posain is common, as is morning stiffness.

Examination often is consistent with lumbosacral instability, and a lumbar capsular pattern (limitation of all movements) may be seen.

## Treatment

Treatment is directed to the instability and to myofascial and vertebral (somatic) dysfunctions, and is often effective. Usually acupuncture, periosteal needling and manual therapy are sufficient. If significant instability is found (usually in the lumbosacral and SI regions), prolotherapy can be considered. Both oral and topical herbs can be used.

## Stenosis

Spinal and lateral foraminal stenosis can be seen in older patients who often are heavy framed, obese and out of shape. Symptoms and signs are variable but often include transient neurological and neurovascular symptoms brought on by activity. Often symptoms are relieved by assuming a forward (flexed) posture (Brown *ibid*).

### Neurogenic Claudication

Neurogenic claudication is due to hypoxia (lack of oxygen) of the nerve roots from compression. Symptoms of burning, weakness and "pins and needles" often are felt first when the patient is walking downhill (because of increased lordosis which results in a reduced foramen space) and are less related to the distance walked. Symptoms are relieved by sitting and leaning forward (Paris *ibid*).

### Vascular Claudication

The onset of vascular claudication is gradual, with a fairly predictable symptomatic pattern—onset of a cramping ache during walking, and ceasing rapidly while standing still (Paris *ibid*).[2]

---

2. Vascular claudication, not an orthopedic disorder, is a cramplike pain caused by poor blood circulation.

## Treatment

The objective of treatment of neurogenic claudication is to open the narrowing of the canal and/or foramen. In mild disorders this can be achieved by reducing the patient's lordosis by using lower or negative heels in their shoes. The obese patient should be encouraged to lose weight and to strengthen the abdominal muscles (Paris *ibid*). Lumbosacral stabilization and ligamentous strengthening may be helpful in some patients. All forward sacral and ERS dysfunctions should be addressed.

In patients with unilateral symptoms placing a heel lift under the opposite leg sometimes is effective, as it produces side-bending to that side, opening the involved neural foramen (Paris *ibid*). In more severe patients, surgery often is necessary. Acupuncture has only a temporary, analgesic effect. Selective nerve blocks and epidural blocks may be beneficial.

Vascular claudication (not orthopedic condition) can be treated with blood thinners or angioplasty. Herbal therapy can be of great help.

## Mushroom Phenomenon

This condition (described by Cyriax) is found in elderly patients that complain of almost immediate severe pain, upon standing up and walking. The pain quickly resolves when the patient is lying down. Radiographic studies show significant disc space narrowing. Cyriax believed that the pain is due to laxity of the posterior longitudinal ligament protruding posteriorly while the patient is weight-bearing. When the patient lies down the ligament is pulled forward or tightened, pressure on the dura is relieved and the pain subsides (Cyriax and Cyriax *ibid*).

## Treatment

According to Hackett et al. (1991) some of these patients benefit from prolotherapy.

Treatments similar to that of spinal or foraminal stenosis may be tried.

## Iliocostal Friction Syndrome

Hirschberg et al. (1992) suggest that patients with iliocostal friction syndrome may have their lower ribs rub against the iliac crest which may cause severe pain at the lower chest margin, or in the low back, hip and groin with radiation into the chest and thigh. Symptoms are aggravated by mobility, such as changing the position of the body from lying to sitting or standing, and are more severe when the patient bends or twists the spine. The syndrome may be detected clinically by palpation of the iliac crests, which are extremely tender and are in contact with the lower ribs.

Pathological conditions that may lead to the reduction of the distance between the ribs and the ilia are severe dorsal kyphosis, scoliosis and compression fracture.

The structures irritated by iliocostal friction are the tendons of the muscles inserting at the iliac crest and the lower rib cage (the abdominal and quadratus lumborum muscles).

### Treatment

Compression of the lower four ribs, pushing them to the inside and away from the iliac crest can be achieved by a strong 3-inch elastic belt. The belt is positioned immediately above the iliac crest and adjusted tightly enough to move the ribs away from the iliac crest. Periosteal acupuncture or proliferant injections at the iliac crest may help.

## Kissing Spine (Basstrap's Disease)

In 1924 Baastrap described the kissing spine condition, in which the spinous processes of the lumbar spine encroach on each other and give rise to arthritis and

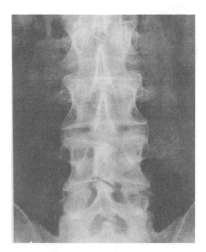

*Figure 9-35:* Kissing spine. Note the closely opposed spinous processes and the articular cortex at their tips.

sclerotic changes, which may be painful, but usually are not. Normal aging and degeneration of the discs can lead to approximation of the spinous processes (which may impinge on one another, especially when the spine is extended) and produce pain that is relieved by forward bending. It is most common in people with large spinous processes, small disc spaces, and excessive lordosis. Other factors may include facet arthrosis, neuromuscular disorders, thoracic kyphosis, thoracolumbar gibbus, obesity, and congenital hip dysplasia (Sartorius, Resnick, and Tyson et al. 1985). Although this syndrome is controversial, surgical intervention has been suggested. Others have also suggested desensitization through prolo injections (Dorman personal communication).

### Treatment

Within the context of this book, treatment includes the correction of any sacral/vertebral dysfunction, especially those that increase lordosis (flexed sacrum and restriction of lumbar flexion i.e., ERS dysfunctions). Tight myofascial layers (especially dorsal) are stretched, and this is followed by strengthening of abdominal and psoas muscles in order to reduce lumbar lordosis. Dry needling using the same principles is appropriate. Often the interspinous ligaments are sensitive and are needled. Negative heels in the shoes can be used to reduce lordosis.

## Short Leg Syndrome

Differences in leg length are common and often are overlooked. A short leg results in an unleveled sacral base and postural compensations. One must differentiate between primary anatomic leg length differences and secondary/functional variations. Leg length discrepancies are seen in asymptomatic populations, as well. Primary (anatomic) leg length discrepancy has been shown to correlate with the frequency of back pain (Friberg 1985). If the difference is larger than 5 mm and symptomatic, it should be treated. Clinical measurement of leg length has been shown to be inaccurate, compared with X-ray measurements (Morscher and Finger 1977). Still, a tape measurement can be helpful (Beattie et al. 1990).

Apparent leg length (secondary to pelvic dysfunction) can be demonstrated after stressing the pelvic ring. This can be accomplished by having the patient perform a "sit-up" and checking for any change in leg length between the sitting and the supine positions.

### Adaptations to Short Leg

Leg length differences generally cause the pelvis to tilt to the side of the short leg, with lumbar sidebending to the opposite side or to the long leg side. Rotation occurs toward the convexity of the curve. However, an opposite adaptation also can be seen, and usually is more symptomatic. The lumbosacral angle is increased by 2-3$^{0}$, and the innominate rotates anteriorly on the side of the short leg and posteriorly on the other side in order to equalize the leg length. Often this compensation masks the

apparent length differences (Basmajian and Nyberg 1993).

The pelvic obliqueness that result from a short leg stresses the ligaments and muscles of the back, pelvis, hip, and possibly as far up as the neck. With time, muscle adaptation, shortening, dysfunction develop and lead to tendon inflammation and ligament insufficiency. The iliolumbar ligament on the convex side is the first to react and show symptoms, since it is affected by both sacral and innominate rotations (Kuchera and Kuchera *ibid*). Often the patient has sciatic-like pain and hip pain on the long leg side.

A short leg often is responsible for recurrent joint dysfunctions anywhere in the spine. It should be suspected if the standing trochanteric plane is unlevel and there is no clinical evidence of shear. Often the PSIS and the iliac crests will be depressed on the side of the short leg. If, after somatic dysfunctions have been treated, the standing flexion test is still positive and sitting flexion is negative, a short leg should be suspected (Kuchera and Kuchera *ibid*).

### Assessment

Short leg syndrome is best assessed by X-ray. The office assessment begins with the patient standing with feet slightly apart. (If the feet are together, the leg that the patient favors may appear longer). The practitioner compares the levelness of both iliac crests, PSISs, ASISs, greater trochanter of both femurs and gluteal folds carefully. He repeats these observations several times to assure that the findings are reproducible, as it is easy to make mistakes. Palpation has been shown to have poor inter-rater reliability in several studies (Potter and Rothstein 1985; Mann, Glassjenn-Wray and Nyberg 1984).

The practitioner compares the levelness of the PSISs when the patient is standing and then when forward bent, as well as when he is seated. If the PSISs become level when the patient is seated, the probability of leg length difference is high. If

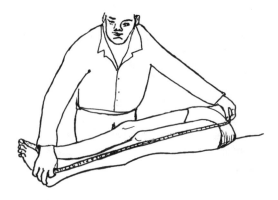

*Figure 9-36:* Tape measurement of leg length.

they remain uneven, pelvic dysfunction is likely. Then with the patient supine, one measures the length between the patient's ASISs and medial malleoli to assess for structural differences and from the umbilicus to the medial malleoli for functional differences (Figure 9-36).

When an anatomic difference is suspected, elevate the patient's heel using a book, and reevaluate all of the findings. In a patient where posture and other findings highly suggest leg length discrepancy, one should elevate the short leg before proceeding with the active lumbar and pelvic examinations.

**Treatment.** Clinically, one should first treat all somatic (mechanical) dysfunctions, including myofascial shortening and spasm, before a final conclusion is made and a heel lift is prescribed.

### Small Hemipelvis

A small hemipelvis is associated with back pain (Lowman 1941). In this condition the pelvis is vertically smaller on one side than on the other, both when the patient is seated and when standing. The patient sits crookedly and leans toward the small side, and often sits cross-legged to cantilever the low side. A seesaw affect tilts the spine in both standing and sitting positions (Travell and Simons *ibid*).

### Assessment

Assessment is done with the patient seated on a hard, flat surface. The feet are supported high enough so that the patient can slip his fingers between his thighs and the front edge of the table. The practitioner observes and checks the same landmarks as when examining for a short leg. Since somatic dysfunction of the pelvis can result in similar findings, the patient is asked to rock and stress his pelvis. If findings do not change, a small hemipelvis should be considered (Travell and Simons 1983).

**Treatment.** If a small hemipelvis is found, the patient should use a sit-pad to compensate while seated.

### Myofascial Syndromes

Muscles of the low back, pelvis and legs generate movement of the back and the legs. The muscular activity and its resulting tensions on the fascial planes may change the vectors of gravitational forces, ligament tension, and lumbosacral stability. Altered myofascial tension may result in strain and instability. Weakness or tightness of muscles results in asymmetrical fascial tension, encouraging somatic dysfunction. Muscular lesions can result from a multitude of causes which should be differentiated.

When pelvic or spinal instability perpetuates myofascial pain, treatment should incorporate all the muscles capable of stabilizing the spine, including exercises for the extension muscles (to include the latissimus dorsi), the torsional muscles (important for the rotatory muscles) and the flexor muscles (abdominal and psoas). Ligaments must be strengthened, as well.

Many myofascial syndromes are secondary to joint dysfunction of the vertebral column and sacroiliac joints. Table 3-6 on page 626 summarize osteopathic categorization of vertebral and sacroiliac joint dysfunctions.

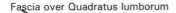

Fascia over Quadratus lumborum

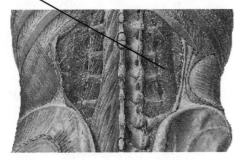

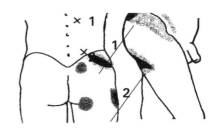

*Figure 9-38:* Referred pain from quadratus lumborum trigger points (After Travell and Simons).

*Figure 9-37:* Quadratus lumborum muscle.

Table 9-16 on page 636 through Table 3-21 on page 641 summarizes myofascial syndromes of the low back.

### Quadratus Lumborum

The quadratus lumborum muscle is one of the most common and overlooked causes of low back pain (Travell and 1992)

**ATTACHMENT.** It attaches superiorly to the TrPs of the lumbar vertebrae and to the medial and anterior surfaces of the 12th rib. Inferiorly the muscle attaches to the anterior iliac crests. The iliolumbar ligament was thought to developed in adulthood from the quadratus lumborum, however newer studies have demonstrated the ligament in babies, as well (Willard *ibid*), (Figure 9-37).

**SYMPTOMS.** Pain from a quadratus lumborum trigger is felt mostly in the L1-2 myotome. It may also be felt to some extent in an L3-4 distribution. Typically the patient has pain over the iliac crests, buttock, hip and groin (Figure 9-38). A lateral bent posture also is common, (although this probably is not due to a lesion of this muscle alone).

The quadratus lumborum muscle often is activated by sudden, unguarded, awkward movements and trauma. Motor vehicle accidents, especially impacts from the driver's side (81% of subjects), activate spasm of this muscle (Baker 1989). Spasm can be caused by heavy lifting or by movements that combine bending and twisting at the same time (this activation is either secondary to SI backward torsional dysfunction, or it could contribute to the formation of a backward torsional dysfunction).

Muscle spasm will restrict movements between the lumbar vertebrae and the sacrum during walking or turning over in bed, and when arising from bed or from sitting (Travell and Simons *ibid*).

**ASSESSMENT.** Flexion, extension and side-bending movements are restricted toward the pain-free side. Rotation may be limited in the direction of the spasm. Tests that use resisted movements are difficult to design, as they will involve other muscles as well.

Tenderness can be demonstrated by palpation, with the patient on the good side and a rolled towel supporting the lumbar spine. It is helpful to have the patient reach up with his arms in order to open up the region and put the muscle into stretch.

**TREATMENT.** Treatment is directed both to the muscle and to vertebral and SI dysfunctions. In acute cases, indirect techniques such as countertension positional release can be followed by muscle energy (direct) techniques to correct vertebral dysfunctions.

In chronic cases, needling of the muscle and its attachment is often necessary. To reach the triggers within the muscle, the patient is placed in the same position used for palpation. A three-inch acupuncture needle is used to needle the muscle, which lies deeply between the kidney and the longissimus dorsi. Spray and stretch and post isometric contraction stretches should follow needling. The muscle attachments are needled, as well.

**ACUPUNCTURE.** Acupuncture points UB-23, GV-4 and Three Emperors are helpful. The Kidney Divergent and Yin Motility (Qiao) channels are treated often.

**COUNTERTENSION POSITIONAL RELEASE.** For countertension positional release (indirect method) the patient lies prone and a pillow is placed beneath the chest to extend the spine. The muscle is shortened by pulling on the patient's ASIS on the dysfunctional side. If needed, sidebending away from the painful side may be used with the legs or toes.

Tenderness is monitored at the myofascial point. When a position that significantly reduces the point's tenderness is found, it is held for 90 seconds and then, without the patient's assistance, the patient is returned to a neutral position.

*Latissimus Dorsi*

The latissimus dorsi is an important and often overlooked source of dysfunction and pain (Travell and Simons *ibid*).

**ATTACHMENT.** The latissimus dorsi attaches to the ilia through the lumbodorsal fascia, to the spines of the lower six thoracic vertebrae, to the lower three to four ribs, and to the intertubercular groove of the humerus (Figure 9-39).

**FUNCTION.** The latissimus dorsi conducts forces to the contralateral ilium, which is an important contributor to force closure of the ilia onto the sacrum, and thereby

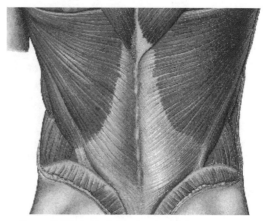

*Figure 9-39:* Latissimus dorsi muscle.

provides stability against shearing. It functions as an extensor, adductor and internal rotator of the arm and shoulder, and it is a strong depressor of the scapula.

It is innervated by the thoracodorsal nerve through the posterior cord and spinal nerves C6, C7 and C8 (Basmajian 1978).

**SYMPTOMS.** When this muscle is shortened, arm extension and elevation are limited. Pain can be felt in the scapular, shoulder and iliac crest regions (Figure 9-40).

**TREATMENT.** Treatment is directed first to all vertebral dysfunctions, at the levels capable of affecting the muscle. If dysfunction continues, the muscle is treated directly. Needling the motor or facilitated points is followed by stretch and spray.

**ACUPUNCTURE.** Acupuncture points SI-6, 11, and Double Child 22.01 are useful.

**COUNTERTENSION POSITIONAL RELEASE.** For countertension positional release, muscle shortening is achieved by having the patient lie supine at the edge of the table, so the arm can be extended without any

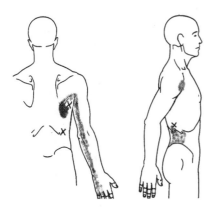

*Figure 9-40:* Referred pain from latissimus dorsi trigger points (After Travell and Simons).

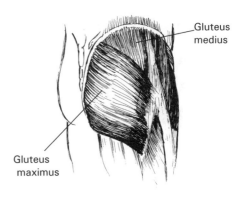

*Figure 9-41:*Gluteus muscles (With permission Dorman and Ravin 1991).

abduction. The patient's arm is extended to 25-30°, and slight internal rotation and slight abduction are added. Then the arm is pulled caudad, side bending the spine. Tenderness is monitored at the myofascial point. When a position that significantly reduces the point's tenderness is found, it is held for 90 seconds. Then, without the patient's assistance, the patient is returned slowly to a neutral position.

### Gluteus Medius

Tenderness of the glutei is almost universal with low back pain. The gluteus medius is situated in the middle of both glutei, sharing its aponeuroses with the gluteus maximus, which also connects to the SI ligaments. The gluteus medius seems to have a regulating function on all of the glutei, and on the SI joint, as well (Brown *ibid*). All of these are important in pelvic stabilization and normal gait.

**ATTACHMENT.** The gluteus medius is a thick, fan-shaped muscle that overlaps the gluteus minimus and is deep to the gluteus maximus. It arises from an area on the lateral upper aspect of the ilium. Its weight is at least twice that of the gluteus minimus, and less than half that of the maximus. It attaches proximally along the anterior

three-fourths of the iliac crest, between the superior and middle gluteal lines, to the gluteal aponeuroses. Distally it is attached to the upper greater trochanter. It is innervated by the L5-S1 roots through the superior gluteal nerve.

**FUNCTION.** The main functions of the gluteus medius are abduction of the thigh, and stabilization of the pelvis during walking or single-limb stance (Travell 1992). The gluteus medius is coupled functionally with the gluteus minimus, maximus, tensor fasciae latae and iliopsoas (Janda 1983). These muscles, together with the quadratus lumborum, function as lateral trunk benders and pelvic supporters and are needed during the swing phase of walking (see gate analysis chapter 4). Once the swing limb is airborne, the muscle action ceases. Then, the contracting ipsilateral gluteus medius allows passage of the leg by abduction of the pelvis on the stationary side. As this pattern is repeated many times each day, any dysfunction within this process (often due to the gluteus medius) can lead to strain and pain. Often SI dysfunction is the root cause of gluteus medius dysfunction and pain (Brown *ibid*).

**SYMPTOMS.** Klein has divided the gluteus medius syndrome into three subconditions, one primary and two secondary. The

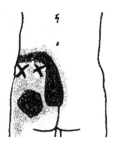

*Figure 9-42:* Referred pain from gluteus
medius trigger points (After Travell and Simons).

first is due to primary muscular injury of
the gluteus medius. The second two are
due to SI ligamentous insufficiency and
nerve root dysfunctions.

Symptoms of pain in the low back,
along the sacroiliac, outer iliac crest, buttocks and outer thigh, are common. Occasionally, in lesions of the uppermost
anterior insertion on the ilium, pain is felt
in the dorsal ankle only. Patients often
complain of pain during walking, sitting
and slumping forward (Figure 9-42), (Travell *ibid*).

**ASSESSMENT.** Weakness or pain of the muscle can be demonstrated with resisted
thigh abduction. The patient lies on his
good side with his leg and lower back
extended. His leg is then abducted, and
the hip is extended about 20° further. The
practitioner then pushes down on the leg
and asks the patient to resist. Weakness is
often reversed immediately after treatment, but may reoccur (Brown *ibid*).

Examination of the standing patient
reveals often a bulkier muscle on the dysfunctional side. During forward flexion,
when maximal muscle effort is required, a
slight muscle quiver may be observed during the first 15° of flexion (Dorman and
Ravin 1991). Muscle tenderness usually
can be demonstrated in the prone position. Flexion and sidebending away from
the dysfunctional side is painful, as it
stretches the muscle. Sit-ups (often prescribed with rehabilitation exercises) can
aggravate gluteus medius pain.

**TREATMENT.** Treatment is directed both at
the cause, if different, and at the muscle.
First, all active trigger points are treated by
needling. The needle is inserted slowly and
gently until a muscle twitch is felt, and
then the needle is removed. The PSIS and
ASIS are needled gently. It is unwise to
needle the muscle vigorously, as aggravation without benefit is common. If necessary, the treatment is repeated.

It is possible to create sacral dysfunctions by needling the gluteus medius and
maximus. Therefore, after needling, this
joint should be reassessed and treated, if
needed. If the condition does not improve
after two to three treatments, the muscle
origins should be needled more vigorously.
If no improvement is still seen, and if all
sacroiliac dysfunction has been cleared,
cortisone injection can be considered.

**ACUPUNCTURE.** Acupuncture points GB-29,
30, 31 and Flower Bone Three And Four
(55.04, 05), and Yang Motility (Qiao) channels are helpful. In unstable patients the
Girdle (Dai) channel is often treated.

**STRETCHING.** To stretch the gluteus medius,
the patient is placed on his good side with
a pillow or a rolled towel under his waist or
hips (whichever is more comfortable), and
his leg and low back extended. Then his
leg is adducted and his hip is extended
about 20° farther. The patient pushes his
leg gently up against the practitioner's
resistance and holds it in that position for
a count of six. Then the patient is told to
relax, and the practitioner stretches the
muscle slightly, until he feels the next barrier of muscle tension. The process is
repeated three to four times. The same is
done with the hip slightly flexed, in order
to stretch the posterior fibers.

**COUNTERTENSION POSITIONAL RELEASE.** For
countertension positional release, muscle
shortening is achieved by having the
patient lie in the prone position while the
practitioner extends the hip and supports
the leg with his thigh. Then the hip is
abducted somewhat, and internally rotated

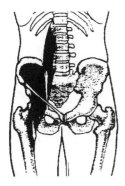

*Figure 9-43:* Iliopsoas muscle.

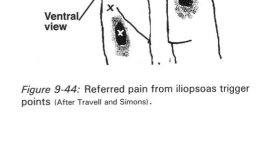

*Figure 9-44:* Referred pain from iliopsoas trigger points (After Travell and Simons).

markedly. Tenderness is monitored at the myofascial point. When a position is found that significantly reduces the point's tenderness, it is held for 90 seconds and then, without the patient's assistance, is returned slowly to a neutral position.

### Iliopsoas

Iliopsoas syndrome, together with quadratus lumborum trigger points, is a common myofascial cause of failed low back surgery (Travell and Simons 1992).

**ATTACHMENT.** The *psoas major* fits like a bowstring from its attachments above, along the sides of the lumbar vertebrae and in the intervertebral discs. Below the muscle runs with the common iliopsoas tendon, joining the lesser trochanter of the femur.

The *iliacus* muscle attaches above to the upper two-thirds of the inner iliac fossa. It connects with the iliolumbar ligaments and the anterior ligaments of the sacroiliac joints. Below, it joins the psoas major tendon, and in addition, some fibers attach directly to the femur near the lesser trochanter. They are innervated by lumbar nerves 2 and 3 (Figure 9-43).

**FUNCTION.** The primary function of the iliopsoas is flexion of the hip when the trunk is fixed. It also can assist in extension and flexion of the lumbar spine, and can influence lumbar lordosis. It is active both during sitting and standing (Janda *ibid;* (Basmajian 1978).

**SYMPTOMS.** Symptoms from the iliopsoas are aggravated by weightbearing activities and relieved by lying down, especially with hips flexed. If one side has increased tone or is shortened, sidebending occurs to that side, slightly shortening and externally rotating the leg.

Pain is felt along the spine ipsilaterally, from the thoracic region to the sacroiliac area, and sometimes to the upper buttock, anterior thigh and groin (Travell and Simons 1992), (Figure 9-44).

Patients with psoas spasm are likely to stand with the torso leaning slightly toward the involved side. When the patient is asked to forward bend, an arc can be seen during approximately the first 20° (they lean farther to the involved side, after which symmetry returns).

**ASSESSMENT.** Examination for muscle length can be done with the patient supine, by testing for hip extension range of movement. Shortness of the quadriceps and tensor fasciae latae must be distinguished from a shortened psoas. When the quadriceps muscle is short, it limits the thigh from dropping down and also keeps the leg flexed. The psoas will limit hip extension only. Resisted movements may be painful (Figure 9-45).

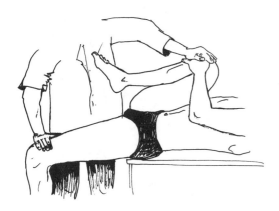

*Figure 9-45:* Assessment of psoas tension.

Tenderness can be demonstrated in the lower muscle between the lesser trochanter and the inguinal ligament, over the iliacus at the inner ilium, or in the upper muscle transabdominally, lateral to the umbilicus.

The psoas syndrome illustrates well the mechanical-linkage of the musculoskeletal system. Since it may involve multiple sites, a good physical and history are necessary to rule out other conditions.

Psoas muscle spasm can cause more disability than a spasm in any other muscle of the back (Kuchera and Kuchera 1992). Summarizing the psoas syndrome, Kuchera says:

> It commonly starts during a prolonged slump sitting on a hard chair or sitting in a very soft chair, while leaning over a desk, while working stooped forward for a long time or while doing sit-ups.

Because in all of these conditions the psoas is shortened, the intrafusal spindle fibers tighten up, so that they can better monitor the muscle length. Then a rapid change in muscle length, usually when the patient returns to his neutral upright position, leads to a protective spasm as the shortened reset spindles try to protect the muscle—which they now monitor as being overstretched.

At first, both psoas muscles are usually involved, causing the patient to forward bend in the typical lumbago posture. If sidebending is introduced during the upright recovery from sitting, a nonneutral (Type II) lumbar dysfunction at L1 or L2 (which is key in the psoas syndrome) can occur, with spasm in one psoas being more evident than in the other. A lumbar list (sidebent) is seen. A compensatory neutral group dysfunction (Type I) is seen in the rest of the lumbar spine.

This dysfunction may result in a non-neutral sacral response. A torsional dysfunction of the sacrum leads to a piriformis muscle irritation, which in turn may cause leg pain and "sciatica."

**Treatment.** All that may be needed in the early stages is to have the patient lie over a towel placed under his lumbar area for a few minutes a day until the condition is relieved. Ice may be helpful. Dry needling with a thin, 36-gauge needle often is helpful. Use only mild stimulation. Needle the lower trigger point areas of the iliopsoas. Also, needle a point level with the symphysis pubis at a triangular intersection of the mid-point between the pubis and the ASIS. It can be needled superficially or deeply. The intervertebral muscles at L1-2 can also be needled, with the patient positioned in the manner appropriate to address the nonneutral dysfunction. Alternatively one corrects the nonneutral dysfunction at L1-2 by manual therapy.

**Acupuncture.** Acupuncture points GV-2, 3 and 26, UB-41, 53, Liv-13 and 14 can be helpful. The Kidney Divergent, the Girdle (Dai), and Penetrating (Chong) channels are often treated.

**Countertension positional release.** For countertension positional release, the patient is placed supine with legs flexed and the psoas muscle relaxed until tenderness over the iliacus or psoas is relieved.

The position is held for 90 seconds and then the leg is slowly extended.

The patient should be educated as to the postural cause of this syndrome. As the patient improves, exercise such as swimming or push-ups may be prescribed. No sit-ups should be allowed. Later on, in chronic patients with a shortened psoas, stretching is indicated. If stretches begin too early, no benefit is gained. Post-isometric contraction stretches can be performed.

**PSOAS WEAKNESS.** A weak psoas with a relatively stronger erector spinae allows the lumbar spine to backward bend, increasing its lordosis. This typical posture of a protruded abdomen and increased lordosis is often blamed on poor abdominal muscle strength, but it can also be due to poor psoas tone alone. This may explain why a person might continue to have a problem holding the abdomen in, even when abdominal exercises have been performed faithfully (Kuchera and Kuchera 1992).

To strengthen the psoas, the patient should lie supine. The practitioner places his palm up, under the patient's mid-lumbar spine, and pushes up against the lumbar spine. The patient is asked to push down his back against the practitioner's hand so that the back is flattened. While holding this position (back flat against the table), the patient is asked to relax his abdomen and hold this position to the count of six. The exercise is performed three to four times, twice a day. Backward sit-ups are helpful, as well.

### Piriformis

The Piriformis Syndrome can be divided into two entities. One involves nerve entrapment, and the other myofascial strain alone. The syndrome is often provoked by SI joint dysfunctions. Piriformis spasm can maintain SI torsional dysfunctions, as well. The syndrome often needs to be differentiated from other conditions affecting the sciatic nerve.

**ATTACHMENT.** The piriformis attaches medially to the anterior surface of the sacrum. It then exits the pelvis through the greater sciatic foramen. Laterally it attaches to the greater trochanter of the femur. It is one of the few muscles that spans two joints, and it is the only muscle to bridge the anterior sacroiliac joint. It also originates from the margins of the greater sciatic foramen and the anterior surface of the sacrotuberous ligament.

**FUNCTION.** The piriformis muscle functions as one of the hip external rotators, together with the superior and inferior gemelli, the obturator internus and externus, and the quadratus femoris. It also assists in abduction when the hip is flexed to 90°. In weight bearing, the muscle restrains excessive medial rotation of the thigh (Basmajian 1978). The piriformis probably is the lower pivot around which the oblique sacral axis rotates. The piriformis can rotate and sidebend the sacrum (Mitchell *ibid*).

The piriformis muscle is innervated by the S1-2 nerves. The nerve trunks branching from the sacral plexus and the branches of the internal iliac vessels all exit the pelvis, together with the piriformis, through the greater sciatic foramen. When the muscle is enlarged due to injury, these structures may get entrapped, giving symptoms of nerve entrapment and/or vascular compromise. In some people the peroneal and tibial portions of the sciatic nerve pass through the piriformis muscle. The reported frequency at which this occurs varies, ranging from 6% to 25% for the peroneal portion, and from 0.5 to 2.1% for both portions (Pecina 1979; Lee and Tsai 1974; Beaton and Anson 1938).

**SYMPTOMS.** Symptoms of the myofascial component of the syndrome usually include low back pain, buttock pain, hip pain, and posterior thigh pain (Travell and Simons 1992). Pain is increased by sitting, especially on a hard surface, by rising from the sitting position or by standing. It may

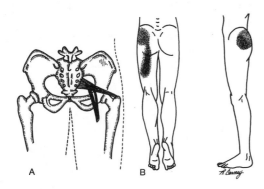

*Figure 9-46:* The piriformis muscle and sciatic nerve—A; pain radiation from trigger points—B (Reprinted with permission Dorman and Ravin 1991).

be related to defecation. Muscle spasm may cause the patient's ipsilateral foot to be everted. Both abduction of the lower extremity and hip internal rotation will be limited. This presentation must be differentiated from somatic dysfunction of the hip and from psoas spasm (Kuchera *ibid*).

Compression of the superior and inferior gluteal nerves and vessels can contribute to buttock pain and atrophy. Pressure on the sciatic nerve gives pain in the distribution of the sciatic nerve, and may project to the calf and foot. Changes in reflexes, reduced muscle power, and paresthesias may be seen (Kopell and Thompson 1960), and easily confused with radiculopathy. If the pudendal nerve is entrapped, the patient may feel peroneal pain and may complain of sexual dysfunction (Figure 9-46).

**PRIMARY CAUSES.** The primary cause of piriformis spasm usually is direct irritation of the muscle. Falls on the buttocks, and sacroiliac region, may produce a bruise and bleeding, which can irritate the muscle. A near slip often strains the piriformis, which is called upon to prevent the fall. Sitting on the toilet seat for a prolonged period ("Reader's Digest syndrome") can activate the muscle. "Billfold syndrome" occurs from sitting on a large billfold in a chair, or in a seat during a long car, train

or airplane ride. Sitting on top of a wallet can also provoke piriformis spasm (Kuchera *ibid*).

**SECONDARY CAUSES.** Secondary causes of piriformis syndrome are; unilateral sacral shear (downslip) on the same side as the piriformis spasm, a psoas syndrome on the opposite side, inflammation of the SI ligaments on the same side, sudden internal rotation of the femur on the same side (commonly seen in athletes), reflex involvement from S1 or S2 lesions, pelvic carcinomas (Kuchera and Kuchera 1992) and sacral torsional dysfunctions. Over pronated foot can result in tension of the piriformis which is then called upon to resist this mechanical dysfunction (Brown *ibid*)

**ASSESSMENT.** Often the straight leg raise (SLR) in these patients is positive. A variant on SLR can be performed by rotating the hip externally, and then internally. One rotation stretches the piriformis. The other relaxes it. If the SLR is more restricted with external rotation, a piriformis syndrome may be considered.

Both with an entrapped nerve and in a myofascial syndrome the areas around the sciatic foramen and over the muscle are quite tender. The entire muscle is palpated, both in the prone position and while the patient is lying on his side. Tenderness may be felt at the muscle insertions, muscle belly and musculotendinous junctions. Related tenderness of the anterior sacroiliac ligament can be palpated, as well.

A myofascial tender point that is always tender in patients with a piriformis syndrome can be found on palpation the practitioner:

**1.** Finds the coccyx (or the ILA) and the PSIS on the side of the piriformis muscle.

**2.** Marks a point midway, intersecting between the ILA and the PSIS.

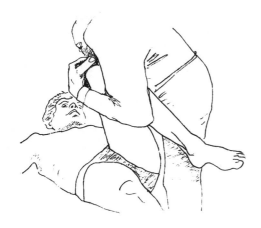

*Figure 9-47:* Assessment of piriformis
tension.

**3.** Finds the superior margin of the greater
trochanter on the side, and mentally
constructs a line between the first point
and the superior margin of the greater
trochanter.

The point is located halfway on that line.

Resisted contraction of the muscle can
be tested with the patient seated by asking
the patient to separate his knees. This may
or may not increase the pain. Testing for
shortness is accomplished with the patient
supine (Figure 9-47).

**TREATMENT OF ACUTE SPASM.** For acute
spasm, countertension positional release
can be used first. With the patient prone,
flexion, abduction and external rotation of
the leg is carried out while monitoring tenderness of the myofascial point. When a
position that reduces the point's tenderness significantly is found, the practitioner
holds for 90 seconds, and then slowly
returns the leg to the neutral position.

**ACUPUNCTURE.** Acupuncture can be applied
at Flower Bone Three and Four (55.04,05)
and GB 30 (or trigger within the muscle).
One may also try to needle the contralateral piriformis. Occasionally this will

release the muscle.

**TREATMENT OF CHRONIC STAGE.** In the
chronic phase direct post-isometric
stretches and needling of the spasmed
muscle are needed often and are quite
helpful.

**ACUPUNCTURE.** Acupuncture is applied at
Flower Bone Three and Four (55.04, 05)
and GB 30. The Girdle (Dai) and Yang
Motility (Qiao) channels are treated often.

**MANUAL THERAPY.** Sacroiliac dysfunction,
especially nonphysiologic (shears), should
be corrected. Torsions are common, as
well.

**ORTHOTICS.** Foot orthotics are commonly
needed to treat the piriformis syndrome
(Brown *ibid*). Correction of rearfoot varus
(or valgus) and inverted forefoot dysfunction often is needed. A functional hallux
limitus commonly is found (with a lax
overpronated foot) and should be treated
with a Kinetic Wedge™. A simple first-ray
(big-toe) cut-out can be used in a patient
with a stable midfoot (Brown *ibid*).

### Paraspinal Muscles

The thoracolumbar paraspinal muscles are
often involved in low back pain. They are
shortened and hypersensitive often, due to
vertebral dysfunctions and neuropathic
activation.

The superficial erector spinae often are
involved in back pain and in neutral type
(group) vertebral dysfunctions. The longissimus thoracis and the more lateral iliocostalis thoracic (Travell and Simons 1992) are
the more commonly involved.

### Longissimus Thoracis

**ATTACHMENT.** The Longissimus thoracis
attaches below to the TrPs of the lumbar
spine, and to the anterior layer of the lum-
bocostal aponeurosis. It unites with the

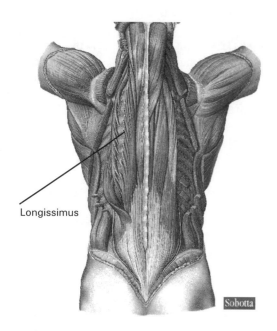

Figure 9-48:   Longissimus muscles.

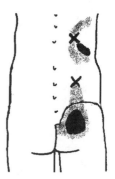

*Figure 9-49:*Referred pain from iliocostalis trigger points (After Travell and Simone).

iliocostalis and spinalis muscles. Above, it attaches to the TrPs of all the thoracic vertebra and to the first to ninth ribs (Figure 9-48).

**FUNCTION.** The superficial lumbar paraspinal muscles produce extension and side-bending of the spine ipsilaterally (Duchenne 1949). They may also produce rotation to the opposite side (Hollinshead 1976). These muscles contract strongly during coughing, and during straining to have a bowel movement (Basmajian 1978).

The superficial muscles are innervated by the lateral branch of the dorsal primary divisions of the spinal nerves.

**SYMPTOMS.** When the longissimus muscles are involved bilaterally, usually at the thoracic-lumbar junction, the patient has difficulty rising from a chair and climbing stairs (Travell and Simons 1992).

Pain from the iliocostalis, at the lower-thoracic area, is felt mostly downward over the lumbar area. It may refer upwards to and across the scapula, and around the abdomen (Travell and Rinzler 1952). Trigger points in the upper lumbar iliocostalis

refer downward and over the mid-buttock and frequently are a source of unilateral posterior hip pain. Trigger points at the lower thoracic level, in the longissimus thoracis, refer pain to the low buttock (Travell and Simons 1992).

### Deep Paraspinal Muscles

The deep paraspinal muscles the *semispinalis thoracis, the multifidi and the rotators* have fibers which become progressively more horizontal, therefore increasingly rotating the spine.

**ATTACHMENT.** The semispinalis thoracis extends below only as far as T10. However, pain from it does extend to the lumbar spine. The deeper multifidi and rotatores lie under the tendons of the more superficial muscles and extend past the lumbosacral junction to the so called "triangle of the sacrum".

The multiarticular semispinalis and multifidi attach laterally and below to multiple TrPs's, the semispinalis to at least 5 vertebra, the multifidi to 2-4 vertebra. The rotators are monoarticular and therefore attach to 2 adjacent vertebrae. Above and medially the multifidi and rotatores muscles attach near the bases of the vertebral spinous processes (Figure 9-50).

The deeper paraspinal muscles are innervated by the medial branch of the

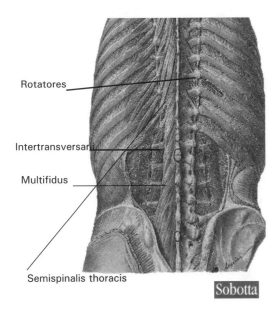

Rotatores

Intertransversari

Multifidus

Semispinalis thoracis

Sobotta

*Figure 9-50:* Deep muscles.

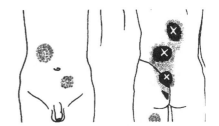

*Figure 9-51:* Referred pain from multifidi trigger points (After Travell and Simons).

dorsal primary division of the spinal nerves (Travell and Simons *ibid*).

**SYMPTOMS.** Pain from the semispinalis distributes in a similar pattern to that of the longissimus. The multifidi refer pain to the region around the spinous process of the vertebra adjacent to the trigger point.

From the L1-L5 level the multifidi also refer pain anteriorly to the abdomen. From the S1 level they refer downwards to the coccyx. The rotatores, throughout the length of the thoracolumbar spine, produce midline pain, and referred tenderness to tapping on the spinous process adjacent to the trigger point (Figure 9-51).

The paraspinal muscles are often activated by sudden overload, sustained contraction for a period of time, awkward movements that combine bending and twisting the back (especially when they are fatigued or cold), whiplash type accident and prolonged immobility (Travell and Simon 1992).

Pain from these muscles often is associated with vertebral and sacroiliac joint dysfunctions and with ligamentous insufficiency.

**ASSESSMENT.** Travell and Simons suggest that palpation of these muscles should be performed after vertebral percussion for tenderness is performed to identify the level of dysfunction—with the patient in the lateral recumbent position (lying on his side).

**TREATMENT.** Treatment to the paraspinal muscle should begin by addressing all vertebral and sacroiliac dysfunctions. The muscles may be needled with the patient positioned to address the appropriate vertebral dysfunction. Post isometric relaxation stretching is helpful. In acutely painful conditions countertension positional release may be used. In chronic lesions the muscle motor points and attachments may be needled.

**ACUPUNCTURE.** Hua Tuo Jia Ji and UB acupuncture channel points can be used. SI-3 and UB-62 are helpful. For unstable patients the Girdle (Dai) channel is often treated.

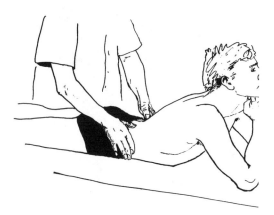

*Figure 9-52:* Evaluation of vertebral extension. Both spinous processes should translate posteriorly. If one side does not there is FRS dysfunction.

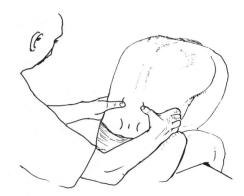

*Figure 9-53:* Evaluation of vertebral flexion. Both spinous processes should translate forward equally. If one side does not, there is ERS dysfunction.

functions of the upper lumbar and lower thoracic regions, the psoas is involved often and should be treated.

## Joint Dysfunctions

*Vertebral Dysfunctions in the Lumbar Spine*

In the lumbar spine, one can find restrictions of flexion and extension that often are due to *nonneutral* (Type II) *dysfunctions* FRS, ERS and *neutral group dysfunctions* (Type I). Figure 9-52 and Figure 9-53 illustrate evaluation methods for assessing joint dysfunctions in the lumbar spine. Table 3-6 on page 626, Table 3-4 on page 475 and Table 3-4 on page 475 summarize joint dysfunctions in the lumbosacral spine.

*Treatment*

Thrust techniques are effective for both Type I and Type II dysfunctions. These may be modified for muscle energy and needling. Flexion restrictions (ERS) and group dysfunctions respond well to needling. Extension restrictions (FRS) respond as well, but not as consistently. With dys-

MUSCLE ENERGY & NEEDLING OF EXTENSION RESTRICTION (FRS DYSFUNCTIONS). The patient is lying on his good side (on examination, when the patient extends his spine, the dysfunctional side is the side in which the transverse process (TrPr) is found to stay anterior).[3] The practitioner:

1. Extends the spine to the feather edge of movement from above and below the dysfunctional segment.

2. Rotates and sidebends the spine by pulling on the patient's uppermost hand and asking the patient to hold onto the table.

3. Needles superficially over the contracted deep intertransverse muscles.

   If needed needles the muscle belly.

---

3. When the spine is extended the transverse processes move backward and posterior. If one side is restricted the transverse process on that side will remain anterior.

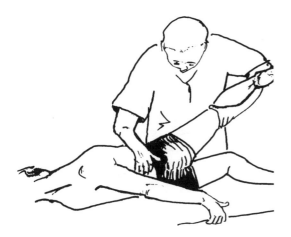

*Figure 9-54:* Muscle energy technique for extension restriction — FRS (lt).

4. Needles the associated channel (i.e. Large Intestine for L5 dysfunctions with the coupled Lung channel).

5. (To use muscle energy), Picks up patient's leg and resists leg adduction (Figure 9-54).

   Localization of the segment must be very accurate (this is less crucial for needling).

**THRUST TECHNIQUES FOR EXTENSION RESTRICTION (FRS DYSFUNCTION).** The patient lies on his side with the dysfunctional side up. The practitioner:

1. Extends the spine to the feather edge of movement at the dysfunctional segment. Standing in front of the patient, the practitioner translates the pelvis forward in order to start extension of the spine.

2. Monitors at the dysfunctional level, in order not to overextend the segment, and then takes the patient's lower leg and moves it backward slowly, extending the hip until the first sense of motion is felt below the dysfunctional segment.

3. (Next, while making sure the patient does not move) brings the uppermost leg forward and places it in front, with the patient's knee flexed and the foot in front of the lower leg.

4. Extends the spine from above by moving the patient's head and upper back backward, until he first feels movement of the segment above the dysfunction.

5. Hooks his left forearm under the patient's axilla (palm down, to minimize painful pressure there) and introduces rotation up to the dysfunctional segment.

6. Places his right forearm over the upper part of the patient's buttock, between the iliac crest and the trochanter.

7. Fine-tunes localization by taking up the slack from below and above, just to the feather edge of movement at the dysfunctional segment (this must be comfortable to both the practitioner and patient).

8. Thrusts forward and slightly superiorly keeping his right forearm down, rotating the ilium and sidebending the spine (Figure 9-55).

This is a facet-closing technique and therefore the familiar popping sound of manipulation may be absent. The same posture can be used for muscle energy by resisting the patient's efforts to sidebend or rotate the spine while the practitioner keeps the same position. Respiratory effort can be used, as well. During inhalation the slack is taken up, and then the patient is asked to exhale forcefully, against the practitioner's attempt to keep the spine in the same position.

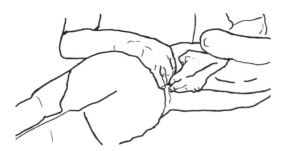

*Figure 9-55:* Thrust manipulation of extension restriction to left — FRS(rt).

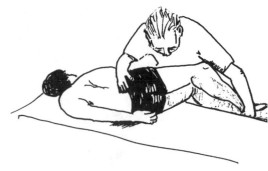

*Figure 9-56:* Muscle energy technique for flexion restrictions — ERS (lt).

**MUSCLE ENERGY & NEEDLING POSITIONS FOR FLEXION RESTRICTION (ERS DYSFUNCTION).** (With the patient prone, the practitioner flexes the patient's knees and rotates the patient toward him, placing the patient in the Sims Position, with the dysfunctional side up (on examination, the side in which the of transverse process is found to remain posterior).[4] The practitioner:

1. Flexes the spine just to the feather edge of movement at the dysfunctional segment, by flexing from below and above, until the restricted barrier is engaged (at the feather edge of the spinous processes' movement).

2. Sidebends the spine by dropping the patient's feet over the edge of the table (as this can be painful to the patient's thighs, a small cushion can be placed between the table and the thigh, or the patient's thigh can be supported by the practitioner).

3. Needles superficially over the deep contracted rotary muscles on the restricted side.

   (If needed) needles the muscle belly.

---

4.  When the spine is flexed the transverse processes
    move forward and anterior. If one side is
    restricted the transverse process on that side will
    remain posterior.

4. Needles the associated channel (i.e. Kidney in L2 dysfunctions).

In muscle energy techniques,

5. Asks the patient to push his feet, lightly, toward the ceiling against the practitioner's resistance. Muscle energy techniques require very accurate localization at the segment's barriers (Figure 9-56).

**THRUST TECHNIQUE FOR FLEXION RESTRICTION (ERS DYSFUNCTION).** The thrust technique is performed with the patient lying on his dysfunctional side (normal side up, the TrPr most anterior when the spine is in flexion). The practitioner stands in front of the patient and:

1. Flexes slowly the lower leg and hip upward until movement is first felt just below the dysfunctional segment. He then flexes from above by translating the patient's head and shoulder forward, until movement is first felt at the superior feather edge of the dysfunctional vertebra.

2. Drops the patient's upper leg just in front of the lower leg, and hooks the foot behind the lower leg.

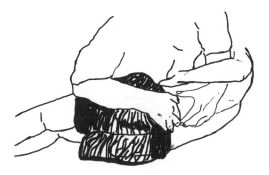

*Figure 9-57:* Thrust manipulation for flexion restriction — ERS(rt).

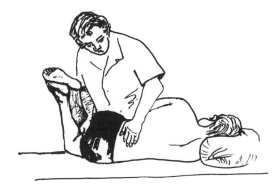

*Figure 9-58:* Muscle energy technique for neutral group dysfunction NR (rt).

**3.** Introduces rotation by sliding his forearm through the patient's upper axilla with fingers over the segment, to monitor motion.

**4.** Moves his own right forearm to and over the buttock, and the fingers of both hands monitor the segment.

**5.** Takes up the slack and fine tunes to the barriers (it must be comfortable to both patient and practitioner).

**6.** Gives a body thrust through his own right arm to the buttock, with the shoulder stable. (excessive pressure of the practitioner's left arm must be avoided, as it may be painful to the patient). The thrust rotates and sidebends the spine to the same side (Figure 9-57).

This position may also be used for muscle energy and respiratory assisted maneuver. The patient attempts to rotate (untwist) the spine against the practitioner's resistance. Sidebending can be resisted by asking the patient to lift his knees against the practitioner's resistance. For respiratory effort during normal respiration the slack is taken up, and then the patient is asked to exhale forcefully against the practitioner's attempt to keep the spine in the same position.

### Neutral Group Dysfunctions

Neutral group dysfunctions are treated with the spine in neutral, sidebending the spine at the apex of the group toward the convex side, and needling the more superficial sidebenders on the concave side.

**NEUTRAL GROUP MUSCLE ENERGY TECHNIQUE.** The patient is placed on his side with the concave side (sidebent group side) down and the spine in neutral, with the apex of the group at maximum ease. The practitioner then:

**1.** Lifts both of the patient's feet toward the ceiling to introduce sidebending.

**2.** Asks the patient to pull his feet down toward the table, against the practitioner's resistance (Figure 9-58).

**THRUST TECHNIQUE FOR NEUTRAL GROUP DYSFUNCTION.** The patient lies with his convex side close to the table.

The practitioner stands in front and monitors the apex of the dysfunctional group. The practitioner:

**1.** Straightens the patient's leg that is closer to the table, until the apex of the group is at a point of maximum ease.

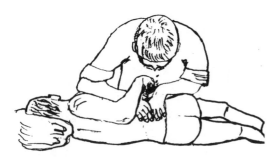

*Figure 9-59:* Thrust manipulation for neutral dysfunction — NR(lt).

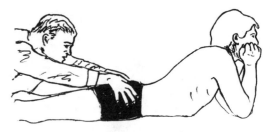

*Figure 9-60:* Assessment of ILA movement in spinal extension

**2.** Flexes the upper leg and drops it in front of the lower leg.

**3.** (While monitoring the segments) Pulls the shoulder out from under the patient, toward his feet, until the barrier is engaged at the upper edge of the group (this sidebends the spine toward the concavity of the group).

**4.** Places one of his forearms on the patient's buttock. The thrust is given by the practitioner's body, through his forearm, in a pure rotational direction, rotating the pelvis forward (Figure 9-59).

This position can be used with needling and with muscle energy. In needling, the sidebenders on the concave side of the group can be needled. For muscle energy, the patient's attempt to change his position in any direction and is resisted by the practitioner.

## Pelvic Dysfunction

Somatic dysfunction in the pelvis is one of the most common causes of back and leg pain. Assessment of ILA movement is important for diagnosis (Figure 9-60).

### Pubic Subluxations

According to Mitchell FL. Jr., pubic shears are the most common subluxation seen in the pelvis. Superior movement of the ipsilateral pube occurs normally in one-legged stance. The pubis can get stuck and result in a superior pubic shear dysfunction. Inferior shears tend to be self-correcting by weightbearing. Pubic shears impair movements of the ipsilateral SI joint. They can be detected by the standing and seated flexion and Stork tests, (Greenman 1989), (Figure 9-6).

In spite of the pubic ligaments the joint does not have intrinsic stability. Absent the aponeurotic extensions of the transversus, obliques, and rectus abdominus and the adductor longus, the pubic symphysis would permit 5-10 mm of vertical shear without much force. Dysfunction of these muscles can result in pubic subluxations. The motor nerves to these muscles originate in the lower thoracic and upper lumbar segments. Dysfunction of the lower thoracic and upper lumbar joints can affect the tone of these muscles. The lower thoracic and upper lumbar joints should be assessed and addressed if needed (Mitchell *ibid*).

**TREATMENT.** Muscle energy is effective to restore normal alignment. A simple shotgun technique, which works on all pubic dysfunctions, is performed with the

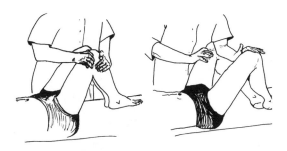

*Figure 9-61:* Shot gun technique for pubic dysfunction.

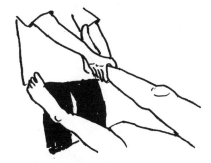

*Figure 9-62:* Manipulation of upslipped innominate on the right (this technique also works for a flexed sacrum).

patient supine. Both the patient's hips and knees are flexed, and feet are flat on the table. The practitioner:

1. Holds both of the patient's knees together and resists the patient's efforts to pull his knees apart.

2. Inserts one forearm between the patient's knees and resists the patient's effort to pull his knees together (Figure 9-61).

Stabilization exercises, sacral belt and, needling are helpful. Prolotherapy can be useful in severe cases.

### Iliosacral Subluxations

According to Mitchell FL. Jr., upslipped innominates are the second most common pelvic dislocation.

**ASSESSMENT.** This vertical shear of the innominate on the sacrum shortens the distance between the sacrococcygeal attachment of the sacrotuberous ligament and its ischial attachment. The ischial tuberosity will be found superiorly on that side, and the sacrotuberous ligament will feel lax (Greenman 1989). Downslipped innominates are a theoretical possibility, but they are rare and usually are self-correcting during weightbearing.[5]

Upslipped innominates occur often during a fall on the buttocks, when stepping into a hole unexpectedly, with car

accidents due to pressure from the brake pedal, or tripping on an unexpected step. Up slips are more common in patients lacking force closure due to soft tissue dysfunctions and therefore soft tissue dysfunctions must be addressed.

Motion testing in these patients usually reveals restrictions on the sheared side during weightbearing. Non-weight bearing tests however, reveal hypermobility. Occasionally the Standing Flexion Test (Figure 4-9 on page 195) is negative on the dislocated side and is positive on the nondislocated side (Mitchell *ibid*).

**TREATMENT.** Manipulative reduction by a longitudinal pull of the lower limb is effective and must be followed by stabilization of the pelvis. The patient is supine, the practitioner is at the base of the table. The practitioner:

1. Abducts and externally rotate the patient's leg.

2. Pulls the leg toward him while asking the patient to cough (Figure 9-62).

Reduction is only stable in about 50% of the cases. A sacral belt can be used to increase force closure of the ilia on the sacrum. If a patient is kept stable for 8 weeks using a belt, the outcome is favorable (Mitchell personal communication). It

5. Although some find inferior shears clinically and treat them with manual therapies.

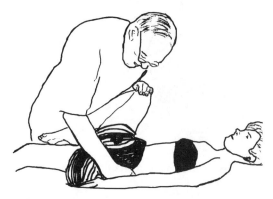

*Figure 9-63:* Muscle energy technique for outflare on the left.

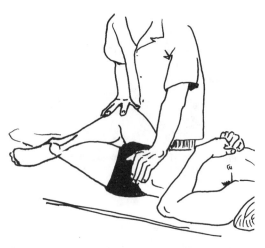

*Figure 9-64:* Muscle energy technique for inflare on right.

may be necessary to teach a family member to evaluate and treat the patient, as subluxations reoccur frequently.

Prolotherapy can be of great help in patients where manipulation, periosteal acupuncture and exercises fail.

### Pelvic Flares

Pelvic flares are the least common type of pelvic subluxation. Flares occur only in patients in whom the shape of the sacroiliac joint is abnormal (Greenman 1996). When the curvature is reversed the iliac side is concave and sacrum side convex. Flares occur with the ilium rotating about a vertical axis. Described as inflares and outflares, they are often associated with pubic dysfunctions.

**ASSESSMENT.** The ASIS is found either lateral or medial from midline in the supine patient (Greenman 1989).

**TREATMENT.** Flares can be treated most effectively with muscle energy techniques, treating the adductor muscles for inflares, and abductor muscles for outflares (Figure 9-63 and Figure 9-64). Needling the hip rotators, abductors and adductors can be beneficial.

### Iliosacral Dysfunctions

If, following successful treatment of pelvic subluxation and SI dysfunctions, the Standing Flexion Test is still positive and the ASISs are still found to be unequal, an iliosacral dysfunction is probable (Greenman 1989).

### Posterior Innominates

Posterior innominates are more common on the left side (Greenman *ibid*).

**ASSESSMENT.** The ASIS will be superior on the side of the positive standing flexion test. The leg on that side will appear to be shorter.

**TREATMENT.** Treatment is directed to the hip flexors, using needling and/or muscle energy. Often post-isometric stretches are useful in chronic cases (Figure 9-65).

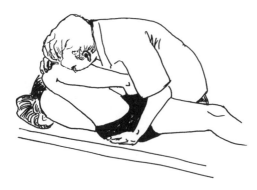

*Figure 9-66:*Muscle energy technique for left anterior innominate.

## Anterior Innominates

Anterior innominates are much more common on the right side (Greenman *ibid*). Here the findings are reversed, and treatment is directed to the hip extenders (Figure 9-66).

## Forward Sacral Torsions

Forward torsional movements are part of the normal walking cycle. Backward torsional movements are a normal sacral response to nonneutral lumbar movements. Torsion dysfunction occurs when

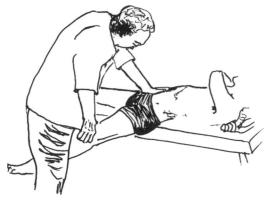

*Figure 9-65:* Muscle energy technique for left posterior innominate.

the sacrum loses the use of one of its oblique axes (Mitchell *ibid*).

Forward torsional dysfunctions are quite common and are described as left-on-left oblique axis, or right-on-right oblique axis sacral torsions.

**LEFT-ON-LEFT.** Left-on-left torsion is quite common and may not cause severe symptoms. Anterior torsional dysfunctions are maintained by the piriformis muscle on one side, and by the sidebenders, principally the quadratus lumborum muscles on the other side. In left-on-left, the affected sidebender muscles are on the left side. *For right-on-right*, which is much less common, the findings are reversed (Mitchell personal communication).

**ASSESSMENT.** In left-on-left, the seated flexion test may be positive on the right. The sacral right base loses its function of posterior nutation. Therefore, malposition and dysfunction (and possibly pain) are exaggerated in forward bending. The ILA and sacral base are posterior (rotated left) on the left in flexion, and become level in extension. The left ILA also is a little inferior, but not as much as in nutation dysfunction (unilaterally flexed sacrum), (Greenman *ibid*).

## Treatment

Treatment can be achieved by needling of the primary involved (spasmed) muscles, preferably with the patient in the lateral Sims position (Figure 9-67) on the involved axis (left, for left-on-left). One can needle the piriformis and quadratus lumborum muscles on the contralateral side, or their antagonists, as well.

**MUSCLE ENERGY.** For exact localization, which is necessary with muscle energy treatment (more precision is necessary than when needing) the patient is in the Sims position on the involved axis side. The practitioner:

**1.** Flexes the patient's hip to a point just before the sacrum begins to move.

**2.** Asks the patient to reach to the floor with his right hand until the practitioner first feels any sign of movement at L5.

**3.** Drops the patient's feet over the edge of the table, without losing any of the localization.

Resists the patient's effort at raising his feet for 3-5 seconds, after which the new barriers are engaged by repeating all of the above steps (Figure 9-68).

*Table 9-3.* **OSTEOPATHIC ILIOSACRAL DISORDERS**

| DYSFUNCTION | GENERAL INFORMATION | FINDINGS |
|---|---|---|
| Iliosacral Dysfunctions General | If, following successful treatment of pelvic subluxation and SI dysfunctions | The standing flexion test is still positive<br>The ASISs are still found to be unequal<br>Then an iliosacral dysfunction is probable |
| Upslipped Innominates | Second most common pelvic dislocation. More common on right side | The ischial tuberosity, Iliac crest, PSIS, ASIS will be found superiorly on that side<br>Sacrotuberous ligament lax on the subluxed side |
| Posterior Innominates (lt) | More common on the left side | The left ASIS will be superior on the side of the positive standing flexion test<br>— the leg on that side will appear to be shorter |
| Anterior Innominates | Anterior innominates are much more common on the right side | The findings are reversed of posterior innominates |
| Iliac Outflare (lt) | Found in pathologic joints | Flexion test positive on left<br>ASIS further from midline on left |
| Iliac Inflare (rt) | Found in pathologic joints | Flexion test positive on right<br>ASIS further from midline on right |

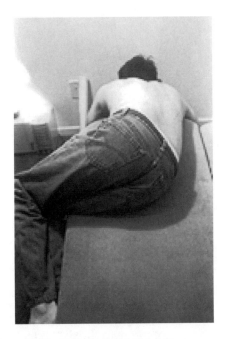

Figure 9-67: Patient treated in the Sims position.

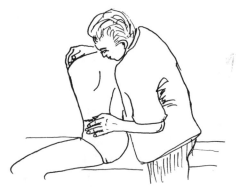

Figure 9-69: Thrust technique for a left on left torsion.

**THRUST MANIPULATION FOR LEFT-ON-LEFT.** A thrust technique can be performed with the patient seated. The seated patient holds his right shoulder with his left hand. The practitioner stands to the right and:

1. Contacts the patient's left sacral base with his left pisiform.

2. (With the other arm over the patient's right shoulder) reaches and grasps the patient's left shoulder.

3. Flexes the patient's spine, including the sacrum, until the first sign of innominate movement is felt.

4. Sidebends and rotates the patient's spine and sacrum to the right until movement is felt first at the innominates.

5. Thrusts his pisiform against the patient's sacrum while the patient is taken further into sidebending and rotation. At the moment of thrust, it is helpful to reduce the lumbosacral flexion (Figure 9-69).

If the condition recurs, muscular re-education, stabilization and stretching often are necessary.

*Backward Sacral Torsions*

Backward torsion dysfunctions, which are less common, are associated with lumbar nonneutral dysfunction, often with extension restrictions (Bourdillon, Day and Brookhout 1992). Backward torsions are described as right-on-left (or left-on-right) oblique axis dysfunctions. Backward torsions often are acute and severely painful. Normal nutation movement of one side of the sacral base is restricted. Therefore,

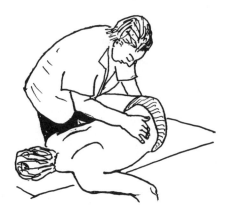

Figure 9-68: Muscle energy technique for left on left.

signs and symptoms are exaggerated by extension of the lumbar spine. Typically, backward torsion dysfunctions occur in patients who have bent forward and then twisted to pick up an object (Greenman *ibid*).

The Ipsilateral co-contraction of the lumbar sidebenders and hip external rotators force the sacrum to rotate its base backward on the oblique axis. The patient's antalgic (fixed, flexed and sidebent) position is indistinguishable from that caused by psoas spasm (Mitchell 1993).

**ASSESSMENT.** In *right-on-left* for example, the standing flexion test is positive on the right. The sacral base and the ILA are posterior on the right in extension, and are level in flexion. The ILA is also slightly displaced inferiorly. Lumbar lordosis and spring are reduced (protective spasm and nonadaptive dysfunction). The accompanying lumbar dysfunction found most commonly is FRS(rt) at L5-S1 (Bourdillon, Day and Brookhout 1992) and should be treated first. Greenman found that 83% of failed back patients have FRS dysfunctions (extension restrictions), of whom 22.4% were at L5. 33% of Greenman's patients had backward torsions.

*Treatment*

Often needling the spasmed piriformis, quadratus lumborum, and if needed the gluteus medius and tensor fascia latae, on the same side, is useful. They may be needled on the opposite side, as well. The patient should be in the lateral recumbent position with the dysfunctional side up and the lumbar spine in extension. The muscles are needled, and after each insertion lumbar extension is increased. The PSIS is needled gently.

**MUSCLE ENERGY.** For muscle energy, localization must be exact. The following example is for right-on-left backward torsion.

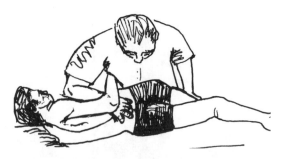

*Figure 9-70:* Muscle energy technique for right on left sacral torsion.

The patient lies on his left side, the side of the involved axis. Standing in front of the patient, the practitioner:

1. Brings the patient's spine into extension by pushing the head backward until movement is first felt at L5.

2. Eases the patient's left leg until the sacrum begins to move.

3. Introduces rotation, by having the patient reach with his right hand holding the edge of the table, just until movement is felt at L5.

4. Drops the patient's upper leg off the table.

5. Resists the patient's effort of raising his leg, and holds for 6 seconds. Then the patient relaxes, and the new barriers are engaged (Figure 9-70).

These procedures are repeated 3-5 times.

**THRUST TECHNIQUE.** Thrust correction is achieved with the patient supine. This is described again, for right on left torsion.

The patient lies supine close to the left edge of the table, holding to the back of his neck with fingers laced.

The practitioner stands on the left side of the patient and:

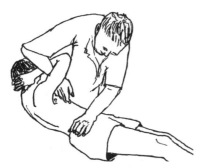

*Figure 9-71:* Thrust manipulation for right of left sacral torsion and unilateral extended sacrum.

1. Moves the patient's feet and head to the other side of the table, producing right sidebending.

2. Threads his right forearm through the patient's right arm and rests it on the patient's chest. With his other hand, he stabilizes the right ilium.

3. Rotates the patient toward him until the ilium begins to lift.

4. Rotates the trunk or thrusts on the right ASIS while holding the trunk flexed, rotated and sidebent.

This technique is effective also for a unilateral extended sacrum (Figure 9-71).

### Sacral Subluxations: Unilateral Flexed Sacrum (Anteriorly Nutated Sacrum)

Unilateral flexed sacrum is also called inferior sacral shear. Bilateral sacral restrictions are rare. Left unilateral flexed sacrum (anterior sacral nutations) are much more common than right-sided dysfunctions (about 9:1), (Greenman *ibid*).

**ASSESSMENT.** In a left unilateral flexed sacrum, often the seated flexion test is positive on the left. The base on that side is restricted in anterior nutation (with loss of counternutation) and will be found anterior to the iliac crest, especially in spinal flexion, but slightly less so in neutral.

In extension it is nearly, but not quite, level. The sacrum is sidebent to the left, and the ILA are inferior on the same side—about 1 cm closer to the feet than the right ILA—and are slightly posterior, but not as much as in torsional dysfunctions (Mitchell *ibid*).

**TREATMENT.** A unilateral flexed sacrum can be maintained by SI joint instability. Therefore it usually is necessary to stabilize this joint. A sacral belt may be helpful, and all muscles contributing to force closure of the ilia must be balanced and strengthened. In case of recurrence, periosteal acupuncture or prolotherapy to the dorsal sacroiliac ligaments may be needed.

This dysfunction can be treated only with manual therapy techniques that often give temporary relief. No lasting effect can be assured. No needling technique is available to correct the dysfunction. Also, since this motion of the sacrum is not muscle-dependent, no true isometric muscle energy treatment is available. A respiratory-assisted isotonic technique is performed with the patient prone, and with his feet hanging over the table. In some patients it is preferable to place a small pillow under the abdomen in order to flex the spine slightly and start sacral counternutation movement.

The practitioner stands at the left side of the patient and:

1. Abducts the patient's leg about 10 to 15°, until the SI joint is loose packed (maximus ease), and asks the patient to point his left toe toward his right side and hold it there.

2. Puts the heel of his hand on the patient's left ILA, and springs it anteriorly. He monitors the sacral sulci for motion and adjusts the angle of the spring hand until maximum motion is felt at the sulci.

3. Asks the patient to take a deep breath and hold it. While he pushes the ILA in the direction found to have the most

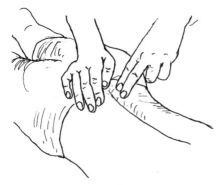

*Figure 9-72:* Muscle energy technique for unilateral flexed sacrum on the left.

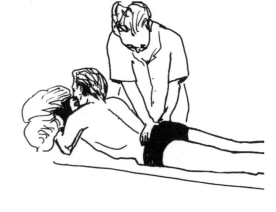

*Figure 9-73:* Muscle energy technique for unilateral extended sacrum.

spring, the patient is asked to attempt to breath even more deeply.

**4.** Holds this position firmly for about 5 seconds and then asks the patient to exhale slowly, while making sure that no pressure is released by the practitioner.

**5.** Repeats this process one or two more times. On the last time, if more force is needed, he asks the patient to cough, and a thrust can be given in the same direction (Figure 9-72).

Because recurrence is common, a relative of the patient can be taught this procedure and should repeat it as necessary.

### Unilateral Extended Sacrum/Posteriorly Nutated Sacrum

The unilateral extended sacrum, in which the sacrum loses its nutation function, is also called a superior sacral shear. Findings are more pronounced in lumbar spine extension. This dysfunction is much more common on the right than the left side. Unilateral extended sacrum probably is created by excessive lumbar lordosis and SI joint instability (Mitchell 1993). However, once dysfunction is established, the lumbar curve and spring are reduced.

**ASSESSMENT.** In unilateral extended sacrum on the right the seated flexion test often is positive on the right. In extension the sacral base is found more posteriorly, and the ILA more anteriorly and superiorly on the right side. In neutral or in flexion they are almost, but not quite, symmetrical. The lumbar lordosis and springiness is reduced (Greenman *ibid*).

### Treatment

**THRUST TECHNIQUE.** Thrust technique is the same as for posterior torsion.

**MUSCLE      ENERGY/RESPIRATORY-ASSISTED TECHNIQUE.** The patient is positioned with the SI loosely packed, as in the case of a unilateral flexed sacrum. The spine is put in extension by asking the patient to hold his elbows together with his chin between his hands (sphinx position). The practitioner then:

**1.** Contacts the patient's posteriorly-stuck sacral base, and supports the pelvis with his other hand under the opposite ASIS.

**2.** Asks the patient to breath out as much as he can while, at the same time, the practitioner is pushing down on the sacral base and pulling on the ASIS.

**3.** Holds for about 5 seconds. Asks the patient to breath in slowly. And he does not ease the pressure.

These steps are repeated 2-3 times. If the conditions reoccur, joint stability should be addressed. The patient should be told to bring his knee to his shoulder on the dysfunctional side (Figure 9-73).

## The Cocktail Syndrome

Chronically recurrent low back pain is often known as the *cocktail* syndrome. This syndrome is characterized by recurrent pain, posain, and nulliness, probably due to ligamentous insufficiency. The patient complains of low back pain which may or may not radiate to the buttock and legs. The pain worsens when the patient stands without being mobile, when sitting or maintaining any position for prolonged duration (posain).

According to Greenman (1996) the osteopathic structural diagnosis findings in this population usually consist of problems on the left side with:

- Left pube being superior.
- Left flexed sacrum.
- Left innominate posterior.
- L5 extended, rotated and sidebent to left.
- Tight erector spinae muscles and weak abdominal muscles.

Treatment often is difficult and patients frequently require a referral to prolotherapy.

## Failed Back Syndrome

Failed back syndrome occurs in patients with persistent pain after conservative and/or surgical intervention. It is toward these patients that this manual is geared, as most other back pain improves on its own, whether treated or not. Patients with failed back syndrome usually represent a mixture of the above-described syndromes, many of which are secondary to ligamentous insufficiency.

Greenman (1992) described the most common somatic dysfunctions found in 183 patients with failed low back syndrome. He reports an increased incidence of restriction of some motions within the SI joint and symphysis pubis. A cluster called the "dirty half dozen" was common. The dirty half dozen are:

- Pelvic obliquities with sacral base unleveling.
- Pubic dysfunctions.
- Anterior nutation restrictions.
- Innominate shears.
- Nonneutral lumbar dysfunctions.
- Muscle imbalances of the lower extremities and trunk.

Greenman found that 62.8% of these patients had significant pelvic unleveling (sacral base unleveling) as a result of leg length inequality. He also found a high incidence of pubic dysfunctions occurring in 45.4% of the patients. Pubic dysfunctions usually were accompanied by an imbalance of the muscle length and strength of the abdominal muscles above, and of the adductors below. Other findings were:

- 33% had posterior torsions and 19% had anterior torsions.
- Innominate shears were found in 23.5% of the patients, with 19.1% having superior shears and 4.4% inferior shears.
- Flexed sacrums were found in 25.1% of the patients; 23% on the left side, 1.6% on the right, and 0.5% bilateral.
- Unilateral extended sacrums were found only on the right in 15.3% of the patients.
- Anterior innominate were 10 times more common on the right.
- Left-on-left torsions were three times more common than right-on-right torsions.

- In post-surgical patients, 58% had posterior torsions and extended sacrums.

As can be seen from the above data, anterior rotation dysfunction on the right, and posterior torsion on the left, are most common and support the "universal pattern" concept (see chapter 4).

Lumbar dysfunctions, including ERS and FRS, were found at the T-12 through L5 levels.
- ERS (flexion restriction) dysfunctions were found in 31.6% of the patients.
- FRS (extension restriction) dysfunctions were found in 83.5% of the patients, of which 47% were at the L4 and L5 levels.
- Neutral dysfunctions of the mid-and upper-lumbar spine were observed frequently, as well.

Overall, 86.3% had two or more dysfunctions, and only 3.7% of the patients had no joint dysfunctions contributing to their pain.

**TREATMENT.** Treatment of failed back syndrome must be comprehensive. These patients often have a multitude of dysfunctions, and the best outcome is obtained by directing treatment to all of them. The patient's posture and functional symmetry must be addressed and corrected. Soft tissue flexibility, strength and movement patterning should be addressed. The patient's global health should also be addressed. Finally, the patient should be educated about perpetuating factors and should be shown ways to avoid them.

*Table 9-4.* OSTEOPATHIC SI DYSFUNCTIONS

| DYSFUNCTION | GENERAL INFORMATION | FINDINGS |
| --- | --- | --- |
| PUBIC SHEARS | The most common subluxation of the pelvis<br>— especially during pregnancy<br>Can be inferior or superior<br>— inferior shears tend to be self-correcting by weightbearing | Positive, standing flexion, seated flexion and Stork tests on the dysfunctional side<br>Superior or inferior pube on the dysfunctional side |
| ANTERIOR TORSIONS | Quite common<br>Often associated with mild symptoms<br>about 4:1. compared to right on right | |
| LEFT-ON-LEFT | | Standing flexion test may be positive on the right<br>Sacral right base loses its function of posterior nutation<br>— therefore malposition and dysfunction (and possibly pain) are exaggerated when patient is forward bent<br>Sacral ILA [a]posterior and inferior on the left<br>Sacral base is posterior (rotated left) on the left in flexion<br>— and becomes level in extension<br>— the left ILA is also a little inferior, but not as much as in nutation dysfunction (unilaterally flexed sacrum) |
| RIGHT-ON-RIGHT | | Findings are reversed from Left-on Left |
| BACKWARD TORSION DYSFUNCTIONS | Less common<br>Described as right-on-left (or left-on-right) oblique axis<br>— associated with lumbar nonneutral dysfunction<br>— often with extension restrictions<br>— often are acute and severely painful | Normal nutation movement of one side of the sacral base is restricted<br>— therefore signs, and usually symptoms, are exaggerated by extension of the lumbar spine |
| RIGHT ON LEFT | More common than Left on Right<br>often with FRS(rt) at L5-S1 that should be treated first | Seating flexion test is positive on the right<br>The sacral base and the ILA are posterior on the right in extension<br>— ILA also slightly inferior<br>— both are level in flexion<br>Lumbar lordosis and spring are reduced |
| LEFT ON RIGHT | | Findings are reversed from Right on Left |

a. Inferior Lateral Angle of sacrum

*Table 9-5.* **OSTEOPATHIC PELVIC DYSFUNCTIONS (CONTINUED)**

| DYSFUNCTION | GENERAL INFORMATION | FINDINGS |
|---|---|---|
| **UNILATERAL FLEXED SACRUM (LEFT)** | Bilateral flexed sacral restrictions are rare<br>Left unilateral flexed sacrum (anterior sacral nutations)<br><br>— are much more common than right-sided dysfunctions (about 9:1)<br>— must be treated with manual therapy | Often the seated flexion test is positive on the left<br>The base on that side is restricted in anterior nutation (with loss of counternutation)<br><br>— base will be found anterior to the iliac crest especially in spinal flexion<br>— but slightly less in neutral<br>— in extension it is nearly, but not quite, level<br>— sacrum is sidebent to the left<br>— ILA is inferior on the same side — about 1 cm, and are slightly posterior, but not as much as in torsional dysfunctions<br>Lumbar compensation is usually rotation of L5 to the right |
| **UNILATERAL EXTENDED SACRUM (RIGHT)** | Sacrum loses its nutation function<br>Findings are more pronounced in lumbar extension<br><br>— Much more common on the right | Often the seated flexion test is positive on the right<br>In extension the sacral base is found more posteriorly on the right<br><br>— the ILA more anteriorly and superior on that side<br>— in neutral or in flexion they are almost, but not quite, symmetrical<br>The lumbar lordosis and spring is reduced<br>Lumbar compensation is usually with L5 rotation to the right |

# General Treatment Techniques

## Acupuncture

Acupuncture can be effective in both acute and chronic low back and leg pain.

### Local & Distal Point Stimulation

An acupuncture treatment may stimulate points that are either local or distal to the injury or painful area.

- Distal points often are preferable, because mobilization and manual therapy of the affected part can be performed simultaneously.
- When local points are used, often it is preferable to treat the patient sitting or standing, and to stimulate the point only for a short time, without needle retention. This may prevent a flare-up.

The practitioner:

1. Generally sedates the local points so as to normalize the flow of Qi and Blood, and to relieve muscle spasm and pain.

2. Aims the needle such that the Qi projects toward the painful site.

3. May use moxa or needle tonification locally (if the patient is deficient or cold).

*Channel Therapy.*

**SINEW CHANNELS.** The Sinew channels are used frequently during the acute phase of low back pain. After activating the channel by stimulation of the Well point and the termination points (SI-18 for Leg-Yang channels and CV-2 or 3 for Leg-Yin channels) local tender points are needled.

**CONNECTING CHANNELS.** Most commonly used are: Urinary Bladder/Kidney, Liver/Gall Bladder, and Spleen/Stomach. If congested (dark) blood vessels are visible the Connecting point of the channel that passes through the region is needled and the vessels are bled. The channels are always used in patients with edema and circulatory problems.

**EAR POINTS.** Common ear points for low back pain are:

- Applicable lumbar vertebrae
- Lumbago.
- Shen Men/Spirit Gate.
- Dermis/subcortex.
- Adrenal/stress control.
- Kidney.
- Sympathetic.
- Thalamus/pain control.

**EXTRA CHANNELS/VESSELS.** The Yin Motility (Qiao) and Conception (Ren) channels are used mainly when low back pain is accompanied with poor abdominal muscle tone and tightness in the lumbar region. The Master points are K-6 and Lu-7, the activating points are K-9 and K-1.

The Girdle (Dai) and Yang linking (Wei) channels are used to treat instability with tenderness in the ASIS and lower abdominal areas. The Master points are GB-41 and TW-5 the activating points are GB-26 and UB-63.

The Governing (Du) and Yang Motility (Qiao) channels are used to treat general weakness of the spine, and patients with palpatory tenderness along the spine, ASIS and K11. The posterior axilla region and the cervical vertebra may be tender as well. The Master points are SI-3 and UB-62, the activating points are GV-1 and UB-62.

Table 9-6 on page 478 through Table 9-11 on page 481 presents points from classical, Tong-style, and modern Japanese style acupuncture.

*Table 9-6.* **POINTS: SPRAIN AND STRAIN**

| Symptom | Points |
|---|---|
| General | GV-26, K-2 and bleeding UB-40 (UB-40-for acute pain) |
| | • next stimulate local ashi (trigger) points quickly |
| | • then needle State H2O, GV-20 and UB-7 ask patient to mobilize the back |
| Pain More Central | SI-3 |
| With Acute Subcostal Pain | Lu-5, LI-11, LI-4, Sp-6, Sp-9, Liv-2, St-36 and LI-10 |
| Acutely Stiff Back and Spine | UB-11, UB-41 and CV-9. |
| | or |
| | GV-11, GV-6, GV-2, GV-1 |
| | or |
| | UB-17, CV-9, GV-4, UB-20, UB-27 and UB-28 |
| | or |
| | UB-47 and GB-25 |
| Low Back Sprain | Lu-5, UB-40, GV-26, UB-60, UB-65, TW-6 and GB-34 |
| Upper Low Back/Thoracic | H-8 |
| Sudden Pain aggravated by deep breath/ cough | Water Gold and Water Passing Through (1010.19-20) |
| Spasm of Quadratus Lumborum (seen often with Kidney deficiency) | Double Child Immortal (internal Hoku, LI4) on the contralateral side |

*Table 9-7.* **Points: Acute and Chronic Disc Pain**

| Points: Acute and Chronic Disc Pain | |
| --- | --- |
| Symptom | Points |
| L2 and L3 Disc Lesions | Passing through Kidney and Upper Back (88.09-11), H-8 |
| L4 and L5 Disc Lesions | GB-31, GB-38, Liv-3, 2 <br> or <br> LI-4 1/2, TW-3 1/2 |
| S1 and S2 Disc Lesions <br> For foot drop | Five Thousand Gold (33.08-09) with UB-40, GB-31, GB-38, H-4 and GV-26 <br> or <br> GB-34, St-36, 38, Liv-3 |
| Acute Flashes of Pain <br> in lumbar spine <br> due to any level disc lesion | GV-26 and UB-40 |
| Pain Radiating to Buttocks | Flower Bone Three and Four (55.04-05) |
| Chronic Disc Lesions | Correct Tendons (77.01-02) <br> GB 30 strong stimulation <br> Hua tuo jia ji in painful areas <br> — Hua tuo points needled with patient sitting, standing or prone, without needle retention |
| Sciatica | Five Thousand Gold (33.08-09) <br> Four Flower Below (77.11) <br> Four Flower (77.10) <br> Bowel Intestine (77.12) <br> with additions of disc points as needed <br> or <br> Stimulate contralaterally to painful side <br> — GB-30, GB-31 and St-36 <br> Stimulate ipsilaterally <br> — UB-27 and UB-25, <br> Follow with moxibustion at <br> — St-36, K-3, UB-23, 59 and 32, and GB31 and 32 |
| Sciatica: other common prescriptions | Pain that radiates down lateral aspect of leg <br> — GB-30, GB-34, GB-39, St-36 and St-4 <br> Pain that radiates down posterior aspect of leg <br> — UB-40, UB-56 and UB-57 <br> For back pain with sciatica <br> — UB-23, UB-30, UB-50, GB-30, UB-51, UB-54 and GB-34 <br> — UB-31, UB-32, UB-49, UB-57, GB-39, UB-60, GB-41 |

*Table 9-8.* **POINTS: OTHER CONDITIONS**

| Symptom | Points |
|---|---|
| Vertebral Hypertrophy | Bleed UB-40<br>Bright Yellow (88.12), Three 9 Miles (88.25-27) and SI- 3½ |
| Coccydynia | GV-20, Hua Tuo points at C5-7<br>If needed, add UB-34, 35 and GB-30 |
| Sacrolliac Dysfunction and Pain | State Waters plus a needle ½-inch laterally to the contralateral side of the painful joint<br>Flower Bone Three and Four bilaterally; mobilize the joint at the same time<br>If needed, palpate and treat Hua Tuo point at T-10 through L1<br>UB-32, 34 contralaterally |
| Pubic Dysfunction and Pain | HuA Tuo Jia Ji at T-12 to through L2 (as needed), CV-6<br>Sp-9. and adductor muscles<br><br>Hormonal dysfunction add Liv-8, 3 Emperors (77.18-21) |

*Table 9-9.* **POINTS: BASED ON LOCATION OF PAIN**

| Symptom | Points |
|---|---|
| Anywhere from Thoracolumbar Junction to Lumbosacral Junction | UB-40, 60 and UB -18 through 25<br>Hua Tuo point at these levels |
| More Central | Moxa UB-67<br>Needles<br>SI-3, GV-16 (or State Waters), LI-4 and 4-1/2, 3 Emperors (77.18-21)<br>Bleeding Flower External (77.14) local Hua Tuo and GV points |
| More Lateral | GB-41, TW-5<br>Beside Three Miles (77.22-23)<br>GB-19, 29, 30, and 31 |
| At Lumbosacral Junction | State Waters (1010.25) plus points ½-1cm lateral to them on the contralateral side of the pain<br>Local points<br>UB-25 through 34, GV-3, 4 |
| More Lateral, at Lumbosacral Area | GB-19,18, 31, Nine Miles (88.25-27)<br>GB-41 with TW-5 |
| At Iliac Crest | GB-31 |

*Table 9-10.* **POINTS: BASED ON MOVEMENT**

| Symptom | Points |
|---|---|
| **Restricted Extension Pain**<br>or<br>Pain<br>Aggravated by Extension | UB-41,53, GV-2,3 and 26, Liv13 and 14, CV-2 through 6 |
| **Pain at Midline** aggravated by<br>Flexion or Extension | GV-26 and SI-3<br>Bleed UB-40<br>K-2. UB 47 and Liv 3 also can be used for extension and or flexion restrictions |
| **Restricted Flexion**<br>or<br>Pain<br>aggravated by Flexion | GV-26, UB- 23, 52<br>Bleed UB- 40<br>Point at sacral base |
| **Restricted Rotation**<br>or<br>**Pain**<br>aggravated by rotation | UB-62 and SI-3 especially with Ion cords<br>or<br>GB-41 and TW-5 |
| Generally Restricted Lumbar<br>Movement | Moxa UB-67, 60<br>Bleed Liv-13, UB-40 |
| **Extension Restrictions** especially with<br>Flaccidity of Muscles<br>of lateral aspect<br>of lower extremity and<br>Spasm of Medial Aspect | K-6 and Lu-7 |
| **Flexion Restrictions** and<br>**Pain** along posterior and lateral aspect<br>of spine, especially if medial aspect of<br>lower extremity muscles are flaccid,<br>and lateral aspect is spasmed | Bl-62 and SI-3 |

*Table 9-11.* **DR. YOSHIO MONAKA'S ION CORD TREATMENT FOR LOW BACK I**

| Symptom | Points |
|---|---|
| Lower Back Pain | UB-47 (black clip)<br>and<br>UB-57 (red clip) |
| Lumbar Pain | UB-23 or UB-47 (black clip) and SI-3<br>or<br>UB-62 (red clip) |
| Lumbar and Thigh Pain | GB-30 or UB-51 (black clip)<br>and<br>GB-35 or GB-34 (red clip) |
| Lateral Low Back Pain | UB-23 (black clip)<br>and<br>GB-29 or GB-34 (red clip) |
| Numbness | Tender points on affected limb, with black clip connected to Yin points and red clip on Yang points |

## Instability

If periosteal needling or prolotherapy is used to treat instability and ligamentous insufficiency, the patient should make movements following the treatment (i.e., bending, walking). In the absence of this kind of movement, random scar tissue will form in the area inflamed by the treatment. But if the patient performs these movements, the result usually is normal-looking ligament fibers (Dorman *ibid*). In the lumbar spine and pelvis periosteal needling does not work as well as in the cervical spine and referral to prolotherapy is needed often.

### Treatment

To treat instability and ligamentous insufficiency, the practitioner:

1. Addresses all vertebral and sacroiliac dysfunctions (before trying to needle the ligaments of the lumbosacral spine).
   Left uncorrected, these dysfunctions will stress the ligaments and will not allow healing to occur. When abnormal mechanical forces are relieved and the ligaments are stimulated, healing and stability are likely to return.

2. Introduces stabilization exercises to the patient.
   These exercises are individualized for each patient, addressing first muscle shortening, and then strengthening.

3. Needles the ligaments.
   Periosteal acupuncture must be integrated with a comprehensive approach. Otherwise, the symptoms are likely to increase, and the needling will have little or no long-term benefit.

4. Instructs the patient to apply an external herbal pack every day during recovery, and to take herbs for Blood circulation and soft tissue strengthening.

**PERIOSTEAL ACUPUNCTURE FOR LIGAMENTOUS**

**INSUFFICIENCY.** Because treatment for instability and ligamentous insufficiency can be painful, the practitioner can give the patient an analgesic before beginning. Yin Hu So Pien (tetrahydropalmatine, 200 mg.[1]) is a good choice, as it is a powerful analgesic with a sedative, of somewhat short duration of action. The practitioner:

1. Prepares the patient's skin and inserts a 30-gage needle, first at midline.

2. Stimulates the interspinous and supraspinous ligaments. Contacts the spine and stimulates the periosteum.

CAUTION: The practitioner must take extreme care not to penetrate the spinal cord.

3. Needles the lumbosacral ligaments.

4. Needles about 1-5 cm from midline down to the base of the lamina, and tries to reach the ligamentum flavum.
   It may be difficult to feel the ligament. However, the small amount of blood spilled probably will reach the ligament and induce inflammation.

5. Pecks the lamina slightly.

6. Needles the iliolumbar ligament attachments at the iliac crest with a thicker needle inserted at the medial end of the iliac crest.

7. "Walks" the needle by repeated insertions until reaching the anterior aspect of the ilia, inserts the needle under the iliac crest, and stimulates the area electrically or manually.

8. Needles the attachments of the sacrotuberous and the sacrospinous ligaments onto the medial edge of the sacrum (with the patient sidelying).

9. Attends to the sacroiliac ligaments, penetrating all superficial nodules.

10. Needles the surfaces of the PSIS and ilia. Stimulates the periosteum.

---

1. No longer available in the US.

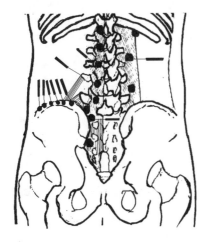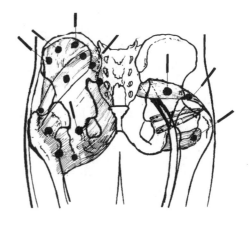

*Figure 9-74:* Important areas to needle for low-back and buttock pain.

**11.** Needles the deeper aspects of the ilia and sacral ligaments. Stimulates the periosteum.

**12.** Selects several 3-inch needles. Needles the anterior superior aspect of the SI joint from above, at a point about two cm lateral to L4, directing the needles downward and slightly laterally toward the sacroiliac joint.

**13.** Leaves the needles in place.

**14.** Places several needles at the midline of the sacrum, directs them toward the attachments of the posterior SI ligaments, and leaves them in place.

**15.** Connects the positive pole (some do better with negative pole) of an electrical stimulator to these needles and leaves it on for as long as conditions allow (the longer the better, up to two hours).

At the end of the treatment, the practitioner must re-evaluate the patient's lumbosacral mechanics, because muscle spasm and vertebral dysfunction may set in due to the strong stimulation of these tissues. The practitioner should correct these conditions before sending the patient home.

The practitioner repeats this treatment one week later. During the week between treatments, the patient must continue stabilization exercises. Lasting results often require 6-15 treatments. If, after eight treatments, no response is evident, the practitioner should stop treatment and refer the patient for injection therapy—prolotherapy.

### Herbal Therapy

A topical herbal formula for ligamentous laxity is:

Os Draconis (Long Gu)

Cornu Bovis Carbcnisatus (Niu Jiao)

Rhizoma Dioscorea Bishie (Bi Xie)

Cortex Kadsurae Radicis (Zi Jing Pi)

Rhizoma Notopterygii (Qiang Huo)

Cortex Albizziae (He Huan Pi)

Sanguis Draconis (Xue Jie)

Rhizoma Bletillae (Bai Ji)

Radix Palygalae (Yuan Zhi)

Copper Pynites (Zi Ran Tong)

Acacia seu Uncaria (Er Cha)

Eupolyphaga seu Opisthoplatia (Tu Bie Chong)

Rhizoma Drynariae (Gu Sui Bu)

## Chronic Myofascial Disorder

Long-term muscular lesions and pain can result in accumulation of waste products. Muscles lose their elasticity and become edematous and tight, and they feel firm and doughy. The practitioner should address all of these aspects. For patients who have had back surgery, often it is important to treat the sacrospinalis tendon attachments to the transverse processes and the spine.

All of the patient's involved muscles should be needled (Figure 9-74). The patient is prone:

- Pillow under abdomen to straighten the lumbar curve.

- Arms hanging by the sides of the table.

- Spine sidebent away from the side to be treated.

The thoracolumbar paraspinal, gluteus medius and piriformis muscles may be assessed and treated with the patient lying on his side.

The practitioner:

1. Palpates for tissue texture and tenderness, marking all additional sites.

2. Performs an electrical diagnostic stimulation, marking all hyperactive sites.

3. Begins treatment centrally and proceeds laterally and distally.

   Both the superficial and the intrinsic muscles of the thorax, lumbar region, buttocks, abdomen and lower extremities should be evaluated and, if necessary, treated.

   The treatment should be aimed at the myofascial groups involved mechanically and neuropathically, according to their myotome patterns.

4. Needles all the following muscles superficially first. If needed needles deeply.

5. Starts, on the nonpainful side, with the superficial layers of the latissimus dorsi and the thoracolumbar fascia.

6. Needles the attachments of the thoracolumbar fascia and the external and internal obliques at the iliac crest.

7. Continues needling the intermediate layers of the erector spinae (when these muscles are released), starting about ½-inch from midline (Hua tuo points).

8. Needles the spinalis perpendicularly.

9. Angles the needle toward the spine and continues needling the longissimus thoracis, about one inch lateral to midline (UB line).

10. Continues to the iliocostalis lumborum, about 2-4 inches from midline (outer UB line).

11. Needles the attachments of the iliocostalis lumborum and longissimus at the iliac crest.

12. Needles the deeper semispinalis, rotators and quadratus lumborum when relaxation of both of the above layers is achieved.

To reach the quadratus lumborum most easily, the practitioner:

- Places a pillow under the sidelying patient.

- Uses a 3-inch needle directed medially.

- Treats the lesion (a tight spasm locus in muscle or fibrotic tissue) by pecking the hard dense fibrous tissue.

   Treats the deeper layers immediately, If no reaction is seen in the superficial muscle.

13. Assesses and treats the buttock muscles using steps 1 and 2.

14. Treats the glutei and piriformis.

15. Treats the muscles of the lower extremities.

   Evaluates and treats, if needed, the:

   - Tensor fascia lata and iliotibial tract.

- Hamstrings (including the biceps femoris).
- Semitendinosus and semimembranosus.
- Quadriceps femoris, including the rectus femoris.
- Vastus lateralis and vastus medialis.
- Adductors.

16. Cups the area (after needling).
If significant trophedema is present, during the first session the cups are left in place. During the second session the practitioner lifts the cups, stretching the fascia further. Later the practitioner performs a moving cup procedure.

### Herbal Therapy

A guiding oral formula for chronic low back pain of myofascial origin is:

Antler glue (Lu Jiao)
Tortosie Plastron glue (Gui Ban Jiao)
Rhizoma Dioscoreae (San Yao)
Fructus Corni (Shan Zhu Yu)
Fructus Lycii (Gou Qi Zi)
Semen Cuscutae (Tu Si Zi)
Cortex Eucommiae (Du Zhong)
Angelica Chinesis (Dang Gui)
Rhizoma Corydalis (Yan Hu Suo) viniger extracted
Myrrh (Mo Yao)
Achyranthes Bidentata (Niu Xi)
Rhizoma Ligustici (Chuan Xiong)
Lumbricus (Di Long)
Eupolyphaga (Tu Bie Chong)
Aconitum Kusenzoffii (Cao Wu Tou)
Poria (Fu Ling)
Semen Plantaginis (Che Qian Zi)
Radix Angelica Pubescentis (Du Huo)
Radix Gentianae (Qin Jiao)
Cortex Lycii Radicis (Di Gu Pi)
Rhizoma Alismatis (Ze Xie)

For a sensetive patient that can not tolerate the above formula an alternative is:

Rhizoma Atractlyodis (Bai Zhu)
Cortex Eucommiae (Du Zhong)
Radix Sileris (Fang Feng)
Angelica Chinesis (Dang Gui)

Squma Manitis (Chuan Shan Jia)

A guiding oral formula for low back pain in a patient with Yin deficiency and Dampness is:

Radix Dioscorea (Shan Yao)
Semen Dolichoris (Bai Bian Dao)
Radix Pseudostellariae (Tai Zi Shen)
Rhizoma Atractylodis (Bai Zhu)
Plumula Nelumbinis (Lian Zi)
Semen Coicis (Yi Yi Ren)
Poria Cocos (Fu Ling)
Rhizoma Alismatis (Ze Xie)
Fructus Corni (Shan Zhu Yu)
Cortex Eucommiae (Du Zhong)
Semen Cuscutae (Tu Si Zi)
Angelica Chinesis (Dang Gui)
Radix Gentianae (Qin Jiao)
Radix Sileris (Fang Feng)

A guiding oral formula for low back pain with sciatica (can be used for sciatica from a disc lesion as well) is:

Treated Rhizoma Arisaematis (Zhi Nan Xing)
Radix Angelicae Dahuricae (Bai Zhi)
Radix Phelodendri (Huang Bai)
Rhizoma Ligustici (Chuan Xiong)
Flos Carthami (Hong Hua)
Rhizoma seu Radix Notopterygii (Qiang Huo)
Radix Clematidis (Wei Ling Xian)
Rhizoma Atractylodis (Cang Zhu)
Semen Persicae (Tao Ren)
Radix Stephaniae (Fang Ji)
Rhizoma Corydalis (Yan Hu Suo)
Radix Angelica Pubescentis (Du Huo)
Radix Gentianae Scabae (Long Dan Cao)
Massa Fermentata (Shen Qu)
Ramulus Cinnamomi (Gui Zhi)
Resina Myrrhae (Mo Yao)
Resina Olibani (Ru Xiang)
Radix Paeoniae (Bai Shao)

# Thrust Techniques

High velocity thrust manipulations have been used throughout the world for centuries. Orthopaedic Medicine techniques and OM manipulative techniques, which are practically identical, can be divided roughly into rotation, distraction and extension methods. Distraction and extension techniques, which also have a rotational component, tend to be nonspecific and are performed away from painful movements. Their goal is to gap the joint and allow it to spring back into place. They also may free any trapped tissues, rupture adhesions, and probably through reciprocal inhibition, may also affect the direct barrier.

### CONTRAINDICATIONS TO THRUST MANIPULATION ARE:

- Cord signs.

- S4 signs (saddle anesthesia, weakness of bladder or anus) and pain in the perineum, rectum or scrotum.

- Bilateral sciatica unaccompanied by backache.

- Spinal claudication.

- Anticoagulant treatment.

Clinical judgement should be used in the following situations: (Muscle energy and indirect techniques are appropriate).

- Pregnancy can be disregarded during the first 4 months, but for the next four months the supine and side-lying techniques are best to use. During the last month, manipulation is best avoided. Some however manipulate to day of delivery.

- Acute pain in patients who roll over slowly and with difficulty during the examination, or in whom gentle pressure sets up unbearable pain.

- In psychologically disturbed patients, manipulation is best avoided.

The following non-specific or semi-specific thrust techniques for lumbosacral spine are useful for the beginner. On occasion they are effective when a more specific technique fails.

## Rotation with Distraction

This technique is an indirect (away from restricted barrier) exaggeration technique. It must be performed on a low treatment table.

The patient lies on his pain-free side (painful side up), spine in neutral without rotation (shoulder square), lower arm comfortable and hand under head. The practitioner stands infront of the patient. The practitioner:

1. Extends the patient's lower leg and flexes the upper leg.

2. Puts his left hand over the patient's trochanteric area, and his right hand over the patient's shoulder, which is rotated toward him.

3. Takes up the slack by rotating the shoulder backward and the hip down and forward.

   The shoulder is mostly stabilized, thereby avoiding excessive pressure on it, which may be uncomfortable to the patient.

4. Keeping his arms straight, has the patient breath in and out several times, continually takes up the slack.

5. Thrusts with his lower arm to the trunk, with an emphasis on a forward and downward direction, so as to both distract and rotate the spine (Figure 9-75).

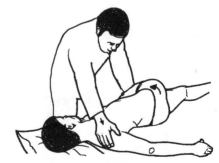

*Figure 9-75:*   Nonspecific rotation distraction technique.

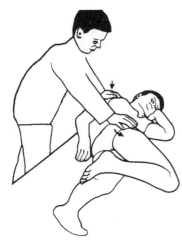

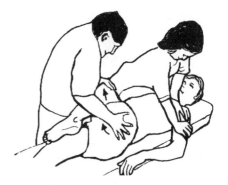

*Figure 9-77:* Lumbar roll.

*Figure 9-76:* Reversed distraction rotation technique.

This technique may be reversed by rotating the hip backward and stabilizing the shoulder forward (Figure 9-76.))

## Lumbar Roll

The lumbar roll, sometimes called the million dollar role, is a nonspecific rotation of the lumbothoracic, lumbar and SI joints. This technique can be performed with or without a helper. The purpose of this manipulation is to gap the spinal and SI joints, to rupture adhesions, to free entrapped tissues and to restore normal alignment. It is a very common technique used by OM, Lauren Berry body work and others. The spine usually is maintained in neutral (no flexion or extension).

The patient lies supine in the center of the treatment table, the height of which is approximately at the level of the practitioner's upper thigh. The practitioner stands on the pain-free side. If an assistant is used, he is on this side, as well.

The patient's shoulder is held down by the assistant, the practitioner or a strap. The practitioner:

1. Flexes the leg on the painful side as far as it will go without causing flexion of the lumbar spine (one can vary the amount of flexion in order to achieve some degree of localization).

2. Places his right arm over the patient's buttock and thigh, both of which are brought forward, thereby rotating the spine until all of the slack is taken up.

3. Asks the patient to breath in and out several times.

4. Takes up the slack further with each breath. When all of the slack is taken up, and at a point where the patient is relaxed, he applies the manipulation thrust along the axis of the femur.

This assures adequate force across both the lumbar and the sacroiliac joints (Figure 9-77).

## Rotation with the Spine in Extension

Manipulation of the spine in extension is performed in patients who have pain with lumbar flexion, either passively or actively. When this nonspecific manipulation is used to treat the SI joint, the placement of the practitioner's hand over the buttock is modified, depending on the position of the PSIS in the standing patient. If the PSIS is caudad at the painful side, the hand is positioned over the ischial tuberosity, mobilizing the ilia upward. If the PSIS is superior on the painful side, the practitioner's arm is placed

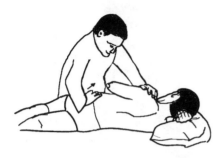

*Figure 9-78:* Rotation extension technique.

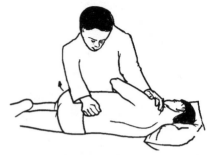

*Figure 9-79:* Rotation flexion technique.

over the iliac crest and mobilization is directed caudad (downward) and anteriorly. Often this manipulation increases lumbar lordosis (extension).

The patient lies comfortably on his pain-free side. The practitioner:

1. Extends the patient's lower leg fully and flexes the upper leg, hooking the foot onto the upper leg.

2. Translates from above the patient's shoulder and head backward, maintaining the shoulder square against the table, thereby increasing the extension of the spine.

3. Stabilizes the patient's shoulder with his hand or forearm (again keeping it, at as much as possible, at a right angle to the table). His other hand is then placed over the patient's buttock, as described above for the position of the PSIS.

4. Takes up the slack while asking the patient to inhale and exhale several times.

5. (At the point of maximal relaxation) thrusts with a scooping movement forwardly, rotating the joints of the pelvis (Figure 9-78).

## Rotation with the Spine in Flexion

Manipulation of the spine in flexion is performed in patients who have pain during lumbar extension, either passively or actively. When this nonspecific manipulation is used to treat the SI joint, the placement of the practitioner's right hand over the buttock is modified, depending on the position of the PSIS in the standing patient. If the PSIS is caudad on the painful side, the hand is positioned over the ischial tuberosity, mobilizing the ilia upward. If the PSIS is superior on the painful side, the hand is placed over the iliac crest and mobilization is directed caudad. This manipulation often increases lumbar kyphosis (flexion).

The patient lies comfortably with his painful side up. The practitioner:

1. Flexes the patient's upper leg and hooks the patient's foot under the lower leg.

2. Flexes slightly the patient's upper trunk.

3. Introduces further flexion and sidebending toward the painless side by pulling the patient's lower arm caudad.

4. Stabilizes the patient's upper trunk with one hand or forearm.

5. Places his other forearm over the buttock according to the position of the PSIS.

6. Asks the patient to inhale and exhale several times and takes up the slack (at the point of maximum relaxation). Thrusts with his body through his forearm, in a downward and forward direction, rotating the joints of the pelvis (Figure 9-79).

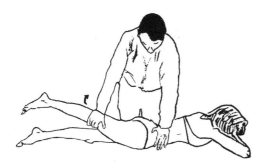

*Figure 9-80:* Prone manipulation.

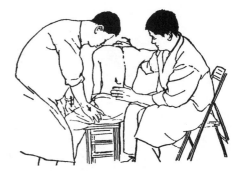

*Figure 9-81:* TCM thrust technique for disc herniation.

If only the lumbar spine is treated, it is best first to flex fully both knees and hips. Then, with the patient's lower leg stabilized by the practitioner's thigh, the thrust is applied along the axis of patient's upper thigh, which is pulled and rotated forward. This will minimize post-manipulation flare.

## Prone Manipulation

This can be used in patients who have central and one-sided pain when the spine is flexed.

The patient is prone, and the practitioner stands on his painless side. The practitioner:

1. Contacts the patient's affected spinous process with the heel of his hand.

2. Lifts and adducts the patient's leg on the affected side. This produces sidebending away from the pain and takes up the slack.

3. (At the point of maximum relaxation) lifts the leg sharply, while stabilizing the segment with the heel of his hand (Figure 9-80).

## Manipulation with the Patient Seated

This is a TCM manipulation for low back pain, especially due to a disc prolapse. This type of manipulation usually is performed only after failure of a manipulation under traction that requires extraordinary force (such a manipulation is performed by a specially trained martial artist/practitioner and therefore is not described in this text). This technique, however, can be performed first.

The following steps describe the manipulation when used for disc prolapse with right sided pain and a displaced spinous process toward the right side of vertebra (vertebra is rotated left).

The patient sits on a stool. An assistant stabilizes the patient's knees between his own. The practitioner stands on the patient's affected side or right side. The practitioner:

1. Slips his right arm under the patient's right axilla, holds onto his neck, and adds slight flexion.

2. Places his left thumb on the left side of the spinous process at the prolapse level.

3. Forcibly pushes on the patient's neck to add flexion, down to 80-90°.

4. Forcefully rotates the upper trunk to the right with his right hand, while he pushes strongly on the spinous process with his left thumb (Figure 9-81).

The typical popping sound of manipulation should be heard. If not, the procedure is repeated. Following the procedure,

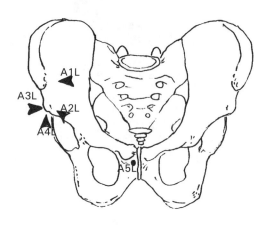

Figure 9-82:   Anterior lower lumbar Jones points (After Jones, Kusunose and Goering 1995).

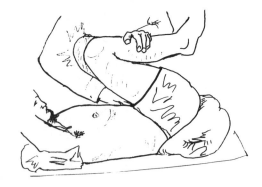

Figure 9-83:   Countertension technique for anterior L1.

the patient must rest for about one week, lying on a firm bed.

# Countertension Positional Release

Countertension positional release is most effective for treatment of facilitated and spasmed muscles. It is particularly helpful during the acute stages of muscle spasms. This section presents examples for muscles that frequently are involved in low back pain.

### Anterior Lumbar Jones Points

Anterior lumbar Jones Points, which are located around the ASIS and over the abdominal wall, indicate anterior vertebral dysfunctions and iliopsoas spasm (Jones *ibid*), (Figure 9-82).

**JONES POINT A1L (AIIS-1) (ILIOPSOAS MUSCLE).** Jones Point A1L (AIIS-1) is located just medial to the ASIS. It is tender in lower thoracic and upper lumbar (L1) vertebral dysfunctions (FRS and some neutral dysfunctions), which accounts for many low back pains that are not associated with local tenderness over the vertebra posteriorly. Pain is felt over the low back, sacral and gluteal areas (iliopsoas spasm). This point is found by approaching in a medial-to-lateral direction, ¾-inch deep.

The patient is supine with the head of the table raised, and pillows under the patient's hips to obtain more flexion of the spine. The practitioner is on the affected side. The practitioner:

1. Flexes and raises the patient's knees and places the patient's legs on his thigh.

2. (To produce the needed spinal flexion) raises the patient's knees farther with one hand, while with the other hand monitors the tender point.

3. Sidebends and rotates toward the tender side until the tenderness is at a minimum.

4. Held for 90 seconds and returns to neutral slowly (Figure 9-83).

**JONES POINT A2L (AIIS-2) (ILIOPSOAS MUSCLE).** Jones Point A2L (AIIS-2) is found medial to the inferior surface of the anterior inferior iliac spine, and is best palpated with the hip flexed. It is sensitive in L2 anterior dysfunctions (FRS) and in iliopsoas spasms.

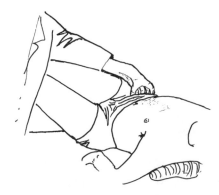

*Figure 9-84:* Countertension technique for Anterior L2.

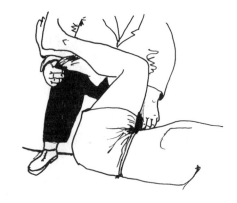

*Figure 9-85:* Countertension technique for anterior L2 (B).

The patient and the practitioner should be located as in the previous example. The practitioner:

1. Flexes the patient's knees and hip to 90°, and rotates 60° away from the tender point.

   In order to avoid pelvic strain from the leverage placed on the thighs during sidebending, only the uppermost leg should be dropped. The spine should be slightly sidebent away from the tender point. Traction on the higher femur, by pulling behind the flexed knee, is helpful.

2. Fine-tunes until tenderness over the point is at a minimum. The resulting position is held 90 seconds.

3. Returns to neutral position slowly (Figure 9-84).

**ABDOMINAL JONES POINT (AB2L) (ILIOPSOAS MUSCLE).** The Abdominal Jones Point (Ab2L) is located about 5cm lateral to the umbilicus and slightly inferior. It is often tender with psoas syndrome or spasm, and with L1, L2 anterior dysfunctions (FRS). Treatment is similar to the one above except that rotation is done to the other side.

The patient and the practitioner are positioned the same as in the above example. The practitioner:

1. Adds more flexion than used with A2L tenderness.

2. Rotates the knees about 60° toward the tender side.

3. Sidebends the spine away by elevating the feet upwards.

4. Fine-tunes until tenderness is minimal.

5. Holds for 90 seconds. Then the patient is returned slowly to neutral position (Figure 9-85).

**JONES POINT A3L (AIIS-3) (ILIOPSOAS MUSCLE).** Jones Point A3L (AIIS-3), located on the lateral surface of the anterior inferior iliac spine, is palpated best with the hips flexed. It is tender with dysfunctions of the 3rd vertebra (FRS) and the iliopsoas muscle.

The patient is placed as in the previous examples. The practitioner stands opposite the tender point. The practitioner:

1. Flexes the patient's legs to approximately 50-90° and rests them on his thigh.

2. Sidebends the patient's spine away from the tender point by pulling the patient's feet toward himself.

3. Rotates the spine slightly, using the patient's legs.

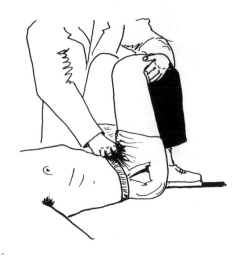

*Figure 9-86:* Countertension technique for anterior L3-4.

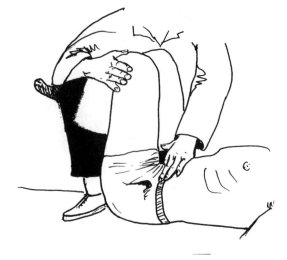

*Figure 9-87:* Countertension technique for anterior L5.

**4.** Fine-tunes until tenderness at the point is minimal.

**5.** Holds for 90 seconds. Then the patient is returned to a neutral position slowly (Figure 9-86).

**JONES POINT A4L (AIIS-4).** Jones Point A4L (AIIS-4), located on the inferior surface of the anterior inferior iliac spine, is best palpated with the hip flexed. It is tender in dysfunctions of the L4 (FRS) and the iliopsoas muscle. Treatment is the same as for A3L (Figure 9-86).

**JONES POINT A5L [A11S-5] (ILIOPSOAS MUSCLE).** Jones Point A5L [A11S-5], located on the anterior surface of the pubic bone approximately 1cm lateral to the pubic symphysis, is tender in anterior L5 (FRS) joint dysfunctions and in iliopsoas spasm. A5L is commonly tender. It also can be tender with bilateral lower pole fifth lumbar dysfunction (LP5L). Treatment of the A5L is effective for this dysfunction, as well.

The patient is placed in the same position as in the previous examples. The practitioner is on the same side as the tender point.

The practitioner:

**1.** Flexes the patient's leg to about 60-90°.

**2.** Sidebends the spine away from the tender point by pushing the legs away.

**3.** Rotates the knees toward the side of the tender point.

**4.** Fine-tunes until tenderness at the point is minimal.

**5.** Holds for 90 seconds. Then the patient is returned to a neutral position slowly (Figure 9-87).

### Posterior Lumbar Jones Points

Jones Points for the posterior lumbar are located in two general areas. One is paravertebral and spinal, and the other is adjacent to and surrounding the PSIS. The paravertebral (PV) and spinal (SP, spinous processes) often are located deeply and are more difficult to monitor than the points around the PSIS (Figure 9-88), (Jones *ibid*).

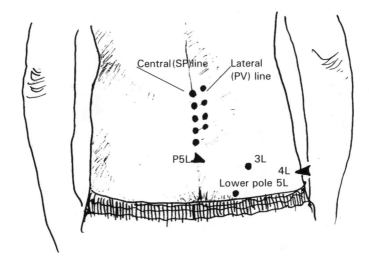

*Figure 9-88:*  Posterior lumbar Jones points (After Jones, Kusunose and Goering 1995).

**JONES POINTS P1L AND P2L. (MULTIFIDUS, ROTATORS AND INTERSPINALIS MUSCLES).** Jones Points P1L and P2L are located on the SP and PV lines. The PV points are located lateral to the spinous process or on the tip of the transverse processes. The SP points are located just below the spinous process. The closer the tender point is to the SP line (midline), the more extension is used for treatment. The more lateral the tender point, the more sidebending away from the tender point is used. The more cephalad (superior) the dysfunction, the greater the need for extension of the upper spine. This treatment is used mostly with posterior (ERS) dysfunctions of the third, fourth and upper pole of the fifth intervertebral joints, and with spasm of the multifidus, rotator, and interspinalis muscles. The third lumbar vertebra usually requires more rotation and less extension than the upper pole of the fifth lumbar. The fourth lumbar area usually requires motion between the two (Jones *ibid*).

The patient is prone, with the head of the table raised, or with his chest propped up with pillows (the degree depends on the level of dysfunction); the practitioner

standing on the opposite side of the tender point. The practitioner:

Option A. Used mostly for the upper lumbar area.

1. Pulls the patient's ASIS on the tender side, posteriorly and medially, creating rotation and sidebending toward the tender side (Figure 9-89).

Option B. Used mostly in the lower lumbar region, and also for P3L tenderness.

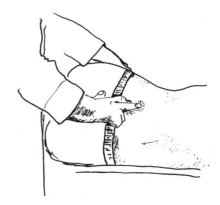

*Figure 9-89:*  Counter tension technique for upper central lumbar points.

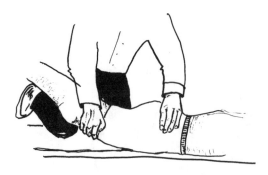

Figure 9-90: Counter tension technique for posterior mid-lumbars.

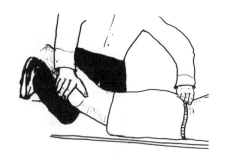

Figure 9-91: Counter tension technique for posterior upper pole L5.

1. Extends the lower leg and adducts on the tender side. The amount of extension and rotation can be controlled by the placement of the hand lifting the thigh. The closer the hand is to the buttock, the greater the rotation and the less the extension.

2. Fine-tunes until the tenderness is at a minimum. Then the patient is returned to a neutral position (Figure 9-90).

**JONES POINT P3L. (MULTIFIDUS, ROTATORS AND INTERSPINALIS MUSCLES).** Jones Point P3L is located about 3cm below the margin of the ilium and about 7cm lateral to the PSIS, and it is about halfway between the PSIS and fourth lumbar tender point. This point is tender with third lumbar posterior dysfunctions (ERS) and spasm in the multifidus, rotator and interspinalis muscles. Treatment is the same as in the above case, using the leg to control rotation, extension and sidebending.

**JONES POINT P4L. (MULTIFIDUS, ROTATORS AND INTERSPINALIS MUSCLES).** Jones Point P4L is located about 4cm below the margin of the ilium and just posterior to the border of the tensor fascia lata. This point is tender with fourth lumbar vertebra posterior dysfunction (ERS) and lesions in the multifidus, rotator and interspinalis muscles. Treatment is the same as for P3L, but with fine-tuning for this point.

**JONES POINT UPL5. (MULTIFIDUS AND ROTATOR MUSCLES).** Jones Point UPL5 (upper pole of fifth lumbar) is located on the superior medial surface of the PSIS. It is best palpated with caudad and lateral pressure toward the PSIS. This point is tender with posterior dysfunction (ERS) of the upper pole of the fifth lumbar vertebra and the multifidus and rotator muscles. Treatment is the same as for PL4, but with fine tuning for this joint (Figure 9-91).

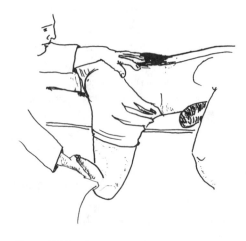

Figure 9-92: Counter tension technique for posterior lower pole L5.

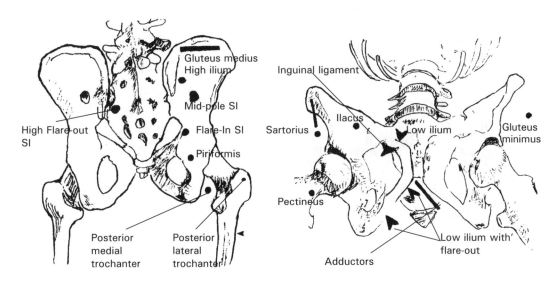

*Figure 9-93:*   Pelvic Jones points (After Jones, Kusunose and Goering 1995).

**JONES POINT LP5L. (MULTIFIDUS AND ROTA-TOR MUSCLES).** Jones Point LP5L (lower pole of the fifth lumbar vertebra) is located about 2cm below the UP5L in a small saddle-shaped depression between the PSIS and posterior inferior iliac spine. This point is tender with posterior (ERS) dysfunctions of the lower fifth lumbar vertebra and with spasm of the multifidus and rotator muscles.

The patient is prone, with his thigh on the side of the tender point suspended over the table by the practitioner, who is seated or standing on the same side. The practitioner:

1. Flexes the patient's hip about 90°, and slightly adducts the knee toward the table. The pelvis rotates about 20°.

2. Holds this position for 90 seconds, and then slowly returns the patient to neutral (Figure 9-92).

*Pelvic Jones Points*

Figure 9-93 illustrates pelvic Johns Points.

**JONES POINT HISI (HIGH ILIUM-SACROILIAC) (GLUTEUS MEDIUS MUSCLE).** Jones Point HISI (high ilium-sacroiliac) is located 3cm lateral to the PSIS and is best palpated by probing medially. This point is tender with dysfunctions of the SI joint in which the ileum is too high and is flared cephalad, and when the gluteus medius is in·spasm.

The patient is prone. The practitioner is standing on the same side of the tender point. The practitioner:

1. Extends the patient's leg and rests it on his thigh.

2. Adds slight abduction to the patient's leg, fine-tuning until tenderness at the point is minimal.

3. Holds this position for 90 seconds, and then slowly returns the patient to neutral (Figure 9-94).

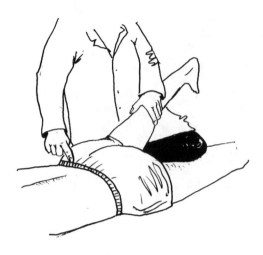

*Figure 9-94:* Countertension technique for high ilium.

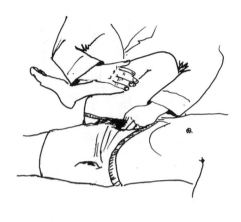

*Figure 9-95:* Counter tension technique for low ilium.

.**Jones Point Low Ilium.** Jones point low Ilium is located on the superior (not anterior) surface of the lateral ramus of the pubic bone, about one and a half inches from the midline. The patient has pain usually in his back or side of the hip and thigh.

The patient is supine. The practitioner is standing on the same side of the tenser point. The practitioner:

1. Flexes the patient's leg and hip markedly.

2. Fine tunes until tenderness at the point is minimal.

3. Holds this position for 90 seconds, then slowly returns the patient to neutral (Figure 9-95).

**Jones Point Flare-In (mid-pole sacroiliac dysfunction), (Gluteus Medius Muscle).** Jones Point Flare-In (mid-pole sacroiliac dysfunction) is located on the buttocks in the slight depression in the musculature. It is best palpated by directing the probing finger medially. This point is tender in dysfunctions of the SI and gluteus medius muscle. This point may help with menstrual cramps.

The patient is prone. The practitioner is standing on the side of the tender point. The practitioner:

1. Abducts the leg and adds slight extension or flexion for fine tuning until tenderness at the point is at a minimum.

2. Holds this position for 90 seconds, then slowly returns the patient to neutral.

**Jones Point HFO-SI (high flare-out sacroiliac dysfunction).** Jones Point HFO-SI (high flare-out sacroiliac dysfunction) is located 4cm below and slightly medial to the lower edge of the PSIS. It is tender in cases of coccygodynia and coccygeus spasm.

The patient is prone. The practitioner stands on the side opposite the tender point. The practitioner:

1. Extends the patient's thigh on the tender point side, just enough to allow abduction over the opposite leg.

2. Fine tunes the abduction until tenderness at the point is minimal.

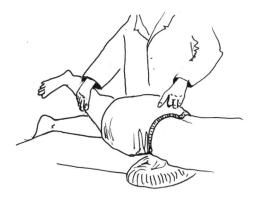

*Figure 9-96:* Countertension technique for high-flar-out.

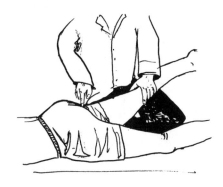

*Figure 9-97:* Countertension technique for posterior lateral trochanter.

**3.** Holds this position for 90 seconds, then slowly returns the patient to neutral (Figure 9-96).

**JONES POINT PLT (POSTERIOR LATERAL TRO-CHANTER), (PIRIFORMIS MUSCLE).** Jones Point PLT (posterior lateral trochanter) is located on the superior lateral surface of the posterior surface of the greater trochanter, at the point of attachment of the piriformis. This point is tender with hip socket dysfunctions, with much hip pain and with spasm of the external rotators of the thigh (i.e. piriformis).

The patient is prone. The practitioner stands on the same side as the tender point. The practitioner:

**1.** Extends the hip on the tender point side and supports the leg on his knee.

**2.** Markedly externally rotates the leg, and abducts it slightly.

**3.** Fine tunes until tenderness at the point is minimal.

**4.** Holds the position for 90 seconds, then returns the patient slowly to neutral (Figure 9-97).

**JONES POINT PMT (POSTERIOR MEDIAL TRO-CHANTER), (GEMELLI AND QUADRATUS FEMO-RIS MUSCLES).** Jones Point PMT (posterior medial trochanter) is located on a line from the lateral inferior surface of the ischial tuberosity to the medial aspect of the posterior surface of the femur. It is tender in many cases of hip socket dysfunctions, (in which the SI joint is often mistakenly blamed), and in cases of spasm of the gemelli and quadratus femoris.

The patient is prone. The practitioner stands on the side opposite the tender point. The practitioner:

**1.** Positions the patient's ankle in the practitioner's axilla and secures it there.

**2.** Grasps the patient's knee.

**3.** Extends the hip moderately, adducts the hip markedly, and rotates the hip markedly into external rotation.

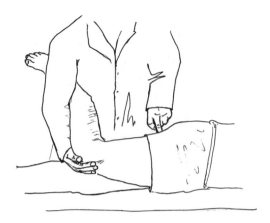

*Figure 9-98:* Countertension technique for posterior medial trochanter.

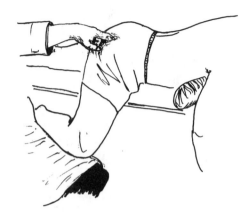

*Figure 9-99:* Countertension technique for piriformis muscle.

**4.** Fine tunes these movements until tenderness at the point is minimal.

**5.** Holds it for 90 seconds, then slowly returns the patient to neutral (Figure 9-98).

**JONES POINT PIR (PIRIFORMIS MUSCLE).** Jones Point PIR (piriformis tender point) is located on the belly of the piriformis muscle, about 8cm medially and slightly cephalad to the greater trochanter. It is tender with SI dysfunctions and piriformis spasm. The treatment is similar to LP5L, except for minor adjustments.

The patient is prone. The practitioner sits or stands on the side of the tender point. The patient's leg on the side of the tenderness is suspended off the table, with the legs resting on the practitioner's thigh. The practitioner:

**1.** Flexes the patient's hip about 120°, and then adds some abduction.

**2.** Fine tunes these movements until the tenderness at the point is minimal.

**3.** Holds this position for 90 seconds, then slowly returns the patient to neutral (Figure 9-99).

**JONES POINT LT (LATERAL TROCHANTER), (TENSOR FASCIA LATA MUSCLE).** Jones Point LT (lateral trochanter) is located 12cm below the greater trochanter, on the lateral side of the shaft of the femur. This point is tender with relatively uncommon hip joint disorders and with tension of the tensor fascia lata.

The patient is prone. The practitioner sits or stands on the tender point side. The practitioner:

**1.** Flexes the patient's hip slightly, and then adds moderate hip abduction.

**2.** Fine tunes with slight amount of external or internal rotation until a position is found in which tenderness at the point is at a minimum.

**3.** Holds for 90 seconds, then slowly returns the patient to neutral position (Figure 9-100).

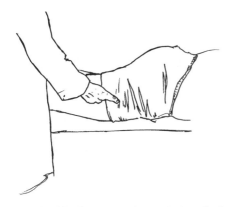

*Figure 9-100:* Countertension technique for lateral trochanter.

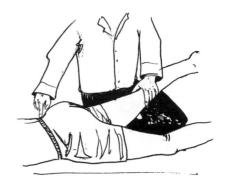

*Figure 9-101:* Counter tension technique for gluteus medius.

**JONES POINT GM (GLUTEUS MEDIUS MUSCLE).** The Jones Point for the Gluteus Medius Muscle (GM) can be found on a line about 1cm below the iliac crest. Often the GM point is tender in reaction to SI dysfunctions and hip pathology.

The patient is prone. The practitioner stands on the tender point side. The practitioner:

1. Lifts the patient's hip and supports the leg on his thigh.

2. Abducts the hip moderately and internally rotates the hip markedly.

3. Fine tunes these motions until tenderness at the point is at a minimum.

4. Holds this position for 90 seconds, then returns the patient slowly to neutral (Figure 9-101).

**JONES POINT FOR QUADRATUS LUMBORUM MUSCLE.** The Jones Point for the Quadratus Lumborum Muscle (QL) can be found on the lateral aspect of the transverse processes of the first through the third lumbar vertebrae. This point is best palpated medially. The QL point is tender with many conditions affecting the lumbosacral spine due to its connection to the ilia, lumbar vertebra and thoracic spine via the 12th rib.

The patient is prone. The practitioner stands on the tender point side. The practitioner:

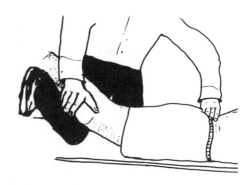

*Figure 9-102:* Counter tension technique for quadratus mumborum.

1. Side flexes the patient's upper torso and lowers the patient's legs to shorten the muscle.

2. Extends the hip on the affected side and supports the patient's thigh on his own leg.

3. Fine tunes by addition of internal rotation of the patient's hip. When a position is found in which tenderness at the point is at a minimum.

4. Held for 90 seconds. Then the patient is slowly returned to neutral position (Figure 9-102).

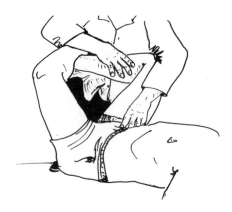

*Figure 9-103:* Counter tension technique for Iliacus muscle.

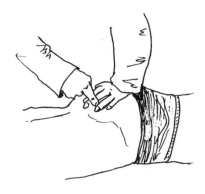

*Figure 9-104:* Countertension technique for PS-1.

**JONES POINT FOR ILIACUS MUSCLE.** Jones point for Iliacus can be found deep in the iliac fossa, about two inches medial and slightly below the ASIS. This point is very likely to be tender with recurring low ilium and low ilium flare-out dysfunctions. Treatment is aimed bilaterally even when tenderness in unilateral. This point is commonly tender in patients with recurring sacroiliac dysfunctions.

The patient is supine. The practitioner is on the tender point side. The practitioner then:

1. Flexes both legs and hips and rests the legs on his thigh.

2. Separates the knees widely and crosses the feet (if one knee is painful it should be on top).

3. Fine tunes flexion, marked external rotation, and abduction of the femoral joint. When a position is found in which tenderness at the point is at a minimum.

4. Held for 90 seconds. Then the patient is slowly returned to neutral position (Figure 9-103).

*Posterior Sacrum Jones Points*

**JONES POINT PS-1 (LEVATOR ANI MUSCLE).** Jones Point PS-1 is located bilaterally at the sacral sides about 1.5 cm medial to the inferior aspect of the PSIS. This point is tender in posterior sacral torsions and spasms of the levator ani.

The patient is prone. The practitioner stands on the side of the tender point. The practitioner:

1. Applies downward pressure to the ILA on the tender point side, toward the corner of the sacrum, opposite of the tender point.

2. Fine tunes the pressure until tenderness at the point is minimal.

3. Holds this position for 90 seconds and then slowly releases the pressure (Figure 9-104).

**JONES POINT PS-2 (LEVATOR ANI MUSCLE).** Jones Point PS-2 is located in the midline of the sacrum between the first and second spinous tubercles. This point often is tender in extended sacrum dysfunction and levator ani spasm.

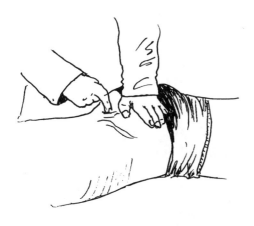

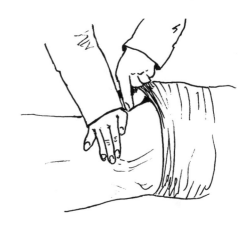

*Figure 9-106:* Countertension technique for PS-4.

*Figure 9-105:* Countertension technique for PS-2.

The patient is prone. The practitioner stands at either side of the patient. The practitioner:

1. Applies a downward pressure to the apex of the sacrum, exaggerating extension (counternutation) of the sacrum.

2. Fine tunes the pressure until the tenderness at the point is minimized.

3. Holds this pressure for 90 seconds, and then releases it slowly (Figure 9-105).

**JONES POINT PS-3 (PUBOCOCCYGEUS MUSCLE).** Jones Point PS-3 is located in the midline of the sacrum between the second and third spinous tubercles. This point often is tender in extended sacrum and spasm of the pubococcygeus muscle. Treatment is the same as for PS-2.

**JONES POINT PS-4 (PUBOCOCCYGEUS MUSCLE).** Jones Point PS-4 is located at the midline of the sacrum, just above the sacral hiatus. It is tender often in flexed sacrum dysfunctions and pubococcygeus muscle spasm.

The patient is prone. The practitioner stands on either side of the patient. The practitioner:

1. Applies a downward pressure to the sacral base until tenderness at the point is reduced to a minimum.

2. Holds this position for 90 seconds and then releases the pressure slowly (Figure 9-106).

**JONES POINT FOR THE COCCYX.** A Jones Point for the Coccyx can be found on the coccyx, on either the lateral edge or the inferior edge of the coccyx.

The patient is prone. The practitioner stands on either side of the patient. The practitioner:

1. Applies downward pressure on the apex of the sacrum in midline.

2. Fine tunes with a twist to the sacrum, clockwise or counterclockwise, most commonly toward the tender point.

3. Holds this position for 90 seconds and then releases slowly (Figure 9-107).

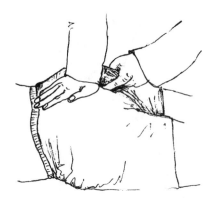

*Figure 9-107:* Countertension technique for coccy.

## Spinal Stretch

The spinal stretch is a Qi Gong (breath, energy and movement) exercise that involves a series of flexion/extension movements. It is a part of a series of exercises in a spinal rehabilitation system. These movements are performed slowly, first elongating the posterior aspect of the spine with flexion, and then, while maintaining the stretch posteriorly, elongating the anterior aspect during extension. The exercise is achieved by a "letting go" meditative stretch, rather then a forceful mechanical stretch. The patient:

1. Stands with knees bent and sacrum slightly tucked under (pelvic tilt,

counternutated sacrum with hip flexion).

2. (Starting the exercise from the bottom) relaxes the lowest vertebra letting go of any tension, and gradually allowing gravity to flex this segment, only.

   The spine above should remain straight and unyielding, especially the neck and head.

3. (When this segment becomes completely relaxed and is flexed as far as it will go) repeats the same process for the next segment.

4. (When the last cervical segment has relaxed and is stretched) lowers the head while at the same time releases the joints of the upper extremities.

5. Lets the arms hang and tries to feel the cranial sacral rhythm (for more detail on cranial sacral rhythm, read osteopathic literature).

6. (Now, starting from below) begins segmental relaxation and extension, opening the front of the vertebral joints.

7. Continues until the last cervical segment has extended, and then raises the head while at the same time pushes together the upper extremity joints.

8. Stands in place and feels the new spinal length.

9. Repeats the exercises a maximum of three times (Figure 9-108; Figure 9-109).

A variation on the spinal stretch can be performed to strengthen and stretch from one to three vertebral segments. A series of local small extensions and flexions is performed with the dysfunctional segment at the apex of the exercises. This can be done sitting or standing.

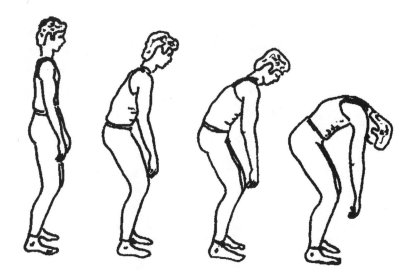

*Figure 9-108:* Spinal stretch part one.

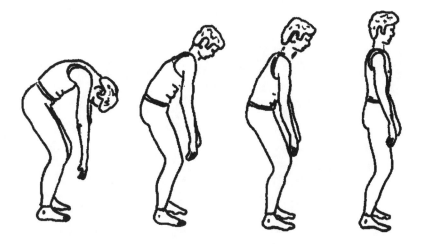

*Figure 9-109:* Spinal stretch part two.

# Chapter 10: *The Upper Extremities*

Pain in the shoulder and upper extremities is common and can be due to either single or multiple pathological processes. The head, neck and upper arms, all highly mobile, are regularly involved in complex movements. These structures often are subjected to heavy weight-bearing and strong physical forces which lead to injury and extremity pain. The responsible pathological processes can be either local or referred from the head, neck, ribs, or cervical or thoracic spine. They can involve muscles, tendons, or support structures such as ligaments and bones. Tendon disorders can be acute, but more often they result from repetitive use. Pain in these areas can originate also from diseased intrathoracic or upper abdominal organs.

The cevicothoracic junction is a major transitional region and the relationship of T1 with the first rib and the sternoclavicular joint is of major significance in upper extremity problems. T1 dysfunctions influence the first rib and can lead to dysfunction there, which then can influence the manubrium of the sternum and sternoclavicular joint. The cervical roots, which are transported through the intertranvesariae muscles, can be affected by chronic passive congestion at these levels. The brachial plexus passes through the scalene muscles which also can result in local pressure. As the plexus traverses laterally, it passes through the costoclavical canal, which can be influenced by the second rib. More laterally, the neurovascular bundle passes under the insertion of the pectoralis minor tendon to the coracoid process of the scapula, all of which can result in pressure on the neurovascular bundle and upper extremity pain (Greenman 1996).

OM disorders of the upper extremities can develop as a result of external pathogenic factors, but more often they are secondary to Liver disorders, Blood stagnation, or weakness of the Nourishing Qi and Blood. Cervical spine disorders also can predispose the upper extremities to obstructive disorders and can leave tissues vulnerable to strain. Acupuncture is a valuable tool for treatment of acute or chronic shoulder and arm pain (Petrie and Langley 1983; Loy 1983; Laitenen 1975; Marcus and Gracer 1994; Gunn 1977).

## The Shoulder

Shoulder pain is a common clinical problem. Many disorders of the shoulder joint respond to treatment described in this text. Acupuncture has been shown to be helpful (Wang et al 1988; Ji 1992; Rong 1986; Marcus and Gracer 1994).

## Anatomy/Biomechanics

The shoulder is an arrangement of three bones held together by muscles, tendons, and ligaments, all of which can become dysfunctional. The shoulder joint proper (glenohumeral joint) is formed by the humerus and the glenoid fossa. The clavicle attaches the shoulder to the rib cage at the sternum, forming the sternoclavicular (SC) joint, and holds the shoulder out from the trunk.

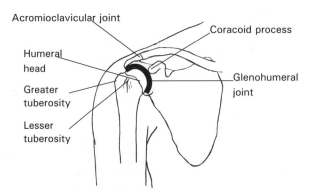

*Figure 10-1:* Shoulder.

The clavicle also connects with the scapula at the acromion, forming the acromioclavicular (AC) joint. The acromion projects from the scapula to form the superior aspect of the shoulder and, with the coracoid process and attached ligaments, contributes glenohumeral stability (Figure 10-1).

Full function and movement of the shoulder and arm depend on mobility of the scapulothoracic mechanism, subacromial mechanism, AC joint, SC joint and glenohumeral joint. Therefore, it is better to think of the entire shoulder girdle as a functional unit. When the arm is fully elevated (to 180°), one-half of the motion takes place at the glenohumeral joint. Additional elevation is due to scapular rotation combined with a final adduction of the humerus (Cyriax *ibid*).

### The Glenohumeral Joint

The glenohumeral joint (shoulder joint proper) is held together by the capsuloligamentous structures and the tendons of the rotator cuff muscles. The ball-like head of the humerus which is cradled in the glenoid fossa forms the glenohumeral joint. The large humeral head, which lies on an almost flat scapular surface, allows for great mobility. The glenohumeral joint is therefore the most mobile joint in the body.

The lax, fibrous portion of the glenohumeral capsule has several recesses which allow for mobility in various directions. Adhesions form often at the inferior recess and lead to the "frozen shoulder syndrome" (Brown 1995). The anterior portion of the capsule has three areas of reinforcement called the superior, middle and inferior glenohumeral ligaments. These ligaments and the rotator cuff muscle contribute to stability of the joint. The rotator cuff tendons reinforce the superior, posterior and anterior capsule.

Movement within the glenohumeral joint takes place on three planes, all of which transverse the head of the humerus (Ombregt, Bisschop, ter Veer and Velde 1995).

Joint play movements at this joint are (Mennell *ibid*):

**1.** Lateral movement of the head of the humerus away from the glenoid cavity.

**2.** Anterior movement of the head of the humerus within the glenoid cavity.

**3.** Posterior shear of the head of the humerus within the glenoid cavity.

**4.** Downward and backward movement of the head of the humerus within the glenoid cavity.

**5.** Outward and backward movement of the head of the humerus within the glenoid cavity.

**6.** Direct posterior movement of the head of the humerus within the glenoid cavity with the arm forward flexed at 90°.

**7.** External rotation of the head of the humerus within the glenoid cavity.

## Muscles

The shallow ball-and-socket (gleno-humeral) joint is held stable by a group of tendons (that become part of the capsule) known as the rotator cuff. All of the rotator-cuff muscles are supplied mainly by the C-5 cervical nerve roots. Table 10-1 summarizes the functions of the muscles.

Each time the arm is raised, the rotator-cuff tendons are squeezed between the acromion and the humerus. The antero-inferior gleno-humeral ligament and infraspinatus muscles function to limit movements that squeeze the rotator cuff).[1] Wear of any rotator-cuff component can create micro-tears and inflammation. One head of the biceps muscle originates in the glenoid fossa and exits through the bicipital groove. It can occasionally be a site of tendinitis.

## Bursae

Between the acromion and the rotator cuff lies the *subdeltoid bursa*, which helps cushion the tendon from the bone. This fluid-filled space can become inflamed, leading to pain and limitation of motion in a noncapsular pattern.

---

1. Disorders of these structures often lead to shoulder instability and recurrent rotator cuff tendinitis.

*Table 10-1.* **ROTATOR CUFF MUSCLES**

| MUSCLE | FUNCTION |
|---|---|
| Supraspinatus | Abduction |
| Infraspinatus | External Rotation |
| Subscapularis | Internal Rotation |
| Teres minor | External Rotation (infrequently affected) |

A second bursa, the *subcoracoid bursa,* is located between the coracoid process and the pectoralis major muscle. Shoulder pain that originates from other sources is often wrongly attributed to bursitis.

# Imaging

Most shoulder problems can be managed without imaging in an orthopedic medical practice. A precise diagnosis usually can be made from a history and examination. Accuracy is not enhanced just because imaging is somehow considered to be sophisticated. (Images often are available or demanded, thus a number of comments are offered here regarding their marginal benefit.)

Plain films of the shoulder can show a dislocation or fracture in acute injuries. If the fracture lines pass through the anatomical neck of the humerus, some bleeding into the glenohumeral capsule will occur. The clinical finding of capsulitis will overlap those of fracture and, as outlined in the section on fractures, this is considered more important in the long run.

It might be possible to show an abnormal degree of mobility at the shoulder joint in cases of recurrent dislocation by having the patient hold 15 pounds of some material and investigate the standing films for excessive depression of the head of the humorous.

In the evaluation of the painful shoulder contrast arthrography to define the presence of tendon and capsular injuries should be considered only as a last resort. A normal communication between the gle-

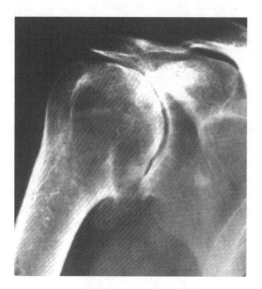

*Figure 10-2:* Degenerative joint disease of glenohumeral joint. Note the nonuniform loss of joint space, sclerosis, and osteophyte formation.

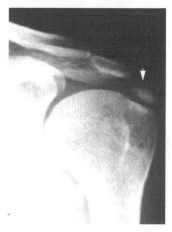

*Figure 10-3:* Calcification over the supraspinous tendon.

nohumeral joint and the subacromial bursa is present in 23% of normal population; therefore, if such a person develops any lesion at the shoulder and is subjected to an arthrogram, the communication is demonstrated and the patient may be erroneously thought to have a ruptured rotator cuff.

Calcification in the tendon (Figure 10-3) or subacromial bursa often is recognized when plain films of the shoulder are obtained. Clinical experience indicates that the presence of calcification is not a barrier to successful management by injection techniques; occasionally, the calcification is seen to regress. In this author's opinion it is not an indication for surgery. Indeed, there are instances of bony disruption of the glenoid from unusual circumstances, and, in these cases, CT scans and MRI scans can demonstrate the disordered anatomy.

Ligament and other soft tissue injuries are the meat of this book. When there is disruption of the continuity of a structure—a tear—it can be visualized with an MRI, provided that the right cut is obtained. A T1-weighted image also can

indicate an increase in the fluid content of tissue and may infer edema. These observations, although true in and of themselves, are not *necessary* for excellent clinical management.

Tears of the glenoid labrum can be seen on MRI (Holt, Helms et al. 1990), and they are best managed expectantly. In the case of athletes, recurrent pain and dysfunction might be present with certain activities. In these instances, prolotherapy at the capsular attachment to the glenoid can be helpful. Parenthetically, it is interesting to note that this treatment was described by Hippocrates (Hippocrates 1988), who used white-hot needles to provoke scar formation in recurrent anterior dislocation of the shoulder in warriors—the first account of prolotherapy.[2]

In general, with plain film examination the radiologist notes: the relation of the humerus to the glenoid cavity, the relation of the clavicle to the acromion process, whether the epiphyseal plate of the humeral head is present and, if so, whether it is normal, whether there are any tendon, bursa or muscle calcifications. The examiner notes any defect on the lateral aspect of the humeral head from

---

2.  Hot-scarring needling is an OM technique as well.

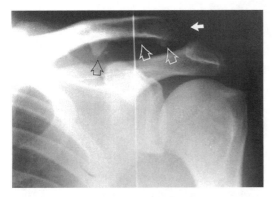

*Figure 10-4:* Antro-posterior view of a chronically subluxing acromioclavicular joint. Note the closed arrow pointing to the elevated and separated clavicle. There is also calcification in the coracoclavicular ligaments (open arrows).

recurrent dislocations—called Hill-Sach lesion. The acromiohumeral interval (the distance between the acromion process and the humerus) is measured. The distance should be 7-14mm—if it is decreased it may indicate rotator cuff tears (Weiner and Macnab 1970).

### Imaging of Acromioclavicular Joint

Laxity of the joint can be demonstrated by taking AP views with the patient standing and holding weights. Separation of the bony images indicates capsular laxity. The degree of laxity is graded in proportion to the separation, each third of the distance of the joint corresponding to a grade, from one to three (Figure 10-4).

It often will be noted that as the clavicle separates from the acromioclavicular joints, a more important gap develops between the clavicle and the coracoid process. On occasion there even may be a fracture of the coracoid itself. This is indicative of injury to the coracoclavicular ligament—which is the primary ligament holding the clavicle in its correct position at the acromion.

Occasionally plain films of the shoulder are helpful in that they will show a loss of bone of the distal clavicle. This osteoly-

sis of the clavicle can be painful, and progressive demonstration by radiography would be a sufficient reason to suggest surgical intervention.

## OM Disorders

The OM view of shoulder physiology is that all arm Yin and Yang channels, and branches of some foot Yang Sinews channels, pass over and through the shoulder. However, only the Yang channels, and to a small extent the Lung, are clinically important.[3] These channels control the shoulder and are individually responsible for complex, multidirectional shoulder movement.

Disorders of the shoulder often are due to disharmony and deficiency of Defensive and Nutritive Qi. When a disorder is acute, the cause often is external pathogenic factor, trauma or sprain, or habitual misuse. Chronic obstruction of local circulation can result in accumulation and transformation to Damp-Heat.

## Biomedical Disorders

Disorders of the inert (noncontractile) shoulder structures are mainly arthritic or involve the bursae. A loose body can develop within the joint, as well.

### Capsular Pattern

The capsular pattern of the shoulder (glenohumeral joint) is characterized by limitation of shoulder movements—external rotation is most affected, internal rotation the least affected, and abduction lies in between the two (Figure 10-5, and Figure 10-6).

---

3. In rare instances, the Lung can become involved in lesions of either the biceps muscle and tendon or the pectoralis major.

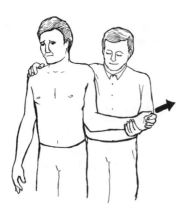

*Figure 10-5:* Assessment of external rotation and end feel.

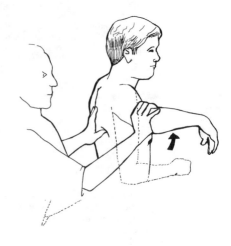

*Figure 10-6:* Assessment of glenohumeral abduction. The scapula should start moving when the arm reaches the horizontal.

The capsular pattern is seen in patients who have arthritis or arthrosis. With arthritis and arthrosis, resisted movements usually are painless.

### Differential Diagnosis

In patients who have a capsular pattern, several conditions should be considered (Ombregt, Bisschop, ter Veer, Van de Velde 1995):

- Septic arthritis.
  Patient with a severely painful, warm, and swollen joint.
- Gout or pseudogout.
  Patient with a history of gout.
- Arthritis from rheumatoid, psoriatic, and systemic lupus erythematosus.
- Traumatic arthritis (Cyriax).
  Patients over 40 years old.
- Hemarthrosis.
  Patient with a bleeding disorder or on blood-thinning medications.
- Shoulder-hand syndrome (RSD).
  Patients with shoulder pain that spreads down the limb, and a bluish and diffusely swollen hand. Distal dystrophy may be seen.
- Metastases.

  Patient with a rapidly increasing pain around the shoulder, radiating to the arm and increasing with all shoulder movements. Muscular wasting, extreme pain and weakness.
- Primary tumor.
  Younger patient with acute pain and stiffness of short duration.
- Tertiary syphilis.
  — Usually painless, sometimes bilateral with neurological signs.
- Aseptic necrosis.
  Patients with moderate or severe pain (especially at night), few other signs, and/or history of steroid use.

### Treatment

Capsulitis is seen in patients with arthritis or arthrosis. Light passive mobilization (within the available joint play), capsular distraction and techniques that stretch the capsule are good treatment methods. Acupuncture techniques are helpful. Injection therapy may be necessary in more severe cases.

**STRETCHING.** Stretching is used in patients who have capsulitis and pain that does not

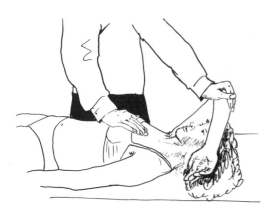

*Figure 10-7:* Shoulder capsule stretch.

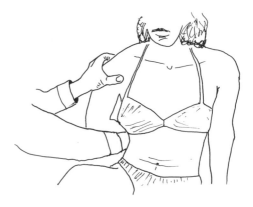

*Figure 10-8:* Apprehension test for the posterior capsule. The test is positive if the patient is apprehensive as pain ensues.

refer below the elbow and does not awaken the patient at night. The amount of force used to stretch the capsule is guided by the patient's response to the treatment. The stretch must be of sufficient magnitude to cause increased pain for two hours following the treatment. However, if the pain does not subside after a couple of hours and continues for a day or two, the force has been excessive. In chronic cases the practitioner may hear and feel a sudden rupture of an adhesion. Usually this type of rupture results in immediate improvement (Ombregt, Bisschop, ter Veer and Va.n de Velde 1995), (Figure 10-7).

**DISTRACTION.** The goal of distraction is to stretch the capsular fibers longitudinally, stimulating mechanoreceptors within the capsule that in turn inhibit nociceptive reflexes. Vibrating the joint slightly may enhance inhibition. It can be used in all stages of capsulitis.

Distraction is done mainly in a lateral and slightly superior anterior direction.

When the joint's ROM begins to increase, the practitioner can slowly introduce external rotation to the joint, as well (Figure 10-10).

**ACUPUNCTURE.** Acupuncture at SI-10, TH-14, LI-15 and St-38 toward UB-57 can be used. The Ear Shoulder point is helpful; a

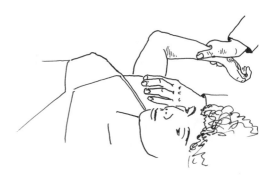

*Figure 10-9:* Apprehension test for the anterior capsule. The test is positive if the patient is apprehensive as pain ensues.

semipermanent needle can be used. For patients over 40, moxa over the needles is often helpful. Local points should be inserted superficially as deep insertion often aggravates the condition. Occasionally however, deep insertion is helpful when superficial insertion does not. Heaven Emperor Quasi may be used while the patient mobilizes the joint.

**INJECTION.** Intra-articular steroid or Sarapin

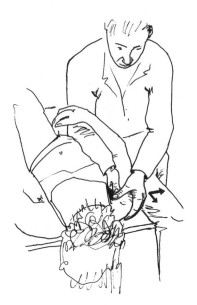

*Figure 10-10:*Distraction technique.

injections often are needed in acute or stubborn chronic cases.

**HERBAL THERAPY.** A guiding oral formula for acute arthrosis (i.e. no or only minor signs of heat and inflammation) with capsular pattern is:

> Rhizoma Curcumae Longae (Jiang Huang)
> Radix Salviae Miltiorrhizae (Dan Shen)
> Rhizoma seu Radix Notopterygium (Qiang Hou)
> Radix Clemetidis Chinesis (Wei Ling Xian)
> Angelica Chinesis (Dang Gui)
> Peoniae Rubra (Chi Shao)
> Radix Ledebouriellae Sesloidis (Fang Feng)
> Herba seu Flos Schizonepeta (Jing Jie)
> Ramulus Cinnamomi Cassiae (Gui Zhi)
> Rhizoma Zingiberis Officinalis Recens (Sheng Jiang)
> Radix Astragali (Huang Qi)
> Radix Glycyrrhizae (Gan Cao)
> Scolpendra (Wu Gong)
> Lumbricus (Di Long)

For arthritis with signs of inflammation and heat:

> Angelica Chinesis (Dang Gui)
> Ramulus Mori (Sang Zhi)
> Herba Impatiens Balsaminae (Tou Gu Cao)
> Rhizoma seu Radix Notopterygium (Qiang Hou)
> Radix Rehmanniae (Sheng Di Huang)
> Rhizoma Cyperi (Xiang Fu)
> Resina Olibani (Ru Xiang)
> Resina Myrrae (Mo Yao)
> Radix Gentinae (Qin Jiao)
> Lumbricus (Di Long)
> Rhizoma Rhei (Da Huang)
> Tripterygium Wilfordii (Lei Gong Teng)
> vitamins B6 and B12 (to prevent possible side effects of Tripterygium)

A guiding herbal formula for topical application is:

> Radix Aconiti Agrestis and Kusenzoffii (Cao Wu Tou and Chuan Wu Tou)
> Pericarpium Zanthoxyli (Hua Jiao)
> Folium Artemisiae Argyi (Ai Ye)
> Herba Artemisiae (Qing Hao)
> Rhizoma Atractylodis (Cang Zhu)
> Ramulus Cinnamomii (Gui Zhi)
> Radix Sileris (Fang Feng)
> Flos Carthami (Hong Hua)
> Herba Impatiens sew Spena (Ji Xing)
> Herba Lycopodii (Shen Qian Cao)
> Rhizoma Curcumae Longae (Jiang Huang)

## Instability

Glenohumeral instability is a common cause of recurrent shoulder pain. Dislocations at this joint are the most common in the body, with anterior subluxations seen most frequently (Dalton and Snyder 1989). Joint laxity can result in a transient subluxation (or sudden weakness) with vague clinical finding. A painful arc (Figure 10-12) may be present (often with a transient weakness). Stress applied to the joint capsule often gives an apprehension sign (Figure 10-8 and Figure 10-9), and drawer tests are positive (Figure 10-11). Mild joint laxity may not result in a positive apprehension test, but the drawer test reveals the pathology. A traumatic history increases the index of suspicion (Brown *ibid*).

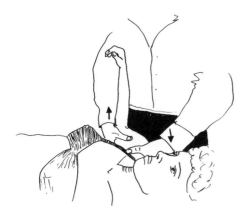

*Figure 10-11:* Drawer test for anterior capsule. The test is positive if there is a lag between humeral and scapular movement.

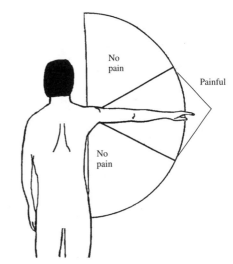

*Figure 10-12:* Painful arc.

## Treatment

Treatment depends on severity of joint laxity and can range from conservative to surgical. Exercises that strengthen the rotator-cuff muscles may be helpful and should be performed with the arm below the shoulder, as this reduces tension at the shoulder ligaments (McCann, Wootte, Kadaba and Bigliani 1993). Often patients who have shoulder instability also suffer from tendinitis which should be addressed before strengthening exercises are started.

For anterior instability (the most common type), the patient exercises the (Ombregt, Bisschop, ter Veer and Van de Velde 1995):

* Subscapularis.
* Pectoralis major.
* Coracobrachialis.
* Long head of biceps.

For posterior instability the patient exercises the:

* Infraspinatus.
* Teres minor.
* Posterior deltoid.

Mild joint laxity can result in superior translation of the humeral head, which then impinges on the rotator-cuff tendons.

Exercises to strengthen the infraspinatus muscle is important to help prevent this complication.

Prolotherapy can be very helpful in the treatment of shoulder instability (Ravin personal communication). Acupuncture techniques are not effective. (Unless hot needle technique is used to scar the capsule).

## Acromioclavicular (AC) Joint

The acromioclavicular (AC) joint is affected often. Passive adduction across the front (Figure 10-13) usually is the most painful movement (Cyriax *ibid*). At times, all passive movements are painful at full range, and a painful arc, may be seen. The pain is in a C-4 distribution (over the shoulder up to the acromial rim). When the deep aspect of the joint is affected, the pain can radiate in a C-5 distribution and then be felt over the deltoid muscle, as well.

AC joint sprains are seen often after a fall on the shoulder with the arm at the side or outstretched. Traumatic AC joint separation can occur, and surgical treatment may or may not be needed, since outcome studies show little benefit from

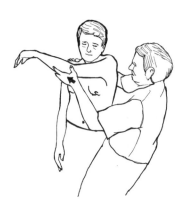

*Figure 10-13:* Assessment of shoulder adduction across the front.

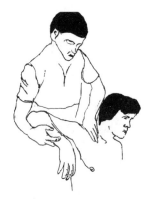

*Figure 10-15:*AC joint manipulation.

surgery as compared to conservative treatments (Bannister et al. 1989). Sprain or instability can also develop with repetitive use (daily activity). Osteoarthritis may be seen.

An AC joint lesion sometimes is difficult to differentiate from either chronic subdeltoid bursitis or early glenohumeral arthritis. A diagnostic injection may be needed (Ombregt, Bisschop, ter Veer and Van de Velde 1995).

Joint play movement at the AC joint is anteroposterior (superoinferior) glide (Mennell *ibid*).

*Treatment*

Sprain of the superficial AC ligament can be treated with cross-fiber massage (Figure 10-14). The deeper aspects are treated with local needling and positive polarity electrostimulation. Mobilization of a subluxed joint can be helpful (Figure 10-15) but should be combined with periosteal acupuncture or prolotherapy to stabilize the joint.

**ACUPUNCTURE.** Treatment to the Lung Sinews channel is helpful.

**INJECTION**. For stubborn cases, intra-articu-lar Sarapin, steroids or prolotherapy may be needed.

**HERBAL MEDICATION.** Topical herbal application is useful. A guiding herbal formula (oral and topical) for chronic ligamentous and tendinous lesions at the shoulder is:

Radix Angelica Chinesis (Dang Gui)

Rhizoma Ligusticum (Chuan Xiang)

Radix Rehmanniae (Shu Di)

Radix Peonae Rubra (Chi Shao)

Semen Persicae (Tao Ren)

Flos Carthami (Hong Hua)

Rhizoma Curcumae Longae (Jiang Huang)

Radix Salviae Miltiorrhizae (Dan Shen)

Cortex Cinnammomi (Rou Gui)

Radix Dipsaci (Chuan Duan)

Cortex Eucommiae (Du Zhong)

Radix Astragalus (Huang Qi)

Rhizoma Zingiberis Officinalis Recens (Sheng Jiang)

Radix Glycyrrhizae (Gan Cao)

Lumbricus (Di Long)

Semen Coicis (Yi Yi Ren)

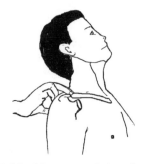

*Figure 10-14:* Massage technique for AC joint sprain.

## Sudeltoid/Subcoracoid Bursitis

Subdeltoid bursitis can be acute or chronic. Passive and active elevation are the most painful movements; resisted movement may or may not be painful. All passive movements often are painful at end range.

When the subcoracoid bursa is inflamed, the pain usually is felt locally in the outer infraclavicular area and does not radiate. Passive external rotation often is painful. The pain disappears when the test is repeated with the arm abducted to the horizontal (Cyriax *ibid*).

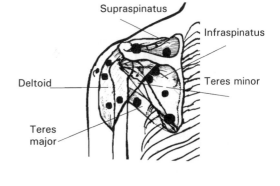

*Figure 10-16:*   Common trigger sites on muscle affecting the shoulder.

*Treatment*

Treatment of bursitis, especially chronic, is achieved with techniques that address all other shoulder dysfunctions. Topical anti-inflammatory soaks are helpful.

**ACUPUNCTURE.** Periosteal needling of the acromial edges (or coracoid process for subcoracoid bursitis) can be helpful. St-38, LI-1, Lu-11, SI-1 and TW-1 can be needled or moxaed. The Lung Connecting and Sinews channels are used often.

**INJECTION.** For stubborn lesions, injection therapy is needed often.

**HERBAL MEDICATION.** A guiding formula for oral and topical use is:

    Rhizoma seu Radix Notopterygium (Qiang Hou)

    Rhizoma Curcumae Longae (Jiang Huang)

    Radix Salviae Miltiorrhizae(Dan Shen)

    Rhizoma Ligusticum (Chuan Xiang)

    Radix Glycyrrhizae (Gan Cao)

    Radix Ledebouriellae Sesloidis (Fang Feng)

    Rhizoma Atractylodes (Cang Zhu)

    Rhizoma Atractylodes Macrocephalae (Bai Zhu)

    Poria Cocus (Fu Ling)

    Radix Stephaniae Tetrandrae (Fang Ji)

    Rhizoma Alisimatis (Ze Xie)

    Semen Coicis (Yi Yi Ren)

    Tripterygium Wilfordii (Lei Gong Teng)

    vitamins B6 and B12 (to prevent possible side effects of Tripterygium)

## Contractile Unit Disorders

Musculotendinous lesion about the shoulder is common. The nature of the lesion is easily identified by selective tension tests. Muscle weakness can be due to neurological lesions, cancer or rupture. Acupuncture has been shown to be helpful in the treatment of tendinitis (Marcus and Gracer 1994).

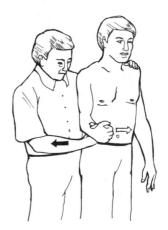

*Figure 10-17:* Assessment of resisted internal rotation, Subscapularis muscle.

## Subscapularis Tendinitis

Subscapularis tendinitis is seen in patients when resisted internal rotation is positive (Figure 10-17). Passive external rotation can be painful at end range. The lesion usually is at the tendon insertion.

NOTE: The pectoralis major, latissimus dorsi and ters major also are internal rotators of the shoulder. However, a lesion in these muscles is less likely, and when present, results in painful resisted adduction as well (since these muscles are both internal rotators and adductors).

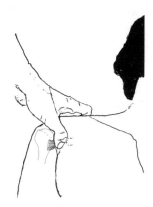

*Figure 10-18:* Massage technique for subscapularis tendinitis.

A lesion in the subscapularis can occur in the superior or inferior aspect of the tendon. A lesion at the:

* Superior aspect results in a painful arc.
* Inferior aspect results in pain on passive horizontal adduction.

### Treatment

The main treatment method is cross-fiber massage. The patient is treated in the supine position, with the arm extended and supinated—for 10-20 minutes. The shoulder is extended slightly to expose more of the tendon. The tendon insertion, at the medial edge of the lesser tuberosity, is massaged (Figure 10-18). Good results are obtained in about two-thirds of patients (Ombregt, Bisschop, ter Veer, Van de Velde 1995). OM Tui-Na mobilization techniques may be helpful in rupturing adhesions (Figure 10-22 on page 282).

ACUPUNCTURE. After activation of the Well and Termination points of the Lung and Small Intestine Sinews channels, needling is performed with the patient in the same position as in massage therapy. This brings the lesser tuberosity of the humerus closer to acupuncture point LI-15 (Figure 10-19). This point is then superficially needled inferiorly and medially toward the lesion. MUE-4 (Jian nei ling) is needled in the direction of the lesion, as well. Ashi (trig-

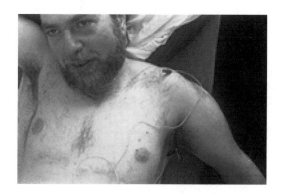

*Figure 10-19:* Acupuncture position for treatment of subscapularis tendinitis.

ger points) are needled superficially (Figure 10-16).

If needed Ashi points at the site of the lesion are needled perpendicularly to the depth of the periosteum. Another needle is inserted through the axilla into the muscle belly.

### Injection

Sarapin or steroid injections can be used in stubborn cases.

## Supraspinatus Tendinitis

Supraspinatus tendinitis is seen in patients when resisted abduction is positive (Figure

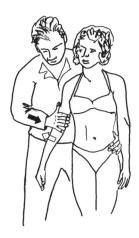

*Figure 10-20:* Assessment of resisted abduction, supraspinatus muscle

10-20). Lesions of the supraspinatus tendon are the most common tendinous lesions at the shoulder (Ombregt, Bisschop, ter Veer and Van de Velde 1995).

**NOTE:** Painful resisted abduction can rarely be due to a deltoid lesion. If resisted abduction is painful and the pain is from the supraspinatus muscle, resisted abduction may be more painful with the arm at 35° of abduction.[4] No painful arc is possible from the deltoid because the muscle is above the acromion.

The supraspinatus tendon can be affected at four sites:

• Superficial tenoperiosteal aspect with a painful arc on active elevation.

• Deep tenoperiosteal aspect with pain on passive elevation.

• Both deep and superficial aspects with a painful arc and painful passive elevation.

• Musculotendinous junction with no localizing signs (Cyriax *ibid*).

4. Older literature stated that the supraspinatus initiates shoulder abduction and the deltoid completes it. However, electrical activity of both the deltoid andsupraspinatus muscles increases progressively throughout abduction.

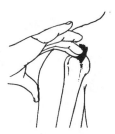

*Figure 10-21:*Massage technique for supraspinatus tendinitis.

*Treatment*

The principal treatment is cross-fiber massage (10-20 minutes). The shoulder is treated with the patient seated and the affected arm in the hammerlock position (arm behind the back). This rotates the shoulder medially, brings the greater tuberosity forward, and exposes the tendon (Figure 10-21).

For massage of the musculotendinous junction the patient's arm rests on a table (Figure 10-22).

**ACUPUNCTURE.** After activating the Large Intestine Sinews channel LI-15 is needled toward the tendon insertion at the humerus. For musculotendinous lesions, LI-16 is needled toward the musculotendinous junction (Figure 10-23).

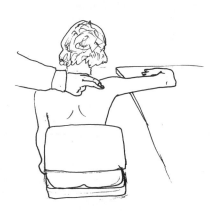

*Figure 10-22:* Massage technique for supraspinatus lesion at the musculotendinous junction.

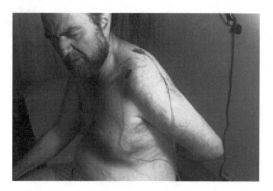

*Figure 10-23:* Acupuncture position for treatment of supraspinatus tendinitis.

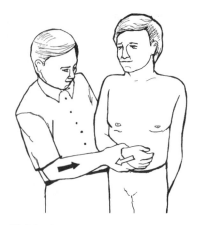

*Figure 10-24:* Assessment of resisted external rotation, infraspinatus muscle.

If needed Ashi points are needled gently down to the periosteum at the site of the lesion (making sure not to further injure the tendon). Another needle is inserted at the motor point.

**INJECTION.** Sarapin or steroid injections may be needed in stubborn cases.

## Infraspinatus Tendinitis

Infraspinatus tendinitis is seen in patients when resisted external rotation is positive (Figure 10-24).

NOTE: Although the teres minor also is an external rotator of the shoulder, it is seldom affected. When it is, resisted external rotation and adduction are painful.

The infraspinatus tendon can be affected in three sites:

• Superficial tenoperiosteal aspect with a painful arc.

• Deep tenoperiosteal aspect with pain on full passive elevation.

Musculotendinous junction with no localizing signs (Cyriax *ibid*).

*Treatment*

The patient sits with the affected arm held at the elbow by the opposite hand. The shoulder is kept adducted and externally rotated (Figure 10-26), (or kept on the treatment table while the patient holds onto the table's edge). This uncovers the head of the humeral tuberosity from under the acromion and exposes the tendon insertion at the posterior aspect of the greater tuberosity. Cross fiber massage is the preferred treatment method (Figure 10-25). OM Tui-Na techniques which integrate movement with massage are helpful.

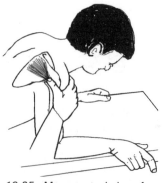

*Figure 10-25:* Massage technique for infraspinatus muscle.

ACUPUNCTURE. After activation the Small Intestine and Triple Warmer Sinews channels SJ-14 and SI-10 are needled superficially toward the lesion. For lesions at the musculotendinous junction, SI-11 is needled perpendicular to, or toward, the lesion (Figure 10-26).

If needed Ashi points over the lesion are needled gently toward the periosteum, making sure not to injure the tendon.

INJECTION. Sarapin or steroid injections may be needed in stubborn cases.

## Teres Minor Tendinitis

The teres minor is involved when resisted adduction and external rotation are painful at the shoulder. Lesions in the teres minor (and major) are extremely rare.

NOTE: Resisted adduction also can cause pain in the pectoralis major, latissimus dorsi and teres major, all of which also are internal rotators of the shoulder. The localization of pain helps differentiate which muscle is involved.

### Treatment

Treatment is similar to that of the infraspinatus tendon, except that localization of the tendon is just below that of the infraspinatus.

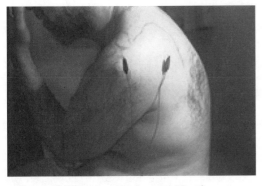

*Figure 10-26:* Acupuncture position for treatment of infraspinatus tendinitis.

## Proximal Biceps Tendinitis

Biceps tendinitis (at the shoulder end) is seen in patients with shoulder pain during resisted elbow flexion. Resisted arm supination usually is painful, as well. This excludes the brachialis muscle. The brachialis is very rarely involved at the shoulder end.

A lesion can develop in two areas: the long tendon at the glenoid origin, and at the bicipital sulcus (groove). Tendinitis at the glenoid origin results in:

- Positive resisted elbow flexion and arm supination.
- Positive resisted adduction with elbow extended, but which becomes negative when the elbow is flexed.

Tendinitis at the bicipital groove area results in:

- Positive resisted elbow flexion and arm supination only (Cyrix *ibid*).

### Treatment

Tendinitis at the bicipital groove responds quickly to massage therapy (Ombregt *ibid*). The patient is supine. At the patient's side, the practitioner:

1. Identifies the biceps tendon in the bicipital groove and presses down hard on the lesion.

2. Holds the patient's flexed and slightly medially rotated arm with his other hand.

3. Rotates the humerus laterally while keeping pressure on the tendon (which achieves cross-fiber stimulation).

4. Releases pressure on the tendon and rotates the arm medially.

5. Repeats the process for 20 minutes (Figure 10-27).

Tendinitis at the glenoid origin requires injection therapy. Needling muscle triggers can be helpful (Figure 10-28).

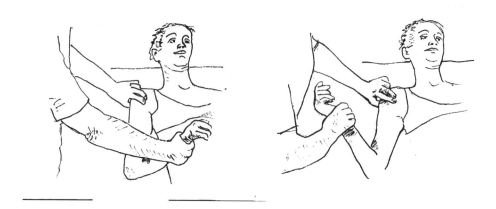

*Figure 10-27:* Massage technique for the biceps tendon.

## Biceps Tendon Rupture

Rupture of the long head of the biceps, at its upper end, is one of the most common tendon ruptures. When the elbow is flexed, a sudden loud pop often is heard, with momentary pain in the upper arm. The condition becomes painless fairly quickly. A muscular nodule, due to the distal displacement of the muscle belly, can be seen, especially during contraction. Usually no treatment is required, although surgical correction can be successful (Ombregt, Bisschop, ter Veer and Van de Velde 1995).

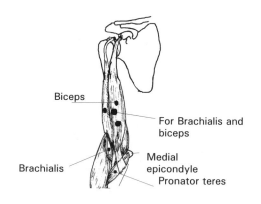

*Figure 10-28:* Common needling site on the biceps

## Snapping Biceps Tendon

The tendon of the biceps long head can slip out of the bicipital groove in some patients. The patient may complain of a feeling of instability when the tendon is displaced. Occasionally tendinitis can develop. Resisted flexion at the elbow with resisted internal rotation of the arm at the same time (Yergason's test) can provoke tendon dislocation (Brown *ibid*).

## Recurrent Shoulder Tendinitis

Recurrent shoulder tendinitis occures most often due to instability of the joint. Instability can be demonstrated by drawer tests. The patient can often be treated effectively with prolotherapy injections (Ravin personal communication).

# The Elbow

Pain at the elbow is common; local disorders are fairly easy to identify. Referred pain from C5 and C6 structures must be considered.

## Anatomy & Biomechanics

The elbow consists of three joints; the humeroulnar, the humeroradial and the upper radioulnar (Figure 10-29). Flexion and extension take place at the humeroulnar and humeroradial joints. Pronation and supination at the upper radioulnar joint occur in close relation to the lower radioulnar joint.

Six ligaments reinforce the capsule: the ulnar collateral ligament, the radial collateral ligament, the radial annular ligament, the quadate ligament, the oblique

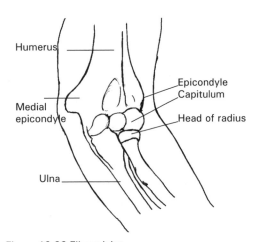

*Figure 10-29:*Elbow joint.

cord, and the interosseous membrane (Kapandji *ibid*). Table 10-2 lists the muscles affecting the elbow.

*Table 10-2.* **MUSCLES AFFECTING THE ELBOW**

| FUNCTION | MUSCLE | INNERVATION |
|---|---|---|
| **EXTENSION** | Triceps | C7-C8 |
| **FLEXION** | Brachialis | C5-C6 |
| | Brachioradialis | C5-C6 |
| | Brachial biceps | C5-C6 |
| | Anconeus | C7-C8 |
| **SUPINATION** | Supinator brevis | C5-C6 |
| | Brachial biceps | C5-C6 |
| **PRONATION** | Pronator teres | C6-C7 |
| | Pronator quadratus | C8-T1 |
| **WRIST AND FINGER EXTENSORS** | Extensor carpi radialis longus and brevis | C6-C7 |
| | | C7 |
| | Extensor carpi ulnaris | C7-C8 |
| | Extensor digitorum communis | C6-C-8 |
| **WRIST AND FINGER FLEXORS** | Flexor carpi radialis | C6-C7 |
| | Flexor carpi ulnaris | C7-C8 |
| | Palmaris longus | C7-T1 |
| | Superficial flexor digitorum | C7-T1 |
| | Flexor pollicis longus | C7-C8 |

Joint play movements at the *superior radioulnar* joint are (Mennell *ibid*):

1. Upward glide of the head of the radius on the ulna.

2. Downward glide of the head of the radius on the ulna.

3. Rotation of the head on the ulna, which is independent of supination and pronation of the forearm.

Movements at the *radiohumeral* joint take place between the articular surface of the head of the radius upon the capitulum of the humerus. There is a change of radial relationship as the elbow is flexed and then extended, and this movement is involuntary in all its phases. This movement is dependent on normal function of the superior radioulnar joint, except when a meniscus is present at the joint (Mennell *ibid*).

Joint play movements at the *humeroulnar* joint are medial and lateral tilt of the olecranon (Mennell *ibid*).

# Imaging

As previously stated the elbow is frequently talked about as an area to be imaged by plain radiography. However the physical examination is so superb, and the imaging modalities relatively imprecise, that the X-rays usually are not needed. In general the examiner notes: the relations of the epicondyles, trochlea, capitulum, radial head, radial tuberosity, coronoid process, olecranon process. Any joint space narrowing, calcification, myositis ossificans, loose bodies, and osteophytes are noted. A "fat pad" sign can occur with joint effusion and may indicate a fracture, acute arthritis, or osteoid osteoma. In a young child the epiphysial plate should be noted to see if it is normal for each of the bones.

# OM Disorders

OM disorders of the elbow are caused by trauma, external pathogenic factors and overuse. Often weakness of Defensive and Nutritive Qi are at the root. Consumption of Qi and Blood leads to malnourishment of tendons and often manifests as lateral epicondylitis. Accumulation of Phlegm and Blood can transform and form a sharp osteophyte at the epicondyle.

# Biomedical Disorders: Inert Structures

Disorders of the elbow's inert (noncontractile) structures are mainly arthritic or involve the bursae around the elbow. A loose body can develop within the joint, as well.

## Capsular Pattern

The capsular pattern at the elbow is characterized by limitation of extension and flexion. Usually flexion is more limited, although equal limitation of both movements can occur. With a loose body in the joint, limitation depends on the site in which the loose body lodges and usually is in one direction only (not a capsular pattern), (Cyriax *ibid*).

## *End Feel*

The normal end feel at the elbow is hard on extension and soft on flexion. In arthritis, the end feel in extension and flexion can be soggy or hard, depending on the amount of edema and muscle spasm. With a loose body, the end feel may become more springy. In arthrosis, the end feel usually is hard in both flexion and extension, and the patient may complain of a slight ache after excessive use of the elbow

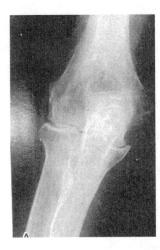

*Figure 10-30:*Rheumatoid arthritis. Note the uniforr loss of joint space.

(Ombregt, Bisschop, ter Veer and Van de Velde 1995).

**DISORDERS TO RULE OUT.** In a patient who has a capsular pattern, the practitioner should rule out traumatic or other types of hemarthrosis, septic arthritis, gout and rheumatoid arthritis (Figure 10-30), (Ombregt, Bisschop, ter Veer and Van de Velde 1995).

## Treatment of Inert Structures

Treatment of inert structures of the elbow usually involve mobilization and application of topical and systemic medication.

### Acupuncture

Points around the joint can be needled. Contralateral St. 36, Beside Three Miles and ipsilateral ear points are helpful.

### Injection

Intra-articular Sarapin or steroid injections may be necessary in stubborn cases.

### Herbal Therapy

A guiding herbal formula for arthrosis at the elbow (for oral and topical use), (mix with warm vinegar when used topically) is:

    Prepared Sichuan Aconite (Zhi Chuan Wu)
    Ramulus Cinnamomi Cassiae (Gui Zhi)
    Radix Angelica Chinesis (Dang Gui)
    Rhizoma Ligusticum (Chuan Xiang)
    Radix Rehmanniae Praeparata (Shu Di Huang)
    Peony Rubra (Chi Shao)
    Semen Persicae (Tao Ren)
    Flos Carthami (Hong Hua)
    Rhizoma Curcumae Longae (Jiang Huang)
    Cortex Eucommiae (Du Zhong)
    Radix Astragalus (Huang Qi)
    Radix Glycyrrhizae (Gan Cao)
    Radix Clemetidis Chinesis (Wei Ling Xian)
    Rhizoma Atractylodes (Cang Zhu)
    Ramulus Mori (Sang Zhi)
    Fructus Chaenomelis (Mu Gua)
    Herba Lycopodii (Shen Jin Cao)

For arthritis with warmth and swelling:

    Take out
    Prepared Sichuan Aconite (Zhi Chuan Wu)
    Ramulus Cinnamomi Cassiae (Gui Zhi)
    Radix Angelica Chinesis (Dang Gui)
    Cortex Eucommiae (Du Zhong)
    Add
    Tripterygium Wilfordii (Lei Gong Teng)
    Cortex Phellodendri (Huang Bai)

## Proximal Radioulnar Joint Laxity

Laxity of the joint can result in recurrent weakness and elbow pain. These symptoms are seen often in patients like construction workers who repetitively pronate and supinate the arm. The patient often develops symptoms of epicondylitis. Limitation of supination and/or pronation is common (Ombregt, Bisschop, ter Veer and Van de Velde 1995).

### Treatment

Manipulative reduction followed by periosteal needling of the annular ligament is helpful. The practitioner:

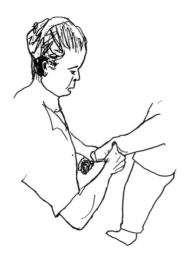

*Figure 10-31:*   Manipulation of radioulnar joint.

1. Supports the patient's elbow with one hand while holding the patient's wrist joint flexed with the other hand.

2. With his or her other hand puts a fulcrum through the joint.

3. Slowly extends the patient's arm while keeping his or her wrist flexed.

4. Quickly hyperextends the elbow (Figure 10-31).

## Dysfunction of the Radial Head and the Capitulum

The head of the radius and the capitulum are separated by a meniscus. Dysfunction at this joint can be manifested with pain in the elbow mimicking, and sometimes associated with, a true tennis elbow. Supination is limited, painful, and is associated with a springy end feel and a noncapsular pattern of limitation of range of movement (Dorman and Ravin 1991).

*Treatment*

Treatment is achieved by manipulative reduction. The technique is similar to the one used for the proximal radioulnar joint laxity. The patient wrist and elbow are flexed fully and then the forearm is fully supinated. The practitioner:

1. Places firm pressure over the head of the radius with the thumb of his upper hand.

2. (Maintaining pressure in an ulnar anterior direction and wrist flexed) extends the forearm until the point at which pain recurs or sensed.

3. Holds this position for a moment and then with a quick thrust of low amplitude extends the elbow fully.

## Pulled Elbow Pediatric Patient

A pulled elbow usually is seen in children under 8 years of age and usually is caused by a forced distal traction at the forearm (pulling a stubborn child by the hand), (Illingworth 1975). The head of the radius is pulled out of the annular ligament, resulting in limited supination.

*Treatment*

Reduction is achieved by gentle mobilization of the elbow into flexion and pronation. Alternatively, with the child standing against the wall or in front of the parent, the practitioner:

1. Abducts the elbow and flexes the child's upper arm.

2. Holds the forearm and pushes the radius upward toward the humerus by pressing the elbow against the wall.

3. (At the same time) gently rotates the forearm back and forth to the end range (Brown *ibid*).

## Pushed Elbow

Pushed elbow is approximately the opposite condition of pulled elbow. Long-axis compression on the forearm is painful at the elbow, as is pronation.

### Treatment

Treatment here is with long-axis traction with slight supination (Dorman and Ravin *ibid*).

## Ulnar Olecranon Block

Trapped synovial fringe at the posterior part of the elbow, between the beak of the olecranon and the posterior humeral fossa, can result in pain on extension with a springy end feel. A boggy, tender mass is often present on palpation.

### Treatment

Treatment is achieved by local needling and anti-inflammatory methods, followed by manipulation. The patient is supine. The practitioner:

1. Holds the patient's elbow at a maximum, comfortable extension.

2. Wobbles the lower humerus to and fro—medially and laterally—with his hand.

3. (With his lower hand) guides the forearm into a controlled, gradual extension (Dorman and Ravin *ibid*).

## Loose Body

Depending on the age group, three clinical pictures of a loose body at the elbow joint can be seen (Ombregt, Bisschop, ter Veer and Van de Velde 1995).

A loose body in the adolescent patient is the only cause of nontraumatic arthrosis in the young, and occurs usually before 14 years of age. A loose body usually is secondary to osteochondritis dissecans of the capitellum, or to an intra-articular chip fracture. Osteochondritis dissecans is more common in the female gymnast, with hyperextension and valgus injuries of the elbow (Singer and Roy 1984).

A loose body in the *adult* patient usually is traumatic, the patient having chipped off a piece of cartilage. Predominance of flexion or extension restriction depends on the location of the loose body. If a loose body lies at the anterior part of the joint it will limit flexion and vice versa. The adult loose body can be treated by manipulation. If recurrent dysfunctions occur surgery may be necessary. A loose body in *middle/old age* patients often is due to multiple factors and can involve multiple loose bodies. Acute attacks often resolve on their own in a few days. Loose bodies in the middle/old age patient usually do not cause arthrosis, therefore surgery usually is not needed.

On examination, a capsular pattern can be seen with decreased passive extension having a soft end feel. A loose body in the adolescent should be treated surgically as it can result in arthrosis of the joint.

### Treatment

Symptoms due to a loose body can be alleviated temporarily by manipulation reduction. The maneuver involves traction together with movement from flexion toward extension and rotation.

## Bursitis

*Epicondylar* and *radiohumeral* bursitis can cause a vague ache at the lateral elbow which can be mistaken for tennis elbow.

*Olecranon* bursitis can occur with repetitive pressure, a fall on a bent elbow, and various other conditions such as gout, rheumatic disease and T.B. Conservative treatment often is not effective (Ombregt, Bisschop, ter Veer and Van de Velde 1995).

### Treatment

Bursitis can be treated with topical and systemic medication and use of Lung and

Large intestine Sinews channels. Ear and
Stomach and Gall bladder points are helpful. For more stubborn lesions injection
therapy can be used.

# Disorders of Contractile Structures

## Lateral Epicondylitis (Tennis Elbow)

Tennis elbow is due to inflammation of the
wrist or finger extensor muscles and often
arises from repetitive or acute trauma to
the tenoperiosteal junction, tendon body,
tendinomuscular junction or muscle belly
(Figure 10-33).

The lesion can occur in 6 locations:

* Type I—occasional—lesion at the tenoperiosteal junction of the extensor carpi
radialis longus at the supraclavicular
ridge.

  — Findings: positive resisted wrist
  extension and radial deviation.

* Type II—by far the most common type
—lesion at the tenoperiosteal junction of
the extensor carpi radialis brevis at the

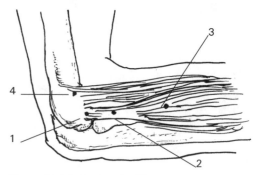

*Figure 10-33:* Lesion sites in tennis elbow: 1,
tenoperiosteal; 2, tendinous; 3, muscular; 4,
supracondylar.

anterior (ridge, roof) aspect of the lateral
epicondyle.

— Findings; positive resisted wrist
extension, tenderness over the
anterior aspect of lateral epicondyle.

* Type III—fairly rare—lesion at the tendon body of the extensor carpi radialis
brevis.

— Findings: positive resisted wrist
extension, tenderness over the
tendon body.

* Type IV—not common—lesion at the
muscle bellies of the extensor carpi radialis and brevis.

— Findings: positive resisted wrist
extension, tenderness at the muscle
bellies near and a few centimeters
distal to the neck of the radius.

* Type V— occasional—lesion at the tenoperiosteal junction of the extensor digitorum, at the anterior distal aspect of the
lateral epicondyle.

— Findings: positive resisted wrist
extension, negative or reduced pain
with resisted wrist extension when
the fingers are held flexed, and
positive resisted extension of the
middle and ring fingers (Figure 10-
32).

* Type VI—occasional—a lesion of the
extensor carpi ulnaris at the tenoperiosteal origin, at the posterior aspect of

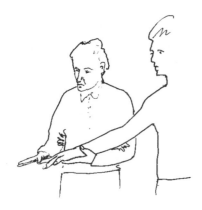

*Figure 10-32:*Resisted wrist and finger
extension.

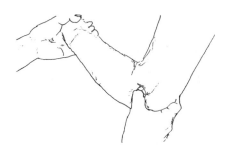

*Figure 10-34:* Massage technique for tennis elbow: at common extensor tendon.

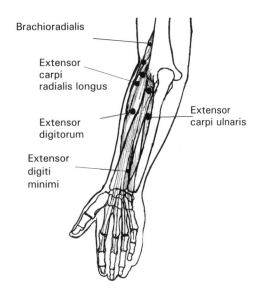

Brachioradialis

Extensor carpi radialis longus

Extensor digitorum

Extensor digiti minimi

Extensor carpi ulnaris

*Figure 10-35:* Common trigger sites on extensor muscles.

the lateral epicondyle, or more rarely at the olecranon.

— Findings: positive resisted wrist extension and positive resisted ulnar deviation. Tenderness at the posterior epicondyle or olecranon.

### Treatment

Treatment of lateral epicondylitis includes a complete evaluation and often treatment of the cervical spine and wrist joints. Manipulation of the cervical spine as been shown to reduce tennis elbow pain (Vicenzino, Collins and Wright 1996). The main local treatment is cross-fiber massage at the appropriate site (Figure 10-34 and Figure 10-33). OM Tui-Na techniques which combine cross-fiber massage with mobilization can be helpful (Figure 10-22 on page 282).

**ACUPUNCTURE.** Acupuncture is effective and compares favorably to cortisone injections (Brattberg 1993; Haker and Lundeberg 1990; Molsberger and Hille 1994). Treatment to the Large Intestine, Small Intestine and Gall Bladder channels are used often. The Liver Organ, Blood and external pathologic factors are addressed frequently, as well. It is helpful to needle Beside Three Miles, and St. 36 contralaterally while the patient stretches the extensor muscle. For disorders of the extensor digitorum and extensor carpi ulnaris,

points on the Small Intestine channels are used. Ashi (triggers) points are needled often (Figure 10-35).

Stretch techniques of the extensor muscles should be taught to the patient and performed every hour for the first week, or during acute exacerbations. Progressive strengthening and stretching has been shown to be more effective than ultrasound (Pienimak et al. 1996).

**RECALCITRANT LESIONS.** For recalcitrant lesions a close look at the cervical spine and wrist joints is warranted. Instability and dysfunction of the lateral wrist joints is a common cause of recurrent tennis elbow (Ravin personal communication).

A manipulative technique to rupture possible adhesions, may be tried. The manipulation is preceded by needling contralateral St-36 and having the patient stretch the tendon. Five to ten minuets of cross fiber massage may be helpful in making the procedure more comfortable as well. The technique should not be tried in patients with limited elbow extension due to capsular pathology. The practitioner should assess the end feel, and, if, extension is limited by pain alone, at the moment of tension buildup at the tendon,

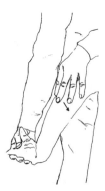

*Figure 10-36:* Manipulation technique to rupture adhesions at the wrist extensors (tennis elbow).

the manipulation may be tried. The patient sits on a chair or lies down. The practitioner stands behind him. The practitioner:

1. Identifies the most sensitive tendinous insertion by testing finger extension of the index, middle and fourth fingers; while at the same time feeling around the lateral epicondyle.

2. (Keeps his thumb at the identified site and) flexes and supinates the patient's wrist.

3. Flexes the patient's elbow.

4. (While continually monitoring the tendon insertion) begins to extend the patient's elbow and flexes and supinates the wrist, until maximum tension builds at the tendon insertion site.

5. (After several seconds) delivers a thrust by quickly extending the elbow (Figure 10-36).

A crack is heard often, indicating rupture of some tendinous fibers. This manipulation is carried out twice a week, for 6-20 times, until no further ruptures are obtained and maximal clinical benefit is achieved (Brown *ibid*).

**HERBAL THERAPY.**

A guiding oral herbal formula for acute tennis elbow is:

> Caulis Milletti (Ji Xue Teng)
> Radix Salviae Miltorrhizae (Dan Shen)
> Ramulus Moriae (Sang Zhi)
> Flos Carthami (Hong Hua)
> Rhizoma Ligustici Wallicii (Chuan Xiong)
> Radix Gentianae Macrophyllae (Qin Jiu)
> Radix Clematidis (Wei Ling Xian)
> Rhizoma Curcumae Longae (Jiang Huang)
> Rhizoma seu Radix Notopterygii (Qiang Huo)
> Paeoniae Rubra (Chi Shao)
> Squma Manitis (Chuan Shan Jia)
> Spina Gleditsiae (Zao Jiao Ci)

A guiding oral herbal formula for chronic tennis elbow is:

> Radix Rehmanniae Praeparata (Shu Di)
> Fructus Corni (Shan Zhu Yu)
> Herba Cistanchis (Rou Cong Rong)
> Cortex Eucommiae (Du Zhong)
> Semen Cuscutae (Tu Si Zi)
> Fructus Psoraleae (Bu Gu Zhi)
> Resina Myrrhae (Mo Yao)
> Flos Carthami (Hong Hua)
> Radix Angelicae Dahuricae (Bai Zhi)
> Fructus Lycii (Gou Qi Zi)
> Radix Angelicae Sinensis (Dang Gui)
> Paeoniae Rubra (Chi Shao)
> Spina Gleditsiae (Zao Jiao Ci)
> Radix Gentianae Macrophyllae (Qin Jiu)
> Cortex Lycii Radicis (Di Gu Pi)

A guiding herbal formula for topical application is:

> Radix Aconiti Agrestis and Kusenzoffii (Cao Wu Tou and Chuan Wu Tou)
> Pericarpium Zanthoxyli (Hua Jiao)
> Folium Artemisiae Argyi (Ai Ye)
> Herba Artemisiae (Qing Hao)
> Rhizoma Atractylodis (Cang Zhu)
> Ramulus Cinnamomii (Gui Zhi)
> Radix Sileris (Fang Feng)
> Flos Carthami (Hong Hua)
> Herba Impatiens sew Spena (Ji Xing)
> Herba Lycopodii (Shen Qian Cao)
> Squma Manitis (Chuan Shan Jia)

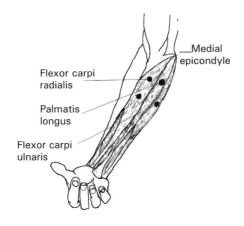

Figure 10-37: Common trigger sites on the flexor muscles

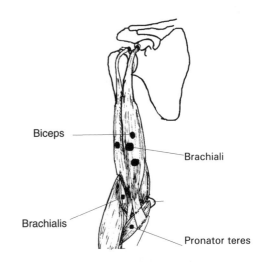

Figure 10-38: Common trigger site on the biceps and brachialis.

## Medial Epicondylitis (Golfer's Elbow)

Medial epicondylitis, also known as golfer's elbow, is seen in patients with painful resisted flexion of the wrist. Resisted pronation is occasionally painful, as well. The disorder is much less common than tennis elbow and usually causes less disability. The lesion can occur in two locations (Cyriax *ibid*):

• Tenoperiosteal junction.
• Musculotendinous junction.

### Treatment

Both varieties are treated with cross-fiber massage and needling of the flexor muscles. Acupuncture to points on the Heart, Pericardium and Lung channels can be used. Needling Ashi (trigger) points can be helpful (Figure 10-37). Topical herbal application is helpful, as well.

## Biceps / Brachialis Disorders

Pain at the elbow with resisted elbow flexion can be due to lesions in the biceps or brachialis muscles. The biceps muscle is at fault if resisted supination is painful as well. Lesions of the brachialis are less common.

The biceps muscle can develop a lesion in four areas (Cyriax *ibid*):

• The tendon in the bicipital groove.
— pain at the shoulder area.
• The muscle belly.
— pain at mid-arm.
• The musculotendinous junction.
— pain in the lower arm.
• The tenoperiosteal insertion.
— pain at the elbow, probably radiating down the forearm.

The brachialis muscle develops a lesion usually at the distal third of the muscle belly.

WARNING: Trauma can result in myositis ossificans at the brachialis muscle, especially following a fracture of the distal end of the humerus. Since many people attribute the development of this condition to previous treatments (such as massage and manipulation) it may be prudent to not give any treatment as long as a full passive range of movement, at the elbow joint, is not present. An X-ray can be ordered before starting any treatment (only positive after several weeks),

(Ombregt, Bisschop, ter Veer and Van de
Velde 1995).

**BICEPS TENDON RUPTURE.** Rupture of the
long head of the biceps, at its upper end, is
one of the most common tendon ruptures.
It normally causes little trouble and treatment usually is not necessary.

The biceps can also rupture at the distal end and often with avulsion of the
radial tuberosity. Surgery is necessary
often (Brown *ibid*).

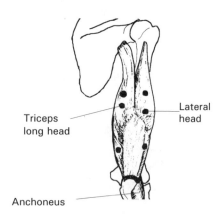

*Figure 10-39:* Common trigger sites on the triceps.

*Treatment*

Lesions at the biceps and brachialis muscles respond to cross-fiber massage. Needling triggers in the muscle can be helpful
(Figure 10-38). Injection may be necessary
in stubborn cases.

## Triceps Tendinitis.

Lesions of the triceps are rare. The muscles
can develop a lesion in the tenoperiosteal
insertion, the body of the tendon or the
musculotendinous junction (Cyriax *ibid*).

*Treatment*

Cross-fiber massage usually is effective
(Ombregt, Bisschop, ter Veer and Van de
Velde *ibid*).

*Treatment*

All three sites respond to cross fiber massage. Usually no other treatment is necessary (Ombregt, Bisschop, ter Veer and Van
de Velde 1995), if needed triggers are needled (Figure 10-39).

## Pronator Teres Tendinitis

Lesions of the pronator teres are quite
rare. They lie usually in the muscle belly
and not the tendon. Symptoms may resemble carpal tunnel syndrome (pronator syndrome), (Brown 1995).

## Supinator Brevis Tendinitis

Lesion in the supinator brevis is very rare.
The patient has pain on resisted supination
but no pain with resisted elbow flexion
which excludes the biceps muscle (Cyriax
*ibid*).

*Treatment*

Cross-fiber massage usually is effective
(Ombregt, Bisschop, ter Veer and Van de
Velde 1995).

# The Wrist & Hand

Disorders of the wrist and hand are complicated, as the anatomy is complex and symptoms can also arise from cervical, shoulder and elbow pathology. Many neural disorders and compressive neuropathies can affect the wrist and hand.

## Anatomy & Biomechanics

The wrist joint has three components: proximal, middle and distal. Proximally, the distal part of the radius (and disc) articulate with the proximal carpal bones to form the radiocarpal joint. In the middle, the intercarpal joints, which are S-shaped, lie between the proximal and distal carpal rows. Distally are the carpometacarpal joints. The distal carpal row consists of:

- Trapezium.
- Trapezoid.
- Capitate.
- Hamate.

The proximal row consists of:

- Scaphoid.
- Lunate.
- Triquetrum.
- Pisiform overlying the triquetrum (Figure 10-40).

A triangular fibrocartilage disc overlies the ulnar head and makes up a portion of the triangular fibrocartilage complex (TFCC). The TFCC acts as a stabilizer of the distal radioulnar joint and is the ulnar continuation to the radius which provides an articular surface for the carpal condyle (Brown 1995).

Functionally the wrists can be divided into three major clinical areas: the midcarpal joint, the radiocarpal, and the ulnomeniscocarpal joint (Mennell *ibid*). For the most part:

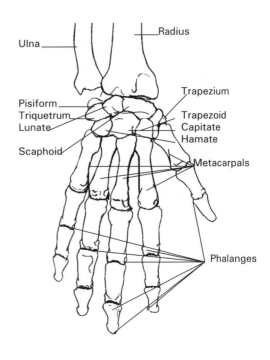

*Figure 10-40:*    Wrist and hand.

- Extension takes place at the midcarpal joint.
- Flexion takes place at the radiocarpal joint.
- Supination and pronation take place at the ulnomeniscocarpal (ulnomeniscotriquetral) joint.

  The inferior radioulnar joint is involved in supination and pronation as well.

The wrist joints are stabilized by many ligaments.

## Imaging

Routine imaging of the wrist should include four views:

**1.** An anteroposterior view.

**2.** A lateral view.

**3.** A view in radial deviation.

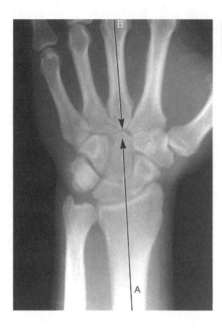

*Figure 10-41:* Wrist with a normal radioulnar relationship. Note the correct alignment of the radius and the third metacarpal bone. Line A and Line B should be in a straight line.

**4.** A view in ulnar deviation.

The AP view requires careful positioning—the wrist and palm should lie flat on the film and the long axis of the third metacarpal should be lined up with the radius. For the lateral view, a guide is helpful to ensure accurate positioning. Attention to these details helps in interpreting problems of alignment (Figure 10-41).

Injuries of the wrist commonly disrupt the distal radioulnar joint, increasing the distance between the distal ends of the forearm bones (Figure 10-43).

The anteroposterior views taken with ulnar and radial deviation are stress views that help to identify the naviculolunate ligament and the radiocarpal ligament laxity, respectively. Because these ligaments contribute to stability at the wrist, it is important to look for abnormal distancing of the relevant bones with stress views (Figure 10-42).

The important manifestations of ligament instability at the wrist have been classified into two groupings:

**1.** Dorsal intercalated segment instability (DISI).

**2.** Volar intercalated segment instability (VISI).

The diagnosis of DISI is made when the angle of dorsiflexion of the lunate exceeds 15°, and a radiographic diagnosis of VISI is made if palmar flexion of the lunate exceeds 20°. The angle formed by the radius and the lunate is measured on the lateral film.

Dorsal intercalated segment instability follows hyperflexion injuries of the dorsal lunatotriquetral ligament. This allows the lunate to tilt toward the volar aspect of the wrist, creating a capitolunate angle of less than 30° (Figure 10-45).

Additional X-ray signs of ligament disruption at the wrist include a slight widening of the naviculolunate joint in the AP view—this abnormality can be brought out in an ulnar stress view—and slight proximal displacement of the capitate, with or without stress. Distal radial fractures and DISI are caused by the same force of injury, thus they often coincide (Figure 10-47).

Ligamentous injuries at the first metacarpophalangeal joint are common among skiers. The collateral ligament on the radial side usually is involved. Laxity can be demonstrated with stress views.

**Cryptic Fractures**

Fractures of carpal bones can be hard to recognize on plain X-rays, thus it is important to identify them early. The management of a fractured navicular bone involves immobilization to ensure union with the distal fragment, the blood supply of which commonly is compromised. The hamate also is subjected to cryptic fractures. Nuclear medicine bone scans identify these conditions within four days of injury (Figure 10-48).

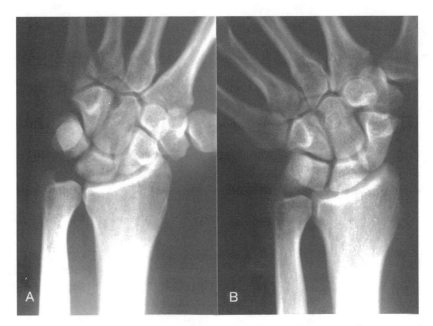

*Figure 10-42:*Radial (A) and ulnar (B) deviation. Normal changes are demonstrated in the proximal row.

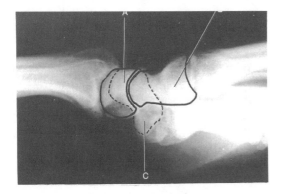

*Figure 10-43:*Lateral view of a normal wrist and the major carpal bones outlined. A = lunate; B = capitate.

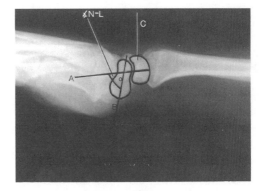

*Figure 10-44:* Wrist demonstrating a navicular somatic dysfunction. Navicular-lunate angle (NL) is greater than 70°.

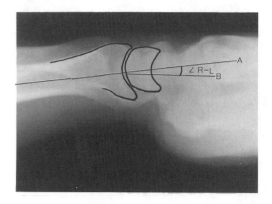

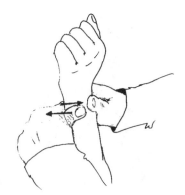

*Figure 10-46:* Anteroposterior glide.

*Figure 10-45:* The radiolunate angle (R-L) demonstrates the presence of somatic joint dysfunction of this joint. Normal is approximately- 5°. Abnormal is greater than 10-20°.

## OM Disorders

Since the wrist and hand lie distally (channels are small in volume), they are susceptible to disorders of accumulation and obstruction. Accumulation of Wind, Damp and Cold obstructs the flow of Qi and Blood. Traumatic causes are common as well.

## Biomedical Disorders

Disorders of the wrist and hand often are articular or involve the ligaments. Lesions at contractile tissues are less common, although both tendinitis and tenosynovitis can be seen. Trauma often results in fracture. Symptoms of local origin do not refer appreciably and the patient usually can recognize the origin. Symptoms of pins and needles in the wrist and hand usually are referred.

### Distal Radioulnar Joint

The distal radioulnar joint allows pronation and supination. Disorders at this joint are uncommon (seen mainly in young women) and usually result in pain at the

wrist. Arthritis can occur and results in painful passive rotations at the wrist (painful pronation and supination with full range of motion—which is the capsular pattern of this joint). Painful supination only, over the distal radioulnar joint, is often due to tenosynovitis of the extensor carpi ulnaris (Cyriax *ibid*).

Mal-united Colles' fracture can result in a decrease of the radius length and cause an irreversible limitation of supination and or pronation (Ombregt, Bisschop, ter Veer and Van de Velde 1995).

Joint play movements at this joint are (Mennell *ibid*):

**1.** Anteroposterior glide.

Assessed by having the practitioner place one thumb posteriorly over the neck of the lower end of the radius. He places his other thumb over the neck of the lower end of the ulna posteriorly with it at a right angle to the long axis of the ulna, and crooks his index finger around the wrist. The practitioner translates the ulna forward upon the radius (Figure 10-46).

**2.** Rotation.

Assessed by using the same examining position as used in anteroposterior glide. The practitioner now wings his forearms at right angles to the patient's forearm. Stabilizing the lower end of the radius, the practitioner rotates the lower end of the ulna on the radius.

## Manual Therapy

Gentle mobilization that moves the radius and ulna backward and forward on each other can often restore normal motion at the joint. The movements used to assess joint play can be used therapeutically except that now a thrust is given at the restricted end range.

## Herbal Medications

A guiding oral and topical herbal formula for early-stage fracture with swelling and pain is:

Radix Angelicae Sinensis (Dang Gui)
Radix Rehmanniae (Shu Di Huang)
Radix Paeoniae Alba (Bai Shao)
Rhizoma Ligustici Wallichii (Chuan Xiang)
Gummi Olibanum (Ru Xiang)
Resina Myrrhae (Mo Yao)
Herba Lycopodii (Shen Jin Cao)
Frctus Liquidambaris (Lu Lu Tong)
Semen Plantaginis (Che Qian Zi)

Flos Loncerae (Jin Yin Hua)
Flos Chrysanthemi (Ju Hua)
Rizoma Paridis (Zao Xiu)

A guiding oral and topical formula for mid-stage fracture (bone union stage) is:

Sanguis Draconis (Xue Jie)
Eupolyphaga seu Opisthoplatiae (Tu Bie Chong)
Squma Manitis (Chuan Shan Jia)
Pyritum (Zi Ran Tong)
Semen Strychnotis (Ma Qian Zi)
Rhizoma Drynari (Gu Sui Bu)
Herba Pyrolaceae (Lu Xian Cao)
Herba Ephedra (Ma Huang)
Animal Bone

A guiding oral and topical formula for late-stage fracture with stiffness and pain is:

Radix Angelica Sinensis (Dang Gui)
Caulis Spatholobi (Ji Xue Teng)
Radix Salviae Miltiorrhizae (Dan Shen)
Ramulus Mori Albae (Sang Zhi)
Flos Carthami (Hong Hua)
Rhizoma Ligustici Wallichii (Chuan Xiong)
Radix Gentianae Macrophyllae (Qin Jiu)
Radix Clematidis (Wei Ling Xian)
Rhizoma Curcumae Longae (Jiang Huang)
Rhizoma seu Radix Notopterygii (Qiang Huo)

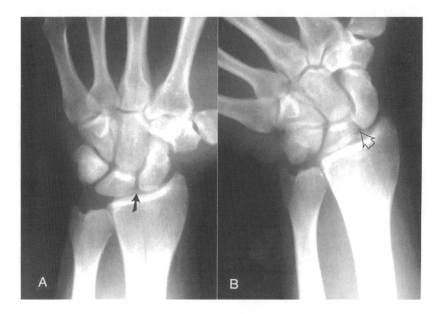

*Figure 10-47:* A and B: Anterior-posterior view of wrist with a wide naviculolunate space (closed arrow). The open arrow points to the naviculolunate space that becomes wider with ulnar deviation. In the normal person, this space remains the same or gets narrower with ulnar deviation.

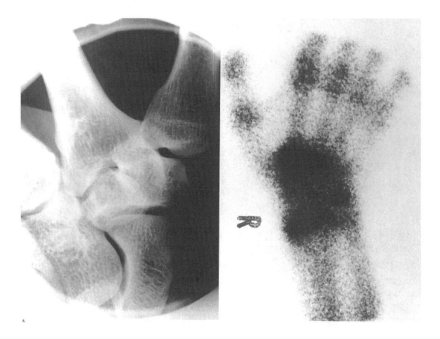

*Figure 10-48:* Radiograph (A) and a Radionuclide scan (B) of a right wrist in a patient with post traumatic hand pain. The x-ray findings are minimal and the fracture of the trapezius is hard to identify. The bone scan of the wrist is quite positive and demonstrates the healing fracture.

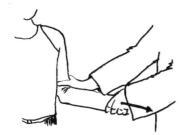

*Figure 10-49:* Long axis extension.

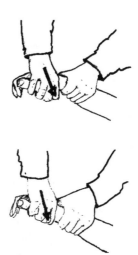

*Figure 10-50:* Anteroposterior glide.

**ACUPUNCTURE.** Acupuncture at the Small Intestines and Triple Warmer channels is helpful. The joint can be needled with SI-6, which lies over the short joint line just radially to the head of the ulna. UB-11 and Beside Three Miles are used often.

## Wrist Joints

The wrist joints are a common source of pain often due to joint laxity.

Joint play movements at the midcarpal joint are (Mennell *ibid*):

**1.** Long axis extension.

Assessed by grasping and pulling the patient's wrist, with his elbow flexed (Figure 10-49).

**2.** Anteroposterior glide.

Assessed by grasping the patient's wrist with one hand at the lower end of the radius, and other hand at the distal carpal row. The patient's wrist is slightly flexed. The proximal carpal row is stabilized and the practitioner's distal hand thrusts forward in an angle of about 45° (Figure 10-50).

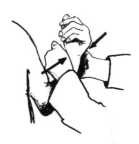

*Figure 10-51:* Backward tilt.

**3.** Backward tilt of the distal carpal bones on the proximal carpal bones.

Assessed by squeezing the patient's midcarpal joints between the practitioner's thenar eminences. The dorsal thenar eminence is over the distal carpal row, and the volar thenar eminence over the proximal carpal row. This movement tilts the patient's distal carpal row backward upon the proximal row. The patient's finger movements are monitored and should extend and spread (Figure 10-51).

## Capsular Pattern

The capsular pattern of the wrist is an equal limitation of both flexion and extension (Cyriax *ibid*). Post-traumatic pain with a capsular pattern that lasts more then a couple of days is most often due to fracture of the carpal bones or of the epiphysis of the radius. The X-ray can be negative in the first two weeks as the fracture can be of a hairline type, and wrist X-rays can be difficult to interpret. Tenderness can often be elicited in the "anatomical snuffbox," which implicates the scaphoid (Ombregt, Bisschop, ter Veer and Van de Velde 1995).

Rheumatoid arthritis often affects the wrists bilaterally and results in limitation of movement in the capsular pattern.

Arthrosis can result from a variety of causes, repetitive use probably the most common. Often ligamentous laxity is a contributing factor. A capsular pattern usually is seen.

## Traumatic & Sports Injuries

Falls onto the outstretched arm more commonly affect the palmar aspect of the hand. However, anything can be injured in a fall and a capsular pattern often is seen. More commonly, falls cause (Ombregt et al. 1995):

- Fracture of the distal radius, with or without disruption of the distal radioulnar joint.
- Fracture of the ulnar styloid.
- Fractures of the waist of the scaphoid.
- Tears of the lunotriquetral or scapholunate ligaments.
- Tears of the triangular fibrocartilage.
- Tears of the volar radiocarpal ligament.
- Transverse fracture of the capitate.

Sport injuries are a common cause of wrist pain (Brown 1995):

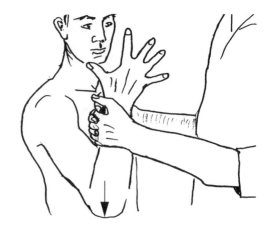

*Figure 10-52:* Nonspecific mobilization of carpal bones.

- Throwing often results in lesions of the tendons and ligaments which support the pisiform.
- Swinging may cause tendinitis of the extensor carpi ulnaris, De Quevain's syndrome (tenosynovitis of the thumb tendon), or occasional sprain of the pisitriquetral ligament.
- Gymnastics (weight-bearing), weight lifting, push-ups, and shot-puts can stress the palmar structures: the flexor carpi ulnaris, pisiform, triquetrum complex and ulnocarpal ligament.
- Hyperextension dorsiflexes the lunate and forces it in a palmar direction. Rupture of the radiocarpal ligaments and intrinsics of the proximal carpal row is possible.
- Twisting of the arm and wrists, seen commonly in martial artists, can result in a tear of the ligaments between the triquetrum and hamate and can cause a midcarpal instability. Disruption of the saddle joint between the hamate and triquetrum causes the hamate to drop palmwards, in supination, and causes the proximal pole of the hamate to cross the articular surface of the lunate, in extreme ulnar deviation.

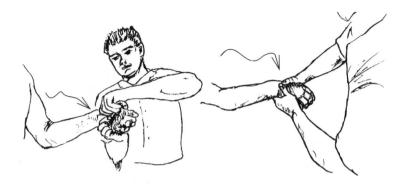

*Figure 10-53:*   Manipulation of carpal joint dysfunctions.

## Limitation in NonCapsular Pattern

Dysfunction and subluxation of the inter-carpal joints occur often. These can result in limitation of either extension or flexion. Occasionally both extension and flexion are limited, but not equally. Dysfunction at the radiocarpal joint often results in limited or painful flexion.

## Painful or Limited Extension

The most common cause of limited or painful extension is a capitate (or other carpal) dysfunction or dorsal subluxation. The capitate, or other involved carpal bone, can be excessively prominent when the wrist is flexed. Ulnar deviation may be limited. The ligaments overlying the joint usually are tender.

Other causes of limited extension can be a ganglion, ligament sprains, ununited fractures, aseptic necrosis of the lunate and isolated arthrosis (Brown 1995).

Periostitis can result in painful passive extension movement, but with full range. This disorder, also called wrist impingement syndrome, usually is caused by repetitive extension movements during weight-bearing, and is seen frequently in

gymnasts. The lesion can be localized by palpation of the inferior border of the radius (Ombregt, Bisschop, ter Veer and Van de Velde 1995).

### Treatment

Carpal dysfunctions and subluxations can be treated with manual techniques. Because subluxations usually are accompanied by ligamentous laxity, the ligaments are treated with periosteal acupuncture and/or laser stimulation. For more severe cases, the ligament should be injected. The same maneuvers used to assess joint play can be used therapeutically, except a thrust is added.

To treat the carpal bones, and the flexor retinaculum and tendons, with the patient seated, the practitioner:

1. Holds the patient's wrist up (elbow pointing to the floor), the practitioner's thumb is overlying the displaced carpal bone.

2. Asks the patient to pull his or her elbow toward the floor.

3. Asks the patient to open his hand wide. A click usually is audible (Figure 10-52).

Alternatively, the practitioner can manipulate the patient's wrist while holding the practitioner's thumb over the displaced carpal bone. A quick, whiplike movement of the patient's arm is induced while pressure is maintained over the displaced bone (Figure 10-53).

**HERBAL MEDICATION.** A guiding topical formula for chronic wrist disorders and ligamentous sprain is:

Radix Angelica Sinensis (Dang Gui)

Rhizoma Ligusticum (Chuan Xiong)

Eupolyphaga seu Opisthoplatiae (Tu Bie Chong)

Cortex Erythrinae Variegatae (Hai Tong Pi)

Rhizoma Dioscoreae (Bi Xie)

Radix Astragali (Huang Qi)

Lignum Pini Nodi (Song Jie)

*Aseptic Necrosis of the Lunate*

Aseptic necrosis of the lunate (Kienbock's disease) is seen usually in a patient in his twenties. The patient complains of wrist pain which may be moderate or severe. Weakness of the hand may be present. Symptoms arise spontaneously or as a result of injury.

Pain is elicited during passive movements with extension usually being the most limited and painful. Early X-rays can be negative but later sclerosis and deformity of the lunate can be seen. MRI is useful for early diagnosis. No effective conservative approach is available (Brown 1995).

**Painful or Limited Flexion**

Painful or limited flexion can result from ventral carpal dysfunctions or subluxations. The lunate is the most commonly affected. Radial deviation may be limited. Symptoms of paresthesia can result and be mistaken for carpal tunnel syndrome (Ombregt, Bisschop, ter Veer and Van de Velde 1995). Three joint play movements can be assessed at the radiocarpal joint (Mennell *ibid*):

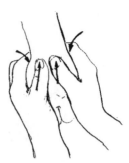

*Figure 10-54:* Backward tilt of the scaphoid and lunate upon the radius.

**1.** Long axis extension.

Assessed in exactly the same manner as long axis extension at the midcarpal joint.

**2.** Backward tilt of the scaphoid and lunate bones on the lower end of the radius.

Assessed by having the practitioner place one thumb over the dorsal aspect of the scaphoid, the thumb being in the long axis of the patient's radius; and his other thumb over the lunate, again being in the long axis of the patient's radius. The practitioner then crooks his index finger around the wrist so that they lie at right angles to his thumbs, but on the ventral surface; their tips are placed over the scaphoid and the lunate in such a manner that the practitioner is grasping the scaphoid with one hand and the lunate with the other hand. The scaphoid and the lunate are gently flexed forward on the lower end of the radius as the forearm is being gently raised by slightly increasing flexion at the elbow. The forearm is then whipped downward toward the floor by sudden ulnar deviation of the practitioner's wrists, the movement being stopped in such a way that, momentarily, the scaphoid and lunate are tilted backward on the lower end of the radius, which tilts the radiocarpal joint open at its ventral aspect (Figure 10-54).

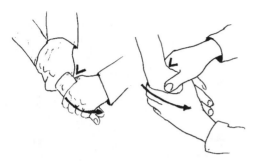

*Figure 10-55:* Side tilt of scaphoid on the radius.

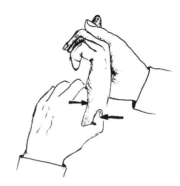

*Figure 10-56:* Anteroposterior glide of the ulna on the triquetrum.

**3.** Side tilt of the scaphoid on the radius.

Assessed by having the practitioner grasp the lower end of the radius and ulna between the thumb and index finger of one of his hands and the proximal carpal row between the thumb and index finger of his other hand, holding the patient's arm in the neutral position and flexed at the elbow. Using the thumb as a pivot, the practitioner stabilizes the lower end of the forearm and by ulnar deviation he tilts the scaphoid away from the lower end of the radius (Figure 10-55).

*Treatment*

Manipulative reduction can be achieved with similar technique to dorsal carpal dysfunctions, except the practitioner's thumb overlies the lunate ventrally. The movements used to assess joint play can be used therapeutically except that now a thrust is used at the restricted end range.

**Painful or Restricted Supination or Pronation**

Painful or restricted supination or pronation can be due to the inferior radioulnar joint or the unlomeniscocarpal (unlomeniscotriquetral) joint. Joint play movement at this joint are (Mennell *ibid*):

**1.** Long axis extension.

Assessed in the same manner as that at the midcarpal joint and the radiocarpal joint.

**2.** Anteroposterior glide.

Assessed by having the practitioner hold the radial half of the patient's hand in one of his hands. He then places the thumb of his other hand over the posterior aspect of the neck of the lower end of the ulna. He next crooks his index finger and places its proximal interphalngeal joint over the patient's pisiform. The practitioner then pinches his thumb and index finger together, thereby carrying the lower end of the patient's ulna forward on the triquetrum as the triquetrum moves backward on the lower end of the ulna and the meniscus which lies between them (Figure 10-56).

**3.** Side tilt of the triquetrum on the ulna.

Assessed by having the practitioner grasp the lower ends of the radius and ulna between the thumb and index finger of one hand and the proximal carpal row between the thumb and index finger of his other hand, holding the patient's arm in the neutral position and flexed at the elbow. Using the practitioner's index finger as a pivot, he stabilizes the lower end of the forearm and tilts the patient's hand into radial deviation (Figure 10-57).

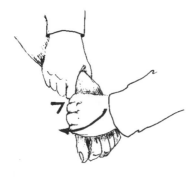

*Figure 10-57:* Side tilt of the triquetrum away from the ulna and the meniscus.

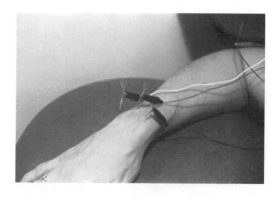

*Figure 10-59:* Periosteal acupuncture to stabilize the dorsal wrist ligaments.

## Disorders of Contractile Structures

Disorders of contractile structures can result in pain over the wrist and hand. Often the lesion is of the tendon or tenosynovial structures. Resisted movements are painful in tendinitis, and stretching the tendon is painful in tenosynovitis.

### Treatment

Treatment consists of cross- fiber massage, acupuncture, topical herbal medication (Figure 10-58) and occasionally injection. De Quevain tenosynovitis may requires injection therapy.

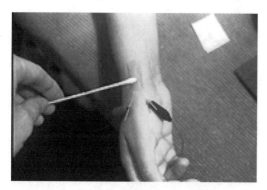

*Figure 10-58:* Topical herbal application with local acupuncture stimulation for De Quevain tenosynovitis.

## Carpal Tunnel Syndrome

Compression of the median nerve in a fibro-osseous canal on the palmar surface of the wrist is known as carpal tunnel syndrome. The median nerve lies superficial to many of the flexor tendons and is the structure most sensitive to pressure within the carpal tunnel. Before the nerve enters the canal, a palmar branch comes off the nerve to supply the skin of the palm and thenar eminence. Within the canal the median nerve may branch into a radial and palmar components. Any inflammation within the canal can result in pressure on the nerve. Some patients have an ulnarly innervated hand (an anomaly) which can result in a nontypical pain distribution (Brown 1995).

Carpal tunnel syndrome must be differentiated from shortening of the pronator teres muscle (pronator syndrome) which also can press on the median nerve and lead to similar symptoms (Brown 1995).

Carpal tunnel syndrome often is secondary to carpal joint dysfunction and ligament laxity. This results in excessive movement, or tension, within the carpal tunnel and pressure to the median nerve.

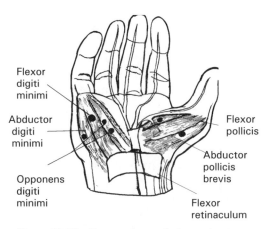

Figure 10-60: Commonly needled muscles to release the flexor retinaculum and carpal tunnel syndrome.

*Treatment*

A therapeutic program can use laser stimulation to the source points of the Yin arm channels (Lu-9, P-7 and H-7) and Well points of all the arm channels (Lu-11, LI-1, P-9, TW-1, H-9 and SI-1) plus P-8 and H-8. Laser therapy, together with microamp TENS, has been reported to effectively treat carpal tunnel syndrome (Naeser 1996).

**HERBAL TREATMENT.** External herbal application can be helpful.

**ACUPUNCTURE TECHNIQUES.** Contralateral Beside Three Miles, ipsilateral Lu-10 and SI-3 (or triggers in the flexor pollicis brevis, abductor pollicis brevis, abductor digiti minimi brevis, and opponens digiti minimi all of which may affect the flexor retinaculum) can be helpful. Superficial stimulation at P-4, 6, 7, TW-4, 5, 7 and Lu-6 is used often. Contralateral Liv-4 and 3 can be tried as the sole treatment. The dorsal wrist ligaments are strengthened by periosteal needling (Figure 10-59).

**MAGNET THERAPY.** Local magnet therapy, north pole at P-6 and south pole at the Well points may be tried.

**INJECTION THERAPY.** In more severe cases

Sarapin or steroid injections can be helpful. To prevent recurrence, any wrist joint dysfunction should be addressed and the ligaments stabilized. Prolotherapy to stabilize the wrist may be needed.

# The Hand

Disorders of the hand often involve the joints and in OM are mainly due to obstructive syndromes.

## Capsular Pattern

The capsular pattern, at any of the fingers, is an equal loss of movement at the beginning and end of the normal range, in either direction. Some movement remains at the midrange. Rotations are painful at the extreme range.

## Arthritis of Metacarpophalangeal & Interphalangeal Joints

Osteo, rheumatoid, traumatic and rarely gouty arthritis can occur at these joints. Rheumatoid arthritis is the most deforming and most incapacitating disorder of the hand. Traumatic arthritis occurs with the typical history of direct contusion and indirect sprains. Osteoarthritis can be secondary to injury, but more often the condition has a spontaneous onset, and affects several joints. It is seen in patients between 40-60 years of age and has a strong familial predisposition. Arthrosis tends to begin at the distal interphalangeal joints while inflammatory arthritis at the proximal joints (Brown *ibid*).

*Treatment*

Treatment is systemic with herbs that address the individual's constitution. Contralateral acupoints can be helpful. The cervical spine should be assessed and treated if necessary.

A guiding formula for pain aggravated by cold weather or with cold extremities is:

Radix Astragalus (Huang Qi)

Ramulus Cinnamomi (Gui Zhi)

Peony Rubra (Qi Shao)

Peony Alba (Bai Shao)

Dry Ginger (Gan Jiang)

Lumbricus (Di Long)

Rhizoma Tumeric (Jiang Huang)

Millettiae (Ji Xue Teng)

Flos Carthami (Hong Hua)

Radix Aconiti Praeparata (Fu Zi)

Gan Cao (Radix Glycyrrhizae)

A guiding formula for inflammatory arthritis is:

Flos Loncerae (Jin Yin Hua)

Wild Chrysanthemum (Ye Ju Hua)

Herba Taraxaci (Pu Gong Ying)

Herba Viola (Zi Hua Di Ding)

Angelica Chinesis (Dang Gui)

Radix Salviae (Dun Shen)

Resina Olibani (Ru Xiang)

Resina Myrrhae (Mo Yao)

Radix Scutellariae (Huang Qin)

Fresh Radix Rehmanniae (Sheng Di)

Gan Cao (Radix Glycyrrhizae)

Tripterygium Wilfordii (Lei Gong Teng)

and vitamins B6 and B12 (to prevent possible side effects of Tripterygium)

## The Thumb

This joint is unusually prone to degenerative changes with recurrent episodes of inflammation, which is a disproportionately painful condition (Dorman and Ravin 1991). Pain may be felt over the radial aspect of the wrist.

### Capsular Lesions

A positive capsular test at the carpometacarpal joint of the thumb is painful or limited backward movement during extension. It is positive commonly with rheumatoid, traumatic, and osteoarthritis.

### Treatment

Treatment is similar to other carpometacarpal joints. Cross fiber massage integrated with traction, at the same time, can be helpful.

## Dupuytren's Contracture

Dupuytren's contacture is a idiopathic, progressive, painless thickening and tightening of subcutaneous tissue of the palm, causing the fourth and fifth fingers to bend into the palm and resist extension. Tendons and nerves are not involved. Although the condition begins in one hand, both will become symmetrically affected. It is found most often in middle-aged males (Brown *ibid*).

### Treatment

Although surgical approaches are usually advocated it has been found that stretching the contracted or contracting fingers is possible. The procedure involves injection of local anesthetic and steroid suspension followed by strong stretching (Dorman and Ravin 1991).

## Trigger Finger

Trigger finger is seen most often in a man that has difficulty with extension of one or more of his fingers. Usually a swelling of the digital flexor tendons forms distally to the metacarpophalangeal joint, with narrowing of the tendon sheath. A snapping sound and feeling accompanies disengagement (Brown 1995).

### Treatment

Trigger finger responds often to massage with active movements in a longitudinal direction.

## Mallet Finger (Tendon Rupture)

Mallet finger is an injury caused by axial compression on an outstretched finger. The extensor tendon is detached from its insertion on the distal phalanx. The distal portion of the tendon may avulse with a small fragment of bone and the injury occasionally is associated with ventral subluxation of the distal phalanx, usually when more than one-third of the joint surface is detached with the fragment (Dorman and Ravin 1991). On examination, the distal joint is held in flexion and the patient is not able to extend it actively. Passive testing is normal.

*Treatment*

Conservative treatment consists of splinting the finger in extension as soon as the injury occurs. The proximal interphalangeal joint is held in full flexion and the distal interphalangeal joint in full extension, to completely relax the extensor tendon until union takes place (Brown 1995).

# Chapter 11: *The Lower Extremities*

Disorders of the lower extremities can be due to various causes and often involve deficiency of the OM Kidneys. Both external and miscellaneous pathogenic factors can be involved. Biomechanical foot disorders often are at the root of lower extremity pain.

## *The Hip & Buttock*

Pain in the hip and buttock areas is seen often. Pain can be due to local disorders, or it can be referred from the spine.

## Anatomy & Biomechanics

The hip joint is a deep ball-and-socket joint formed by the femoral head and acetabulum. A fibrocartilaginous ring, the labrum acetabulum, is attached to the ace-tabulum and deepens the joint surface further (Figure 11-1). The central part of the joint is nonarticular and houses the ligamentum teres, a flat fibrous band embedded in adipose tissue and lined by a synovial membrane. The joint is supported by three ligaments anteriorly which together are arranged in a Z shape. In the erect position all the ligaments are tightened because of the obliquity of their fibers. Posteriorly, the capsule is strengthened by the ischiofemoral ligaments. The femoral head and neck receive vascular supply by a branch of the obturator artery (which runs through the center of the ligamentum teres) and the capsular vessels that arise from the medial and lateral circumflex arteries (Kapandji *ibid*). Movements at the hip are flexion, extension, abduction, adduction, and internal and external rotations. The muscles which affect the hip are summarized in Table 11-2 on page 548 through Table 11-6 on page 549, (Figure 11-15). Joint play movement at the hip joint is long axis extension (Mennell *ibid*).

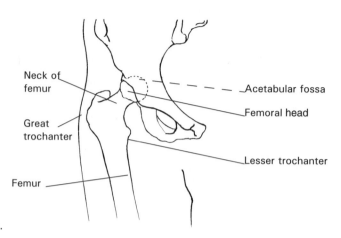

*Figure 11-1:* Hip joint.

*Table 11-1.* **FLEXOR MUSCLES OF HIP**

| MUSCLE | INNERVATION |
| --- | --- |
| Iliopsoas | L2-L3 |
| Sartorius | L2-L3 |
| Pectineus | L2-L3 |
| Adductor longus | L2-L3 |
| Adductor brevis | L2-L3 |
| Rectus femoris | L3 |
| Adductor magnus | L3-L4 |
| Gluteus medius | L5 |
| Gluteus minimus | L5 |
| Tensor fascia lata | L5 |

*Table 11-2.* **EXTENSOR MUSCLES OF HIP**

| MUSCLE | INNERVATION |
| --- | --- |
| Gluteus maximus | S1 |
| Semimembranosus | S1-S2 |
| Semitendinosus | S1-S2 |
| Biceps femoris | S1-S2 |

*Table 11-3.* **ABDUCTOR MUSCLES OF HIP**

| MUSCLE | INNERVATION |
|---|---|
| Gluteus medius | L5 |
| Gluteus minimus | L5 |
| Tensor fascia lata | L5 |
| Gluteus maximus | S1 |

*Table 11-4.* **ADDUCTOR MUSCLES OF HIP**

| MUSCLE | INNERVATION |
|---|---|
| Adductor longus | L2-L3 |
| Pectineus | L2-L3 |
| Gracilis | L2-L4 |
| Adductor magnus | L3-L4 |
| External obturator | L3-L4 |
| Quadratus femoris | L4-S1 |
| Semimembranosus | S1-S2 |
| Semitendinosus | S1-S2 |
| Biceps femoris | S1-S2 |

*Table 11-5.* **EXTERNAL ROTATOR MUSCLES OF HIP**

| MUSCLE | INNERVATION |
|---|---|
| Iliopsoas | L2-L3 |
| Sartorius | L2-L3 |
| External obturator | L3-L4 |
| Adductor magnus | L3-4 |
| Quadratus femoris | L4-S1 |
| Gluteus medius | L4-S1 |
| Gluteus maximus | L5-S2 |
| Biceps femoris | S1-S2 |
| Piriformis | S1-S2 |

*Table 11-6.* **INTERNAL ROTATOR MUSCLES OF HIP**

| MUSCLE | INNERVATION |
|---|---|
| Tensor fasciae lata | L5 |
| Gluteus medius | L5 |
| Gluteus minimus | L5 |
| Semimembranosus | S1-S2 |
| Semitendinosus | S1-S2 |

## Bursae

The hip area has several important bursae:

- The trochanteric bursa, the most superficial, is lateral to the gluteal bursae between the greater trochanter and iliotibial tract.

- The gluteal bursae are located deep beneath the gluteus medius and maximus.

- The psoas bursa lies deep to the iliopsoas muscle just in front of the hip joint.

- The ischial bursa lies distally to the ischial tuberosity and is covered by the edge of the gluteus maximus.

# Imaging

The radiographic evaluation of the hip can be divided into two components. The first is the evaluation of the bony architecture as it applies to the knowledge of this weightbearing structure—how the bones of the acetabulum and the femur interact, which is important in understanding how and why degenerative joint disease begins and progresses. The second is the evaluation of degenerative joint disease of the hip. The basic evaluation of hip joint disease is relatively simple, and visible changes closely follow the clinical presentation. The following paragraphs will briefly explore the basics of these changes.

As with any joint disease there are many possible changes for the images to reflect, but for the nonradiologist health care provider there are only a few changes that they will see frequently. These changes are for the most part moderate to severe degenerative joint disease in the adult. In order to place these radiographic changes in perspective an understanding of the basics of the bony anatomy of the hip would be helpful.

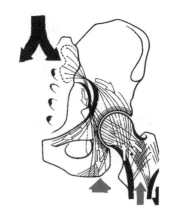

*Figure 11-2:* Trabecular arches (after Kapandji).

## The Hip Bone

The pelvic bone forms the connection between the spine and the legs. The need to accommodate both movement and spinal stability places unique demands on this structure. At first, the hip seems like just a simple ball-and-socket joint, but there are a few anatomic relationships of the bony structures that when evaluated can alter clinical decision making. Forces of walking upright lead to the evolution of bony architecture of the hip and femur that are both light and strong. These bones contain several internal "arches" created by the trabeculae, and the similarity of these arches to the gothic arch of buildings are seen in at least three sites. There is a trabecular arch between the sacroiliac joint and the acetabulum, an arch between the sacroiliac joint and the ischium, and the classic arch in the head of the femur (Figure 11-2).

The trabeculae support the stresses of walking particularly about the weightbearing zone on the apex of the hip joint itself. This framework of lamellae forms a triangle, the base of which corresponds to the weightbearing surface and looks like an eyebrow on radiographs. The sides of the triangle are formed by condensed arch-like bone lamellae. In the normal hip, the apex

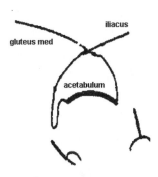

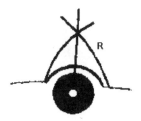

Figure 11-4: Anatomic relationship of femoral head and the acetabulum.

Figure 11-3: Muscle forces affecting the lateral group of lamella (after Bomelli).

of this triangle is directly above the mid portion of the semilunar weightbearing zone and the center of rotation of the femoral head. This triangular structure is one of the "Gothic arches" of the pelvis. The lamella that forms the sides of the gothic arch does not end at its apex but extends cephalad. The medial lamella coming from the lamina quadrilateral is directed towards the anterior inferior and superior iliac spines. The lateral lamella extends from the lateral acetabular ridge to the sacroiliac joint. Together they form an hourglass configuration. This lamella represents the reaction of the bone to muscular activity. The direction of the lateral group of lamella corresponds to the resultant force of the abductors, the glutei and piriformis muscles arising from the lateral side of the pelvis, and inserting distally into the greater trochanter. The medial groups of lamella reflect the direction of the iliacus arising from the medial surface of the pelvis and insert distally into the lesser trochanter. Bombilli graphically illustrates how these forces work (Figure 11-3).

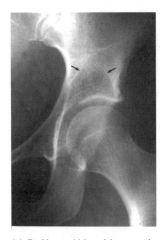

Figure 11-5: Normal hip with normal gothic arch (arrows).

thickness and smooth configuration of the acetabular roof is evidence of the equal distribution of the stresses of walking. The anatomic relationships of the femoral head to the acetabulum are summarized in Figure 11-4. Figure 11-5 is a hip X-ray that shows how the "gothic arch" is directly above the center of rotation of the femoral head, and in the center of the acetabulum.

*Femoral Head*

The head, neck and shaft of the femur are known as an "overhang" in engineering terms. To prevent the shearing of the base of the femoral head, the femur has a special structural pattern that can be easily seen on a radiograph. Figure 11-6 is

*Acetabulum*

At the top of the acetabulum there is a curved area of dense bone. It develops as a response to the stress imposed on the femoral head by the counter thrust of the ground. In the normal hip, the uniform

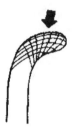

*Figure 11-6:* Femoral overhang with trabecular pattern (after Kapndji).

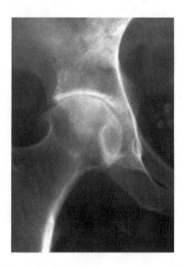

*Figure 11-7:* Early degenerative arthritis.

adapted from Kapandji and illustrates the general outline of the trabecular pattern.

In general, with plain films the radiologist notes:

**1.** The joint spaces and pelvic line.

**2.** The neck-shaft angle.

**3.** The shape of femoral head.

**4.** Are the femoral head and acetabulum equal and normal on both sides.

**5.** Is there any evidence of fracture or dislocation.

**6.** Is there any pelvic distortion.

**7.** Is there any bone disease.

## Hip Joint Disease

### Congenial Abnormalities

Congenital dislocation of the hips, and other congenital boney problems of the infant usually are found on early physical examinations and followed up by X-rays for confirmation. If this problem is missed in the first year and the infant begins to walk on the abnormal hip, serious long term hip disease is assured. This problem should not be initially diagnosed by X-ray but rather by a good physical exam and infant gait observation.

### Slipped Capital Femoral Epiphysis

This is a slip of the capital femoral epiphysis usually in a downwards and backwards direction. In a teenager with hip pain and limping and some varus positioning of the leg and outward rotation of the femur obtaining an X-ray of the hip is very important. This also is mostly a clinical diagnosis with radiographic conformation.

### Adult Degenerative Joint Disease

In the abnormal hip the direction of the weightbearing surface is not horizontal, it is inclined either laterally or medially. This abnormal inclination of the weightbearing surface affects the orientation of the gothic arch, and therefore the resultant forces of the abductors and iliopsoas. The loss of the normal anatomic relationships makes the hip joint unstable and the development of degenerative joint disease will progress with varying degrees of speed. The speed and degree of degenerative joint disease often is compounded by the degree of ligamentous laxity of the hip capsule. Referring to Figure 11-5 will remind the reader about the normal anatomic relationships and when evaluating any pelvis or hip films, if this normal relationship is not present and there are developing osteophytes from the acetabular rim or the edges of the femur, then the diagnosis of degenerative joint disease can be made on the films alone.

The degenerative joint disease initially presents as a very subtle joint space narrowing with hard to identify osteophytes (Figure 11-7), and progresses to gross space narrowing with massive osteophytes (Figure 11-9). Radiographs in chronic hip disease and pain can help confirm the diagnosis of the process and can be used to clinically grade the process. There is a word of caution however; physical examination of the hip with loss of range of motion and associated muscle weakness generally correlate well with the radiographs, but the pain complaints can be deceptive with minimal radiographic changes causing considerable pain; and also individuals with significant degenerative changes are able to function well with minimal pain.

### Avascular Necrosis

Avascular necrosis of the hip joint is fairly common. Late in the disease process the femoral head collapses and shows an irregular contour and osteonecrosis (Figure 11-16). If one suspects avascular necrosis a CT or MRI should be ordered.

## OM Disorders

Hip, buttock and leg pain is caused mainly by Painful Obstruction (Bi) disorders. Trauma or strain can injure the channels and collaterals and can result in stagnation of Qi and Blood. In the chronic stage malnourishment of soft tissues can lead to atrophy, numbness or pain.

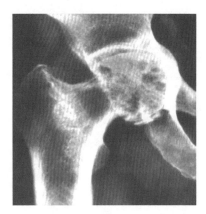

*Figure 11-8:* Rheumatoid arthritis of hip. Note the uniform loss of joint space

## Biomedical Disorders

Pain in the hip and buttock areas can result from any lesion in the L1, L2, L3 and S2 nerve roots, as these supply the hip and buttock, as well. Most hip and buttock pain results from lesions of the spine, sacroiliac joints (Ombregt, Bisschop, ter Veer and Van de Veldeand *ibid*) and ligaments.

The *capsular pattern* at the hip joint is gross limitation of internal rotation (Figure 11-10), abduction and flexion; less limitation of extension; and little or no limitation of adduction and external rotation (Cyriax *ibid*). Fabere Patrick's maneuver is

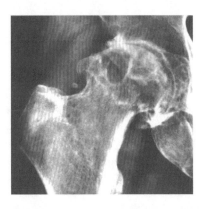

*Figure 11-9:* Degenerative joint disease of the hip. Note the lack of uniformity in the joint space loss.

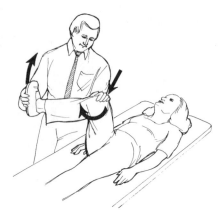

*Figure 11-10:* Assessment of internal rotation and end feel at the hip (Reproduced with permission Dorman and Ravin 1991).

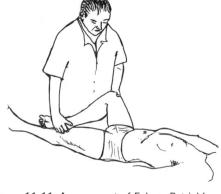

*Figure 11-11:* Assessment of Fabere Patrick's maneuver to test flexion, abduction and external rotation.

limited often and may result in pain (Figure 11-11).

## Capsular Pattern

Capsular limitation can result from arthritis (traumatic, osteo, rheumatoid, septic and crystalline), (Figure 11-8 and Figure 11-9) and arthrosis of the hip. A capsular pattern in a child or adolescent always suggests a serious disorder (Ombregt, Bisschop, ter Veer and Van de Veldeand 1995).

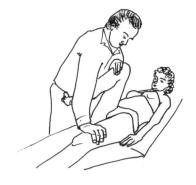

*Figure 11-12:* Stretching hip; flexion technique.

*Treatment*

Treatment can include stretch techniques, mobilization, acupuncture, injection therapy and herbal therapy.

**STRETCH TECHNIQUES**. Techniques that stretch the capsule are important in the early stages of arthrosis. The decision whether to use stretch techniques depends on the clinical findings. In patients with an early capsular pattern and a more or less elastic end feel stretch techniques usually are very helpful. Stretch techniques are not helpful in advanced arthrosis with gross limitation of movements, a hard end

feel and crepitus.

Stretch techniques should be started as early as possible. If delayed, further progression and degeneration is likely (Ombregt, Bisschop, ter Veer and Van de Velde 1995).

Treatment is given two to three times a week for 10-20 sessions. Three planes are stretched—flexion, extension, and internal rotation—for 5-10 minutes each (Figure 11-14 through Figure 11-12). Treatment often results in increased pain for 1-2 hours. If pain lasts for 1-2 days, the joint was stretched too strongly (Ombregt, Bisschop, ter Veer and Van de Velde 1995).

**ACUPUNCTURE**. Acupuncture is helpful in

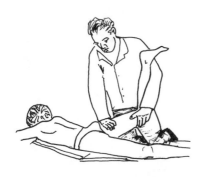

*Figure 11-13:* Stretching hip; extension technique.

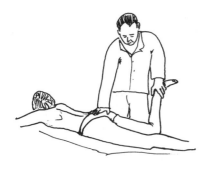

*Figure 11-14:* Stretching hip; internal rotation technique.

mild arthritis or arthrosis of the hip joint. Treatment applied to the Gall Bladder and Urinary Bladder channels, Sinews channels and local points is appropriate. UB-43 can be bled and cupped in most disorders of the hip and lower extremities. For groin and inner thigh pain, Heart Door (33.12) on the opposite side can be used. LI-4 1/2 and LI-3 can be used for treatment of pain in the ischial area.

**HERBAL THERAPY.** A guiding oral formula for arthrosis of the hip is:

    Loranthus (Sang Ji Sheng)

    Prepared Cortex Eucommiae (Chao Du Zhong)

    Angelica Pubescens (Du Hou)

    Peony Rubra (Chi Shao)

    Ligusticum (Chuan Xiong)

    Angelica Chinesis (Dang Gui)

    Ramulus Cinnamomi (Gui Zhi)

    Zaocys Khumnades,—Black-striped Snake (Wu Shao She)

    Semen Coix, frash (Sheng Yi Ren)

    Radix Aconiti Praeparata (Fu Zi)

    Achyranthes bidentata Blume (Huai Niu Xi)

    Radix Ledebouriella (Fang Feng)

    Poria Cocos (Fu Ling)

For arthritis (active inflammation),

**Takeout:**

    Radix Aconiti (Fu Zi)

    Ramulus Cinnamomi (Gui Zhi)

**Add:**

    Cortex Phellodendri (Huang Bai)

    Rhizoma Atractylodis (Cang Zu)

    Tripterygium Wilfordii (Lei Gong Teng)

    and vitamins B6 and B12 (to prevent possible side effects of Tripterygium).

**INJECTION THERAPY.** Injection therapy can be helpful in more severe cases. Prolotherapy can be helpful in chronic mild to moderate osteoarthritis (Dorman personal communication).

## Noncapsular Pattern

A limitation in a noncapsular pattern is associated with both articular and nonarticular disorders. A loose body in the joint, aseptic necrosis of the femoral head (Figure 11-16), bursitis and muscular lesions can give rise to limitations in a noncapsular pattern.

## Bursitis

Bursitis can result in noncapsular limitation. Several bursae around the hip joint can be affected clinically:

- Gluteal bursae (involved most frequently).
  Pain is felt at the gluteal or trochanteric area, spreading to outer or posterior thigh. The pain is not related to sitting

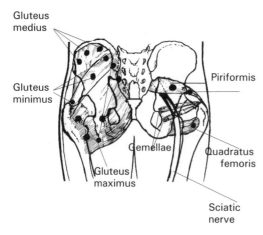

*Figure 11-15:* Common trigger sites in the buttock area.

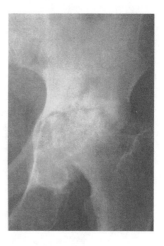

*Figure 11-16:* Complications from avascular necrosis. Note the collapse of the femoral head with an irregular contour and osteonecrosis.

but increases with walking and stair-climbing.

Typically, painful passive internal rotation and passive abduction are seen. Resisted external rotation or resisted abduction may be painful, as well.

• Trochanteric bursa.

Pain felt at trochanteric area, spreading to lateral aspect of knee especially while running or stair-climbing.

External rotation with hip and knee flexed is very painful and sometimes limited.

• Psoas bursa

Pain is felt in the groin area.

Passive adduction in flexion is most painful. External rotation and flexion are painful at end range.

• Ischial bursae.

Pain is felt at the ischial area as soon as the patient is seated (Ombregt, Bisschop, ter Veer and Van de Velde 1995).

*Treatment*

Bursitis can respond to treatment directed at the muscles that surround the hip (Gunn *ibid*) and correction of sacroiliac and upper lumbar joint dysfunctions.

Occasionally, steroid or Sarapin infiltration by ionophoresis or injection is needed.

**HERBAL THERAPY.** A guiding oral and topical formula for bursitis of the hip is:

> Radix Stephaniae (Fang Ji)
> Semen Coix (Yi Yi Ren)
> Semen Plantaginis (Che Qian Zi)
> Herba Plantaginis (Che Qian Cao)
> Aconitum Carmichaeli (Chuan Wu Tou)
> Aconitum Kusnezoffii (Cao Wu Tou)
> Lumricus (Di Long)
> Gan Cao (Radix Glycyrrhiza)
> Achyranthes Bidentata (Niu Xi)
> Fructus Lycii (Gou Qi Zi)
> Flos Carthami (Hong Hua)
> Tripterygium Wilfordii (Lei Gong Teng)
> Vitamins B6 and B12 (to prevent possible side effects of Tripterygium)

**Myofascial Pain**

Primary myofascial involvement in hip or buttock pain is uncommon. The hip muscles often are involved in disorders of the spine or pelvis. Table 11-7 on page 557 summarizes the muscles involved most commonly when pain occurs due to disorders of the hip and spine.

Table 11-7. CONTRACTILE LESIONS OF THE HIP

| MUSCLE | SIGNS | SIGNS MAY BE DUE TO |
|---|---|---|
| Iliopsoas | painful resisted hip flexion | rectus femoris, sartorius, avulsions, obturator hernia, cancers |
| Gluteus medius | painful resisted hip abduction, and external rotation or internal rotation | SI joint, fracture |
| Piriformis | painful resisted external rotation of hip | quadratus femoris, bursae, gluteus |
| Adductor longus | painful resisted adduction of hip | fracture, cancer, SI joint, hip joint |
| Rectus femoris | painful resisted flexion of hip | iliopsoas, sartorius avulsions, obturator hernia, cancers |
| Quadratus femoris | painful resisted external rotation of hip | piriformis, bursae, gluteus |
| Semimembranosus | painful adduction and internal rotation of hip | adductors longus, fracture, cancer, SI joint, hip joint |
| Semitendinosus | painful adduction and internal rotation of hip | adductors longus, fracture, cancer, SI joint, hip joint |
| Hamstrings | painful resisted flexion of knee, pain in the buttock area | sacrotuberous ligament, bursae |

## Sign Of The Buttock

*Sign of the buttock* is a clinical finding, described by Cyriax, which is seen in major disorders of the buttock. Sign of the buttock is characterized by more limitation and/or pain in hip flexion with the knee flexed than with the knee extended (SLR). Other hip movements are limited in a non-capsular pattern. This sign can be seen in fractures, neoplasms, abscesses and septic bursitis (Cyriax *ibid*).

## Aseptic Necrosis

Aseptic necrosis is characterized by a rapidly progressive destruction of the femoral head due to trauma or unknown cause. Aseptic necrosis is seen more often in patients who have a history of corticosteroid or alcohol use, which suggests a toxic origin (Figure 11-16), (Vreden et al. 1991; Matsuo et al. 1988).

Aseptic necrosis, usually seen in patients between the ages of 30 and 50, presents often with sudden groin pain or pain in L3 dermatomal distribution during weight-bearing. Occasional night pain occurs, as well. The patient often walks with a limp, even though the hip examination shows only a slight limitation in a non-capsular pattern. As the condition advances the limp intensifies (the patient often needs a cane) and a capsular pattern is seen.

Early necrosis does not show on X-ray; CT or MRI are recommended. Early diagnosis is imperative as the condition responds to core decompression (a surgical procedure) with rest. Once gross necrosis occurs, osteotomy or joint replacement is necessary (Ombregt, Bisschop, ter Veer and Van de Velde 1995).

## Loose Body in the Hip Joint

A loose body in the hip joint can be seen occasionally in patients who complain of sudden twinges of sharp pain in the groin or trochanteric area. A sudden twinge or giving-way is felt often while walking or

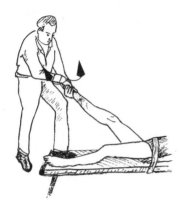

*Figure 11-17:* First manipulative technique for a loose body.

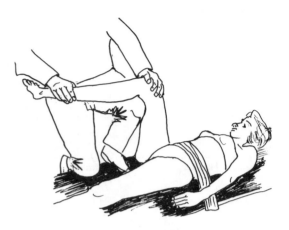

*Figure 11-18:* Second manipulation technique for a loose body in the hip.

descending stairs. The pain can last for a while or disappear quickly.

A capsular pattern can be present if the patient also suffers from hip arthrosis (common). Flexion and external rotation usually are painful (Cyriax *ibid*).

### Treatment

Manipulative reduction usually results in immediate and lasting relief of symptoms. Two techniques can be used.

**FIRST TECHNIQUE.** The patient lies supine and is strapped to the table or held by an assistant. The practitioner:

1. Stands on the end of the table and holds the patient's ankle with both hands.

2. Raises the leg to about 75° and leans backward.

3. (As soon as the muscles are relaxed) moves gradually off of the table while extending the leg he jerks the leg to full internal rotation and then returns it to neutral (Figure 11-17).

**SECOND TECHNIQUE.** The second technique is used if the previous manipulation did not work. The patient is supine and strapped down to the table or held by an assistant. The practitioner:

1. Places one of his feet on the table and puts the patient's leg over his thigh.

2. Holds the patient's knee with one hand and ankle with the other.

3. Raises his thigh and pushes down on the patient's lower leg in order to apply traction to the patient's hip.

4. (When muscles are relaxed) moves the patient's leg (to either side per patient comfort) in order to rotate the patient's femur (Figure 11-18).

# The Knee

Knee pain is common and often is associated with OM deficiency syndromes. Acupuncture has been shown to be helpful (Petrou 1988; Christensen 1992).

## Anatomy & Biomechanics

The knee is a compound diarthrodial hinge joint between the femur and tibia (Figure 11-19). The knee must remain both stable and mobile transmitting axial compression under the action of gravity and during gait. This is accomplished by a complex arrangement of ligaments, menisci, muscles and tendons. When standing, the line of force passes just in front of the horizontal axis of the hinge. Stability is maintained mechanically by a locked joint supported by the tightened posterior ligaments (Kapandji *ibid*).

Joint play movements at the *femorotibial* joint are (Mennell *ibid*):

**1.** Side tilt medially (valgus strain).

**2.** Side tilt laterally (varus strain).

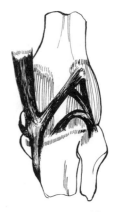

*Figure 11-20:* Posterior view of ligaments of the knee (With permission Dorman and Ravin 1991).

**3.** Anteroposterior glide.

**4.** Rotation.

These are assessed in the same manner as the usual orthopedic examination.

Joint play movements at the *patellofemoral* joint consist of (Mennell *ibid*):

**1.** Patellar excursion cephalad.

**2.** Patellar excursion caudad.

**3.** Patellar excursion medially.

**4.** Patellar excursion laterally.

Joint play movement at the superior tibiofibular joint is anteroposterior glide (Mennell *ibid*).

### Menisci

The menisci function as spacers between the femoral and tibial condyles. The superior and inferior surfaces are in contact with the femoral and tibial condyles, respectively, and the peripheral surfaces are adherent to the synovial membrane of the capsule. Movement between the tibial surface and the menisci is limited by the coronary ligaments that connect the outer meniscal borders with the tibial edge. The

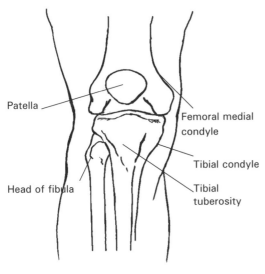

Patella

Femoral medial condyle

Tibial condyle

Head of fibula

Tibial tuberosity

*Figure 11-19:*   Knee joint.

medial collateral ligament is attached by its deep fibers to the outer border of the medial meniscus. A few fibers of the popliteus muscle are attached to the posterior border of the lateral meniscus, and some fibers of the semimembranosus muscle are attached to the posterior border of the medial meniscus (Ombregt, Bisschop, ter Veer and Van de Velde 1995).

## Ligaments

The knee joint is kept stable by an ingenious arrangement of ligaments. The col-

lateral ligaments provide lateral and medial stability. The cruciate ligaments provide anteroposterior stability and, with the collateral ligaments, prevent rotational movement during extension. The posterior capsule is strengthened by the oblique popliteal and the arcuate popliteal ligaments (Figure 11-20), (Kapendji *ibid*).

## Muscles

Figure 11-8 summarizes muscles that act on the knee.

*Table 11-8.* **Muscles Affecting the Knee**

| Muscles | Function | INNERVATION |
|---|---|---|
| Gracilis | Flexion<br>also Internal rotation | L2-L4 |
| Sartorius | Flexion<br>also Internal rotation | L2-L3 |
| Biceps femoris | Flexion<br>also External rotation | L5-S1 |
| Tensor fascia lata<br>(Iliotibial tract) | Flexion<br>also External rotation | L4-L5 |
| Gastrocnemius | Flexion<br>also Internal / External rotation | S1-S2 |
| Popliteus | Flexion<br>also Internal rotation | L4-S1 |
| Quadriceps | Extension | L2-L4 |
| Semitendinosus | Flexion | L5-S2 |
| Semimembranosus | Flexion<br>also Internal rotation | L5-S2 |

## Knee Movements

The main movement at the knee is flexion-extension with secondary movement of internal and external rotations. During gait, for the knee to unlock in the first few degrees of flexion, the tibia must first rotate internally about 20°. During terminal extension the tibia rotates externally to lock the joint. With knee flexion the femoral condyles roll backward and slide forward on the tibia. With extension movement the process is reversed (Kapandji *ibid*).

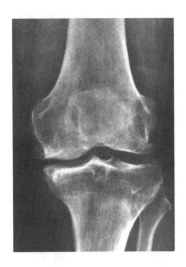

*Figure 11-22:* OA of the knee.

# Imaging

Imaging of the knee has changed significantly with the advent of CT scanning and MRI imaging. In fact, CT scanning has replaced the plain film for the evaluation of disease processes such as osteochondritis dissecans, patellar chondritis, and degenerative changes. The MRI scan easily can image the cruciate ligaments and the menisci. The MRI also can display tears in the menisci and, along with it, tendinitis and partial ligament tears sometimes can be shown.

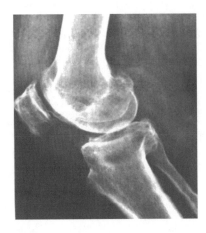

*Figure 11-21:* Lateral view of the knee joint with OA.

Patellar tendinitis can be recognized on occasion by the presence of an imaging inconsistency within the peripatellar ligaments, hence the MRI helps in the differential diagnosis of patellar pains.

The use of MRI to define and specifically identify ligamentous injuries of the knee is well known. This technique and the more careful observation and analysis of the status of the posterior cruciate ligament, however, seem to be important reasons for looking at these images more closely. It has been demonstrated many times in the past that most significant ligamentous injuries to the anterior cruciate ligament also cause some stretching and some tearing of the posterior cruciate ligament. The entire capsule also is usually distorted and stretched under these circumstances, and its evaluation by CT or MRI scanning is more difficult.

Evaluation of osteochondritis dissecans in its many forms in the knee is best diagnosed clinically, but with MRI, the inflammatory changes of bursitis around the knee can be recognized. (For a number of the uses of modern imaging techniques see Figure 11-23 through Figure 11-26).

In general, with plain film imaging the radiologist notes:

1. Any fractures (osteochondral).

2. Epiphyseal damage.

3. Lipping.

4. Loose bodies.

5. Alterations in bone texture.

6. Abnormal calcification.

7. Tumors.

8. Accessory ossification centers,

9. Varus or valgus deformity.

10. Patella alta or baja.

11. Asymmetry of femoral heads.

12. Degenerative disease (reduced joint space, bony cyst etc.).

13. The presence of the fabella, which is found in 20% of the population and often mistaken for a loose body.

14. Osteochondritis dissecans.

15. Osgood-Schlatter disease.

## OM Disorders

Knee functions are controlled by the foot Sinews channels. The Kidney Organ and channel are said to relate to the knee joint. Disorders of the knee joint can be caused by external pathogenic factors, by Independent factors (injuries), or by weakness of Nourishing Qi. External pathogens invade the knee when the Defensive Qi is weak. Accumulation of Cold and Damp can lead to stagnation of Qi and Blood. Dampness often transforms to Heat and results in swelling and warmth at the knee.

Alternatively, a weak constitution or chronic illness weakens the Kidneys and damages the Nourishing Qi and Blood. The knees become vulnerable to External pathogenic factors. When dysfunction lasts for extended periods, the Qi and Blood are further exhausted, and the Kidneys and Liver are depleted. This results in local joint deformity, muscle weakness and emaciation. The knee develops the "Crane's knee" syndrome.

## Biomedical Disorders

In disorders of the knee a good history is important, as it can often point to a diagnosis. The knee is innervated by L2 and L3 at the front and S1 and S2 at the back. Disorders at these levels can refer pain to the knee. Hip disorders and lesions of the third lumbar nerve root often refer pain to the front of the knee. Disorders of the sacroiliac joint and first and second sacral nerves often refer pain to the back of the knee. Referred pain usually is more vague; however, the patient may insist that the pain originates in the knee.

Three cardinal symptoms must be evaluated in patients with knee pain:

- Locking—sudden painful limitation of one movement while the other remains fairly unaffected—is seen often in disorders of the menisci.

- Painful twinges—sudden sharp and unexpected pain that usually disappears quickly so that normal gait is regained— is seen often with a loose body within the knee joint.

Giving way—sudden weakness, with or without pain—is seen often with instability or painful twinges (Ombregt, Bisschop, ter Veer and Van de Velde 1995).

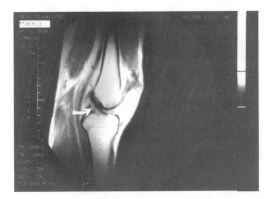

*Figure 11-23:* Arrow points to the normal cruciate ligament.

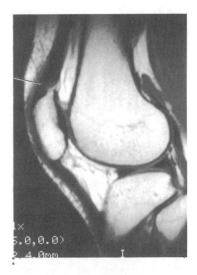

*Figure 11-24:* This is an MRI scan of a jumper knee. The quadriceps and the patellar tendon being low in water content are almost black in this type of scan. The presence of edema in the tendon causes the image to become "white" (closed arrow).

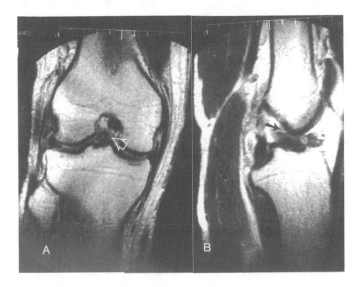

*Figure 11-25:* A and B: MRI scan of a knee with a torn anterior cruciate ligament. The lateral view (B) of the same knee shows the torn incomplete anterior cruciate ligament (closed arrow).

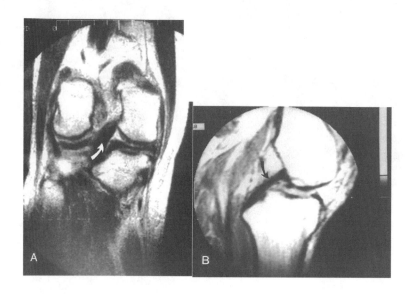

*Figure 11-26:* A and B MRI scan of a normal knee. The frontal view (A) shows the normal posterior cruciate ligament (closed arrow). The lateral view (B) also demonstrates the posterior cruciate ligament (open arrow). The ligament is the black arcing structure.

## Capsular Pattern

The capsular pattern at the knee joint is gross limitation of flexion, and slight limitation of extension at a ratio of about 10:1. The capsular pattern can be seen in patients with arthritis or arthrosis of the knee joint (Cyriax *ibid*).

Disorders such as rheumatoid arthritis, gonococcal arthritis, Reiter's syndrome and Crohn's disease can result in arthritis with a capsular pattern. Septic arthritis can result from a primary infection or from other infections such as cystitis, urethritis, dental abscesses and skin infection which also result in the capsular pattern of limitation (Ombregt, Bisschop, ter Veer and Van de Velde 1995). Septic knee infections must be treated aggressively with intravenous antibiotics.

Injuries to the medial collateral and coronary ligament also can result in a capsular pattern, as these communicate with the joint capsule (Ombregt, Bisschop, ter Veer and Van de Velde 1995).

*Treatment*

Treatment of capsular disorders is accomplished by combination of manual therapies, acupuncture and herbal medication. Occasionally, injection therapy is needed.

Since a capsular pattern can be found with a variety of disorders, manual techniques vary according to the cause. In chronic osteoarthritis, treatment is directed toward gaining maximal joint range of movement. This can be achieved by direct stretches in restricted directions, or by gentle joint movements in the direction of tissue preference (toward maximal joint play or tissue relaxation).

**ACUPUNCTURE.** Acupuncture at St-35, Xiyan (extra point), St-36, St-34, Liv-8, Sp-9 and GB-34 is helpful. P-6 can be needled on the opposite side and Great Space (11.01), Small Space (11.02), and Middle Space (11.05) can be needled on the left side. UB-43 can be bled, especially in the elderly. For medial knee pain Heart Door (33.12) can be used. The Kidney and Liver are strengthened in weak patients and in patients with joint deformity, the Divergent channels are used. For swelling, the Connecting channels of the Liver, Spleen/pancreas and Stomach are used.

**HERBAL THERAPY**. A guiding herbal formula for arthrosis (noninflammatory arthritis) of the knee joint is:

    Radix Aconitum Carmichaeli Debs (Zhi Chuan Wu)
    Radix Ephedrae (Ma Huang)
    Radix Achyranthes Bidentata (Niu Xi)
    Radix Peony Alba (Bai Shao)
    Rhizoma seu Radix Notopterygium (Qiang Huo)
    Radix Angelica Pubescens (Du Hou)
    Ramulus Cinnamomi (Gui Zhi)
    Angelica Sinensis (Dang Gui)
    Rhizoma Ligustricum (Chuan Xiong)
    Radix Stephaniae Tetrandrea (Fang Ji)
    Cortex Eucommiae (Du Zhong)
    Ramulas Loranthus (Sang Ji Sheng)
    Radix Glycyrrhizae (Gan Cao)

A guiding formula for arthritis with warmth and swelling is:

    Cortex Phellodendri (Huang Bai)
    Rhizoma Atractylodes (Cang Zhu)
    Tripterygium Wilfordii (Lei Gong Teng), (with vitamins B6 and B12)
    Angelica Sinensis (Dang Gui)
    Radix Stephaniae Tetrandrea (Fang Ji)
    Achyranthes Bidentata (Niu Xi)
    Rhizoma Dioscore (Bei Xie)
    Caulis Loncerae (Ren Dong Teng)
    Radix Scutellariae (Huang Qin)
    Cortex Mountan Radicis (Dan Pi)
    Peony Rubra (Chi Shao)
    Frash Rehmanniae (Sheng Di)
    Clematis (Wei Ling Xian)

A formula for "Crane's Knee" is:

    Prepared Rehmannia (Shu Di)
    Achyranthes Bidentata (Niu Xi)
    Angelica Sinensis (Dang Gui)
    Angelica Pubescent (Du Hou)
    Tripterygium Wilfordii (Lei Gong Teng), (with vitamins B6 and B12)
    Fructus Corni (Shan Zhu Yu)
    Fructus Lycii (Gou Qi Zi)

    Poria Cocos (Fu ling)
    Cortex Eucommiae (Du Zhong)
    Rhizoma Ligustricum (Chuan Xiong)
    Fructus Psoraleae (Bu Gu Zhi)
    Loranthus Parasiticus (Sang Ji Sheng)
    Radix Glycyrrhizae (Gan Cao)

## NonCapsular Pattern

Non-capsular disorders can involve the menisci, ligaments, muscles and bursae of the knee.

## Meniscal Lesions

Meniscal lesions result most often from trauma that involves torsion of the knee. Meniscal tears can occur in a vertical or longitudinal direction. Vertical tears tend to have a traumatic origin, while horizontal tears occur often in middle-aged patients and are degenerative in character (Smillie 1967). MRI and arthroscopic findings must be related to clinical findings because meniscal lesions are common and are not always clinically important. The symptoms often are secondary to ligament lesions (Ravin personal communication).

### Medial Meniscus

The medial meniscus is most vulnerable to traumatic injury as it is less mobile. The medial collateral and medial coronary ligaments can be affected, as well. Meniscal injuries can result in the so called locked knee, with limited extension.

### Anterior Horn Lesions

In injuries with displacement of part of the anterior meniscal horn (or impacted synovial membrane), the patient gait is affected, and the knee can be warm and slightly swollen. Flexion is normal or slightly limited by secondary arthritis. Extension is limited with a springy end feel. Rotation away from the painful side is painful (Ombregt, Bisschop, ter Veer and Van de Velde 1995).

### Posterior Horn Lesions

Posterior horn meniscal lesions may not result in a locked knee, and the patient may report giving way and sudden twinges. Some extension limitation can follow; however, self mobilization (shaking of leg) often results in immediate relief. Flexion often is painful and limited (Ombregt, Bisschop, ter Veer and Van de Velde 1995).

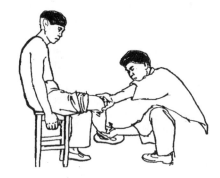

*Figure 11-27:* Meniscal manipulative reduction technique.

### Other Meniscal Disorders

The meniscus can be affected by metabolic conditions, the most important of which is chondrocalcinosis. A cyst can develop, most often in the lateral meniscus (Brown *ibid*).

### Treatment

Meniscal lesions can be treated with manipulation, cross-fiber massage and needling. Topical herbs are helpful. In more severe tears, injection or surgery may be necessary.

**MANIPULATIVE REDUCTION**. Manipulative reduction of a displaced meniscus (or impacted synovial membrane) often results in immediate restoration of extension movements. Reduction can be achieved with the patient seated or supine. If the knee is swollen or several movements are painful, acupuncture and application of a topical analgesic take place prior to the manipulative reduction (ultrasound or electrical stimulation can be used to drive the medication deeper).

With the patient seated, the practitioner holds the patient's ankle on the affected extremity with one hand, and with the thumb of his other hand he presses on the lateral end of the affected meniscus.

The practitioner:

**1.** Flexes the patient's knee to 90°.

**2.** Induces a valgus pressure (for medial meniscus, varus for lateral meniscus) in

order to open up the space over the meniscus.

**3.** Rotates the knee (with his hand on the ankle) internally (externally for lateral meniscus).

**4.** Keeps his thumb pressed on the meniscus, and extends the leg. A click is audible usually. (Do not extend the knee through a painful barrier. Instead perform this process repeatedly).

**5.** (If needed) rotates the leg to-and-fro while repeating extensions (Figure 11-27).

**DEEP FRICTION AND PERIOSTEAL NEEDLING**. Deep friction or local periosteal needling (with monopolar (+) electric stimulation) to the coronary ligaments is often needed as they usually are sprained (Figure 11-28).

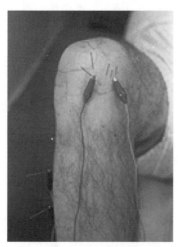

*Figure 11-29:* Electro-periosteal-acupuncture for medial meniscus and coronary ligaments.

**HERBAL THERAPY.** Herbal therapy is helpful. A guiding topical herbal formula for a sprained meniscus is:

Rhizoma Bletillae (Bai Ji)

Radix Paeoniae Alba (Bai Shao)

Semen Melo (Hu Gua Zi)

Cortex Albizziae (He Huan Pi)

Rhizoma Homalonemae (Qian Nian Jian)

Eupolyphagae (Tu Bie Chong)

Rhizoma Dioscoreae (Bi Xie)

Radix Angelicae Dahuricae (Bai Zhi)

Radix Dipsaci (Xu Duan)

Radix Polygalae (Yuan Zhi)

Radix Glycyrrhizae (Gan Cao)

Egg White

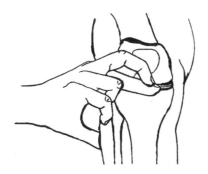

*Figure 11-28:* **Massage technique to coronary ligaments.**

A guiding topical formula for sprained meniscus complicated by partly torn coronary ligament is:

Cortex Erythrinae (Hai Tong Pi)

Cortex Kadsurae Radicis (Zi Jing Pi)

Radix Aucklandiae (Yun Mu Xiang)

Eupolyphagae (Tu Bie Chong)

Achyranthes Bidentata (Niu Xi)

Rhizoma Notopterygium (Qiang Huo)

Radix Angelica Pubescentis (Du Huo)

Radix Dipsaci (Xu Duan)

Acacia seu Uncaria (Er Cha)

## Loose Body

A loose body in the knee presents often with symptoms similar to those of a torn meniscus. However, it usually lacks a traumatic onset and the knee can lock in extension (limited flexion—which must be differentiated from a posterior horn meniscal lesion). A history of sudden (for no reason) and temporary painful twinges, swelling, warmth and localized pain, usually when the patient walks downstairs or plays sports, is seen. The knee may or may not be locked. More often, either flexion or extension is painful at end range, and the end feel is springy.

In the teenager and young adult a loose body usually is the result of osteochondritis dissecans, but sometimes arises from chondromalacia patella (Figure 11-43), or a small osteochondral chip fracture. Treatment for teens and young adults is surgical, as arthrosis of the knee can result if the loose body is not removed. In middle-aged or elderly patients, conservative treatment usually suffices (Ombregt, Bisschop, ter Veer and Van de Velde 1995).

### Treatment

Treatment for a loose body (in the middle-aged or elderly patient) is manipulative reduction. If accompanied by ligamentous laxity, which is common, stabilization of the knee is achieved by exercise, periosteal needling or prolotherapy.

Three basic techniques (the technique used for the meniscus can be tried as well) are designed to open the joint and allow the loose body to shift to a less obstructive location. Recurrence is common, although episodes can be far apart (Ombregt, Bisschop, ter Veer and Van de Velde 1995).

**FIRST TECHNIQUE.** Patient is prone on a low treatment table with knee flexed and the affected thigh strapped to the table or held by an assistant. The practitioner stands level with the knee, with one foot on the table, and holds the patient's foot and ankle. The foot is kept in dorsiflexion during the entire procedure. The practitioner then:

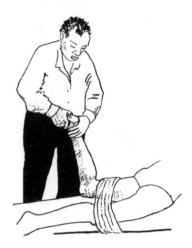

*Figure 11-30:* First manipulation technique for a loose body in the knee.

1. Places the patient's foot on his knee and raises his own knee to induce traction to the patient's knee. He holds this for several seconds until he feels the patient's knee relax and in traction.

2. Keeps the patient's knee distracted while he lowers his foot from the table.

3. Extends the leg (does not force through pain and restriction) while he rotates the knee internally. Rechecks knee.

4. Repeats steps one and two, this time rotating the knee externally. Rechecks.

5. Repeats 10-20 times (Figure 11-30).

**SECOND TECHNIQUE.** If only partial reduction has been achieved by the first technique, and flexion is still limited, the second technique can be tried.

While patient is supine, the practitioner places one of his own fists (or an assistants fist) behind the popliteal fossa (back of knee) while his other hand holds the patient's distal leg. The practitioner:

1. Flexes the patient's knee as far as it can go to take up all the slack in the joint.

2. (When the patient is relaxed) applies a quick over flexion. This usually results in an audible click. Rechecks.

3. (If flexion is still limited), repeats the maneuver with the addition of rotation (Figure 11-31).

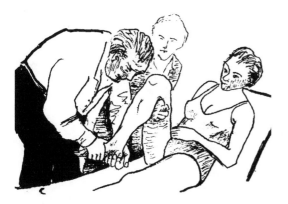

*Figure 11-31:* Second manipulation technique for a loose body in the knee.

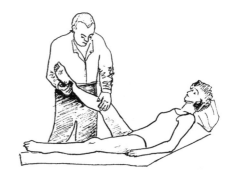

*Figure 11-32:* Third manipulation technique for a loose body in the knee.

**THIRD TECHNIQUE.** If only partial reduction has been achieved by the first technique and extension is still limited or painful, the third technique can be tried. The patient is supine. The practitioner stands level with the knee. He then:

1. Flexes the patient's knee and hip.

2. Externally rotates the hip.

3. Places one hand over the knee while the other hand supports the underside of the distal leg. He then applies strong varus pressure to the knee joint.

4. Asks the patient to actively and slowly extend the knee while he keeps varus pressure.

5. Maintains varus pressure while the patient's leg is near full extension, and adds a quick final jerk toward extension (Figure 11-32).

6. Instructs the patient to do this type of movement on his own while sitting.

## Bursitis

Many bursae are found around the knee; all can become inflamed (Brown *ibid*). The *prepatellar* bursa is the most frequently affected. Prepatellar bursitis is seen most often in patients who kneel repeatedly, as brick layers do. The front of the knee is swollen between the skin and the patella. Severe swelling can limit flexion due to pain that results from stretching the bursa.

Another common location of bursitis is under the *medial collateral ligament*. Here the pain is over the medial joint line. It gets worse with activity and eases with rest. Flexion can be limited with a soft end feel. Valgus strain and lateral rotation are painful. A solid swelling, that can be mistaken for bone, can be palpated under the ligament.

A bursitis over the medial collateral ligament also can occur in the space between the tendons of the sartorius, gracilis and semitendinosus—*Pes anserinus bursitis*.

Finally a bursa between the *iliotibial tract* and the *lateral epicondyle* can form in long-distance runners, skiers and cyclists. When inflamed, pain is felt over the lateral aspect of the knee while walking or running. A painful arc can be seen at 30° of flexion. Swelling can be felt between the condyle and the iliotibial tract.

*Treatment*

Treatment of bursitis around the knee requires addressing all the muscles around the bursa. The inflamed bursa can be drained. Bleeding and cupping techniques can be used. Topical and oral herbs are helpful. The formula for hip bursitis can be used both orally and topically (page 556). In more severe cases Sarapin or steroid injections may be needed.

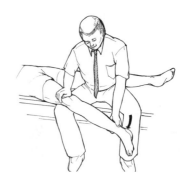

*Figure 11-33:* Valgus over pressure to assess medial collateral and coronary ligament (With permission Dorman and Ravin 1991).

## Ligamentous Disorders

Ligamentous disorders at the knee are very common. They can have a traumatic origin, or can result from degenerative processes.

## Coronary & Medial Collateral Ligaments

The coronary and medial collateral ligaments are affected quite often and can result in much disability. Symptoms often are mistaken for those of a meniscus lesion. In more severe trauma both the meniscus and anterior cruciate ligament can be affected.

With lesions of the medial coronary and medial collateral ligaments, the pain usually is at the medial knee. Valgus strain (Figure 11-33) is painful and rotation of the knee to the opposite side is painful, as well. In the acute stage sprain can result in traumatic arthritis and a capsular pattern. Swelling can be palpated. In chronic lesions the pain comes on after use, and the knee feels stiff after it has been motionless for some time (posain). Ligament adhesions can develop (Ombregt, Bisschop, ter Veer and Van de Velde 1995).

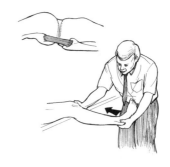

*Figure 11-34:* Varus over pressure to assess the lateral collateral and coronary ligaments (With permission Dorman and Ravin 1991).

.Lateral Collateral Ligament

The lateral collateral ligament is affected much less frequently. The pain is felt over the lateral knee. Varus strain (Figure 11-34) is painful. When acute, it can result in traumatic arthritis that can last about two weeks (Ombregt, Bisschop, ter Veer and Van de Velde 1995).

## Cruciate Ligaments

Lesions of the anterior and posterior cruciate ligaments can result from trauma or degenerative processes. When torn or lax they can cause anteroposterior or posterioranteror instability. The drawer tests are positive (Figure 11-35).

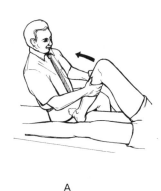 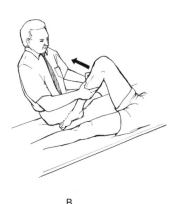

A                                                                                 B

*Figure 11-35:* (A) Assessment of posterior cruciate ligament. (B) Assessment of anterior cruciate ligament. Movement should be minimal and symmetric on the symptomatic and non-symptomatic side (With permission Dorman and Ravin 1991).

*Treatment*

Treatment of ligamentous lesions depends on location and severity. In the acute stage ice and compression together with anti-inflammatory and hemostatic herbs are used. Light cross fiber massage is started as soon as possible (to prevent adhesions).

Disorders of the cruciate ligaments are more difficult to treat, and depending on severity, surgery may be necessary. Milder lesions often resolve with injection therapy (Ravin personal communication).

In the chronic stage the coronary, medial and lateral collateral ligaments can be treated by cross fiber massage, periosteal needling, and topical herbal application. A manipulative rupture of adhesions may be needed.

*Contractile Structures*

Both muscular and tendinous lesions can result in pain about the knee. Muscle weakness can be caused by a neurological disorder or a torn muscle or tendon.

## Quadriceps Strain & Patellar Tendinitis

The patella sits within the superficial and deep fibers of the quadriceps muscle, making it a sesamoid bone within the tendon (Figure 11-37). Tendinous lesions can occur at the superior, inferior, medial and lateral aspects of the patellar edges. The pain comes on usually after exertion and is felt at the front of the knee. Walking upstairs and getting up from a deep chair are painful often. Resisted knee extension (Figure 11-36) is painful. Local tenderness can be palpated (Cyriax *ibid*).

Lesions of the quadriceps expansion result in tenderness at either side of the patella. In rare cases the lesion is at the insertion of the infrapatellar tendon on the tibial tuberosity, which is seen more often in athletes. Osteochondrosis of the tibial tuberosity in boys between 10 and 15 years old is known as *Osgood Schlatter Dis-*

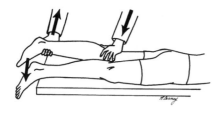

*Figure 11-36:* Assessing resisted extension of knee for quadriceps lesions (With permission Dorman and Ravin 1991).

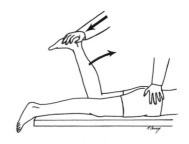

*Figure 11-38:* Assessing resisted flexion of the knee for hamstring lesion (With permission Dorman and Ravin 1991).

*ease* (Ombregt, Bisschop, ter Veer and Van de Velde 1995).

## Hamstring Strain & Tendinitis

Hamstring (Figure 11-39) strains are quite common, especially in athletes. Resisted knee flexion is painful (Figure 11-38). In lesions of the muscle belly straight-leg raising is limited by pain. Resisted external

rotation or internal rotation can help the practitioner differentiate between a biceps lesion and a lesion in the medial hamstring —resisted external rotation is painful with biceps lesions. Biceps lesions are more common, and the pain is felt over the outer side, especially with tendinitis (Ombregt, Bisschop, ter Veer and Van de Velde 1995).

Painful resisted flexion can be seen also from a lesion in the upper tibiofibular joint, which results from the biceps muscle pulling on the tibiofibular joint. However, resisted flexion with the knee in almost full extension is painless, because the fibular head is now being pulled upward instead of backward (Ombregt,

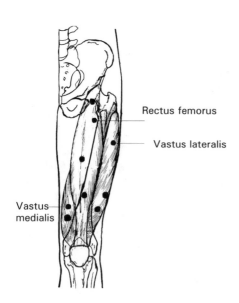

*Figure 11-37:* Common trigger sites on the quadriceps femoris.

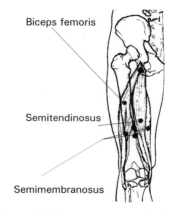

*Figure 11-39:* Common trigger sites on the hamstrings.

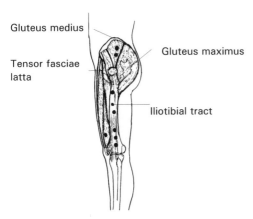

Gluteus medius

Tensor fasciae latta

Gluteus maximus

Iliotibial tract

Figure 11-40: Common trigger sites on the iliotibial tract.

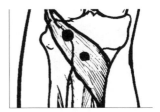

Figure 11-41: Common trigger sites on popliteus.

Bisschop, ter Veer and Van de Velde 1995).

## Iliotibial Strain

The iliotibial band has fiber connections to the gluteus maximus and is an extension of the fascia latta muscle (Figure 11-40). The band inserts at the tibial tubercle of Gerdy. Symptoms arising from the iliotibial band are common in people suffering from hip and low back disorders. Strains also can develop in long distance runners due to rubbing of the iliotibial band on the prominent lateral epicondyle—a painful bursa can form. Resisted extension and external rotation may be uncomfortable (Ombregt, Bisschop, ter Veer and Van de Velde 1995).

## Popliteus Strain

The popliteus (Figure 11-41) is an important active stabilizer of the lateral and posterolateral aspects of the knee joint preventing a sliding forward of the lateral femoral condyle on the fixed tibia during the stance phase of gait (Barnett and Rich-

ardson 1953). The muscle is strained often in long distance runners and skiers.

Popliteus strain can result in pain at the lateral or posterolateral areas of the knee. Resisted flexion and internal rotation may be painful. The practitioner must differentiate between disorders that cause pain at the posterolateral knee, such as medial hamstring lesion (pain in the medial side), cysts, posterior horn meniscal lesions, bursitis, etc. (Brown 1995).

### Treatment

Contractile unit disorders about the knee respond to massage (Figure 11-42), needling of motor, trigger, and acupuncture points. Post-isometric stretches are helpful in chronic cases. Herbs can be helpful, especially in tendinitis. Activation of the

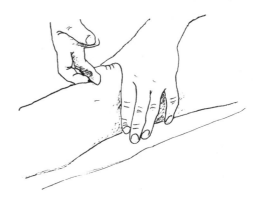

Figure 11-42: Massage technique for infrapatellar tendinitis.

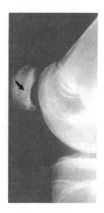

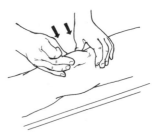

*Figure 11-44:*  Assessment of patellar mobility.

*Figure 11-43:* Chondromalacia patellae. Note the small localized area of radiolucency on the retropatellar surface. This lesion is infrequently seen in this disorder.

appropriate Sinews channel is particularly important. Laser acupuncture has been shown to be useful in the treatment of patellar tendinitis (Aigner et al. 1996).

### Anterior Knee Pain

Many conditions can result in anterior knee pain. Chondromalacia patellae and recurrent patellar subluxations, among others, should be considered (Brown 1995).

### Chondromalacia Patellae

Chondromalacia patellae is a degenerative condition of the articular surface of the patella (and softening of the patellar cartilage) from unknown cause. The condition is associated with increased Q angle[1] and abnormal patellar tracking (Huberti and Hayes 1984).

Chondromalacia patellae is more common in women who complain of anterior

knee pain precipitated by kneeling, or during and after bending the knee. The routine examination shows nothing. Inspection may reveal increased Q angle, decreased patellar mobility (Figure 11-44), infacing patella, and a thickened and palpable lateral retinaculum.

*Treatment*

Since chondromalacia patellae is associated with abnormal patellar tracking, treatment to improve tracking is essential. Rehabilitating the vastus medialis, infrapatellar strapping (to displace the patella upward and slightly anteriorly) can be used. Foot orthotics are often helpful. Herbal and acupuncture treatments are similar to those used for other degenerative knee disorders.

### Recurrent Patellar Subluxation

Recurrent patellar subluxation affects mostly girls and usually begins at puberty with a sudden onset. If patellar dislocation occurs the patient often falls to the ground suddenly and feels as if something is out of place at the lateral aspect of the knee. When the knee is straightened there is a loud click and extension is possible again.

---

1.  The angle at the center of the patella between imaginary lines, from the anterior-superior iliac spine (ASIS) to the center of the patella and from the tibial tuberosity to the center of the patella. Normal Q angle is about $20^{\circ}$.

Patients with recurrent patellar subluxations often report a family history of knee pain; decreased Q angle, weak and atrophied vastus medialis muscle, and enlarged fat pad can be seen (Reider, Marshall and Warren 1981). Increased lateral mobility of the patella can be demonstrated.

*Treatment*

Intensive strengthening of the vastus medialis muscle is the most important aspect of treatment.

Both active rehabilitation and electrostimulation can be used. Patellar bracing and taping is helpful. In more severe cases surgery may be considered (Brown *ibid*).

## *Lower Leg, Ankle & Foot*

Disorders of the lower leg, foot and ankle are numerous and have widespread effects, as they can affect gait and the entire musculoskeletal system. The importance and contribution of the feet to the body's mechanics and as a primary initiator of myofascial pain often is overlooked.

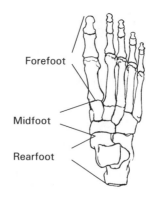

*Figure 11-45:* The foot.

# Anatomy/Biomechanics

The foot and ankle are made of three functional parts which together are formed by 26 bones, 36 joints, 13 intrinsic muscles, and 12 extrinsic muscles. The rearfoot is formed by the ankle and subtalar joints, the midfoot formed by five tarsal bones, and the forefoot formed by the phalanges and metatarsal bones (Figure 11-45). The foot's three architectural arches form a tripod with the talus distributing the body weight and other loads throughout the foot. About 17% of the time we spend walking, our entire weight is supported by a single foot. More detail is given in the appropriate section of this chapter. Table 11-9 summarizes lower leg muscles.

# Imaging

Ankle imaging is as equally important as wrist imaging. Sprained ankles, any inversion injury and almost any ankle injury is capable of creating a tremendous number of somatic dysfunctions and ligamentous injuries. Injuries to the ligament holding the tibia and fibula together (the syndesmosis) are frequent, particularly in sprained ankles. This slight widening of the ankle mortise creates a moderate amount of ankle instability that can sometimes be treated by conservative measures—ie prolotherapy.

*Table 11-9.* LOWER LEG MUSCLES

| MUSCLE | FUNCTION | INNERVATION |
| --- | --- | --- |
| Tibialis anterior | Dorsiflexion/Inversion | L-4 (5) |
| Extensor digitorum longus | Dorsiflexion/Eversion | L-4, L-5 |
| Extensor hallucis longus | Dorsiflexion/Inversion | L-4, L-5 |
| Peronei | Eversion/Plantarflexion | L-5, S-1 |
| Tibialis posterior | Inversion/Plantarflexion | L-4, L-5 |
| Flexor digitorum longus | Plantarflexion/Inversion | L-5, S1 |
| Flexor hallucis longus | Plantarflexion/Inversion | L-5, S1 |
| Triceps surae | Plantarflexion | S-1, S2 |

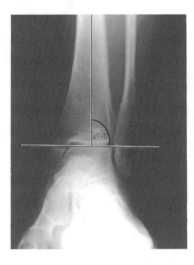

*Figure 11-46:* Anterior-posterior view of the foot with normal horizontal and vertical lines drawn on it. The (T-T) should be close to 90°.

## X-Rays

The posture of the foot and ankle is maintained by ligaments. In the presence of ligament attenuation, the position of the bone is changed with stress. It goes without saying the foot and ankle should be examined in a standing position and X-rays should be taken with the patient standing as well. Ligament injuries are common and important (Subotnick 1975).

The standing AP films of the foot and ankle reveal the position of the talus, the calcaneus, and the distal tibia. They should be seen to lie in a straight line, the top of the talus being horizontal, the long axis of the tibia being vertical (Figure 11-46).

The distal ends of the leg bones are not normally at the same level. The tip of the lateral malleolus hangs half-a-finger breath below the medial on the average. With ligament laxity, typically an inversion injury, the lateral malleolus tends to lie even lower and the mortise widens (Figure 11-47 and Figure 11-48)

If the fibula lies low, it should be assumed that ankle joint dysfunction exists, but the width of the joint may *seem* less abnormal than it really is.

Left uncorrected, fibular dysfunction can persist and become chronic. Slight resorption of bone at the fibulotalar space can develop, particularly on the fibular side; later, the other changes characteristic of osteoarthritis may appear, including osteophytes, subchondral bone sclerosis, and cyst formation (Figure 11-49).

A distally displaced fibula also is seen with subluxation of the cuboid. This is a common clinical problem and the radiograph can be helpful in explaining persistent foot pain. The talus is one of the bones supported only by ligaments; hence it is subject to asymlocation. When the ankle mortise is sprung from ligament attenuation, the talus rolls on weightbearing. The usual tendency is for its medial side to descend. On AP standing films, the instability can be judged by observing the angle between the bottom of the tibia and the top of the talus. The normal vertical line of tibia to talus to calcaneus will be replaced by a line seeming to go from lateral to medial, or from "outside to inside" (Figure 11-50). A line drawn through the long axis of the tibia on lateral standing films should be seen to pass just behind the mid portion of the subtalar joint. The dome of the talus is expected to fit snugly under the tibia. In ligament attenuation, there is a tendency for it to slip backward (Figure 11-51).

The relative positions of the bones of the foot, as seen in the lateral weightbearing view, indicate the condition of several important ligaments of the midfoot. A convenient visual aid is the S-shaped *cyma line*. It is formed by the anterior surfaces of the talus, the calcaneum with the cuboid, and navicular bones. A break in the cyma line represents somatic joint dysfunction(s) of the subtalar joint and the forefoot (Nielsen 1987). The position of the cuboid should be noted; when subluxed, the cyma line is discontinued. A subluxed cuboid moves medially and inferiorly, the lateral malleolus descends, and the fifth metatarsal bone seems to be in

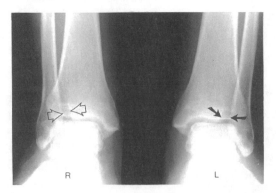

*Figure 11-47:* Anterior-posterior view of the ankles with widened left tibiofibular joint and distally displaced left fibula. The closed arrows point to the widened joint space, and the open arrows to the more normal joint space.

contact with the table. (Ordinarily it should appear a little elevated), (Figure 11-52 through Figure 11-54).

Additional stress films can be obtained by pushing the foot into adduction/inversion and by taking AP standing views. Laxity of the mortise (Kaartinen 1988) and attenuation of the calcaneofibular ligament allow abnormal tilting of the talus within the tibiofibular mortise (Lindstrand 1977; Grace 1984).

Anteroposterior instability of the tibiotalar joint can be demonstrated on lateral stress X-rays. The patient is asked to lean forward on the foot, as if in the middle of a stride. Displacement represents laxity of the anterior tibiofibular ligament, the fibulotalar ligament, and the interosseous membrane. The patient's pain may be reproduced.

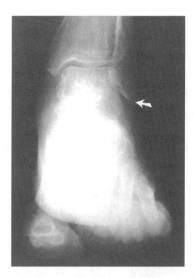

*Figure 11-48:* Standing anterior-posterior view of the ankle with an inferiorly displaced fibula. Note the arrow points to the displaced fibula. It is abnormal if it is more than one finger width below the tip of the medial malleolus.

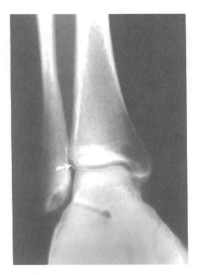

*Figure 11-49:* Anterior-posterior view of the ankle. At the arrow tip there is an area of bony resorption. This is the first sign of a degenerative osteoarthritis of tibiofibular joint.

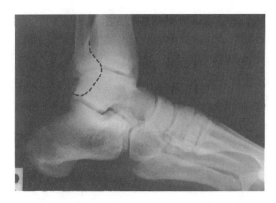

*Figure 11-51:* Lateral view of the foot with tibia displaced backward over the talus.

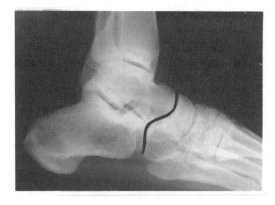

*Figure 11-52:* Lateral x-ray of foot with cyma line drawn on it.

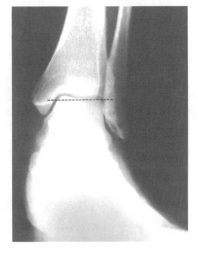

*Figure 11-50:* Anteroposterior view of the ankle with "outside to inside" axis of tibia.

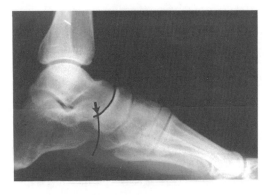

*Figure 11-53:* Lateral x-ray of foot with abnormal cyma line.

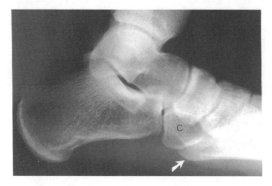

*Figure 11-54:* Lateral x-ray of foot with dropped first fifth metatarsal. The cuboid ("C") has rotated medially, causing the peroneal groove of the cuboid to disappear.

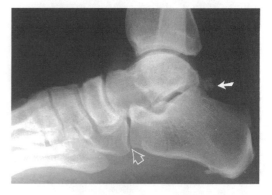

*Figure 11-56:* Lateral view of an ankle with a prominent os trigonum (closed arrow). The ankle also has a broken cyma line which reflects multiple somatic joint dysfunctions. The normally smooth inferior junction between the cuboid and the calcaneus is broken, also an indication of a joint dysfunction (open arrow). The head of the fifth metatarsal is also low. Compare this image with figure 11-52.

Anteroposterior instability of the talocalcaneal joint is demonstrable on the AP stress views if the usually strong talocalcaneal ligament is attenuated, as in inversion injuries. In this condition the talus is seen to glide forward and beyond the normal range (Figure 11-57).

If there has been a rupture of the posterior fibulotalar ligament, during gait, the tibia slides forward unrestrained on the talus and comes to a stop along the neck of the talus. This area of contact is subject to irritation, and may be the site of an anterior osteophyte (Hamilton 1984), (Figure 11-55).

Clever techniques for holding the patient for stress views and even the use of contrast have been added (Black 1978), but they are not necessary in normal practice. A stress X-ray is complex and should be used only in conjunction with a careful clinical evaluation.

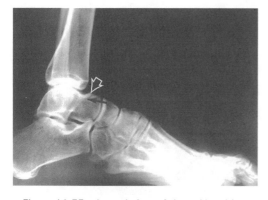

*Figure 11-55:* Lateral view of the ankle with osteophytes (open arrow) and sclerosis (closed arrow) at the neck of the talus. This is a late sign of ankle ligament laxity.

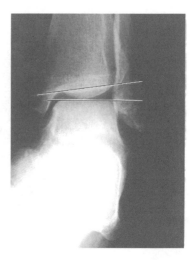

*Figure 11-57:* Anterior-posterior view of the ankle with stress demonstrating the widening of the tibiotalar joint. This represents laxity of the fibulocalcaneal, fibulotalar, and the talocalcaneal ligaments.

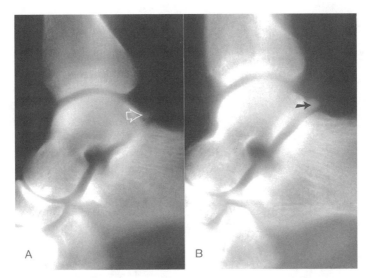

*Figure 11-58:* A and B lateral tomogram demonstrating two separate structures in the region of the posterior talus. The open arrow points to the osteophyte from the Steida process. The closed arrow points to the "os trigonum." The distance between these two images is 5mm and demonstrates that they are two separate structures.

## Magnetic Resonance Imaging & Computed Tomography

The ankle and foot have not been denied the wonders of computer image reconstruction. As in other parts of the body, MRI is altered in the ankle when inflammation increases the water content of ligaments and tendons (Rosenberg 1988; Daffner 1986). The astute clinician might continue to recognize most of these entities by examination.

Pain at the back of the heel may be caused by a cryptic fracture of the talus in the region of the Stieda's process, where the talofibular ligament is attached. Stieda's process is subject to avulsion fracture that may need to be distinguished from an os trigonum, which is an occasional extranumerary sesamoid. Multiplanar tomography is used for this purpose. In an avulsion fracture or in chronic irritation of the "beak", there may be subchondral bone sclerosis and osteophyte formation. After an injury, a bone scan may help separate a Stieda process fracture from an injury to the talofibular ligament (Figure 11-56 and Figure 11-58).

The interosseous talocalcaneal ligament restrains the talus from sliding forward on the calcaneum when walking. It is subject to damage in inversion injuries and can be responsible for chronic pain when walking on rough ground. With MRI it has become possible to image this ligament and recognize damage on occasion (Bower 1989). The talocalcaneal ligament calcifies once in a while and the bony bar itself can fracture.

# OM Disorders

Disorders of the lower extremity and foot are due mainly to; external pathogenic factors, Independent factors (sprains/strains) that can result in deficiency of Qi and Blood, and disorders of the Kidney and Liver Organs.

The main pathogenic factor affecting the feet is Dampness, as Dampness is "heavy" and tends to descend. Occasionally, Dampness transforms to Damp-Heat with signs of inflammation. Sprains/strains block the flow of Qi and Blood, resulting in swelling and pain. When sprains are not treated appropriately, obstructive malnourishment of the sinews results in tissue weakness and chronicity. Congenital weakness, prolonged illness, or excessive lifestyles and sexual activity can result in insufficiency of the Liver and Kidney. This leads to malnourishment of sinews and bones.

# Biomedical Disorders: Lower Leg

Disorders of the lower leg are mainly myofascial, and often arise from mechanical dysfunction of the foot and ankle. Medical conditions such as *intermittent claudication, Baker's cyst, deep venous thrombosis, compartment syndromes, radicular and pelvic disorders* should be considered. In patients with persistent localized pain and few clinical findings, disorders such as metastases, primary bone tumors, osteomyelitis and Paget's disease can be considered (Ombregt, Bisschop, ter Veer and Van de Velde 1995). Since mechanical foot dysfunctions are common, foot orthotics can be very helpful and are used often.

## Plantiflexor Lesions

Lesions of the plantiflexors mostly involve the gastrocnemius muscle or achilles tendon. Rising on tiptoe usually is diagnostic (Ombregt, Bisschop, ter Veer and Van de Velde 1995).

## Tennis Leg

Tennis leg is a term commonly used to describe a tear in the triceps surae complex. It occurs mostly in the medial belly of the gastrocnemius muscle, just above the musculotendinous junction (Figure 11-60). Usually the patient feels a sudden

severe pain in the calf during vigorous activity. Resisted plantiflexion is painful but not weak. Foot dorsiflexion is limited with the knee extended, but normal with the knee flexed (Brown *ibid*).

The condition should be differentiated from lesions in the Achilles tendon, deep venous thrombosis, intermittent claudication, ruptured Baker's cyst, compartment syndrome and referred pain (Ombregt et al. *ibid*).

*Treatment*

Tears in the triceps, as in all other muscles, should not be treated by immobilization because it leads to adhesions that in time give rise to painful restrictions. Blood should be aspirated as soon as possible, to decrease inflammation and irritation. Cross-fiber massage, topical oils, spirits, oral herbal medications and electrical stimulation are helpful and should be applied daily for the first few days. A heel raise should be used during the recovery stage or until a good scar is formed. The patient is encouraged to perform mild (non weight-bearing) movements. Later the muscle is stretched and reeducated. Infiltration with a local anesthetic is helpful.

## Achilles Tendinitis

The Achilles tendon (the common tendon of the triceps surae complex) has relatively poor blood supply, consisting mostly of longitudinal arterioles which course the length of the tendon, supplemented by vessels from the mesotendon (midtendon). Studies have shown the area of least vascularity to be 2-6 cm above the tendon insertion. The tendon fibers rotate laterally as they descend, which leaves the fibers vulnerable to injury and wear. Inflammation can develop within the tendon or around the tendon—peritendinitis (Brown 1995).

Achilles tendinitis is seen most often in runners and other athletes. It can also develop after simple overexertion, such as a long walk. Achilles tendinitis often results from training errors such as:

- Increase in training mileage.

- Increased running intensity.

- Single severe running session.

- Running of hills.

- Training in uneven or slippery terrain.

- Recommencement of training after an extended time of inactivity.

Anatomical factors contributing to the development of Achilles tendinitis are;

- Excessive pronation.

- Forefoot varus.

    In a runner with a hindfoot and forefoot varus, the Achilles tendon is forced to go from lateral to median as the foot goes from foot strike to midstance. This causes a "whipping" action of the tendon. In addition, shear forces are established between the gasro and soleus muscles, creating an area of stress.

- Tight heel cord.

- Tibia vara.

Initially, inflammation involves the peritendinous structures such as the bursae and tendon sheath. As the severity of inflammation progresses, the tendon itself becomes involved. The lesion lies usually at the mid-tendon. It can be found also at the tenoperiosteal junction and at the musculotendinous junction (Brown 1995).

The patient usually complains of heel pain during or after walking or running. The pain can present at the beginning of exertion and improve during the activity. When severe, the pain is continuous. Asking the patient to rise on tiptoe brings on the pain.

The possibility of tendon microtears must be kept in mind (as can eventually result in tendon rupture) and an MRI or bone scan can be ordered. When the Achilles tendon ruptures, the patient can not rise on tiptoe. Passive movements become painless, and there is an excessive range of ankle extension (dorsiflexion). Neurologi-

cal disorders should be differentiated (Brown *ibid*).

### Treatment

The most important aspect of treatment of achilles tendinitis is correction of biomechanical foot dysfunctions. An orthotic is often needed. It is helpful to raise shoe heels and /or use a wide-heeled running shoe for increased stability (Ombregt, Bisschop, ter Veer and Van de Velde 1995).

The athlete should decrease the intensity of training, stop hill running and increase cross-training with low-impact exercise (pool, bike etc.) to maintain cardiovascular fitness. The triceps surae complex is stretched before and after exercise. As soon as the pain is under control and exercise can be done without difficulty, an eccentric program can be initiated to increase tendon strength and prevent future problems. This is done by having the patient perform a toe raise on a 4-inch step. Both legs perform the toe raise. Once maximum plantar flexion is achieved, the patient lifts the uninvolved leg and lowers the involved leg into dorsiflexion.

In chronic cases a longer period of rest should be prescribed. Rest and immobilization may range from 2-6 weeks, depending on severity of inflammation (usually 3 weeks). In some patients a 1 week period in a walker boot or cast can be helpful. The athlete cross-trains to maintain cardiovascular fitness (Brown 1995).

Cross-fiber massage (Figure 11-59) is often effective in the acute and chronic stage, but must be very specific to the lesion. Careful palpation can identify the appropriate site which usually lies 2-6 cm above the tenoperiosteal junction (the area with a critical zone—reduced vascularity). Usually, treatment lasts 15 minutes and performed three times a week for 2-4 is weeks. Cryotherapy, cryokinetic massage, iontophoresis, microcurrent stimulation and massage and ultrasound are helpful (Brown 1995).

Needling the calf motor points and topical oils or spirits are helpful. Steroid

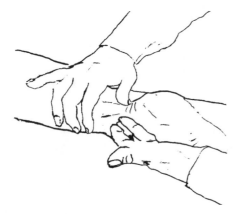

*Figure 11-59:* Massage technique for a lesion at the anterior aspect of the Achilles tendon.

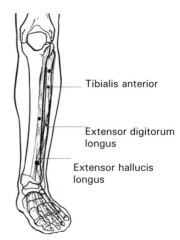

Tibialis anterior

Extensor digitorum longus

Extensor hallucis longus

*Figure 11-61:* Common trigger sites on the Dorsiflexor muscles.

and other injection therapies are controversial, as some cases of resulting tendon rupture have been reported (although a pre-existing pathology may have been the cause). Treatment of tendon rupture usually is surgical.

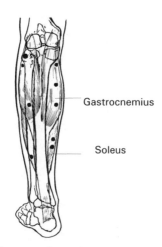

Gastrocnemius

Soleus

*Figure 11-60:* Common trigger sites on the calf for treatment of achilles tendinitis.

### Dorsiflexor (Exensors) Lesions

Lesions of the dorsiflexors usually are seen when resisted dorsiflexion is painful. These can be due to lesions in the extensor hallucis and digitorum longus, the tibialis anterior, and fascia of the anterior compartment (Figure 11-61). Testing resisted dorsiflexion of the foot, hallux, and toes identifies the muscle. The cause often is dysfunction of the midtarsal joints. The condition should be differentiated from compartment syndrome, which is rare. If the muscles are weak a neurological cause should be considered (Ombregt, Bisschop, ter Veer and Van de Velde 1995).

### *Treatment*

Treatment follows the general rules for myofascial syndromes. Orthotics often are helpful. Surgery may be needed in anterior compartment syndromes.

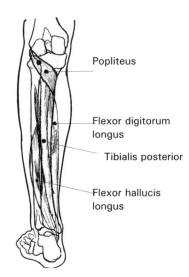

Popliteus

Flexor digitorum longus

Tibialis posterior

Flexor hallucis longus

*Figure 11-62:* Common trigger sites on the evertor muscles.

## Invertor Lesions

The main invertor muscle is the posterior tibialis and is assisted by the anterior tibialis, flexor hallucis longus and triceps (Figure 11-62). Posterior tibialis tendinitis can arise from overuse and often is due to a valgus deformity at the subtalar joint. Resisted inversion of the foot is painful, and resisted dorsiflexion is not. Rising to tiptoe can be painful, as well (Ombregt, Bisschop, ter Veer and Van de Velde 1995).

The lesion can be palpated at the insertion on the navicular bone, at the tendon body (distal or proximal to, or under the medial malleolus—which must be differentiated from tarsal tunnel syndrome), at the muscle belly or at the proximal musculotendinous junction.

*Treatment*

Treatment follows the general rules for myofascial syndromes. Cross- fiber massage usually is effective. Often, orthotics that support the heel and the longitudinal arch are needed to prevent recurrences.

## Shin Splints

The term shin splints has been used to describe a wide variety of disorders, including stress fractures, periostitis, soleus syndrome, compartment syndromes and other soft tissue inflammations. The American Medical Association subcommittee on sports injuries restricts the term to musculotendinous lesions of the tibialis anterior muscle (AMA 1976). Some, however, consider shin splints to apply only to pain along the inner (medial) distal two-thirds of the tibial shaft due to lesions in the posterior tibialis muscle (Travel and Simons 1982). Shin splints are seen most often in athletes and long-distance runners who put pressure on the musculotendinous and fascial tissues of the deep flexor muscles. The patient usually complains of pain or a dull ache at the medial tibial border during, or after, exertion. A patient with a stress fracture often has pain which can be elicited by striking the heel; or the bone is tender to direct pressure.

Resisted inversion of the foot can be slightly painful. The musculotendinous junction of the tibialis posterior usually is tender and indurated (most often between the upper and medial thirds). X-ray, ultrasound or bone scan may be necessary to differentiate simple shin splints from a stress fracture.

A rupture of the tibialis posterior muscle can lead to a progressive, unilateral, acquired flat foot, with increasing valgus of the heel, plantar flexion of the talus and subluxation of the talonavicular joint (Ombregt, Bisschop, ter Veer and Van de Velde 1995).

*Treatment*

Shin splints can be treated by cross-fiber massage, periosteal needling of the medial edge of tibia (or prolotherapy), and needling of tibialis trigger and motor points (Figure 11-63). Often Ashi points on the Stomach channel and anterior tibialis muscle are needled. As foot dysfunctions usually are present orthotics are used often.

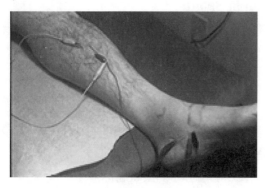

*Figure 11-63:* Electroacupuncture for shin splints with medial deep approach to reach tibialis triggers and bony insertion.

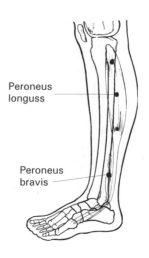

*Figure 11-64:* Common trigger sites on the evertor muscles.

Conservative treatment for muscle rupture include an orthotic with a medial heel wedge and a longitudinal arch support (Ombregt, Bisschop, ter Veer and Van de Velde 1995). Surgical intervention should be considered.

### Evertor Lesions

Lesions of the evertors mostly involve the peroneal muscles (Figure 11-64). Tendinitis can develop anywhere between the lower fibula to the cuboid and the fifth metatarsal base. Peroneal tendinitis can result from overuse and ankle sprains. Loosening of the peroneal tendon in its grove on the posterior surface of the fibula can result in a snapping feeling at the outer side of the ankle. Peroneal lesions often result from talocalcanean and mid-tarsal joint dysfunctions. Weakness is mostly a result of neurological lesions (Ombregt, Bisschop, ter Veer and Van de Velde 1995).

#### Treatment

Treatment follows the general rules for myofascial syndromes. Cross-fiber massage for 2-4 weeks often results in full recovery (Ombregt, Bisschop, ter Veer and Van de Velde 1995). The patient must not stress the muscle during the treatment phase. Taping the foot in eversion can be helpful. Orthotics are needed often to avoid reinjury.

# The Rearfoot

The rearfoot is composed of the ankle and subtalar joints.

# The Ankle

The ankle is a simple joint made of the superior surface of the talus which sits between the fibular and tibial malleoli, forming the ankle mortise (Figure 11-65). Stability of the tibiofibular mortise is provided by the anterior and posterior tibiofibular ligaments and the interosseous ligament (Kapendji *ibid*).

Movement at the ankle joint is of plantiflexion and dorsiflexion. The wedge-shaped talus, with its wider portion anteriorly, prevents any varus or valgus move-

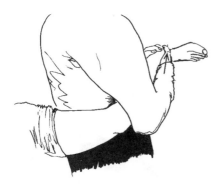

Figure 11-66: Long axis extension.

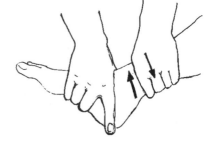

Figure 11-67: Anteroposterior glide of tibia and fibula on the talus

ment when the ankle is held in extension (dorsiflexion), unless the mortise is unstable due to ligamentous injury.

Joint play movements at the mortise joint are (Mennell *ibid*):

**1.** Long axis extension.

Assessed by having the seated practitioner cradle the supine patient's foot, as close to the ankle as possible (the patient's leg is flexed at 90°) with both hands from the front and back. Long axis extension is then applied by leaning backward of the patient's thigh (Figure 11-66).

**2.** Anteroposterior glide.

Assessed by having the patient lie supine with hip, knee, and ankle all at 90° angle. The practitioner grasps the patient's lower leg around the ankle just

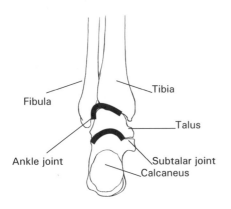

Figure 11-65: Rearfoot.

above the malleoli with one hand; and the dorsum of the foot with the other hand, which will stabilize it during the performance of the movement. The mobilizing hand then pulls forward and pushes backward alternately (Figure 11-67).

# The Subtalar Joint

The subtalar joint (STJ) is formed by the talus and calcaneus bones, divided by the tarsal canal. The lateral end of the canal is easily palpated (at GB-40 point) in front of the fibular malleolus, between the talus and calcaneus. In the canal a strong interosseous talocalcaneal ligament binds the two bones. The main movements in the subtalar joint are varus and valgus movements (Kapandji *ibid*).

Joint play movements are (Mennell *ibid*):

**1.** Talar rock.

Assessed by having the patient lie supine with hip, knee and ankle at 90°. The practitioner grasps the lower leg some 6 inches above the malleoli with one hand and supports the sole of the foot with his other hand. The patient's foot rests upon the posteroinferior

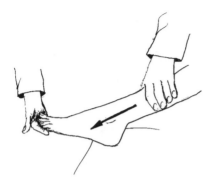

*Figure 11-68:* Talar rock.

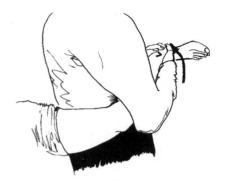

*Figure 11-70:* Rock of the talus on calcaneus.

Assessed by adopting the same examination position has in the mortise joint. The practitioner now rocks the calcaneus forward and backward (Figure 11-70).

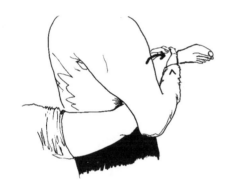

*Figure 11-69:* Side tilt.

angle of the calcaneus. The practitioner now pushes the foot by pushing downward on the tibia producing a rock of the talus on the calcaneus (Figure 11-68).

**2.** Long axis extension.

Assessed by adopting the same examination position in the mortise joint.

**3.** Side tilt.

Assessed by adopting the same examination position in the mortise joint. The practitioner performs long axis extension and then tilts the calcaneus medially and laterally (Figure 11-69).

**4.** Rock of the talus on calcaneus.

## Effects of Rearfoot Positioning

Rearfoot positioning is important for normal gait. The subtalar joints (STJ) function differently in open (nonweight-bearing) and closed (weight bearing) kinetic chain movements. During the first half of the swing phase of gait the STJ pronates. During the last half of the swing phase of gait the STJ supinates. In open kinetic chain the calcaneus moves around the talus, which functions as an immobile extension of the leg. This contrasts with open kinetic chain in that both the talus and calcaneus move (Brown *ibid*).[2]

The energy expended to accomplish ground clearance is minimized by STJ pronation. Without STJ pronation it would be necessary to use the hip and thigh muscles even more, to accomplish the same ground clearance. Therefore, if the rear-

2. An important factor to remember is that tibial rotation is intimately related to closed kinetic chain function and the STJ. This motion has significant importance in evaluating many lower extremity problems (patella). The tibia rotates internally with pronation and externally with supination.

foot is unstable or the subtalar joint malfunctions, gait becomes inefficient, with far-reaching effects throughout the body.

Factors that can affect rearfoot position include (Brown 1995):

- STJ axis and its relationship to adjacent muscles.
- Effects of muscular dysfunction on the rearfoot.
  Such as imbalance of the supinator and pronator muscles. Peroneal spastic flatfoot.
- Charcot-Marie-Tooth disease.
- Subtalar varus and valgus.
- Rearfoot varus and valgus (Figure 11-71).
- Tibial varum and valgum.
- Tarsal coalition (abnormal union between two or more tarsal bones).

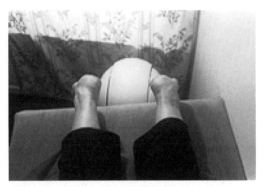

*Figure 11-71:* Patient with rearfoot varus that resulted in piriformis irritation. Note the inward pointed direction of the rearfoot.

## Capsular Pattern

The capsular pattern of the ankle is slightly more limitation of flexion (plantiflexion) than extension (dorsiflexion) (Cyriax *ibid*). The joint can be affected by traumatic, rheumatoid, and osteoarthritis. Hemarthrosis can result from inversion sprains. X-ray is recommended in patients with severe ankle sprains to exclude osteochondral fractures (Ombregt, Bisschop, ter Veer and Van de Velde 1995).

The capsular pattern of the subtalar joint results in progressive limitation of varus movements. The subtalar joint can also be affected by arthritis (Cyriax *ibid*).

*Treatment of Disorders Resulting in Capsular Pattern*

Treatment of foot arthrosis includes oral medications, foot soaks and local needling. Bleeding UB-43 and foot orthotics can be helpful.

**HERBAL THERAPY**. A guiding oral formula for arthrosis is:

Rhizoma et Radix Notopterygium (Qiang Hou)

Radix Angelicae Pubescentis (Du Huo)

Ramulus Cinnamomi (Gui Zhi)

Achyranthes Bidentata (Niu Xi)

Loranthus Parasiticus (Sang Ji Sheng)

Radix Gentianae (Qin Jiao)

Cortex Erythrinae (Hai Feng Teng)

Radix Angelica Sinensis (Dang Gui)

Rhizoma Ligusticum (Chuan Xiong)

Herba Asari (Xi Xin)

Radix Glycerrhizae (Gan Cao)

For Kidney and Liver deficiency add Restore the Left Pill (Zuo Gui Wan).

For active arthritis remove:

Ramulus Cinnamomi (Gui Zhi)

Rhizoma et Radix Notopterygium (Qiang Hou)

Add:

Tripterygium Wilfordii (Lei Gong Teng) (with vitamins B6 and B12)

Cortex Phellodendri (Huang Bai)

Rhizoma Atractylodes (Cang Zhu)

Radix Stephaniae Tetrandrea (Fang Ji)

## Non Capsular Patterns — Sprains

The most common cause of limitation in the noncapsular pattern in the rearfoot is sprain of the ankle joint. Approximately 23,000 inversion ankle sprains occur each day in the U.S. (Broods 1981) and ankle sprain is the most common injury in sports

(Drez 1996). The most frequently sprained structures are the (Ombregt et al. 1995; Brown 1995):

1. Fibular origin of the anterior talofibular ligament.

2. Fibular origin of the anterior calcaneoufibular ligament.

3. Talar insertion of the anterior talofibular ligament.

4. Distal posterior tibiofibular ligament and interosseous ligament.

5. Interosseous talocalcaneal ligament.

6. Lateral fibers of the calcaneocuboid ligament.

7. Peroneal tendons.

8. Anterior tibiotalar ligament.

9. Tendons of the extensor digitorum longus.

10. Ligaments of the cuboid-fifth metatarsal joint and cuboid-fourth metatarsal joint.

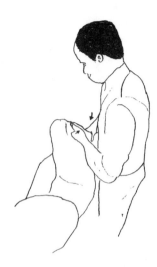

*Figure 11-72:* Mobilization of fibula.

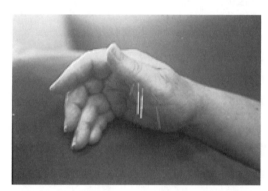

*Figure 11-73:*Five Tigers treated for ankle sprain.

*Treatment: Acute Stage*

Treatment of ankle sprain follows the general rules for management of acute injuries (see chapter 6). Local bleeding techniques, compression, electrostimulation and herbal compresses are particularly important. In the first 48 hours compression and icing are especially significant. Mobilization of the fibula is often necessary at a later stage, because the fibula can sublux from ankle inversion sprains (Figure 11-72).

**ACUPUNCTURE.** The appropriated Sinews channels are activated by needling the Well points and the termination points, CV-2 or 3 for leg Yin channels and SI-18 for leg Yang channels. Contralateral Five Tigers can be needled and the foot mobilized (Figure 11-73). The Connecting channels are used to treat swelling and local congested vessels are bled.

**COMPRESSES/TAPING.** A horseshoe-shaped (and herbal soaked) pressure pad is fitted under the lateral malleoli, open end upward. The ankle is then wrapped in slight eversion, from the base of the toes (tightly) to above the ankle (more loosely). This allows the blood and serous exudates to move out of the injured tissues and maximize healing.

**BLEEDING.** Bleeding techniques can be very helpful in reducing edema and having analgesic effects (Figure 11-74).

**HERBAL THERAPY.** A guiding herbal formula

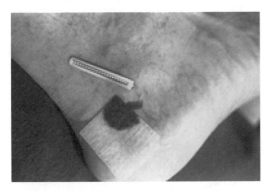

*Figure 11-74:* Bleeding congested vessels around the ankle.

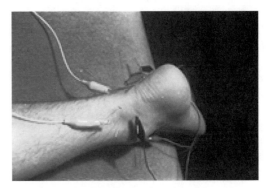

*Figure 11-75:* Patient's posterior tibiofibular ligament treated for post-sprain instability.

(for oral and topical use) for acute ankle sprain is:

> Flos Carthami (Hong Hua)
> Resina Olibani (Ru Xiang)
> Resina Myrrhae (Mo Yao)
> Dragon's Blood (Xue Jie)
> Acacia seu Uncaria (Er Cha)
> Rhizoma Ligusticum (Chuan Xiong)
> Radix Angelica Sinensis (Dang Gui)
> Semen Persiae (Tao Ren)
> Radix Rhubrab (Da Huang)
> Rhizoma Corydalis (Yan Hu Suo)
> Fructus Aurantii (Zhi Qiao)
> Radix Glycerrhizae (Gan Cao)

**TREATMENT: CHRONIC STAGE.** In the chronic stage, manual techniques are used to restore function and local needling or injection therapy of sprained ligaments is used to restore stability. Bleeding techniques are helpful. Foot orthotics are helpful. Prophylactic ankle taping can be used to prevent reinjury. Muscular straightening with isometrics, isotonics, isodynamic, isokinetic, and proprioceptive training are used.

**HERBAL THERAPY.** A guiding oral and topical formula for the chronic stage is:

> Prepared Sichuan Aconite (Zhi Chuan Wu)
> Flos Carthami (Hong Hua)
> Resina Olibani (Ru Xiang)
> Resina Myrrhae (Mo Yao)
> Radix Salviae (Dan Shen)
> Radix Peony Alba and Rubra (Bai Shao, Chi Shao)

> Radix Angelica Sinensis (Dang Gui)
> Lumbricus (Di Long)
> Radix Angelicae Pubescentis (Du Huo)
> Rhizoma et Radix Notopterygium (Qiang Hou)
> Herba Lycopodii (Shen Jin Cao)
> Cortex Cinnamomi (Rou Gui)
> Psoralea (Bu Gu Zhi)
> Fructus Chaenomelis (Mu Gua)
> Loranthus Parasiticus (Sang Ji Sheng)
> Radix Gentianae (Qin Jiao)
> Radix Glycerrhizae (Gan Cao)

For Kidney and Liver deficiency add Restore the Left Pill (Zuo Gui Wan).

### Sinus Tarsi Syndrome

Sinus tarsi syndrome is characterized by pain and tenderness over the lateral opening of the sinus tarsi (GB-40) along with a feeling of instability (giving way) of the ankle. The syndrome usually is associated with inversion sprains. However, it can develop insidiously secondary to the cumulative effects of biomechanical faults and gait abnormality. The pain arises from the interosseous ligament (Brown 1995).

The patient complains of pain at the lateral side of the foot, which increases with firm pressure over the lateral opening of the sinus tarsi (GB 40). Pain is worse standing, walking on uneven ground, and with supination and adduction of the foot.

The pain can be reduced by taping the foot in pronation.

A routine clinical exam and stress X-ray do not demonstrate any significant instability (Taillard, Meyer and Garcia 1981). Subtalar joint dysfunction is common (Mennell *ibid*).

### Treatment

Local needling (inserting several needles with electrical stimulation into the sinus tarsi canal—GB-40), re-education of the peroneal and calf muscles, and orthotics are usually very helpful. Prolotherapy (Brown 1995) usually is curative. Movements used to assess joint play can be used therapeutically.

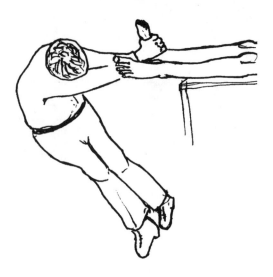

*Figure 11-76:* Manipulation under strong traction for a loose body in the ankle joint.

## Loose Body

A loose body in the ankle joint can cause limitation in the noncapsular pattern. It usually is secondary to inversion ankle sprains which result from a transchondral fracture (osteochondritis dissecans) of the dome of the talus. The patient complains of twinges in the ankle during walking, especially when plantiflexing the foot (as when walking downstairs), (Ombregt, Bisschop, ter Veer and Van de Velde 1995).

A loose body in the subtalar joint results in painful twinges provoked by walking on uneven surfaces. This condition should be differentiated from a sinus tarsi syndrome and ankle instability (Ombregt, Bisschop, ter Veer and Van de Velde 1995).

### Treatment

Treatment of a loose body is by manipulation. If the joint is unstable, periosteal needling or prolotherapy is used to stabilize the joint.

**MANIPULATION OF ANKLE JOINT**. For manipulation of a loose body in the ankle joint,

the patient lies supine and is held down by an assistant or strapped down. The practitioner:

1. Holds the patient's foot with one hand under the heel, and the other encircling the dorsal side as close to the ankle as possible, and with the thumb on the planter aspect of the foot.

2. Applies slight extension to the foot on the ankle.

3. Applies strong traction to the joint by leaning backward.

4. Performs a cirumduction movement (under traction), clockwise for the right foot and counterclockwise for the left foot.

5. Repeats cirumduction movements several times (Figure 11-76).

**MANIPULATION OF SUBTALAR JOINT**. To treat subtalar joint dysfunctions (also for a loose body at the joint) the patient lies prone with his foot just over the table, the dorsum of his foot touching the table (foot slightly plantarflexed). The practitioner stands behind, and holds the patient's heel

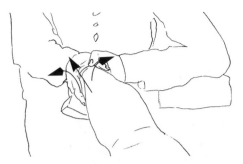

*Figure 11-77:* Manipulation technique of subtalar joint.

with two hands, thumbs on top. He then:

1. Leans backward applying traction to the joint.

2. Performs a varus-valgus movement at the joint.

3. Repeats this several times (Figure 11-77).

## Painful Heel

Most types of heel pain are due to local disorders. However, a lesion from an S1 structure (nerve root, sacroiliac joint, especially sacrotuberous ligament) can refer pain to the heel.

**PLANTAR HEEL PAIN MAY BE DUE TO** (Ombregt et al. 1995):

- Plantar fasciitis / plantar fascia rupture.
- Calcaneal spur (rarely).
- Fat pad syndrome.
- Calcaneal periostitis.
- Compression of the nerve to the abductor digiti quinti.

**MEDIAL HEEL PAIN MAY BE DUE TO:**

- Tarsal tunnel syndrome.
- Medial calcaneal neuritis.
- Posterior tibial tendon disorders.

**LATERAL HEEL PAIN MAY BE DUE TO:**

- Lateral calcaneal neuritis.

- Peroneal tendon disorders.

**POSTERIOR HEEL PAIN MAY BE DUE TO:**

- Retrocalcaneal bursitis.
- Calcaneal apophysitis (peds).
- Haglund's deformity.
- Calcaneal exostosis.
- Achilles tendinitis.
- Os trigonum.

**DIFFUSE HEEL PAIN MAY BE DUE TO:**

- Calcaneal stress fracture.
- Calcaneal fracture.

**OTHER CAUSES OF HEEL PAIN ARE** (Brown 1995):

- Systemic disorders (often bilateral).
- Reiter's syndrome.
- Ankylosing spondylitis.
- Lupus.
- Gouty arthopathy.
- Pseudogout.
- Rheumatoid arthritis.
- Systemic lupus erythematosus.

Occasionally a loose body at the ankle or subtalar joint refers painful twinges to the heel (Ombregt et al. 1995).

## Achilles Bursitis

Achilles bursitis can cause limitation in the noncapsular pattern. Pain is elicited when the bursa is squeezed between the posterior side of the tibia and the upper surface of the calcaneus at the extreme of passive plantiflexion. The condition should be differentiated from a posterior tibiotalar impingement of the trigonum (a large posterior tubercle of the posterior talus or an accessory bone) and Achilles tendinitis (Ombregt, Bisschop, ter Veer and Van de Velde 1995).

*Treatment*

Treatment of Achilles bursitis includes local needling and herbal packs (the formula for bursitis in the knee can be used). If pain persists, local infiltration with Sarapin or steroid usually resolves the problem (the dangers of steroids about the Achilles tendon must be kept in mind).

## Plantar Fasciitis

Plantar fasciitis is a common cause of heel pain. The patient usually complains of heel and medial foot pain, especially in the morning or during the first few steps after sitting or lying down. The condition is more common in people with valgus or flat feet (Katoh, Chao and Morrey 1984) (although some say the condition is found equally in high arched and flat feet; Horwitz personal communication). Plantar fasciitis seems to be more common in people who stand for prolonged periods, as well (Ombregt, Bisschop, ter Veer and Van de Velde 1995).

Disorders of the calf muscle and Achilles tendon are seen often in patients with plantar fascia pain, possibly due to pulling up of the heel by the Achilles tendon, which can increase tension on the plantar fascia. Heel spurs are commonly seen on X-ray, however there is little correlation between heel spurs and the amount of pain (Horwitz personal communication).

*Treatment*

Raising the heel can afford immediate relief from symptoms. A shock absorption device in the shoe, heel cups, and orthotics to control pronation are helpful. A heel cushion can be modified by a medial cut-out, or an orthotic with accommodations (cut-outs) can be used when a nerve is suspected of being compressed or irritated (Ombregt, Bisschop, ter Veer and Van de Velde 1995).

Periosteal needling with electrical stimulation at the plantar fascia insertion can

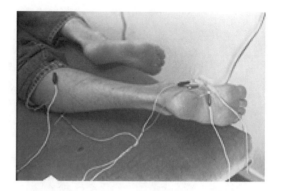

*Figure 11-78:*Electroacupuncture treatment of plantar fasciitis. Patient's gastrocnemmii and spring ligament are treated as well.

be helpful. Correct Tendons and triceps surae (soleus and both gastrocnemii) muscle triggers can be needled on the affected side (Figure 11-78, Figure 11-79). These muscles should be stretched and strengthened. For persistent lesions, local Sarapin, steroid or prolotherapy usually is effective (Brown personal communication).

## Tarsal Tunnel Syndrome

Tarsal tunnel syndrome is caused by pressure on the tibial nerve as it passes around the medial malleolus in the tarsal tunnel. The tarsal tunnel is formed by an osteofibrous space bordered by the medial malleolus, the medial aspect of the talus and

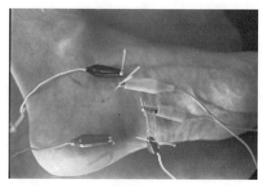

*Figure 11-79:*Insertion sites for the plantar fascia and spring ligament.

calcaneus and flexor retinaculum. The tunnel contains the tibialis posterior, the flexor hallucis longus, the flexor digitorum longus, arteries, and posterior tibial nerve. Inflammation of any of these or any space-occupying lesion can result in pressure on the tibial nerve. The syndrome is seen more often in patients with rearfoot valgus and overpronated forefoot (Brown *ibid*).

The patient complains of pins and needles, burning pain and numbness over the medial and plantar forefoot, sometimes rising up the leg. Pressure over the deep peroneal nerve (anterior to the talar joint) can produce pain and pins and needles in the big toe. Occasionally, submaleolar swelling can be palpated. Tinel's sign is positive often. Planiflexion and inversion may reproduce the symptoms (Ombregt, Bisschop, ter Veer and Van de Velde 1995).

### Treatment

Treatment is achieved by correcting foot mechanics. Muscles that pass through the tunnel are assessed and treated when needed. Injection therapy with Sarapin or steroids can be tried (Brown *ibid*). Surgical release of the flexor retinaculum may be needed in patients who do not respond to conservative treatment.

## Posterior Periostitis/Dancer's Heel

Posterior periostitis (dancer's heel) or bruising of the periosteum at the back of the lower tibia is seen commonly in ballet dancers due to excessive flexion (plantarflexion) at the ankle joint. The patient complains of pain at the back of the heel during plantiflexion. The condition should be differentiated from Achilles bursitis, pinching of the os trigonum, bone-spurs, fractures and partial tears (Ombregt, Bisschop, ter Veer and Van de Velde 1995).

### Treatment

Local needling at the posterior articular margin of the tibia and herbal soaks are helpful. For severe symptoms, Sarapin or steroid infiltration is needed.

## Anterior Periostitis

Anterior periostitis or bruising of the anterior margin of the tibia and pressure of the tibia on the talar neck during extreme dorsiflexion can be seen in gymnasts landing flat on the feet, but with the knees bent so that the ankle is forced into extreme dorsiflexion. This type of injury also can cause subtalar and cuboid subluxations, and tendinitis in the posterior tibialis muscle (Ombregt, Bisschop, ter Veer and Van de Velde 1995).

### Treatment

Local needling at the anterior articular margin of the tibia and herbal soaks are helpful. For severe symptoms, Sarapin or steroid infiltration is needed.

# The Midfoot

The midfoot is formed by the five tarsal bones: navicular, cuboid and the three cuneiforms. Together they form the midtransverse arch, with the navicular functioning as the keystone (Figure 11-80).

## Movements of the Midtarsal Joints

Passive movements at this joint are: flexion/extension, pronation/supination, and abduction/adduction. For normal and efficient toe-off the midfoot or midtarsal joints are loose packed during the swing phase of gait. This results in energy accumulation, and allows the foot to clear the ground and become close packed with supination as the foot begins to plant for

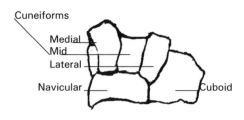

*Figure 11-80:*  Midfoot.

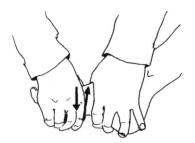

*Figure 11-82:*  Tarsometatarso anteroposterior glide.

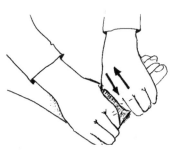

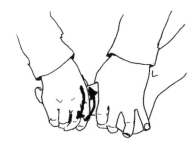

*Figure 11-83:*  Tarsometatarso rotation.

*Figure 11-81:*  Midtarsal anteroposterior glide.

normal and stable weight-bearing (Brown 1995).

Joint play movement at the *midtarsal* joints is anteroposterior (superoinferior) glide (Mennell *ibid*), (Figure 11-81).

At the *tarsometatarsal* joints joint play movements are (Mennell *ibid*):

**1.** Anteroposterior glide.

Assessed by having the practitioner stabilize the midtarsal bones and mobilize the metatarsal bones, plantarward (Figure 11-82).

**2.** Rotation.

Assessed by having the practitioner stabilize the midtarsal bones and mobilize the metatarsal bones into eversion and inversion (Figure 11-83).

### Capsular Pattern

The capsular pattern at the midtarsal joints (talonavicular, calcaneocuboid and tarsometatarsal) is increasing limitation of inversion (adduction, supination, plantiflexion) more than dorsiflexion. Peroneal muscle spasm can result and lead to a fixed abducted and pronated midfoot. A capsular pattern is seen in patients with acute, subacute or chronic arthritis. Often the patient who has degenerative arthritis is overweight and about 50 years old. An isolated strain can be the cause, as well (Ombregt, Bisschop, ter Veer and Van de Velde 1995).

### *Treatment*

Treatments are similar to those used for arthritis in the ankle joints. Taping the

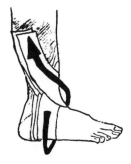

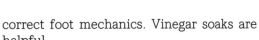

*Figure 11-85:* Manipulation technique for subluxed cuboid.

*Figure 11-84:* Taping technique for the midtarsal joint.

correct foot mechanics. Vinegar soaks are helpful.

heel in varus and midtarsal joint in supination (by a figure-of-eight strap) is helpful (Figure 11-84). An orthotic with a medial wedge can be helpful, as well (Ombregt, Bisschop, ter Veer and Van de Velde 1995).

## Noncapsular Pattern

Sprains and degenerative instability are a common cause of midfoot disorders, frequently resulting from movement of the talus due to ankle and foot sprains. The talus can move forward, straining the midtarsal joints and ligaments and leading to cuboid and navicular subluxations. This pattern also can result from wearing high-heeled shoes. Midtarsal dysfunction often results in strain of the halucis longus and tibialis posterior muscles (Ombregt, Bisschop, ter Veer and Van de Velde 1995).

### Treatment

Joint dysfunctions and ligamentous adhesions are treated by manual techniques. Ligaments are often inflamed, and oral and topical medications are helpful. To increase stability, periosteal needling or prolotherapy is used. Electrical stimulation is used to train the short plantiflexor and invertor muscles, and orthotics are used to

## Cuboid Subluxation

Subluxation and rotation of the cuboid on the calcaneus is the most common midfoot dysfunction. It can result from traumatic sprains or a short and tight peroneus longus muscle which pulls on the cuboid, rotating the lateral side upwards (Ombregt, Bisschop, ter Veer and Van de Velde 1995). The tibialis posterior, which inserts in part at the plantar medial cuboid, often needs attention as well.

### Treatment

Treatment is by manipulative reduction. The calcanous-cuboid and spring ligament (in patients with a flat foot) are needled or injected.

Manipulation is performed with the patient prone and with the dysfunctional leg off the side of table. The practitioner stands at the side of table, holding the patient's foot. The practitioner:

1. Grips the forefoot with two hands and with thumbs over the plantar surface of the cuboid. He then reinforces one thumb with the thumb of his other hand.

2. Engages the barrier, and with a slight whipping motion, pushes dorsally with his thumbs (Figure 11-85).

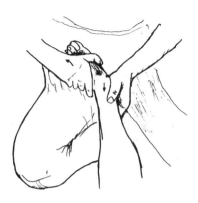

*Figure 11-86:* Manipulation technique for subluxed navicular.

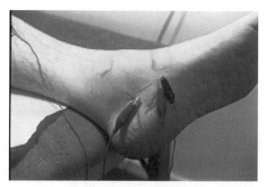

*Figure 11-87:* Treating the plantar ligaments.

Performing the maneuver in a standing patient may be preferable with a stiff joint.

## Navicular Subluxation

Rotation of the navicular on the talus can result in medial arch dysfunction. A weak calcanous-novicular ligament (spring ligament) can result in a flat foot (Ombregt, Bisschop, ter Veer and Van de Velde 1995), and increase tension on the tibialis posterior which also lends some support the spring ligament and arch.

### Treatment

For manipulative reduction the patient is supine with the foot at the edge of table. The practitioner is at the end of the table. He:

1. Grasps the neck of the talus between the web of the thumb and the index finger.

2. Surrounds the tasal navicular joint with the thumb web of his other (distal hand) hand.

3. (When engaging the joint barrier) Makes a quick movement of the distal hand against the proximal hand to mobilize the joint (Figure 11-86).

**PERIOSTEAL ACUPUNCTURE**. Stabilizing the planter ligaments with periosteal acupuncture or prolotherapy is needed often in recurrent dislocations of the navicular or cuboid (Figure 11-87).

## Forwardly Talus Subluxation

For manipulative reduction the patient is supine with the hip and knee flexed to 90°. The practitioner:

1. Adducts the patient's leg slightly, holding the lower leg.

2. Grasps the neck of the talus between the web of the thumb and the index finger, with his other hand.

3. Finds the loose pack position and thrusts with the hand over the talus posteriorly (Figure 11-66 on page 587).

Alternatively, the patient lies prone and the knee and ankle are flexed to 90°. The practitioner:

1. Cups his hands around the talus.

2. Applies some effort to extend and distract the joint.

3. Rocks the talus within the ankle joint posteriorly (Figure 11-89).

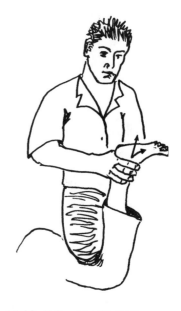

*Figure 11-89:* Talar and ankle joints mobilization.

# The Forefoot

The forefoot is composed of the metatarsals, phalanges and soft tissues of the forefoot (Figure 11-88).

Disorders are mainly related to arthritic lesions. The first ray commonly develops a hallux valgus deformity, probably due to breakdown of foot mechanics and tension in the flexors and long extensors of the big toe which pull the big toe into further adduction. Increased tension on the joint results in an inflamed bursa (bunion), (Brown *ibid*).

Joint play at the *distal intermetatarsal* joints is (Mennell *ibid*):

1. Anteroposterior glide.

2. Rotation.

## Capsular Pattern

The capsular pattern of the first metatarsophalangeal joint is slight limitation of flexion and marked limitation of extension. The capsular pattern in the outer four metatarsophalangeal joints is more limita-

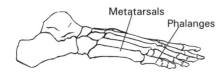
Metatarsals
Phalanges

*Figure 11-88:* Forefoot.

tion of flexion than extension. The joints can be affected by traumatic, osteo, rheumatoid and gouty arthritis (Cyriax *ibid*).

### Treatment

Local needling, herbal soaks, medications and orthotics are helpful in the treatment of capsular disorders.

**HERBAL THERAPY.** For acute inflammatory condition (gout, rheumatoid arthritis etc.) a guiding formula for oral and topical use is:

> Flos Loncerae (Jin Yin Hua)
> Wild Chrysanthemum (Ye Ju Hua)
> Herba Taraxaci (Pu Gong Ying)
> Herba Viola (Zi Hua Di Ding)
> Radix Angelica Sinensis (Dang Gui)
> Resina Olibani (Ru Xiang)
> Resina Myrrhae (Mo Yao)
> Radix Salviae (Dan Shen)
> Peony Rubra (Chi Shao)
> Radix Scutellaria (Huang Qin)
> Achyranthes Bid (Niu Xi)
> Radix Rhemanniae (Sheng Di)
> Tripterygium Wilfordii (Lei Gong Teng) (with vitamines B6 and B12)

Radix Glycyrrhizae (Gan Cao)

A guiding formula for arthrosis and bunions is:

Radix Astragali (Huang Qi)

Radix Codonopsis (Dang Shen)

Radix Angelica Sinensis (Dang Gui)

Radix Salvia (Dan Shen)

Radix Achyranthes Bidentata (Niu Xi)

Radix Peony Rubra (Chi Shao)

Radix Peony Alba (Bai Shao)

Ramulus Cinnamomi (Gui Zhi)

Fructus Chaenomelis (Mu Gua)

Radix Ophiopogonis (Mai Dong)

Loranthus Parasiticus (Shang Ji Sheng)

Radix Morindae (Ba Ji Tian)

Fructus Lycii (Gao Qi Zi)

Radix Rehmannia praeparata (Shu Di)

Ramulus Mori (Sang Zhi)

Radix Glycyrrhizae (Gan Cao)

## Sesmoiditis

Sesmoiditis or inflammation at the sesmao-first-metatarsal joint can result from over-use or traumatic causes. Patients with rigid feet and shortened calf muscles are at risk. Resisted flexion of the hallux can be painful (Ombregt, Bisschop, ter Veer and Van de Velde 1995).

### Treatment

Treatment is with anti-inflammatory methods. Supporting the metatarsal joint and raising a horizontal heel is helpful. A forefoot and rearfoot valgus post can be used to prolong weight-bearing on the lateral foot (Horwitz personal communication).

## Hallux Valgus

Hallux valgus (Figure 11-90) is a static subluxation of the first metatarsophalangeal joint. Hallux valgus is characterized by valgus deviation of the great toe and varus deviation of the first metatarsal and is seen most frequently in shoe-wearing societies, especially in females. Pronation of the foot has been implicated in the development of the hallux valgus, which can result in increased pressure on the medial border of the hallux and deformation of the capsular structures. Other, less common causes are congenital, stroke, and collagen diseases (Ombregt, Bisschop, ter Veer and Van de Velde 1995).

No correlation between the degree of valgus deformity and the severity of symptoms exists. The condition may be aggravated by high heeled and pointed shoes. Imbalance between the adductor hallucis and abductor hallucis and contraction of the flexors and long extensor muscles of the toe, which act like a bowstring, shift the toe into adduction. This results in shifting of toe-off phase of gait to the second toe. A painful bursa can form (bunion) (Brown 1995).

### Treatment

An orthotic that limits pronation together with medial forefoot posting can elevate the first ray off the foot, so that the toe can drop into a more correct position and help take the stress off the second toe (Ombregt, Bisschop, ter Veer and Van de Velde 1995). Needling and stretching the adductor hallucis, flexors and extensors of the big toe are helpful (Figure 11-91). The abductor hallucis is strengthened by electrical stimulation.

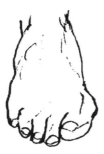

*Figure 11-90:* Hallux valgus.

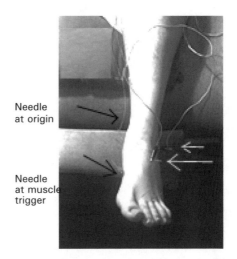

Needle
at origin

Needle
at muscle
trigger

*Figure 11-91:* Strengthening of the abductor hallucis muscle by deep medial approach electroacupuncture (black arrows). Strengthening the extensor hallucis (white arrows).

## Functional Hallux Limitus & Hallux Rigidus

Functional hallux limitus is a momentary locking of the first ray joint (great toe) just at the time when the body moves past the planted foot, resulting in limited extension of the toe during the propulsion phase of gait. This limitation results from a deformity of the first metatarsophalangeal joint (MTP), in which the base of the proximal phalanx of the hallux is subluxed plantarly upon the first met-head, on weight-bearing. Further trauma to the joint can result in proliferative changes which ultimately can lead to ankylosis of the first MTP—called hallux rigidus (Brown 1995).

### THE POSSIBLE CAUSES OF HALLUX LIMITUS ARE:

• Hypermobility of the first ray, in conjunction with eversion of the foot caused by abnormal subtalar joint pronation.

• Immobilization of the first ray.

• Excessively long first metatarsal.

• Dorsiflexed first ray.

• Degenerative joint disease.

• Trauma.

A hallux limitus results in secondary alterations and adaptations which have profound abnormal biomechanical effects up the lower kinetic chain, causing problems at the hip, pelvis, and lumbar spine (Brown 1995).

### Treatment

The most common cause of mild to moderate hallux limitus is everted forefoot relative to the ground by abnormal subtalar joint pronation. The first ray is hypermobile, and ground reaction maintains it in a dorsiflexed position during propulsion. A functional orthotic with a Kinetic Wedge™,, which is designed to restore normal timing and sagittal plane function on the first MTP joint, is said to be effective. When the first MTP joint becomes stiff (in weight-bearing), mobilization may be required (Figure 11-92).

## Chronic Metatarsalgia

Chronic metatarsalgia results in pain at the plantar aspects of the foot. It affects the middle and three toes and arises when the metatarsal heads have to bear a disproportionate amount of the body's weight. The condition occurs in patient's with:

- Splay foot.
- Plantar deformity.
- High heels.
- Pes cavus deformity.
- Weak flexor muscles.
- Dancer's metatarsalgia (Ombregt et al. *ibid*).

The patient usually complains of pain at the plantar aspect of the forefoot on standing and walking, relieved by rest.

Examination shows pain at the end of dorsiflexion, sometimes at the end of both dorsiflexion and plantiflexion. The met-heads are tender.

### *Treatment*

Treatment consists of reducing stresses on the forefoot. High heels must have a horizontal surface which will bring more weight onto the rearfoot and prevents the foot from sliding forwards. A metatarsal pad is fitted into the shoe, or orthotic, with the thickest part stopping just behind the met-heads.

In patients with splay foot or after a long stay in bed, vigorous strengthening of the short flexor muscles of the toes by exercises and electrical stimulation is necessary, so that the toes flex properly at each step in order to take most of the body weight during walking (Ombregt, Bisschop, ter Veer and Van de Velde 1995).

Anti-inflammatory methods are helpful, as well.

## Interdigital Neuritis, Morton's Metatarsalgia (Neuroma)

In the later part of the stance phase preceding toe-off, extension occurs at the metatarsophalangeal joint. A compression of the interdigital nerves can occur under the intermetatarsal ligament leading to interdigital neuritis. Morton's metatarsalgia is caused by a neuroma at the interdigital nerve between the third and fourth toes (it may be found between the fourth and fifth toe as well). The patient complains usually of sudden sharp and unexpected pain at the outer side of the forefoot. The pain resolves on its own after several minutes. The patient may experience many or few such episodes; frequency tends to increase with time (Ombregt, Bisschop, ter Veer and Van de Velde 1995).

### *Treatment*

Any underlying mechanical dysfunctions are addressed. A metatarsal pad positioned just proximal to the metatarsal heads can prevent hyperextension and spread the transverse arch, therefore reducing pressure on the nerve. Alternatively, a small support under the head of the fourth toe which lifts the bone keeping it out of line with the third toe may be helpful.

## Stress Fractures

A stress fracture is defined as a partial or complete fracture of bone due to its inability to withstand nonviolent stresses applied in a rhythmic, repeated and sub-threshold manner. The clinical diagnosis of stress fracture is especially important since histopathologic and radiographic findings may not correlate with the clinical symptoms. It is commonplace to have normal radiographs but with a positive bone scan.

Stress fractures occur in the metatarsals, lateral malleolus, medial malleolus, calcaneus, talus, navicular and sesamoid.

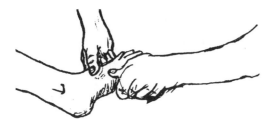

*Figure 11-92:* Mobilization of first ray.

The metatarsals are by far the most commonly affected.

Diagnosis is achieved by history, physical exam (with tenderness revelling the most), X-ray, bone scan (the gold standard), tomography and CT scans (Brown 1995).

### Treatment

Most stress fractures are treated by rest and partial immobilization. Since abnormal stresses often are due to foot mechanics, an orthotic usually is helpful. Local needling with electric stimulation and herbal medication are helpful.

# High & Low Arch Feet[3]

Biomechanics and foot structure have long-reaching effects on the entire body frame.

## Talipes Equino Varus

Dr. Horwitz has named the Talipes Equino Varus foot by the name "Heidi" because it is a high arch foot and the name Heidi is easy to remember. According to Dr. Horwitz, a patient who has a Heidi foot can present with some of the following physical characteristics and complaints:

- Occipital or frontal headaches.
- Stiff neck with limited and painful forward bending.
- Extended neck that sits forward on the thoracic spine.
- Slouched stance with a hyperkypotic thoracic spine.
- Reduced and painful shoulder movement on extension.
- Internally rotated shoulders.
- Bilateral tight iliopsoas and piriformis muscles.
- Hyperlordotic lumbar spine.
- Coccyx pain that mimics a sciatic lesion by radiating down the back of the legs.
- Posterior knee pain.
- Chronic Achilles tendinitis.
- Balanced stance over the balls of feet (standing on the toes and having difficulty bringing heels to the ground).
- Shortened plantar fascia.
- Burning in the balls of the feet.

A patient who has a Heidi foot tends to be muscularly stiff, probably a good runner, comfortable in high heel shoes and unlikely to stand for any period of time. X-rays show calcaneal inclination angle of greater than 18°. This angle is measured weight-bearing, with the beam aimed at the talo-navicular joint.

### Treatment

The goal of foot treatments is to bring the ground to the body, as opposed to bringing the body to the ground.

**EXERCISE.** The patient should stretch his/her tight muscles daily to correct the muscles' pull on the osseous frame. The essential muscles are the *gastrocnemius* of the leg, *biceps* of the thigh, *psoas* of the pelvis, upper *trapezium* of the shoulder and *short*

3. This section is written by Lennord Horwitz DPM.

*deep extensor* of the neck. Strengthening of synergistic muscles can only be done after lengthening and stretching of the tight muscles. The practitioner must pay particular attention to muscles that move the scapula posteriorly and stretch the anterior chest wall. A simple, but effective, home exercise that moves the scapula back and stretches out the deltoid muscle is lifting a broom handle, or weighted barbells, or even a chair from behind the back, several times a day.

For Janda's *Untercross lesion,* standing with balls of the feet on stairs while letting the heels sink to the floor (for at east 90 seconds) can release the *golgi mechanism* in the posterior muscle column. This exercise allows the calf muscles to relax and stretch. The hip joint comes in line with the coronal plane of the body and centers the pelvis and the head over the feet. In addition, it brings the head over the spine by allowing the body to balance over the *calcaneal-cuboid* joint of the foot.

To keep the plantar muscles and joints supple, the patient can use a rolling pin covered with foam to stroke the bottoms of the feet. This massage stroke should be soft and go from the toes to the heel. It has an additional benefit of stimulating the lost pedal skin reflexes necessary for normal proprioception.

**MANIPULATION.** Heidi's ankle architecture results in reduced extension range of motion. To increase the range of motion at the ankle joint, an extension and distraction manipulation maneuver is important. The patient lies prone and the knee and ankle are flexed to 90°. The practitioner:

1. Cups his hands around the upper part of the ankle.

2. Applies some effort to extend and distract the joint.

3. Rocks the ankle from extension into flexion several times while still distracting the joint (Figure 11-89 on page 599).

This places the talus in the ankle mortise and allows for better foot and ankle movement in the toe-off phase of walking.

**NEUROTHERAPY.** Neurotherapy is an effective treatment of some of Heidi's back and leg complaints. This is because the nerve branch in the area between the third and fourth toes contains all the elements of the sciatic nerve. Most nerves in the foot are either of the S-1 or L-5 dermatome, sclerotome pattern. The third plantar intermetatarsal nerve picks up fibers from both nerve branches and possibly being the end nerve (of the end nerve) of the sciatic nerve. Multiple acupuncture and reflex points exist in this general region of the foot.

**NERVE BLOCKS.** The injection of 1% procaine into the perineural tissues on the affected limb often affords relief from sciatic and muscular-type pain. The practitioner must keep in mind that this pain between the toes, and the positive Tinnel's sign, are probably not a true Morton's neuroma. If surgery is performed, the post operative review usually indicates that this is a hypertrophy of the neurolemma of the involved nerve. In a case study done during the Korean War, a large percentage of the postmortem-studies showed that the hypertrophied neurolemma was a frequent finding, even in normal feet. The practitioner's aim should be to keep Heidi out of the hands of the surgeon.

**ORTHOTIC THERAPY.** Orthotic therapy can be used either by itself or with all or some of the other treatment regimes. The purpose of the orthotics is to bring the ground to the body and to increase the lack of shock absorption in Heidi feet. This can be accomplished by using an orthotic that raises the heel cephalically with materials that absorb the shock generated by the foot striking the ground. A *Pelit* and *Crepe* combination orthotic, or a semi-rigid plastic orthotic, ending behind the metatarsal heads, generally accomplishes both goals.

Shoes and sneakers in which the heel is higher than the ball of the foot are recommended. Women can wear highheeled shoes and men can wear cowboy boots with a riding heel.

## Pes Valgo Planus

Pes Valgo Planus the counterpart to the Heidi foot was named Lois by Dr. Horwitz. Lois is a low arch foot which is often referred to as a falling arch foot. Although a Lois foot looks like a low arch or falling arch foot, it should never be considered a flat foot.

The patient who has a Pes Valgo Planus or Lois foot has physical manifestations of:

• Temporal headaches.

• A one-sided stiff neck that at times is painful when bent.

• Stands straight.

• Hypokyphotic thoracic spine.

• One shoulder that is anteriorly rotated and sometimes painful.

• Unilaterally tight Iliopsoas and piriformis muscles.

• Hip and mid-back pain, lumbar 2-5 pain that radiates down the outside of the leg.

• Torqued pelvis.

• Medial knee pain.

• Chronic shin splints.

• Chronically sprained ankles.

• Arch pain or *plantar fasciitis*.

• Heel pain.

Lois's center of gravity is higher on the back than Heidi's. In modern times the Lois foot presents with reduced skin proprioception and ligamentous resiliency. With loss of proprioception and the reciprocal ground reaction force, the muscles fatigue more quickly and become irritable easily. As the ligaments lose strength the Lois foot weakens. The muscles that hold up the arch also weaken, and then the arch collapses. The internal collapse of the long-limb arch allows the pelvic girdle to internally sublux and rotate on the sacrum. In response to the sacral torque, the back, neck and head become unstable.

For a Lois patient to pull his/her legs from the ground while walking, he or she must hyper-rotate and sidebend the middle lumbar spines. This movement weakens the lumbar ligaments and causes the *costa-lumbar fascia* and associative muscles (*quadratus lumborum and erector spinalis*) to become spastic and shortened on the long-limbed side, as a means of lifting the other leg from the ground. A predictable domino effect in the upper torso causes a sidebend and misalignment to the osteoarticular and ligamentous structure of the lumbar and lower thoracic spines, shoulder and neck.

The implosion of the medial or spring arch causes protective muscular splinting, plantar fasciitis, and other muscle imbalances. These are often associated with Janda's *Untercross lesion*. As the foot structure slides forward and downward, the navicular can no longer act as the keystone to the foot. This causes the following in the foot's domelike structure:

• The cuboid-calcaneal joint rotates, subluxes and collapses on itself.

• The peroneus bravis, tertius and longus muscles no longer have the necessary fulcrum in the foot to help stabilize the leg and low back.

• The results are gluteus maximus weakness and lateral bant or tensor fascia pain.

Myofascial and structural disorganization are almost always associated with this foot lesion.

X-ray examination of a Lois foot reveals a calcaneal inclination angle of 12 to 18°, measured on a weight bearing X-ray with the beam aimed at the talo-navicular joint.

*Treatment*

Lois-type body structure is very amenable to repair and stabilization. The goal of the treatment is to strengthen the dorsal muscle groups and reestablish foot motion and spatial proprioception, which in turn helps effect more efficient body movements.

**MUSCULAR TREATMENT.** Muscular treatment should focus on strengthening the postural muscles:

- *Peroneal* of the leg.
- *Tensor fascia lata* of the thigh.
- *Psoas* of the pelvis.
- Lower *trapezium* of the shoulder.
- Short, deep, *extensor muscles* of the neck.

Faradic current to the involved muscles can reintroduce the twitch reflex. This reflex has decayed due to muscle overuse and fatigue. It has been reported that after treatment of 6 to 10 minutes, Russian Stimulation current (a variation of faradic current) can strengthen the muscle fibers for up to nine months.

Patients benefit from exercise programs using isotonics, isometrics, and free weights. Although running and swimming might increase endurance, they are not helpful in the overall muscle patterning or posture.

Proprioceptive training by the use of the rebounder or minitramp is particularly helpful. This returns visual and postural integration while improving posture and muscle strength.

**MANIPULATION.** The foot's mid-tarsal architecture has an increased rotary range of motion. A *cuboid-calcaneal* dysfunction and an excessive rotation of the talus and ankle joint are seen. The *superior fibulotibial* joint is subluxed, and the ASIS is anteriorly displaced and externally rotated. Appropriate manipulative procedures and flexible restrictive bandaging are important and necessary parts of the treatment. Dr. John Mennel describes these procedures well in his book, *Foot Pain*, as does Phill Greenman, D.O., who shows these techniques in his videotapes.

**PROLOTHERAPY.** Prolotherapy of the involved ligaments of the foot and ankle is both beneficial and essential. The foot ligaments which are most lax are those that correspond to the control of excessive motions and their associated muscle fatigue. These ligaments and associative muscles are:

- Talo-navicular or short spring ligaments. Anterior and posterior tibial muscles.
- Plantar mid-tarsal ligaments. Peroneus longus and post tibial muscles.
- Plantar mid-tarsal ligaments. Plantar fascia and halluces brevis muscle.

Special attention should be given to the *dorsal cuboid cuneiform* articular ligament. Also involved is the *peroneus brevis* muscle. The breakdown of the synergism between the *peroneus brevis* and *gluteus medius* muscles produces hip pains.

During examination the practitioner might find other ligaments that are lax in the foot, leg and ankle that may need to be treated.

**ORTHOTIC THERAPY.** The purpose of orthotics for a Lois foot is to stabilize the mid-tarsal joint of the foot and realign the body's coronal plane. This helps in weight transference and muscle balance. Ideally, the feel of the foot ground is imitated, helping restore the lost proprioception. The orthotics should end at the toe's sulcus and should be made from a combination of Pelite and Crepe, cork, or thin elastic plastic. Many podiatry physicians use a more rigid orthotic, (e.g. rigid plastics, etc.) which is useful if the practitioner does not use prolotherapy. However, the use of rigid orthotics can result in three unwanted effects:

1. Disuse atrophy of the intrinsic muscles of the foot from the immobilization.

2. Loss of the skin's proprioception from the unyielding concrete-like composite of the orthotic.

**3.** Loss of shock absorption causing unrecognized symptoms (e.g., knee, hip, and back pain).

There has been much discussion and advertisement about shoe gear. A Lois foot can wear any shoe that is comfortable, new, and long enough to accommodate the orthotics. The best way to regain pedal proprioceptive response is to go barefoot at every opportunity.

*Summary*

The two types of feet presented here can be considered to be pure types. However, rarely do we ever see mechanical problems that do not have mixed physical findings. In practice the practitioner sees feet and body types that have some essential components of both High Arched and Low Arched feet. This can be due to the body's compensation for the long limb, versus the short limb, syndrome. Table 11-10 on page 607 summarizes the Heidi and Lois foot types.

*Table 11-10.* **TALIPES EQUINO VARUS (HEIDI) AND PES VALGO PLANUS (LOIS)**

|  | **TALIPES EQUINO VARUS (HEIDI)** | **PES VALGO PLANUS (LOIS)** |
|---|---|---|
| Coronal Plane | Frontal | Posterior |
| Cranial | Inhalation | Exhalation |
| Vision | Skyward | Earthbound |
| Teeth | Over-Bite | Under-Bite |
| Ligaments | Tight | Loose |
| TMJ | Bilateral | Unilateral (long side) |
| Neck | Egyptian | Centered |
| Shoulder | Inward | Squared |
| Upper Back | Hyperkyposis | Straight |
| Lower Back | Hyperlordotic | Torque |
| Lower Back | Hyperlordotic | Torque |
| Pelvic Girdle | Narrow | Wide |
| Gait | Straight or Toed in | External or Toed out |
| Thigh Muscles | Tight Biceps Femoris Spastic Rectus Femoris; Tight Pectineus | Tight Adductors and Vastus Lateralis Painful Tensor Fascia Lata |
| Knee | Posterior and Lateral Pain | Anterior and Medial Pain |
| Leg Muscles | Tight Triceps Surri Spastic Posterior Tibial Muscle | Weak Peroneal; Overused Post Tibial Weak Anterior; Tibial Muscle |
| Ankle Joint | Talus Posterior and Superior in Mortise | Anterior and Medial Plantar Rotation |
| Weight-Bearing | Ball of Foot | Heel |
| Toes | Nonfixed Hammer Toes | Fixed Hammer Toes |
| Foot Pain | Ball of Foot | Heel |
| Applied Kinesiology | Strong with Heel Raise Bilateral | Strong with Unilateral Heel and Opposite Toe Raise |

# Appendix A: *Nutrition*

Nutrition plays an important role in musculoskeletal disorders. Not only in keeping the body's tissues and systems healthy, but also therapeutically. Table AP-1 through Table AP-10 summarizes some of the literature on nutritional and botanical medicine.

*Table AP-1.* **ANALGESIA**

| | |
|---|---|
| THIAMINE | At very high doses (10-30gm) produces ganglionic blockade and suppresses the transmission of neural stimuli to skeletal muscles (Lenot 1966). Oral supplementation may be beneficial as well (Quirin 1986) |
| PYRIDOXINE | Necessary for making serotonin and supplementation may be effective (Bernstein1990)<br>May be beneficial in chronic pain patient as they often have decreased serotonin levels |
| VITAMIN B12 | May be beneficial in vertebral pain and degenerative neuropathy (Hieber 1974;Dettori, Ponari 1973)<br>Reported effective in the treatment of bursitis |
| ASCORBIC ACID | Supplementation may have analgesic effects (Hanck, Weiser 1985; Creagan et al. 1979) |
| VITAMIN E | Supplementation may have analgesic effect by activating the endorphin system(*ibid*) |
| VITAMIN K1 | Supplementation may have analgesic effects (Hanck, Weiser 1985) |
| GERANIUM SESPUIOXIDE | May enhance morphine analgesia (Hachisu M et al. 1983) |
| SELENIUM | Deficiency may be associated with muscle pain (Van Rij et al. 1979) |
| COPPER | Deficiency may lower enkephalin levels affecting pain perception (Bhathena S et al. 1986) |
| D-PHENYLALANINE (DPA) | Inhibits carboxypeptidase A which is involved in enkephalin degradation. May be potentiated by prostaglandin inhibitors. DPA supplementation may be beneficial and potentiate acupuncture analgesia (Balagot et al. 1983; Kitade T et al.1988) |
| L-TRYPTOPHAN | Is a precursor to serotonin which is one of the neurotransmitters involved in pain perception. Supplementation may have analgesic effects (Liberman et al. 1983) |

*Table AP-2.* **ANALGESIA (BOTANICALS)**

| | |
|---|---|
| **CAPSICUM FRUTESSCENS** | The active ingredient in hot pepper. Shown effective in neuropathic pain by blocking small-diameter pain fibers (C-fibers) by depleting them of substance P. Used in treatment of post-herpetic neuralgia, trigeminal neuralgia and diabetic neuropathy and arthritis (Cordell, Araujo 1993) |
| **TUMERIC** | The active ingredient called curcumin, may work in similar ways as capsicum. Used for its analgesic, anti-inflammatory and enhancement of micro-circulation (Patacchini, Maggi and Mel 1990) |
| **CIMICIFUGA HERACLEFOLIA** | H2O extracts of the herb show analgesic effects with visamnol being the strongest. (Shigata 1977) |
| **CORYDALIS TURTSCHANINOVII** | The entire herb has analgesic effects. d-corydaline and L-coridalis showing analgesic properties. dl-tetrahydropalmatine an alkaloid found in the herb is a potent analgesic being approximately 50% as effective as morphine (Jiang et al. 1958) |
| **GINGER (ZINGIBER)** | Administration may be effective in chronic muscular (rheumatic) discomfort (Srivastava and Mustafa 1992). Often used for pain that increases with cold rainy weather |
| **ACONITUM CHINESE** | Ethanol extracts have marked analgesic effects (Su et al.1959) Crystalline delvaconitine developed from the alkaloids has local surface anesthesia twice the strength of cocaine (Jin et al. 1957). Aconitum is used often both topically and orally in many painful disorders |
| **BUFO GARGARIZANS (TOAD VENOM)** | 80% ethanol extract of the venom has a strong local anesthetic effect. Stronger and more persistent than that of cocaine, Bufalin being approximately 90 times stronger then cocaine (Suga 1976) Extracts can be used as an alternative local anesthetics |
| **ANGELICA SINENSIS** | Aqueous extract has anti-inflammatory/analgesic effects 1.1 stronger then sodium acetylsalicylate (type of aspirin). Like sodium acetylsalicylate it suppressed the release of inflammatory factors (e.g., 5-HT) from platelets (Yi 1980) |
| **ANGELICA PUBESCENS** | Shows analgesic and anti-inflammatory effects in animal models (Feng Jiangxi and Yirao 1961) |

*Table AP-3.* **ARTHRITIS**

| | |
|---|---|
| **NIACINAMIDE** | Effective in osteoarthritis (Kaufman 1955) |
| **PANTOTHENIC ACID** | Together with B complex may be beneficial in the treatment of arthritis (Annand 1962, although a larger study did not show benefit (63% of patients with osteoarthritis) (General Practitioner Research Group 1980) |
| **VITAMIN C** | May be beneficial based on the pathophysiology (Bland, Cooper 1984) |
| **VITAMIN E** | May inhibit prostaglandins (White 1977) |
| **BORON** | Intake may be inversely related to incidence of osteoarthritis (De Fabio 1990), supplementation may be beneficial (Travers, et al 1990) |
| **SELENIUM** | Levels measured as glutathione peroxidase (a selenium-containing enzyme) may be low in patients with osteoarthritis (Jameson et al. 1985). Supplementation with vitamin E may be beneficial (Jameson S et al 1985) |
| **SULFUR** | A sulfur containing amino-acid (Sullivan and Hess 1935).<br>May be reduced as measured by cystine<br>Supplementation may be beneficial (woldenberg 1935 |
| **ZINC** | Serum levels may be low in patients with arthritis (Greenman et al. 1980) |
| **GLUCOSAMINE SULFATE** | A building block of proteoglycans, the ground substance of articular cartilage. Inhibits the degradation of proteoglycans in contrast to NSAID's which can facilitate such degradation (Vidal, Plana et al 1978). The sulfate component appears to potentiate its therapeutic effect (D'Ambrosio et al 1981). Shown in several studies to be effective in osteoarthritis (especially of the knees) (Werback 1995) |
| **CHONDROITIN SULFATES** | Long-chain polymers of a repeating disaccharide unit; galactodamine sulfate and glucuronic acid. In quantitative amounts they are the major GAG (see below) found in cartilage. Chondroitin sulfate may inhibit degenerative enzymes and reduce atherosclerosis. This may improve nutrient supply to cartilage (Bucci 1984). The oral absorbtion of chondroitin sulfate is still unclear as there are conflicting reports (Andermann, Dietz 1982; Prino 1989). Both oral and intramuscular injections were found effective in osteoarthritis (Prudden and Balassa 1987) |
| **GLYCOSAMINOGLYCANS (GAG)** | Found in cartilage tissue and may be effective both in osteo and rheumatoid arthritis. High Molecular weight GAG-peptide complex is effective (Rejhole 1987). Dried shark cartilage is effective (Jose 1989) |
| **CARTILAGE EXTRACTS** | Inhibit neovascularisation (Moses, Subhalter, Langer 1990), thought to be involved in osteoathritic process (Brown and Weiss 1988) |
| **FATTY ACIDS** | Supplementation may be beneficial. Omega-3 are used most frequently (Stammers T et al 1989) |
| **S-ADENOSYL-METHIONINE (SAME)** | Produced from L-methionine and ATP through the action of methionine-adenosyl-trasferase may be as effective as NSAID's with less side-effects.(Padova 1987) |
| **SOD** | Unpublished studies by a manufacturer have shown some benefit by oral administration. Other studies have shown benefit when SOD was injected (Flohe et al 1980) |

*Table AP-4.* **ARTHRITIS (BOTANICALS)**

| | |
|---|---|
| **BOSWELLIA SERRATA (SEE INFLAMMATION)** | Effective in a variety of animal models of arthritis (Reddy, Chandrakasan and Dhar 1989; Singh and Atal 1986) |
| **BROMELAIN (ALSO SEE INFLAMMATION)** | A sulfur containing proteolytic enzymes or proteases obtained from the stem of pineapple plant may be beneficial (Cohen and Goldman 1964) |
| **CAPSAICIN** | see pain |
| **DEVIL'S CLAW (HARPAGOPHYTUM PROCUMBENS)** | May be beneficial, although reports are contradictory and may reflect the model being studied. Several studies have shown the herb not to have an anti-inflammatory effect (Moussard 1992; Mcleod, Revell and Robinson 1979; J Medecine Actuelle 1985) |

*Table AP-5.* **Inflammation (Vitamins, Minerals and fatty acids)**

| | |
|---|---|
| **Vitamin B12** | Has beneficial effects on inflammation used in bursitis (Hanck and Weiser 1985; Kelmes1957) |
| **Vitamin C** | Has anti-inflammatory activity in animals (Hanck, Wiser 1985). Supplementation may be beneficial in the treatment of subtalar bursitis (Biskind, Marin 1955). However, may worsen the stability of lysozomal membranes, allowing the enzymes to leak out of the lysozomes thus aggravate inflammation |
| **Vitamin E** | May reduce inflammation as it can inhibit both chemotaxis and chemiluminescence of activated neutrophilic granulocytes (Blankenhorn 1988). May protect lysosome and other membranes which may inhibit histamine liberation from granules of mast cells and serotonin liberation (Kamimura 1972) |
| **Vitamin K** | A strong stabilizer of the lysozome membranes in the rheumatoid synovium. Oral, IM and IV administered to rats shown to have a significant anti-inflammatory effect (Hanck and Weiser 1985) |
| **Copper** | Diminished superoxide dismutase (SOD) activity, a copper containing enzyme may contribute to development of inflammatory diseases (Sorenson 1989). Copper supplementation with copper salicylate complex may be more effective than aspirin alone (Sorenson 1980) |
| **SOD** | Anti-inflammatory when taken in adequate amounts. In equivalent weight it is more potent than dexamethazone. This enzyme is present in all red cells and many other cells in the body. It is non-toxic, even in high doses. Oral absorbtion of SOD is controversial (Werback 1988) |
| **Fatty acids** | Several fatty acids been reported to be beneficial in inflammation including Omega3, Omega 6, and $\gamma$-linolenic acid-enriched oils. They are recursors to prostaglandins a hormone like mediator of inflammation. Supplantation may change the balance of prostaglandins and leukotrienes |
| **Borage oil** | Preferable as it contains the highest amount of GLA which seems to be the most beneficial. GLA should be take with fish oils on a 1 to 10 ratio (Lee et al. 1985; Ziboh Va and Fletcher1992). Evening primrose, blackcurrent, fish, and flax seed (which also contain omega-9 fatty acids) are uses as well. |

*Table AP-6.* **INFLAMMATION (FLAVONOID COMPOUNDS AND BOTANICALS)**

| | |
|---|---|
| **HESPERIDIN METHYL CHALCONE, AND GLYCOSIDE** | Commonly used in musculoskeletal medicine. Reduce the incidence of athletic injuries (Cragin 1962) |
| **CATECHIN AND PYCNOGENOLS** | Flavonoids that affect collagen metabolism, including an increase in cross-linkage formation in normal and lathyritic collagen (Orloff, Krieg and Muller 1982; Tixier et al 1984) |
| **QUERCETIN** | Inhibits the lipoxygenase pathway of arachidonic acid metabolism (Bauman et al. 1980) |
| **ANTHOCYANOSIDES** | Extremely powerful antioxidant vascular stabilizer and anti-inflammatory compound (Lietti et al. 1976) Bilberry extracts can be used in cases of inflammation and neuropathy. |
| **PROTEOLYTIC ENZYMES** | May be beneficial for treatment of inflammation (Cichoke and Marty 1981) |
| **BOSWELLIN** | Contains oils, terpenoids and gum resin that are potent anti-inflammatory compounds that inhibit 5-lipoxygenase. In contrast to ketoprofen (an NSAID) does not affect glycosaminoglycans negatively and thus may not increase joint degeneration (Ammon and Mack et al. 1991) |
| **CURCUMIN** | Stabilizes lysosomal membranes, acts as an uncoupler of oxidative phosphorylation, releases cortisol from the adrenals and inhibits prostaglandin synthesis (Srivastava and Srimal 1973) |
| **PLANTAGO SEED** | Several extracts especially plantaglucide reduce inflammatory edema elicited by dextran (Obodencheva, Farmakologiia and Tokisikologiia 1966) |
| **EUCOMMIA ULMOIDES** | H20 extracts have anti-inflationary effects, the mechanisms of which are thought to involve enhancement of adrenocortical function (Guizhou Institute 1962). |
| **ACONITUM CARMICHAELI** | Extracts have potent anti-inflammatory effects Some studies suggest mediation of adrenal cortex (Yang et al. 1966) |
| **STEPHANIA TETRANDRA** | Extracts especially tetrandrine and demethyltetrandrine have strong anti-inflammatory action (Lu et al. 1957) |
| **TRIPTERYGIUM WILFORDII** | Extracts especially the terpenes have very strong anti-inflammatory action (Tripterygium Wilfordii Coordiating Research Group 1979). Has been shown effective in rheumatoid arthritis (Rheumatoid Arthritis Coordinating Research Group 1977) |
| **ACHYRANTHES BIDENTATA** | The alcohol extracts are anti-inflammatory and analgesic (Song et al. 1963) |
| **GENTIANA MACROPHYLL** | The entire herb has anti-inflammatory effects the mechanisms of which are thought to activate the pituitary-adenocortical function via the nervous system (Song et al. 1958). Effective in both osteo and rheumatoid arthritis (Editorial Department. National Medical Journal of China 1978) |
| **LICORICE (GLYCYRRHIZA)** | Contains about 6% glycyrrizin, which is converted into glycyrrhetinic acid, which has many pharmacological activities including anti-inflammatory properties. It can both bind to cortisol receptors and prevent degradation, thus extending the half life of endogenous cortisol. Glycyrrhizine can inhibit prostaglandin synthesis (Okimasa et al. 1983; Ohuchi et al. 1981) |

*Table AP-7.* **MUSCLE SPASM**

| | |
|---|---|
| **MINERALS** | **Calcium and Magnesium** have been used empirically in the treatment of spasm. Some individuals with carbohydrate intolerance may manifest metabolic acidosis thus. The calcium, magnesium and zinc are both excreted in the urine and deposited in the growing hair to buffer the organic acids. This leads to functional deficiency of these minerals leaves the muscles more excitable (Jonathan Write lecture) |
| **ALANGUM CHINESE** | The extracts of the herb especially its alkaloids have a significant striated muscle relaxant effects (Alangium chinese Research Group, 1970) |
| **MENISPERUM DAURICUM** | The daurisoline alkaloid isolated from the herb has a significant muscle relaxant effect on skeletal muscles (Long el al. 1979). The sinomenine alkaloid is used in neuralgias, myalgias, and acute and chronic rheumatic arthritis (Zhu 1958) |
| **STEPHANIA TETRANDRA** | All the alkaloids are striated muscle relaxants (Basic Research Group 1972). Mostly used in conditions affecting the low back and lower extremities |
| **CORYDALIS TURTSCHANINOVII** | The methyltetrahydropalmatine bromide alkaloid has significant muscle relaxant action. It acts postsynaptically and is antagonized by neostigmine (a cholinergic agonist) (Chen et al. 1978) |
| **KAVA KAVA** (PIPER METHYSTICUM) | The extracts have muscle relaxant activity. This action may be due to central and peripheral action (Lindenberg, Pitule-Scodel 1990; Singh 1983) |

*Table AP-8.* **WOUND HEALING AND TISSUE STRENGTH (VITAMINS, MINERALS, HERBS)**

| | |
|---|---|
| **PANTOTHENIC ACID** | Supplementing may hasten the normal healing process, it may increase aponeurosis strength post surgically and increase the fibroblast content of the scars (Aprahamian et al. 1985) |
| **THIAMINE** | Deficiency may interfere with formation of granulation tissue affecting collagen synthesis (Alvarez and Gilbereath 1982) |
| **VITAMIN A** | Supplementation may increase the tensile strength of scar tissue (Seitfer et al. 1975); topical application may counter the inhibitory effect of corticosteroids on healing of open wounds (Hunt et al. 1969) |
| **ASCORBIC ACID** | Supplementation may promote collagen and elastin formation (Murad et al. 1981) |
| **VITAMIN E** | Supplementation may be beneficial in increasing the breaking point and strength of connective tissue in wounds (Taren et al. 1987) |
| **COPPER** | A co-factor for the action of lysyl amino oxidase in the aldehyde reactions which generate strong covalent bonds in collagen (Miller 1975) |
| **MANGANESE** | Necessary for the glycosylation of hydroxyproline residues in the formation of collagen (Mille 1975) |
| **ZINC** | Supplementation may stimulate wound healing but only in pts with zinc deficiency (Fulgham 1969). Topical application may assist the healing of open wounds (Williams et al. 1969) |
| **ARGININE** | A constituent of wound proteins and is the penultimate substrate for polyamine synthesis that signels scar tissue proliferation. Arginine may also relax vascular smooth muscle, causing fluids and some cells to accumulate in the wound sites (Seifter 1989) |
| **ESSENTIAL FATTY ACIDS** | Necessary for the transport of substances across cell membranes. Deficiency may be associated with poor wound healing (Dowling et al. 1985) |
| **GLYCOSAMINOGLYCANS** | Topical application may accelerate wound healing and increase the tensile strength of the scar (Prudden and Allen 1965) |
| **GLUCOSAMINE SULFATE** | Supplementation may speed the healing of chondropathia patellae and prevent cartilage destruction (Bohmer et al. 1984) |
| **EPIMEDIUM** | Strengthens tissues and inhibit MAO B (Dai et al. 1987) |
| **LEUKOCYNAIDINS** (PYCNOGENOLS, GRAPE SEED EXTRACT) | Support collagen structure and preventing collagen destruction; cross-link collagen fibers; prevent free radical damage; inhibit enzymatic cleavage of collagen by enzymes secreted by WBC; prevent the release and synthesis of compounds that promote inflammation, such as histamine, serice proteases, prostaglandins, and leukotrienes. (Werback 1984) |
| **CENTELLA ASIATICA** (GOTU KOLA) | The total triterpenoid fraction (TIFCA) may increase collagen synthesis in a dose-dependent fashion whereas a simultaneous decrease in the specific activity of neosynthesized collagen (Maquart et al. 1990) |
| **CERVUS NIPPON** (DEER HORN) | Pantocrine can promote granulation tissue and healing of fractures, increasing bone torsional strength (Reshentinkova 1954) |
| **PLANTAGO ASIATICA** | Extract injected into synovial cavity leads to hyperplasia of connective tissue (Lin 1954) |

*Table AP-9.* **Peripheral Circulation (Vitamins and Minerals)**

| | |
|---|---|
| **Vitamin A** | Supplementation may be beneficial in peripheral vascular disease (Acta 1982) |
| **Vitamin B6** | Excessive homocysteine was seen in patients with occlusive arterial disease. B6 may reduce homocysteine levels (N Eng J Med 1985) |
| **Inositol Nicotinate** (A type of niacin) | Supplementation may be beneficial for intermittent claudication. (O'Hara 1985) |
| **Vitamin C** | Supplementation may improve periperal circulation. (Willis 1954) |
| **Vitamin E** | Supplementation may reduce symptoms of intermittent claudication (Piesse 1984) |
| **Magnesium** | Supplementation may be beneficial in magnesium deficient patient with PVD (Howard 1990) |
| **Zinc** | Supplementation may be beneficial in intermittent claudication (Jenzel (1968) |
| **Carnitine** | Supplementation may be helpful in intermittent claudication (Brevetti et al. 1988) |
| **Hydroxyethylrutoside** | Administration may improve arterial blood flow in the extremities (Jelnes et al. 1986) |
| **Omega-3 Fatty Acids** | Supplementation may be beneficial in intermittent claudication (Kamada et al. 1986) |
| **Omega-6 Fatty Acids** | Supplementation may improve symptoms in patient with intermittent claudication (Christie et al. 1986) |
| **Bilberry** (Vaccinium myritillus) | Can improve microcirculation and protect the vascular endothelium. Supplementation may improve arterial function and symptoms of periperal vascular insufficiency (Colantuoni S et al. 1991) |
| **Bromelain** | The fibrinolytic activities may be beneficial in thrombophlebitis (Taussig and Batkin 1988) |
| **Centella asiatica** | The total triterpenoid fraction seem to have regulatory affects on connective tissue of the vascular wall. Administration may be helpful in venous insufficiency (Arpaia et al. 1990) |
| **Ginkgo biloba** | Extract containing 24% ginkgoflavonglycosides may be beneficial in PVD (Kleijnen and Knipschild 1992) |
| **Hawthorn** (Crataegus) | The procynidins extracts may be beneficial in the treatment of PVD. (Di Renzi et al. 1969) |
| **Procynidolic oligomers** (pycnogenols) | Supplementation may be helpful in veno-lymphatic insufficiency (Henriet 1993) |
| **Carnitine** | Supplementation may be helpful in intermittent claudication (Brevetti et al. 1988) |
| **Hydroxyethylrutoside** | Administration may improve arterial blood flow in the extremities (Jelnes et al. 1986) |
| **Ligusticum rhizome** | The total alkaloids and tetramethylopyraxine can decrease vascular resistance in anesthetized dogs, and increase blood flow to the brain, femoral artery, and lower limbs (Yu 1979) |
| **Angelica sinensis** | A 25% extraction of the total herb is commonly used as injection therapy in various peripheral vascular conditions (Health J of Jubei 1977) |

*Table AP-9.* **PERIPHERAL CIRCULATION (VITAMINS AND MINERALS) (CONTINUED)**

| | |
|---|---|
| **SALVIA MILTIORRHIZA** | Aqueous extractions have a vasodilatory action (Zhang et al. 1965) |
| **CARTHAMUS TINCRORIUS** | Alcohol extracts have a vasodilatory action. When applied externally on local contusions and sprains it causes a local hyperamia and rapid subsidence of swelling. It can also be used in subacute tenosynovitis (Yu et al. 1959) |

Table AP-10. **ANXIETY, INSOMNIA, DEPRESSION AND STRESS DISORDERS**

| | |
|---|---|
| **ASHWAGANDHA** (WITHANIA SOMIFERA) | A methanolic extract inhibits specific binding of GABA and TBPS and enhances the binding of flunitrazepam (a valium like medicine) to receptor sites. Can mimic GABA activity (Mehta 1991);A reduction in 5-hydroxytryptophan, circulating monoamine oxidase and GABA seen in patients with anxiety, treatment results in decreased psychological complaints (Upadhaya et al. 1990) |
| **BUPLEURUM CHINESE** | Several preparations, especially the alkaloids have significant sedative effects. The herb also has analgesic and antipyretic effects. (Shibata 1973) |
| **CRATAEGUS PINNATIFIDA** | Extracts been shown to inhibit MAO B in mice (Dai and Yin 1987) |
| **GARUM ARMORICUM** (STABILIUM) | Garum armoricum may be effective for anxiety and depression (Dorman et al. 1995; Crocqu et al. 1980) |
| **GINKGO BILOBA** | The 24% ginkgoflavonglycosides may be effective for depression, especially in cases with cerebrovascular insufficiency (DeFeudis 1991) |
| **KAVA KAVA** (PIPER METHYSTICUM) | The extract been shown effective for anxiety (Kinzler, Kromer and Lehamann 1991) |
| **LIGUSTICUM RHIZOME** | The volatile oils have significant sedative effects which can potentiate the sedative effects of sodium pentobarbital (Zang et al. 1964) |
| **PANAX GINSENG** | The herb has a adaptogenic and anxiolytic properties (Bhattacharya and Mira 1991);also been shown to inhibit monoamine oxidase (Dau and Yin 1978) |
| **PASSION FLOWER** (PASSIFLORA INCARNATA): | The extracts have a mild sedative effects (Sopranzi et al 1990) |
| **PANTOCRINE** (DEER HORN EXTRACT) | Is a potent monoamine oxidase inhibitor (MAOI) yielding 80% reduction of MAO-B activity in mice (Dai and Yin 1987) |
| **POLYGONUM MULTIFLORUM:** | Extracts yielded 80% reduction of MAO activity in mice (Chenet et al.1991) |
| **SALVIA MILTIORRHIZA** | Extracts have been shown to inhibit MAO (Dain and Tin 1987) |
| **ST. JOHNS WORT** | Standardized extracts containing hypericin may be effective in the treatment of depression, anxiety and insomnia. (Woelk 1992) |
| **VALERIAN** (VALERIANA OFFICINALIS) | The fat soluble valepotriates and the water-soluble components are thought to have a sedative hypnotic activity (Houghton 1988) |
| **UNCARIA RHYNOPHYLLLA** | The ethanol extract has significant sedative and anti-convulsion activity Fan et al. 1965) |
| **ZIZIPHUS JUJUBA** | Reported to have excellent sedative and hypnotic effects, which synergized with many sedatives and hypnotics. (Hu 1957) |

# Appendix B: *Tables*

*Table 2-1.* **THE CENTRAL NERVOUS SYSTEM (CNS)**

| | |
|---|---|
| **BRAIN** | Brainstem<br>• gives rise to 10 of 12 pairs of cranial nerves<br>• controls basic bodily functions such as respiratory and heart rates<br>• determines general level of alertness<br>• warns of important incoming information<br>• directs attention to specific events<br>Cerebellum<br>• maintains posture, balance and skeletal muscle function<br>• attached to rear of brainstem<br>• mainly involved with motor system<br>Cerebrum<br>• largest part of human brain<br>• each hemisphere controls opposite side of body<br>Cortex<br>• frontal, temporal, parietal, occipital lobes<br>• important in organizing, remembering, communicating, understanding, appreciating, creating thoughts.<br>Limbic System<br>• involved in many self-regulating systems of body and in emotional reactions<br>• group of cellular structures rather than single brain region<br>• located between brainstem and cortex<br>• interconnects structures within cerebrum and with pathways that connect to all parts of brain |
| **SPINAL CORD** | Center (H-shaped area):<br>• anterior portion (ventral horn) motor system<br>• posterior portion (dorsal horn) processing of sensory information from somata and viscera<br>Receives about 31 pairs of spinal nerves:<br>• divided into layers (laminae) each organizes differential connection<br>• spinal segment defined by level at which associated nerve enters cord<br>• lamina V somatic and visceral input converge with descending fibers<br>  — Cells in this lamina contribute to referred pain<br>  — Laminae V and I contribute significantly to the perception of pain<br>• can vary in response to different circumstances<br>• can function in<br>  — normal control state<br>  — suppressed state (higher-end pain threshold)<br>  — sensitized state (lower pain threshold) |

*Table 2-2.* SYMPATHETIC INNERVATION

| REGION | LEVEL | COMMENTS |
|---|---|---|
| Entire Body | T1-T12 | Sympathetic Innervation<br>Originates in thoracic spine, except for those innervated by sympathetic cell bodies originating at L1 and L2 |
| Mucous Membranes<br>Vessels of Head<br>Vessels of Neck and Eyes | T1-T3 | |
| Upper Limbs | T3-T7 | |
| Heart and Lungs | T1-T5 | |
| GI Tract | T6-T10 | |
| 50% of upper Legs | T10-T12 | |
| Other 50% of lower Legs | L1, L2 | |
| Kidneys<br>Adrenals<br>Gonads<br>Bladder<br>Uterus | T11-L2 | |

*Table 2-3.* EMBRYONIC SEGMENTAL DERIVATIONS

| ORGAN | DERIVATION | ORGAN | DERIVATION |
|---|---|---|---|
| Heart | C8-T4 (left)<br>(C-3?) | Small Intestine | T9-10 |
| Lungs | T2-T5 | Appendix and ascending colon | T10-L1 |
| Esophagus | T4-T6 | Epididymis | T10 |
| Diaphragm | C3-C4 | Kidney | T10-L1 |
| Stomach & duodenum | T6-T10 | Ovary, testis & suprarenals | T11-L1 |
| Liver and gallbladder | T7-T9(right) | Bladder fundus, colonic flexure, uterine fundus | L1-L3 |
| Spleen | T7-T10(left) | Sigmoid colon, | S3-S5 |
| Pancreas | T8 (left) | Rectum, cervix, neck of bladder, prostate, and urethra | S2-S5 |

*Table 3-4.* **OSTEOPATHIC ILIOSACRAL DISORDERS**

| DYSFUNCTION | GENERAL INFORMATION | FINDINGS |
| --- | --- | --- |
| Iliosacral Dysfunctions General | If, following successful treatment of pelvic subluxation and SI dysfunctions | The standing flexion test is still positive. The ASISs are still found to be unequal.<br>Then an iliosacral dysfunction is probable |
| Upslipped Innominate | Second most common pelvic dislocation. More common on right side | The ischial tuberosity, Iliac crest, PSIS, ASIS will be found superiorly on that side.<br>Sacrotuberous ligament lax on the subluxed side |
| Posterior Innominate (lt) | More common on the left side | The left ASIS will be superior on the side of the positive standing flexion test. The leg on that side will appear to be shorter |
| Anterior Innominate | Anterior innominate are much more common on the right side | The findings are reversed of posterior innominate |
| Iliac Outflare (lt) | Found in pathologic joints | Flexion test positive on left<br>ASIS further from midline on left |
| Iliac Inflare (rt) | Found in pathologic joints | Flexion test positive on right<br>ASIS further from midline on right |

*Table 3-5.* OSTEOPATHIC SI DYSFUNCTIONS

| DYSFUNCTION | GENERAL INFORMATION | FINDINGS |
|---|---|---|
| PUBIC SHEARS | The most common subluxation of the pelvis<br>— especially during pregnancy<br>Can be inferior or superior<br>— inferior shears tend to be self-correcting by weightbearing | Positive, standing flexion, seated flexion and Stork tests on the dysfunctional side<br>Superior or inferior pube on the dysfunctional side. |
| ANTERIOR TORSIONS | Quite common, Often associated with mild symptoms | |
| LEFT-ON-LEFT | about 4:1. compared to right on right | Standing flexion test may be positive on the right<br>Sacral right base loses its function of posterior nutation<br>   — therefore malposition and dysfunction (and possibly pain) are exaggerated when patient is forward bent<br>• Sacral ILA [a]posterior and inferior on the left<br>• Sacral base is posterior (rotated left) on the left in flexion<br>   — and becomes level in extension<br>   — the left ILA is also a little inferior, but not as much as in nutation dysfunction (unilaterally flexed sacrum) |
| RIGHT-ON-RIGHT | | Findings are reversed |
| BACKWARD TORSION DYSFUNCTIONS | Less common<br>Described as right-on-left (or left-on-right) oblique axis<br>   — associated with lumbar nonneutral dysfunction<br>   — often with extension restrictions<br>   — often are acute and severely painful | Normal nutation movement of one side of the sacral base is restricted<br>   — therefore signs, and usually symptoms, are exaggerated by extension of the lumbar spine |
| RIGHT ON LEFT | More common than left on right<br>   — often with FRS(rt) at L5-S1 that should be treated first | Seating flexion test is positive on the right<br>The sacral base and the ILA are posterior on the right in extension<br>   — ILA also slightly inferior<br>   — both are level in flexion<br>Lumbar lordosis and spring are reduced |
| LEFT ON RIGHT | | Findings are reversed |

*Table 3-5.* **OSTEOPATHIC SI DYSFUNCTIONS (CONTINUED)**

| | | |
|---|---|---|
| **UNILATERAL FLEXED SACRUM (LEFT)** | Left unilateral flexed sacrum (anterior sacral nutations, inferior shear on left)<br><br>— are much more common than right-sided dysfunctions (about 9:1)<br>— must be treated with manual therapy | Often the seated flexion test is positive on the left<br>The base on that side is "stuck" in anterior nutation (flexion) (with loss of counternutation)<br><br>— base will be found anterior to the iliac crest especially in spinal flexion<br>— but slightly less in neutral<br>— in extension it is nearly, but not quite, level<br>— sacrum is sidebent to the left<br>— ILA are inferior on the same side — about 1 cm, and are slightly posterior, but not as much as in torsional dysfunctions<br>Lumbar compensation is usually rotation of L5 to the right[b] |
| **UNILATERAL EXTENDED SCRAM (RIGHT)** | Sacrum loses its nutation function<br>Findings are more pronounced in lumbar extension<br><br>— much more common on the right | Often the seated flexion test is positive on the right<br>In extension the sacral base is found more posteriorly on the right<br><br>— the ILA more anteriorly and superior on that side<br>— in neutral or in flexion they are almost, but not quite, symmetrical<br>The lumbar lordosis and spring is reduced<br>Lumbar compensation is usually with L5 rotation to the right |

a.  Inferior Lateral Angle of sacrum.
b. Greenman says to left.

*Table 3-6.* OSTEOPATHIC VERTEBRAL DYSFUNCTIONS

| ARIA AND DYSFUNCTION | FINDINGS, AND GENERAL INFORMATION |
|---|---|
| Lumbar and Thoracic Spine | Restrictions of flexion or extension that often are due to:<br>— Nonneutral (Type II) dysfunctions called FRS and ERS<br>— Or neutral (Type I) dysfunctions called NR |
| Neutral group dysfunction NR(side) | • Usually a compensatory reaction to a nonneutral dysfunction<br>• N represents neutral, R represents the rotation the direction of the rotation in the parentheses<br>• Sidebending is to the side opposite of rotation<br>• Motion is restricted toward the convex side of the group and rotation is restricted in the opposite direction<br>• Total range of flexion and extension usually will be reduced<br>• Neutral restriction i.e., rotated and sidebent to opposite sides can occur in one motion segment (not a group dysfunction) |
| FRS(side) | Describes a segment as flexed, rotated and sidebent to one side (the side is marked in parentheses)<br>• Restrictions of movements and provocation of pain will often be in the opposite directions<br>• Usually the total range of extension and flexion will be reduced |
| ERS (side) | Opposite of FRS<br>• Restricted motions and often the provocation of pain will be in flexion, rotation and sidebending to the opposite side<br>• Spinous process and the supraspinous ligament will be tender<br>• TrPs and/or the articular capsule often are very tender |

*Table 4-7.* **Symptoms: Pain**

| Symptom | Indication |
|---|---|
| **Abdominal Pain** | |
| In general | Can be referred from spine, thorax, pelvic organs and/or genitalia. Can be caused by exogenous, endogenous, metabolic or neurogenic disorders (Marcus 1991). |
| Rhythmic increase unrelated to movement, or any severe pain felt ventrally | Internal medical disorders, especially when pain is at the same level as the back pain. |
| Concomitant abdominal and back pain (abdominal pain lower than back pain) | Suggests orthopedic origin. |
| **Coughing, Pain Aggravated by** | |
| In general | Suggests intraspinal lesion. |
| Upper limbs | Especially suggests intraspinal lesion. |
| Sacroiliac joints | Momentary rise in intra-abdominal pressure due to coughing also causes broadening of sacroiliac joints and can increase painful conditions there. |
| Upper back | Can increase upper back pain if cause is pleuritis. Can be caused/aggravated by mechanical lesion in chest wall and thoracic cage. |
| **Organic Origin, Pain of** | |
| Low back | Can be due to kidney, bladder, prostate or intestinal diseases. |
| Sacrum | Can be due to pelvic or rectal diseases. |
| Upper back and shoulder | Can be due to disorders of the gallbladder, liver, heart, lung, pancreas or stomach, and ectopic pregnancy. |
| Neck, jaw, arm, or back | Can be referred due to esophagus and heart disorders. |
| **Posture, Activity, Rest, Exertion** | |
| Pain that is | |
| Relieved by rest | Can be caused by overuse syndromes, disc disease. |
| Relieved by rest in absence of discrete pathology | Can be caused by joint dysfunction. |
| Aggravated by activity | Suggests joint (somatic) dysfunction. Typically, certain movements are more painful than others. Also suggests muscle pathology, overuse syndromes, disc disease. |
| Initially alleviated by activity, later aggravated by activity | Can be due to pathological joints. |
| **Also See** | |
| Table xref, Paresthesias Table xref, Medical Considerations Table xref, Timing of Symptoms | |

*Table 4-8.* **SYMPTOMS: PARESTHESIA, HYPERESTHESIA**

| SYMPTOM | INDICATION |
| --- | --- |
| **PARESTHESIA (PINS AND NEEDLES)** | |
| | Suggests nervous system involvement. |
| In the feet | An early symptom of pressure on the spinal cord. Can be experienced before the plantar response becomes extensor (Babinski sign). |
| **VAGUE NUMBNESS**[A] | |
| Alleviated by stroking | Suggests a ligamentous source. |
| **TINGLING** | |
| | Suggests ligament, neurological or vascular involvement, diabetes, metabolic causes, vitamin deficiency or toxicity, heavy metal toxicity. |
| | If due to peripheral nerve involvement, affects the area supplied by that nerve, such as meralgia paraesthetica (a lesion of the lateral cutaneous nerve), which affects only the skin it innervates directly. |
| Vague tingling with numbness, pins and needles and/or pain | Suggests peripheral nerve, nerve root, nerve trunk, or central nervous system disorders. |
| **OTHER NEUROLOGICAL SYMPTOMS** | |
| Spontaneous Burning or Aching Pain, Hyperesthesia (excessive sensitivity to pain) Dysesthesia (numbness) Other Abnormal Sensations | Characteristic of central nervous system pain (upper motor neuron). |

a. Nulliness is a subjective numbness that occurs with ligamentous lesions. Rubbing/stroking alleviates nulliness momentarily, whereas rubbing/stroking can aggravate neurological pain.

*Table 4-9.* SYMPTOMS: TWINGES, GIVING 'WAY, LOCKING

| SYMPTOM | INDICATION |
|---|---|
| **TWINGES WITH GIVING 'WAY** | |
| In general | Can suggest instability, joint block or tendinitis. |
| **LOCKING WITH SUDDEN TWINGES WITH HISTORY OF RECURRENCE** | |
| | Suggests internal derangement of joints. |
| | In internal derangement of facets or disc, joint most commonly locks in flexion. |
| | This typical antalgic posture also can be due to spasm of psoas and of deep aspect of quadratus lumborum, FRS spinal dysfunctions, and backward torsions of SI joint. |
| **PAINFUL TWINGES** | |
| In general | Suggests loose body in the joint space. |
| | Also suggests neurological origin, such as post-herpetic neuralgia and Morton's neuroma. |
| with momentary loss of strength | Suggests joint instability. |
| with transitory loss of strength | Suggests tendinitis, which frequently follows overuse. (May be due to mechanical stress by adhesion or a lesion). |

*Table 4-10.* MEDICAL CONSIDERATIONS

| HISTORY | INDICATION |
|---|---|
| **HEART DISEASE** | Suggests rheumatic disease. |
| **CONSTITUTIONAL SYMPTOMS** SUCH AS WEAKNESS, FATIGUE, LOSS OF WEIGHT, PERSPIRATION | Suggest serious conditions. |
| **RICH DIET** | Suggests possibility of gout. |
| Recent Travel | Suggests possibility of symptom arising from infection. |
| **PAINFUL CONDITIONS** AMBIGUOUS ORIGIN OR SHORT DURATION | Suggest internal medical condition. Also common in orthopedic conditions. |
| History of Swelling | Can occur due to autoimmune disorder. (Indicative of inflammatory process). |
| Subcutaneous, from soft tissue inflammation | Feels soft. |
| From bleeding | Feels somewhat harder. |
| Family History | Can suggest similar condition. |

*Table 4-11.* SYMPTOMS OF CANCER

| SYMPTOM/SIGN | INDICATION |
|---|---|
| **CAUTION ACRONYM** | |
| Symptoms and signs per the acronym CAUTION:<br>**C**hanges in bowel/bladder habits<br>**A** sore that does not heal<br>**U**nusual bleeding/discharge<br>**T**hickening/lumps<br>**I**ndigestion or difficulty swallowing<br>**O**bvious changes in wart or mole<br>**N**agging cough or hoarseness | |
| Excessive Perspiration[a] | |
| In general | Suggests<br>• heart and/or other serious medical conditions, especially lymphoma.<br>or<br>• sympathetic nervous system involvement. |

a. Lung disorders, Heat, Yin deficiency, or disharmony of Defensive Qi and Nutritive Qi

*Table 4-12.* SYMPTOMS: TIMING

| SYMPTOM TIMING | INDICATES |
|---|---|
| **PAIN** | |
| Initially | Initially felt close to culprit lesion.<br>Account of where pain started and to where it has progressed is helpful. |
| Later | More likely to be referred. |
| At onset | Occurs in traumatic injuries (such as fractures and dislocation) and/or internal derangements. |
| Develops progressively, several hours | Suggests sprained ligaments. |
| Sudden, during particular movement | Can be due to muscle or tendon tears. |
| Following overuse | Can be due to a tendinous disorder. |
| Insidious onset | Can be due to repetitive microtrauma such as overuse tendinitis. |
| At night, especially w/insidious onset | Suggests inflammation and serious conditions. |
| **SWELLING** | |
| Occurs several hours after trauma | Suggests effusion of serous fluid. |
| Of joints quick-filling with fluid or sudden swelling | Suggests presence of bleeding.<br>(Should be aspirated when possible.) |

*Table 9-13.* **BioMedical Causes of Back Pain**

| **Urinary System** | Urinary infection and stones are common. |
|---|---|
| | — renal disease may result in pain at flanks and upper lumbar regions which may be sensitive to percussion and may radiate to the thigh |
| | — calculi (stones) or other obstructive diseases often radiate pain to the groin, testes and thigh |
| | — prostatitis commonly refers pain to the back and sacrum |
| | — calculi, the Urinalysis often reveals blood |
| | — in other obstructions, usually there is proteinuria |
| **Retroperitoneal Masses** | Lymphomas, GYN disorders and aneurysms may refer pain to the back. |
| | — excessive perspiration often an early sign of lymphoma |
| | — a bruit (a friction-like sound) may be heard over an aneurysm, and often a pulsating mass is felt during palpation. |
| | — gynecological diseases often refer pain to the lumbosacral regions. |
| **Rectosigmoid Diseases** | Can refer an ache to the low back. |
| | — often the character of such pain may change with defecation. |
| **Urinary System** | Urinary infection and stones are common. |
| | — renal disease may result in pain at flanks and upper lumbar regions which may be sensitive to percussion and may radiate to the thigh |
| | — calculi (stones) or other obstructive diseases often radiate pain to the groin, testes and thigh |
| | — prostatitis commonly refers pain to the back and sacrum |
| | — calculi, the Urinalysis often reveals blood |
| | — in other obstructions, usually there is proteinuria |
| **Infectious Conditions** | Gonococcal, staphylococcal, syphilitic, tubercular and viral infections should be kept in mind. |
| | — osteomyelitis (often seen in younger patients) |
| | — brucellosis (farm workers), |
| | — tuberculosis (in immune deficient patients) |
| **Inflammatory Conditions** | Rheumatoid arthritis can involve the spine. |
| | — although usually spinal involvement does not occur in the early stages<br>Reiter's syndrome (a triad of arthritis with fever, conjunctivitis and urethritis)<br>Psoriatic arthritis<br>Ankylosing spondylitis |
| **Malignant Diseases** | Usually seen in patients over 50 years of age.<br>Most common are metastatic carcinomas from. |
| | — prostate, breast, lung, uterus, colon and bladder<br>Primary spinal tumors. |
| | — most commonly osteosarcomas, affect younger patients |
| | — Multiple myelomas (the most common primary malignant bone tumor), and chondrosarcomas are seen in older patients, as well |
| **Neurofibromatosis (von Recklinghausen's disease)** | Tumors of nervous tissue that may appear on the skin or in the optic and acoustic nerves.<br>other manifestations include: |
| | — multiple soft tissue, pendunculated fleshy tumors, and café-au-lait-pigmented macules (café-colored plaque or patches) |
| | — associated with pain confined to radicular pattern |
| | — symptoms often start in the periphery and progress proximally |

*Table 9-13.* **BioMedical Causes of Back Pain (Continued)**

| METABOLIC DESTRUCTIVE PROCESSES | Osteoporosis and osteomalacia suspected in:<br>— elderly, kyphotic patients<br>— or in patients in whom minor injuries cause severe, localized pain<br>Paget's disease (osteitis deformans) seen in 3% of adults over 40 years.<br> — ninety per cent of patients are asymptomatic<br>Ochronosis.<br>— a rare condition marked by dark pigmentation of cartilage, ligaments, fibrous tissue, skin and urine |
|---|---|
| DEPRESSION, ANXIETY DISORDERS | Common cause of back pain.<br>Patients diagnosed with fibromyalgia syndromes<br>— score much higher on anxiety and depression scales<br>— although not thought to be a psychogenic disease these patients are helped with treatment for depression<br>— pain tends to be variable and is associated with fatigue, sleep disorders, head and other aches and inability to cope with stress |

*Table 9-14.* **D**ISC **L**ESIONS WITH **R**OOT SIGNS

| RADICULAR SIGNS | SYMPTOMS AND SIGNS | DIFFERENTIAL DIAGNOSIS |
|---|---|---|
| **L1** | Pain from the low back to <br> — the groin and above the trochanter <br> Numbness <br> — can be sensed in the groin. <br> Superficial cremasteric and abdominal reflex may be absent | Lesions of the iliolumbar ligament and the quadratus lumborum |
| **L2** <br> **D**ISC PROTRUSION LESIONS AT **L1** AND **L2** ARE VERY RARE | Pain may extend from the back anteriorly <br> — as far as the inner thigh and knee <br> — It is aggravated by standing and alleviated by sitting <br> Numbness <br> — may be sensed in the groin and knee <br> Weakness <br> — may be seen with hip flexion (psoas) <br> Superficial cremasteric and abdominal reflex may be absent | Iliolumbar ligament, posterior superior SI ligament and quadratus lumborum lesions <br> Secondary malignant deposits can cause gross weakness in the psoas and can disturb spinal movements <br> Pain in the front of the thigh also can be caused by lesions of the psoas, hip, quadriceps and abductor muscles, lumbar facets and SI ligaments |
| **L3** | Pain starts locally and extends <br> — to the upper buttock, the whole front of the thigh and knee, extending to just above the ankle <br> — Extension stretches the nerve root and aggravates the leg pain <br> — Flexion may or may not alleviate the pain <br> — The SLR may be limited, and it may be painful at full range <br> Numbness <br> — can occur from the knee to the ankle <br> Weakness <br> — of the psoas may be demonstrated by resisted hip flexion, <br> — quadriceps by knee extension <br> Prone-lying knee flexion <br> — (Nachlas Test or L3 stretch) stretches the L3 root and is painful <br> A sluggish or absent knee reflex may be seen | Other conditions, as mentioned in L2, also should be excluded <br> Knee dysfunction in lower leg pain or numbness <br> Iliopsoas syndrome must be ruled out |

*Table 9-14.* **DISC LESIONS WITH ROOT SIGNS (CONTINUED)**

| L4 | Pain often starts at the mid-lumbar region or the iliac crest | Lesion of the gluteus medius /minimus and quadratus lumborum syndromes |
|---|---|---|
| | — radiates to inner quadrant of the buttock and the outer aspect of the thigh and legs, and crosses over the dorsum of the foot to the big toe | Lesions of tibialis anterior<br>SI joint and the superior and middle portions of the posterior ligaments |
| | — Marked trunk list (lateral deviation) can be seen on occasion | |
| | — SLR may be limited and painful bilaterally | |
| | Numbness | |
| | — in the lateral side of the thigh and leg, including the knee | |
| | — crosses to the anterior part of the shin, often into the medial side of the foot and to the big toe | |
| | Muscle weakness | |
| | — of the tibialis anterior, extensor hallucis | |
| | Patellar reflex may be affected | |
| L5 | Lumbar list may be seen | Piriformis, gluteus medius/minimus and quadratus lumborum myofascial syndromes |
| | — Lumbar movements are painful | SI joint and ligament dysfunctions |
| | — SLR is limited unilaterally and painful, with dural tension signs | Patients with leg pain only, and weakness or numbness but no back signs, consider |
| | Weakness | • impingement of the peroneal nerve from fibular, tibial and surrounding soft tissue dysfunctions |
| | — of the gluteus medius, peronei and the extensor hallucis | • foot symptoms may be caused by impingement of the superficial peroneal nerve at the ankle or foot |
| | Numbness | |
| | — may follow a similar path, as in L4 lesions | |
| | — however, the first three toes are involved | |
| | Ankle reflex is sluggish or absent | |

Table 1-15. SACRAL ROOT SIGNS

| ROOT LEVEL | SYMPTOMS AND SIGNS | DIFFERENTIAL DIAGNOSIS |
|---|---|---|
| S1 | Pain felt<br><br>— at the posterior leg muscles, the lateral foot and the 4th and 5th toes, but does not involve the buttock<br><br>— SLR is unilaterally limited and painful<br>Weakness<br><br>— of the hamstrings, calf and the peroneal muscles<br><br>— wasting of the gluteal muscles or inability to contract the gluteal mass may be seen<br>Numbness<br><br>— may affect the outer leg, foot and outer two toes.<br>Sluggish or absent ankle reflexes | Sacrotuberous ligament lesion<br>Posterior gluteus medius lesion<br>Piriformis syndromes |
| S2 | Same as S1<br><br>— excluding the peroneal muscles<br>— numbness ends at the heel | Sacrospinous ligament<br>Gluteus minimus and medial piriformis lesions |
| S3 | Pain felt<br><br>— at the groin, running down the inner thigh to the knee<br>However, no muscle weakness is seen<br>No changes in the reflexes or in bladder functions<br><br>— SLR not limited | Iliolumbar ligament<br>Quadratus lumborum and psoas muscles |
| S4 | Pain<br><br>— in the saddle area (perineum and genitals)<br>Weakness<br><br>— bladder and rectal weakness<br>Numbness<br><br>— of the anus<br>— "pins and needles" in the genitals | Note: this is a surgical emergency |

*Table 9-16.* **MYOFASCIAL SYNDROMES— QUADRATUS LUMBORUM MUSCLE**

| MUSCLE | INNERVATION | DESCRIPTION |
|---|---|---|
| Quadratus lumborum | Lumbar plexus, T-12 through L-4 | **FUNCTIONS**<br>• Stabilizer of lumbar spine<br>• Lateral flexor<br>• Hip hiker<br>**SYMPTOMS**<br>One of the most common and overlooked causes of low back pain<br>• Typically pain over the iliac crests, buttock, hip and groin<br>• Often activated by sudden, unguarded, awkward movements and trauma<br>  — spasm will restrict movements between the lumbar vertebrae and the sacrum<br>  — during walking or turning over in bed<br>  — when arising from bed or from sitting<br>Examination<br>• Flexion, extension and sidebending toward the pain-free side are restricted<br>• Rotation may be limited in the direction of the spasm<br>• A lateral list also is common<br>**TREATMENT**<br>• Muscle energy<br>• Post-isometric techniques<br>• Countertension-positioning<br>• Dry needling<br>• Acupuncture Yin Qiao, Kidney and Urinary channels |

*Table 9-17.* **Myofascial Syndromes Piriformis Muscle**

| Muscle | Innervation | Description |
|---|---|---|
| Piriformis | S1-S2 | **FUNCTION:**<br>• Lateral rotation of thigh in non-weight bearing with hip extended<br>• Abduction when hip flexed 90°<br>**SYMPTOMS:**<br>Syndrome can be divided into two entities<br>Of myofascial component of the syndrome usually include<br>• Buttock pain, hip pain, and posterior thigh pain<br>• Pain is increased by sitting, especially on a hard surface, by rising from the sitting position or by standing<br>• It may be related to defecation<br>Nerve Compression Type<br>• Compression of the superior and inferior gluteal nerves and vessels can contribute to buttock pain and atrophy<br>• Pressure on the sciatic nerve gives pain in the distribution of the sciatic nerve, and may project to the calf and foot<br>**Examination:**<br>• Resisted contraction may or may not increase the pain<br>• Muscle spasm may cause the patient's ipsilateral foot to be everted<br>• Both abduction of the lower extremity and hip internal rotation will be limited<br>• Must be differentiated from somatic dysfunction of the hip and from psoas spasm<br>With nerve compression<br>• Changes in reflexes, reduced muscle power and paresthesias may be seen<br>• Often the SLR is positive<br>• SLR can be performed by rotating the hip externally, and then internally<br>　— If the SLR is more restricted with external rotation, a piriformis syndrome may be considered<br>• If the pudendal nerve is entrapped, the patient may feel peroneal pain and may complain of sexual dysfunction<br>TREATMENT<br>• Muscle energy<br>• Post-isometric techniques<br>• Countertension-positioning<br>• Dry needling<br>• Acupuncture GB, UB and Yang Qiao channels<br>• Foot orthotics |

*Table 9-18.* **MYOFASCIAL SYNDROMES GLUTEUS MEDIUS**

| MUSCLE | INNERVATION | DESCRIPTION |
|---|---|---|
| Gluteus Medius | L4-S1 | **FUNCTIONS**<br>• Abduction of thigh<br>• Stabilization of pelvis during single-leg stance<br>**SYMPTOMS**<br>Tenderness of the glutei is almost universal with low back pain<br>Three syndromes<br>• One primary and two secondary<br>— the first is due to primary muscular injury<br>— the second two are due to SI ligamentous insufficiency and nerve root dysfunctions.<br>• Pain felt in the low back, along the sacroiliac, outer iliac crest, buttocks and outer thigh<br>• Pain during walking, sitting and slumping forward<br>• Occasionally, in lesions of the uppermost anterior insertion to the ilium<br>— pain is felt in the dorsal ankle only<br>Examination<br>• Weakness or pain with resisted thigh abduction<br>• Flexion and sidebending away from the dysfunctional side is painful<br><br>**TREATMENT**<br>• Muscle energy<br>• Post-isometric techniques<br>• Countertension-positioning<br>• Dry needling<br>• Acupuncture Dai and Yang Qiao vessel<br>• Foot orthotics |

*Table 9-19.* MYOFASCIAL SYNDROMES ILIOPSOAS MUSCLE

| MUSCLE | INNERVATION | DESCRIPTION |
|---|---|---|
| Iliopsoas | Lumbar plexus, L1-L4 | FUNCTION<br>• Flexion of thigh and hip<br>• Extension of lumbar spine<br>• Abduction of thigh<br>SYMPTOMS<br>• Iliopsoas syndrome, together with quadratus lumborum is a common myofascial cause of failed low back syndrome<br>• Psoas spasm can cause more disability than any other muscle of the back<br>• Pain is felt along the spine ipsilaterally, from the thoracic region to the sacroiliac area<br>• Pain sometimes to the upper buttock, anterior thigh and groin<br>Examination<br>• Patient likely to stand with the torso leaning slightly toward the involved side<br>• When bending forward an arc can be seen during approximately the first 20°<br>• The psoas will limit hip extension<br>• Resisted movements may be painful<br>• Tenderness at the lower muscle between the lesser trochanter and the inguinal ligament, over the iliacus at the inner ilium<br>  — or above transabdominally, lateral to the umbilicus<br>  — a nonneutral (Type II) lumbar dysfunction at L1 or L2 can occur<br>  — compensatory neutral group dysfunction (Type I) is seen in the rest of the lumbar spine<br>TREATMENT<br>• Muscle energy<br>• Post-isometric techniques<br>• Countertension-positioning<br>• Dry needling<br>• Acupuncture Chong, K and Liv channels |

*Table 9-20.* MYOFASCIAL SYNDROMES — THORACOLUMBAR PARASPINAL MUSCLES

| MUSCLE | INNERVATION | DESCRIPTION |
|---|---|---|
| Thoracolumbar paraspinal | Branches of the dorsal primary divisions of the spinal nerves | **FUNCTION:**<br>• Extension and rotation of spine<br>**SYMPTOMS:**<br>• Often involved in low back pain<br>• When the longissimus muscles are involved bilaterally<br>  — usually at the thoracic-lumbar junction<br>  — the patient has difficulty rising from a chair and climbing stairs<br>• Pain from the iliocostalis at the lower-thoracic felt mostly downward over the lumbar area, it may refer upwards and across the scapula, and around the abdomen<br>• Trigger points in the upper lumbar iliocostalis refers<br>  — strongly downward and over the mid-buttock and are a frequent source of unilateral posterior hip pain<br>• Trigger points at the lower thoracic level in the longissimus thoracis<br>  — refer pain strongly to the low buttock<br>Result from:<br>• Awkward movements that combine bending and twisting the back<br>• Whiplash type accident and prolonged immobility<br>  — Pain in these muscles is often associated with vertebral and sacroiliac joint dysfunctions and with ligamentous insufficiency<br>TREATMENT<br>• Muscle energy<br>• Post-isometric techniques<br>• Countertension-positioning<br>• Dry needling<br>• Acupuncture Jia Ji points and UB channels |

*Table 9-21.* MYOFASCIAL SYNDROMES — LATISSIMUS DORSI MUSCLE

| MUSCLE | INNERVATION | DESCRIPTION |
|---|---|---|
| Latissimus dorsi | C6-C8 | FUNCTIONS |
| | | • Adduction and internal rotation of arm |
| | | • Depression of scapula |
| | | • Stabilizes lumbar spine |
| | | **SYMPTOMS** |
| | | • Frequently-overlooked contributor to lumbosacral dysfunction and pain |
| | | • Pain can be felt in the scapular, shoulder and iliac crest regions |
| | | Examination |
| | | • When shortened, arm extension and elevation often is limited |
| | | TREATMENT |
| | | • Muscle energy |
| | | • Post-isometric techniques |
| | | • Countertension-positioning |
| | | • Dry needling |
| | | • Acupuncture Yang Qiao and UB channels |

# Appendix C: *Resources*

## Educational & Professional Organizations

**AMERICAN ACADEMY OF COMPLEMENTARY ORTHOPEDICS (AACO)**. The Academy, with which the author is associated, gears their courses towards allied-health practitioners and teaches the management of musculoskeletal disorders with techniques that are similar to those shown in this text.

AACO can be reached at 6137 North Thesta # 101A, Fresno, Ca 93710. Phone (209) 435-9745, Fax (209) 435-9748.

**AMERICAN ACADEMY OF PAIN MANAGEMENT (AAPM)**. AAPM is an inclusive organization that offers professional certification and education in pain management.

AAPM can be reached at 13947 Mono Way #A, Sonora, CA 95370. Phone (209) 533-9744, Fax (209) 533-9750, E-Mail: aapm@aapainmange.org

**AMERICAN ASSOCIATION OF NATUROPATHIC PHYSICIANS (AANP)**. AANP provides information for both professionals and the public on naturopathic medicine.

AANP can be reached at 601 Valley St., #105, Seattle, WA 98109. Phone (206) 298-0126, Fax (206) 298-0129, Web-www.naturopathic.org

**AMERICAN ASSOCIATION OF ORIENTAL MEDICINE (AAOM)**. AAOM is the oldest and largest professional organization of Oriental Medicine. It offers information on Oriental Medicine and is associated with the American Academy of Complementary Orthopedics.

AAOM can be reached at 433 Front Street, Catasauqua, PA 18032-1832. Phone (610) 433-2448, Fax (610) 433-1832.

**AMERICAN ASSOCIATION OF ORTHOPAEDIC MEDICINE (AAOM)**. AAOM is an inclusive organization (accepts allied-health memberships) and offers training in orthopaedic medicine mainly for allopathic and osteopathic physicians.

AAOM can be reached at 90 S Cascade Avenue, Suite 1190, Colorado Springs, Colorado 80903. Phone (800) 922-2063, Fax-(719) 475-8748.

**AMERICAN CHIROPRACTIC ASSOCIATION (ACA)**. ACA has approximately 19,000 members and is a source for information for both professionals and the public.

ACA can be reached at 1701 Clarendon Blvd., Arlington, VI 22209. Phone (703) 276-8800, Fax (703) 273-243-2598, Web-www.amerchiro.org

**AMERICAN OSTEOPATHIC ASSOCIATION (AOA)**. AOA provides information for both professionals and the public on osteopathic medicine.

AOA can be reached at 142 East Ontario St., Chicago, IL 60611. Phone (800) 621-1773, Fax (312) 280-3860, e-mail osteomed@wwa.com

**THE INTERNATIONAL ALLIANCE OF HEALTHCARE EDUCATORS**. The International Alliance is a source for seminars, books, videos and tapes on many types of somatic therapies.

The Alliance can be reached at 11211 Prosperity Farms Rd., #D-325, Palm Beach Gardens, FL 33410. Phone (800) 311-9204.

# Herbs & Acupuncture Supplies

**LHASA MEDICAL, INC.** Lhasa medical carries a variety of acupuncture needles (including Korean needles), Korean hand-acupuncture supplies, moxa supplies (including smokeless needle moxa), cupping equipment, magnets, acupuncture models, electrostimulators (including an inexpensive micro-TENS unit), lasers, heat lamps, massage aids and homeopathic medicines.

Lhasa medical can be reached at 539 Accord Station, Accord, MA 02018-0539. Phone (800) 722-8775, Fax (617) 335-6296. Website: www.LhasaMedical.com

**MED SERVI-SYSTEMS CANADA LTD.** MED Servi is a family enterprise that provides auricular medicine, acupuncture and educational supplies. They carry: Chinese & Japanese moxibustion supplies and accessories, lasers, a variety of acupuncture needles (Japanese & Chinese styles), stimulators, point finders, books, educational seminars, videos and magnets.

MED Servi-Systems Canada can be reached at 8 Sweetnam Dr., Stittsville ON K2S 1 G2. Phone (800) 267-6868 (Canada & US.). Website: http://www.medserv.ca/, Email: info@medserv.ca

**NUHERBS CO.** Nuherbs carries Chinese herbal products in bulk (row herbs), powders, extract powders, patent formulas, liniments, plasters and ointments. Nuherbs is the sole distributor of Herbal Times, a GMP certified, sugarless concentrated classical formulas (including many of the classic formulas mentioned in the text). Herbal Times manufacture herbal concentrates and standardized extracts. Of particular interest in musculoskeletal medicine Nuherbs carries: Chin Koo Tieh Shang Wan, Shi Hui San, Yunnan PaiYao (in liquid, powder and capsules) and Gu Zhe Cuo Shang San for the treatment of injuries. They carry Notoginseng Herbal Analgesic Liniment and a proprietary product for the same purpose, Wan Hua oil for use with Gua Sha scraping and a sugar and alcohol free Tian Ma Shou Wu Chih tonic. They also carry a large variety of medicated plasters. Nuherbs can custom grind herbal formulas and produce honey pills. Nuherbs also carries acupuncture, cupping and moxa supplies and books.

Nuherbs Co. can be reached at 3820 Penniman Ave., Oakland, CA 94619. Phone (800) 233-4307, Fax (800) 550-1928.

**(DRALINE TONG HERBS** is a retail store that carries Nuherbs products. Draline Tong can fill prescriptions and mail them to the patient. Draline Tong is located at 1002 Webster St. Oakland, CA 94607. Phone (510) 465-6544, Fax (510) 465-4690).

**OMS MEDICAL SUPPLIES INC.** OMS carries acupuncture, chiropractic, medical and physical therapy supplies. Including: a large variety of acupuncture needles, magnets, cupping instruments, acupuncture hand probes, ion pumping equipment, moxa supplies and accessories, electrical stimulators (including high quality Japanese instruments), office supplies, massage aids, acupuncture models and diagnostic instruments.

OMS can be reached at 1950 Washington St., Braintree, MA 02185. Phone (800) 323-1839, Fax (781) 335-5779. Website: www.omsmedical.com

**QUALIHERBS.** QualiHerbs herbs carry Sheng Chang herbs, which are GMP certified herbal extracts, in both single herb powders and classical formulas. They also carry some formulas in tablet and honey pill form. Besides having a very large selection of single herbs, classical and other formulas (including most of the classic formulas mentioned in the text) they also carry a topical spray and plasters for external use in musculoskeletal injuries. QualiHerbs herbs can custom manufacture and label formulas. They also carry books.

Finemost herbs can be reached at 13839 Bentley Place, Cerritos, CA 90703. Phone (800) 533-5907, Fax (562) 802-0625, E-mail: qualiherb@worldnet.att.net

**Tashi Enterprises.** Tashi enterprises carries Min Tong GMP certified herbal extracts, in both single herb granules and classical formulas (including most of the classical formulas mentioned in the text). They also carry acupuncture equipment (needles, magnets, moxa supplies, electric stimulators, heating lamps, and a Qi-gong massager), nutritional supplements, books and videos.

Tashi Enterprises can be reached at 5221 Central Ave., #105, Richmond, CA 94804. Phone (800) 538-1333, Fax (800) 875-0798, Email: http://www.tashi.com/acu

# Nutritional Supplements

**Allergy Research Group/Nutricology, Inc.** Allergy research carries a variety of nutritional products including products that are helpful in musculoskeletal therapy such as: "live mesenchyme and shark cartilage proteins", Arthred (hydrolyzed collagen) and Matrixx for support of connective tissue, Cytolog (colostrum pepties) for arthritis, SAM and Stabilium for fibromyalgia, anxiety and depression. They also manufacture a large variety of products for gastrointestinal, immune and glandular support.

Allergy Research/Nutricology can be reached at 418 Mission St. San Rafael, CA 94901. Phone (888) 563-1506, Fax (415) 453-1483, Email: arg@nutricology.com

**Douglas Laboratories.** Douglas Laboratories carries a large variety of nutritional products including products that are helpful in musculoskeletal therapy such as: Uni-Joint, and Arthred-Forte for joint support, Proteozyme Forte for injuries, P.I. Pack (cold/hot pack, blue gel and proteozyme) for post-traumatic initial visitl, "live mesenchyme and shark cartilage cells". They manufacture a large variety of products for gastrointestinal, immune and glandular support. Douglas Laboratories

can custom pack and label products for the practitioner.

Douglas Laboratories can be reached at Boyce Rd., Pittsburgh, PA 95205. Phone (800) 245-4440, Fax (412) 494-0122, e-mail nutrition@douglaslabs.com

**Terrace International Distributors, Inc. (TID).** TID is the first nation-wide firm to distribute products from multiple companies, exclusively to health professionals. TID represents over 60 leading nutritional supplement producers (including Thorne research and Allergy Research/Nutricology). They offer convenient one stop shopping for those who choose to purchase products from a variety of companies. TID also offers technical information.

TID can be reached at 2015 W. Park Ave., #4, Redlands, CA 92373. Phone (800) 824-2434, Fax (909) 307-2111.

**Thorne Research, Inc.** Thorne research carries a variety of nutritional products including proprietary products that are helpful in musculoskeletal therapy such as: copper and boron picolinate, AR-Encap for joint inflammation, Collag-En for soft tissue support, water soluble quercetin for inflammation, Myorel for muscle spasm and Sedaplus for anxiety. They also manufacture a large variety of products for gastrointestinal, immune and glandular support. Thorne research is the publisher of *Alternative Medicine Review a Journal of Clinical Therapeutics* (an excellent journal).

Thorne Research can be reached at P.O. Box 3200, Sandpoint, Idaho 83864. Phone (800) 228-1966, Fax (208) 265-2488, Email: info@thorne.com

# Therapy & Orthotic Supplies

**Orthopedic Physical Therapy Products (OPTP).** OPTP carries many exclusive products including books and supplies to be used with the McKenzie system. They also carry many books and video tapes on musculoskeletal therapy, a non-elastic SI belt, manipulation straps, wedges, massage aids, gym balls, proprioception training equipment, stretching and strengthening aids.

OPTP can be reached at P.O. Box 47009, Minneapolis, MN 55447-0009. Phone (800) 367-7393, Fax (612) 553-9355, Email: OPTP@worldnet.att.net

**ORTHO—RITE, INC.** Ortho-Rite manufactures a variety of foot custom orthotic devices at reasonable prices. They are familiar with Dr. Horwitz's Heidy and Lois concepts.

Ortho-Rite can be reached at Westchester county NY. Phone (800) 473-6682, Fax (914) 235-9697, Website: orthorite.com

# *References*

## **Works Cited**

Auaisha BB et al. Acupuncture for the treatment of Chronic Painful Peripheral Diabetic Neuropathy: A long-Term Study. *Diabetic Research and Clinical Practice* 39:115, 1998.

Adams MA, Dolan P, Hutton WC The lumbar spine in backward bending. *spine.* 13:1019, 1988.

Adems MA, Dolan P.: Posture and spinal mechanisms during lifting. *2ed interdisciplinary world congress on low back pain.* The integrated function of the lumbar spine SI joins 1995.

Aigner N et al. Laseracupuncture for Patellar Tendinitis in Performance Athletes. *Akupuncktur Theorie und Praxis* 24:11, 1996.

Akai M, Oda H, Shiraski Y, Tateishi T. Electrical stimulation of ligament healing: An experimental study of the patellar ligament of rabbits. *Clin Orthop.* 235:296, 1988.

Akeson WH, Amiel D, Woo SL-Y. Immobility effects on synovial joints, the pathomechanics of joint contracture. *Biorheology.* 17:95, 1980.

Aldman B. Injury Biomechanics. Government/Industry Meeting and Eposition. Washington, DC: *Society of Automotive Engineers*, 1987; SP-731.

Alvarez OM, Gilbereath RL. Thiamine influence on collagen during the granulation of skin wounds. *J Surg Res* 32:24,1982.

Alvarez OM, Gilbereath RL. Thiamine influence on collagen during the granulation of skin wounds. *J Surg Res* 32:24,1982.

Alvarez OM, Gilbereath RL. Thiamine influence on collagen during the granulation of skin wounds. *J Surg Res* 32:24,1982Alves WM et al.: Understanding posttraumatic symptoms after minor head injury. *J Head Trouma Rehabil.* 1:1, 1986.

Alves WM. Motor vehicle head injuries: damage and outcome. *In: Crash Injury Impairment and Disability*: Long Term Effects. International Congress and Exposition; paper 860423. Detroit, Mich: Society of Automotive Engineers; SP-661:167-176, 1986.

American Medical Association. *Standard Nomenclature of Athletic Injuries.* AMA Chicago, 1976.

Amiel D, Woo S et al. The effects of immobilization on collagen turnover in connective tissue. *Trans Orthop Res Soc* 6:85, 1981.

Ammon HPT, Mack T, et al. Inhibition of Leukotriene B4 Formation in rat Peritoneal Neutrophils by Ethanolic extract of the Gum Resin Exudate of Boswellia Serrata. *Planta Medica* 57:203, 1991.

Andermann G and Dietz M. The influence of an endogenous macromolecule: Chondroitin Sulfate (CSA), *Eur.J.Drug Metabol. Pharmacol.,* 7,11,1982.

Angelica sinensis research unit, Second Teaching Hospital of Hubei Medical College. *Health J of Jubei* 5:64, 1977.

Annand JC. Pantothenic acid and osteoarthritis. Letter. Lancet 2:1168,1963;

Annand JC. Osteoarthrosis and pantothenic acid. Letter. *J coll Gen Pract* 5:136,1962.

Aprahamian M et al. *Am J Clin Nutr* 578:89,1985.

Aprill C, Bogduk N.:High-intensity zone: a diagnostic sign of painful lumbar disc on magnetic resonance imaging. *Br J Radiol.* 65:361, 1992.

Aprill C. et al: Discografic outcomes predicted by centralization of pain and directional preference. A prospective study. *Presented at the Eighth Annual International Intradical therapy Society Meeting*, San Diego, Calif, 1995.

Arpaia MR et al. Effects of Centella asiatica extract on mucopolysaccharide metabolism in subjects with varicose veins. *Int J Clin Pharmacol Res* 10:229-,1990.

Asmundson GJ, Taylor S. Role of anxiety sensitivity in pain-related fear and avoidance. *J Behav Med* 19:577, 1996.

## **B**

Baker BA: The muscle trigger: evidence of overload injury. *J Neurol Orthop Med Surg* 10:129, 1989.

Baker d, Daito M.: *Proc. R Soc. Land. B.* 212,1981.

Baker DM. Penniculitis. *Lancet. 2: 75,* 1951.

Balagot RC et al. Analgesia in mice and humans

by D-phenylalanine: Relation to inhibition of enkephalin degradation and enkephalin levels. *Adv Pain Res Ther* 5:289,1983.

Baldry PE. Acupuncture, *Trigger Points and Musculoskeletal Pain* (2ed ed) Churchill Livingstone 1993.

Balgent, Michael, Leigh, Richard. *The Dead Sea Scrolls Deception.* Simon and Schuster, New York, 1991.

Balla, J., Karnaghan, J. Whiplash Headache. *Clin Exp Neurol* 23:179, 1987.

Brand P. Pain--it's all in your head: a philosophical essay. *J Hand Ther* 10:59, 1997.

Banks AR. A rationale for prolotherapy. *J Orthop Med* 13:54, 1991.

Bann RT, Woods PH: An attempt to estimate the size of the problem. *Rheumatol Rehabil* 14:121,1975.

Bannister G et al. The management of acute acromioclavicular dislocations. *J Bone Joint Surg* 71:848, 1989.

Barnsley L, Lord SM, Wallis BJ, Bogduk N. The prevalence of chronic cervical zygapophyseal joint pain after whiplash. *Spine* 20:20, 1995.

Barnett C, Richardson AT. The postural function of the popliteus muscle. *Ann Phys Med* 17:179, 1953.

Barnsley L, Lord SM, Wallis BJ, Bogduk N Lack of effect of intra-articular corticosteroids for chronic pain in the cervical zygapophyseal joints. *N Engl J Med* 330:1047, 1994.

Barson PK, Solomon JD. Blood Serotonin in Chronic Pain Syndromes. *Am J Pain Mang* 8:49, 1998.

Basford JR. Low-energy laser therapy: Controversies and new research findings. *Lasers Surg Med* 9:1,1989.

Basic Research Group. Xian Medical Collage *Shaanxi Med J* 1:28,1972.

Basmajian JV. *Muscles Alive.* 4th Ed. Williams & Willkins, Baltimore, 1978.

Basmajian JV and Nyberg R. *Rational Manual Therapies* edi Williams & Wilkins 1993.

Bates CJ, Levene CI. The effect of ascorbic acid deficiency on the glycosaminoglycans and glycoproteins in connective tissue. Biol Nutr Dieta 13:131, 1969.

Battié MC et al. Smoking and lumbar interverte-

bral disc degeneration: as MRI study of identical twins, *spine.* 16:1015, 1991.

Bauman J et al. *Prostaglandins* 20:627,1980.

Beaton E, Anson BJ: The sciatic nerve and the piriformis muscle: their interrelationship a possible cause of coccygodynia. *J Bone Joint Surg* [Br] 20:686, 1938.

Beattie P et al. Validity of derived measurements of leg length differences obtained by use of a tape measure. *Phys Ther* 70 150, 1990.

Becker RO, Selden G. *The Body Electric: Electromagnetism and the Foundation of Life.* New York: William Morrow and Company, 1985.

Becker RO and Marino AA. *Electromagnetism and life,* State University of NY Press, 1982.

Beforre GH J et al. Heterozygosity for homocystinuria in premature peripheral and cerebral occlusive arterial disease. *N Eng J Med* 313:709,1985.

Beighton, P., R. Grahame, and H Brode: *Hypermobility of Joints.* Berlin, Pringer-Verlag, 1983.

Beneliyahu DJ. Chiropractic management and manipulative therapy for MRI documented cervical disk herniation. *J Manipulative Physiol Ther* 17:177, 1994.

Bennett GF. Neuropathic pain In: *Textbook of pain* Wall and Melzack (ed). Churchill Livingstone (3ed ed), 1994.

Bensoussan A. *The Vital Meridian, A modern Exploration of Acupuncture.* Churchill Livingstone UK 1991.

Bettany JA, Fish DR, Mendel FC. Influence of high voltage pulsed galvanic stimulation on edema formation following impact injury. *Pys Ther.* 69:301, 1988.

Bernstein IH, Jaremko ME, Hinkley BS. On the utility of the West-Haven-Yale-Multidimensional pain inventory. *Spine* 20:956, 1995).

Bernstein Al. Vitamin B6 in neurology. *Ann N Y Acad Sci* 585:250,1990.

Bhathena S et al. Decreased plasma enkephalins in copper deficiency in man. *Am J Clin Nutr* 43:42,1986.

Bhattacharya SK and Mira SK. Anxiolytic activity of Panax ginseng roots: an experimental study. *J Ethnopharmacol* 34:87,1991.

Biering-Sorenson F. Physical measurements as risk factors for low back trouble over a one year period. *Spine* 9:106, 1984.

Binkley and Peat.: The effects of immobilization on the ultrastructure and mechanical properties of the rat medial collateral ligament. *Clin Orthop* 203:30, 1986.

Biochem Pharm 38:3527-34;1989.

Biskind MS, Marin WC. The use of citrus flavonoids in infection. II. *Am J Digest Dis* 22:4145, 1955.

Black HN. An improved technique for the evaluation of ligamentous infer in severe ankle sprains. *Am J Sports Med* ^:276, 1978.

Bland JH. The cervical spine: from anatomy to clinical care. *Med Times*. 9:15, 1989.

Blankenhorn G. Vitamin E: Clinical research from Europe. *Nutr Dietary Consult*. June 1988.

Bland JH, Cooper SM. Osteoarthritis: A review of the cell biology involved and evidence for reversibility. Management rationally related to Known genesis and pathophysiology. *Semin Arthritis Rheum* 14:106,1984.

Blau JN, MacGregor EA. Migraine and the neck. *Headache* 2:88, 1994.

Blum LW et al. Peripheral neuropathy and cadmium toxicity. *Pa Med* 92:54,1989Baker D. Banks R. The muscle spindle. In: Engel A, Benker B. eds. *Myology*. NY: McGraw-Hill, 1986.

Bridgman C, Eldred E., *Science* 143,481,1964.

Bogduk, N., Aprill, C. On the Nature of Neck Pain, Discography and Cervical Zygapophyseal Joint Blocks. *Pain* 54:213, 1993.

Bogduk N, Tynan W, Wilson AS. The nerve supply to the human lumbar intervertebral discs. *J Anat* 132:39,1981.

Bogduk N. A reappraisal of the anatomy of the human erector spinae. *J Anat* 131:525, 1980.

Bogduk N, Macintosh JE, Pearcy MJ.: A universal model of the lumbar back muscles in the upright position. *Spine* 17:897, 1992.

Bogduk N, Windsor M, Inglis A. The innervation of the cervical intervertebral discs. *Spine*. 13:3, 1988.

Bogduk N, Twomey LT.: *Clinical Anatomy of the Lumbar Spine*. 2nd Ed. Churchill Livingstone, Melbourne, 1991.

Bogduk N.:Pathology of lumbar disc pain. *J Manu Medi*. 5:72,1990.

Bogduk, N. The anatomical Basis for Cervico-

genic Headache. *J Manipulative Physiol Ther*. 1:67, 1992.

Bogduk N. A reappraisal of the anatomy of the human erector spinae. *J Anat* 131:525, 1980.

Bogduk N. *The zygapophyseal joints—the most common source of neck pain*. American Back Society 1997.

Boline PD, Kassak K, Bronfort G, Nelson C, Anderson AV. Spinal manipulation vs. amitriptyline for the treatment of chronic tension-type headaches: a randomized clinical trial. *J Manipulative Physiol Ther* 3:148, 1995.

Bombelli R. *Structure and function in normal and abnormal hips*. 3ed ed. Springer-Verlag NY 1993.

Bonica J.J., *The Management of Pain*. lea & febinger 1990.

Borsook H et al. The relief of symptoms of major trigeminal neuralgia (tic douloureux) following the use of vitamin B1 and concentrated liver extract. *JAMA* April 13, 1940.

Bourdillon JF, Day EA, Brookhout MR. *Spinal Manipulation Butterworth Heinemann 5th edi. 1992.*

Bourguignon GJ, Bourguignon LYW. Electric stimulation of protein and DNA synthesis in human fibroblasts. *FASEB J*. 1:198, 1987.

Bower BL. Rigid subtalar Joint—a radiographic spectrum. *Skeletal Radiol* 17:583, 1989.

Bowsher D. The physiology of stimulation-producted analgesia. *J of the British Med Acupuncture Society* 2:58, 1991.

Brandmuller J. Fivefold symmetry in mathematics, physics, chemistry, biology and beyond. In *Fivefold Symmetry*, Hargittai I, editor. World Scientific Singapure 1992.

Brattberg G. Acupuncture therapy for tennis elbow. *Pain* 16:283, 1983.

Brevetti G et al. Increases in walking distance in patients with peripheral vascular disease treated with L-carnitine: A double-blind, crossover study. *Circulation* 77:767,1988.

Brighton CT, Pollack SR. Treatment of recalcitrant nonunion with a capacitively coupled electrical field. *J Bone Joint Surg*. 67-A:577, 1986.

Brodsky AE, Khalil MA. Update of experience with electrical stimulation for enhancement of lumbar spine fusion. *Tras Biol Repair Growth*

*Soc.* 8:25, 1988.

Brooks PM, Potter SR, Buchanan WW. NSAID and osteoarthritis help or hindrance. J Rheumatol 9:3, 1985.

Brouillette DL, Gurske DT. Chiropractic treatment of cervical radiculopathy caused by a herniated cervical disc. *J Manipulative Physiol Ther* 17:119, 1994.

Brown M. American Academy of Oriental Orthopedics. *Lectures* 1995; 1996.

Brown CW, Orme TJ, Richardson HD. The rate of pseudoarthrosis (surgical nonunion) in patients who are smokers and patients who are nonsmokers: a comparison study. *Spine.* 11:943, 1986.

Brown RA. Weiss JB. Neovascularisation and its role in the osteoarthritic process. *Ann Ruem Dis* 47:881,1988.

Burns et al. Linking symptom-specific physiological reactivity to pain severity in chronic low back pain patients: a test of mediation and moderation models. Health Psychol 16:319, 1997.

Bucci LR. Chondroprotective Agents Glucosamine Salts and Chondroitin Sulfates. *Townsend Letter for Doctors*, Jan 1994 Cohen A, Goldman J. Bromelains therapy in rheumatoid arthritis. *Pennsyl Med J* 67:27,1964.

Byers CM et al. Pyridoxine metabolism in carpal tunnel syndrome with and without peripheral neuropathy. *Am J Med* 75:887,1983.

C

Cailliet R. *Neck and Arm Pain*. 3ed ed. Philadelphia: FA Davis Co; 1991.

Cailliet R. Neck and Arm Pain 12th (ed). FA Davis Company, Philadelphia, 1977.

Cailleit, R. *Low Back Pain Syndromes*. 3st Ed. Philadelphia, F.A. Davis, 1981.

Calabro, J.J., et al.: Classification of anterior chest wall syndrome. JAMA, 243:1420,1980.

Campbell SM. Clinical characteristics of fibrositis. *Arthritis and Rheumatism.* 26:817,1983.

Carey PF A report on the occurrence of cerebral vascular accidents in chiropractic practice; *J of the Canadian Chiro Ass*; 37:104, 1993.

Cats-Baril WL, Frymoyer JW. Identifying patients at risk of becoming disabled because of low-back pain. *Spine* 16:605, 1991.

Cervero F. Afferent activity evoked by neural stimulation of the biliary system of the efferents. *Pain.* 13:137, 1982.

Cervero F, Laird JMA, Pozo MA.: Selective changes of receptive field properties of spinal nociceptive neurons induced by noxious visceral stimulation in the cat. *Pain* 51:335-342, 1992.

Chan SHH. What is being stimulated in Acupuncture: Evaluation of the existence of a specific substrate. *Neurosci Biobehav Rev* 8:25, 1984.

Chen GS. The effect of acupuncture treatment on carpal tunnel syndrome. *Amer J of Acup* 18:5, 1990.

Chen XG, et. al. Effects of the extract of Polygonum multiflorum on some biochemical indicators related to aging in old mice. *Chinese Traditional and Herbal Drugs*;22:357, 1991.

Chen JM et al. *Zhongma Tongxun* (communications of Chinese Traditional Anesthesia) 3:30, 1978Calcium pantothenate in arthritis conditions. A report from the General Practitioner Research Group. *Practitioner* 224:208,1980.

Chiang CY, Liu JY, Chu TH, Pai YH, Chang SC. Studies on spinal ascending pathway for effect of acupuncture analgesia in rabbits. *Sci China* 18:651, 1975.

Chiang CY, Chiang CT and Chu HL. Peripheral afferent pathways for acupuncture analgesia. *Sci China* 16:210, 1973.

Christensen BV et al. Acupuncture treatment of severe knee osteoarthritis: a long-term study. *Acta Anaes Scand* 36:5, 1992.

Christie SBM et al. Observations on the performance of a standard exercise test by claudicants taking gamma-linolenic acid. *J Atheroscler Res.* 8:83,1986.

Chung JM, Lee KH, Hori Y, Endo K, Willis WD. Factors influencing peripheral nerve stimulation produced inhibition of primate spinothalamic tract cells. *Pain* 19:277, 1984.

Chusid JG. *Correlative Neuroanatomy & Functional Neurology*. 18th edition Lang Medical Publications Los Altos 1982.

Cichoke AJ, Marty L. The use of proteolytic enzymes with soft tissue athletic injuries. *Am Chiropractor*, Oct 1981.

Clark K. et al, Aged-related hearing loss and

bone mass in population of rural women aged 60-85 years. Annals of Epidemiology, 5:8-4, 1995.

Clark CR. Atlanto-axial rotatory fixation with compensatory counter occipito-atlantal subluxation. *Spine* 12:488, 1987.

C T.: Experimental models of osteoarthritis: the role of immobilization. *Clin Biomech* 2:223, 1987.

Cobb JR. Outline for the study of scoliosis. *Am Acad Orthop Surg* 5:261, 1958.

Cohnheim JF. Lectures on general pathology (English translation) London 1889.

Colantuoni S et al. Effects of Vaccinium myritillus anthocyanosides on arterial vasomotion. *Arzneim Forsch* 41:905,1991.

Colachis SC, Worden RE, Bechtol CO et al. Movement of the sacro-iliac joint in the adult male: A preliminary report *Archiv Phys Med Rehabil* 44, 1963.

Cook SP, Vulchanova L, Hargreaves KM, Elde R, McCleskey EW. Distinct ATP receptors on pain-sensing and stretch-sensing neurons. *Nature* 387:505,1997.

Cordell GA, Araujo OE. Capsaicin: Identification, Nomenclature, and pharmacotherapy. *Ann Pharmacother* 27: 330,1993.

Cragin RB.: The use of Bioflavonoids in the Prevention and Treatment of Athletic Injuries. *Medical Times* Vol 90,No 5 May 1962.

Creagan ET et al. Failure of high-dose vitamin C therapy to benefit patients with advanced cancer. *N Engl J Med* 301:687,1979.

Crocq L et al. Treatment of astheno-depressive conditions by Manprine, Multi-center study of 248 cases assessed by Fatigue. *Psychologie Medicale* 12:643, 1980.

Cyriax JH, Cyriax PJ. *Cyriax's illustrated manual of orthopaedic medicine*, Oxford Butterworth Heinemann 1993.

Cyriax, J. *Textbook of Orthopaedic Medicine, Vol I* 8th ed. Baillère Tindall 1982.

**D**

Daffner RH. Stress fractures: current concepts. *Skeletal Radiol*.

Dai YR and Yin Y. Inhibition of MAO B activity by Chinese medicinal materials. *Chinese Journal of Geriatrics* 6:27, 1987.

Dai YR and Yin Y. Inhibition of MAO B activity by Chinese medicinal materials. *Chinese Journal of Geriatrics* 6:27, 1987.

Dain TR and Tin Y. Inhibition of MAO B activity by Chinese medicinal materials. *Chinese Journal of Geriatrics* 6:27, 1987.

DeFeudis FV. Ginkgo biloba extract (EGb 761). *Pharmacological Activities and Clinical Applications*. Paris, Elsevier, 1991.

Daffner RH. Magnetic resonance imaging in acute tendon ruptures. *Skeletal Radiol* 15:619, 1986.

Dettori Ag, Ponari O. Effetto antalgico della aobamimide in corso di neuropatie periferche di diversa etopatogenesi. *Minerva Med* 64:1077,1973Dalal, B., Harrison, G. Psychiatric Consequences of Road Traffic Accidents, *BMJ* 307:1282, 1993.

Dalton S, Snyder S. Glenohumeral instability. *Balliere's Clin Rheumatol* 3:511, 1989.

Dau TR and Yin Y. Inhibition of MAO B activity by Chinese medicinal materials. *Chinese Journal of Geriatrics* 6:271978.

de Duve C. *A guided tour of the living cell.* Scientific American Books, New York 1984.

De Fabio A. Treatment & prevention of osteoarthritis. *Townsend Letter for Doctors*. February-March, 143, 1990.

De Vernejoul P, Albaréde P, Darras JC. Etude des Méridiens D'acupuncture Par Les Traceurs Radioactifs. *Bull Acad Nat Méd* 169:1071, 1985.

Deans et al. Neck sprain: a major cause of disability following car accidents. *Injury*18:10, 1987.

Deburge A, Mazda K, Guigui P. Unstable degenerative spondylolisthesis of the cervical spine. *J Bone Joint Surg Br* Jan 77:122, 1995.

Deng Y-C, Goldsmith W. Response of a human head/neck/upper-torso replica to dynamic loading. I: physical model. *J Biomechanics* 5:741,1987.

Denslow, JS., Korr IM.,Krems AD. Quantitative studies of chronic facilitation in human motoneuron pools, *Amer. J. Phsiol.* 105: 229, 1947.

Derby R. Interadiscal Radio-Frequency Thermocoagulation - A Prospective Pilot Study. *Proceedings of the American Back Society* SF 1997.

Dettori AG, Ponari O. Effetto antalgico della

cobamamide in corso di neuropatie periferiche di diversa etiopatogenesi. *Minerva Med* 64:1077,1973.

Deyo RA, Diehl AK, Rosenthal M.: How many days of bed rest for acute low back pain?. *N Engl J Med*. 315:1064, 1986.

D'Ambrosio E et al. Glucosamine sulphate: A controlled clinical investigation in arthrosis. *Pharmatherapeutica* 2:504,1981.

Di Renzi L et al. [On the use of injectable crataegus extracts in therapy of the lower extremities]. *Voll Soc Ital Cardiol* 14:577,1969.

Dieck GS et al. An epidemiologic study of the relationship between postural asymmetry in the teen years and subsequent back neck pain. *Spine* 10:872, 1985.

Dihlmann Wolfgang. *Diagnostic Radiology of the Sacroiliac Joint*. Yearbook Medical Publishers Inc.: Chicago and london 1980.

Donelson R, Silva G, Murphy K. Centralization phenomenon: Its usefulness in evaluating and treating referred pain. *Spine* 15:211,1990.

DonTigny R L. Sacroiliac dysfunction: Recognition and treatment. First Interdisciplinary *World Congress on Low Back Pain and its Relation to the Sacroiliac Joint* San Diego. November 5-6, 1992.

Dorman TA, Ravin TH. *Diagnosis and Injection Techniques in Orthopedic Medicine*. Williams & Wilkens, 1991.

Dorman TA. Failure of self-bracing at the sacroiliac joints: The slipping clutch syndrome. *J of Othrop Med*. 16:49, 1994.

Dorman T A, Buchmiller JC, Cohen RE, Lively AJ, Peffall SM Stein JB Brown R. Energy Efficiency During Human Walking. *J Orthop Med*. 1993.

Dorman TA. *A new understanding of whiplash*. American Back Society 1997.

Dorman, T.A., Cohen R E., Dasig D., Jeng S., Fischer N., Dejong, A. Energy Efficiency During Human Walking; Before and After Prolotherapy. *J Orthop Med* 17:1, 1995 (accepted).

Dorman T, et al. The effective of Garum Amoricum (Stabilium) on Reducing Anxiety in College Students. *J of Advan in Med* 8:193, 1995.

Dorman HL, Gage TW. Effects of electroacupuncture on the threshold for eliciting the jaw depressor reflex in cats. *Arch Oral Biol* 23:505, 1982.

Dowling RJ et al. Use of fat emulsions, in M Deitel, Ed. *Nutrition in Clinical Surgery*. Baltimore, Williams and Wilkins, 1985.

Dragomirescu C, et al. L'action de l'acupuncture sur les composants sanguins et les principales fonctions de défense organique. *Revue Internationale d'Acupuncture*, 2:16, 1961.

Dreyfuss P, Michaelsen M, Fletcher D. Atlanto-occipital and lateral atlanto-axial joint pain patterns. *Spine* 19:1125, 1994.

Duchenne GB. *Physiology of motion*, translated by E.B. Kaplan. J.B. Lippincott, Philadelphia, 1949.

Dung HC: Anatomical features contributing to the formation of acupuncture points. *Amer J Acup* 12:139, 1984.

Dvorák, J., Schmeider, E., Rahn, B. Biomechanics of the Cranio-cervical Region: the Alar and Transverse Ligaments. *J. Orthop. Res.* 6:452, 1988.

Dvorák j. CT-Functional diagnostics of the rotary instability of upper cervical spine. *Spine* 12:197, 1987.

Dvorák, J.M., Panjabi, M., Grber, M., Wichmann, W. CT-Functional Diagnostics of the Rotary Instability of Upper Cervical Spine. I: An Experimental Study on Cadavers. *Spine* 12:195, 1987.

Dvorák, J., Dvorák, V. *Manual Medicine Diagnostics*, 2nd ed. Thieme Medical Publishers, Inc. 1990.

Dvorák J, Baumgartner J, Antinnes JA: Frequency of complications of manipulations of the spine. *Eur Spine*. 2;136, 1993.

**E**

Eguchi K, Origuchi T, Takashima H, Iwata K, Katamine S, Nagataki S. *Arthritis Rheum* 39:463, 1996.

Egund, N. et al.: Movements in the sacroiliac joints demonstrated with Roentgen stereophotogrammetry. *Acta Radiol. Diagn* 19:5, 1978.

Egund N, Olsson TH, Schmid H et al. Movement in the sacro-iliac joints demonstrated with Roentgen stereophotogrammetry. *Acta Radiologica Diagnosis* 19:83345, 1978.

Ehrenpreis S. Potentiation of acupuncture analgesia by inhibition of endorphin degradation. *Acupunct Electrother Res Int J.* 8:310, 1993.

Eliyahu DJB. Disc herniations of the cervical spine. *Am j Chiro Med.* 3:93, 1989.

Epstein NE. Technical note: "Dynamic" MRI scanning of the cervical spine. *Spine* 13:937, 1988.

Ernst M, Lee MHM. Sympathetic vasomotor changes induced by manual and electrical acupuncture of Hoku Point visualized by thermography. *Pain*, 21:25, 1985.


**F**

Fam A G et al.: Stress fractures in rheumatoid arthritis. J. Rheumatol., 10:722, 1983.

Fan YJ et al. Information on Medical Sciences and Technology, *Guangxi Institute of Medical and Pharmaceutical Bulletin* 11:56, 1965.

Fan SG, Qu ZC, Zhe QZ, Han JS. GABA: antagonistic effect on electroacupuncture analgesia and morpine analgesia in rat. *Life Sci* 31:1225, 1982.

Farfan H F. *Mechanical Disorders of the low back*. Philadelphia, Lea&Feber, 1973.

Fassbender HG. Der rheumatische Schmerz, *Med.Welt* 36:1263, 1980.

Feng GH. *Jiangxi Yirao* (Jiangxi Medical J) 6:26, 1961.

Fiexner, Abraharn. *Medical Education in the United States and Canada* A report to the Carnegie Foundation for the Advancement of Teaching, 1910.

Fitz-Ritson D. Phasic exercises for cervical rehabilitation after "whiplash" trauma. *J Manipulative Physiol Ther* 18:21, 1995.

Fitzmaurice R, Cooper RG, Freemont AJ: A histo-morphometric comparison of muscle biopsies from normal subjects and patients with ankylosing spondylitis and severe mechanical low back pain. *J Pathol* 163:182, 1992.

Flohe L. Superoxide dismutase for therapeutic use: clinical experience, dead ends and hopes. *Mol Cell Biochem* 84: 123,1988).

Flohe L et al. Effectiveness of superoxide dismutase in osteoarthritis of the knee joint. Results of a double blind multi-center clinical trial, in WH Bannister, JV Bannester, Eds. *Biological and Clinical Aspects of Superoxide and Superoxde Dismutase*. New York, Elsevier/North Holland,1980.

Foreman RD, Ohata CA. Effect of coronary artery occlusion on thoracic spinal neurons receiving viscerosomatic inputs. *Am. J. Physiol.* 238:H666, 1980.

Foreman SM. *Whiplash Injuries*. Williams & Wilkins, 1988.

Foreman SM, Croft AC. Whiplash Injuries, *The Cervical Acceleration/Deceleration Syndrome*. Williams & Wilkins 1988.

Forese RV et al. Licorice-induced hypermineralocorticoidism. *N Engl J Med* 325:1223,1991.

Franson RC, Saal JS, Saal JA. Human disc phospholipase A2 is inflammatory. *Spine.* 17:S129, 1992.

Friberg O. Clinical symptoms and Biomechanics of lumbar spine and hip joint in leg length inequality. *Spine* 8: 643, 1985.

Frost FA, Jessen B, Siggaard-Andersen J. A controlled, double-blind comparison of mepivacaine injection versus saline injection for myofascial pain. *Lancet* 1:499, 1980.

Fukui S, Ohseto K, Shiotani M, Ohno K, Karasawa H, Naganuma Y, Yuda Y. Referred pain distribution of the cervical zygapophyseal joints and cervical dorsal rami. Pain 68:79, 1996.

Fuller RB. *Synergetics*. New York 1975.

Fulgham DD. Ascorbic acid revisited. *Arch Dermatol*, 113:91,1977Fairbank et al.: The Oswestry Low Back Pain Index, *Physiotherapy* 66:271, 1980.

Furtado D, Chicorro V. *Rev Clin Espan Madrid* 5:516,1942.


**G**

Gargan MF, Mannister GC. Long term prognosis of soft tissue injury of the neck. *JBJS* 72-B:901, 1990.

Garrick JG, Ebb DR. *Sports Injuries: Diagnosis and Management*. Saunders Comp 1990.

Gatchel RJ et al. Million Behavioral Health Inventory: its ability in predicting physical function in patients with low back pain. *Arch Phy Med Rehab* 67:878, 1986).

Gattett NE et al. Role of substance P in inflammatory arthritis. *Ann Reum Dis* 51:1014, 1992.

Gedhey EH. Hypermobile joint *Osteopathic Profession* 4:30, 1937.

Greenman DM et al. Serum copper and zinc in rheumatoid arthritis and osteoarthritis. *N Z Med J* 91:47,1980.

Gelberman et al. The effects of mobilization on the vascularization of healing flexor tendons in dogs. *Clin Orthop* 153:283, 1989.

Gerlach. H.L. Über die Bewegung in den Atlas-gelenke unde deren Beziehungen du der Butsrömmung an den vertebral Arterien. *Beitr. Morpbol*, 1:104, 1984.

Gilmer W, Anderson L. Reaction of the somatic tissue which progress to bone formation. *South Med J*. 52:1432, 1959.

Gleick J. *Chaos*. Penguin Books New York 1988.

Glogowski G, Wallraff J. Ein beitrag zur Klinik und Histologie der Muskelharten (Myo-gelosen). *Z Orthop* 80:237, 1951.

Gogia PP, Sabbahi MA. Electromyographic analysis of neck muscle fatigue in patients with osteoarthritis of the cervical spine. *Spine* 19:502, 1994.

Gordon JE. *The science of structures and materials*. Scientific American Library. New York, 1988.

Gordon JE. *Structures: or Why things don't fall down*. De Capa Press, New York 1978.

Grace DL. Lateral ankle ligament injuries. *Clin Orthop* 183:153, 1984.

Gracovetsky S. *The Spinal Engine*. Springer-Verlag, New York 1988.

Grant, R. Dizziness Testing and Manipulation of the Cervical Spine, in *Physical Therapy of the Cervical and Thoracic Spine*. ed.: R. Grant 1988.

Greenman PE. *Principles of Manual Medicine*. Williams & Wilkins 1989.

Greenman PE. *Principles of Manual Medicine* (2ed edi). Williams & Wilkins 1996.

Greenman P.E. Sacroiliac Dysfunction In The Failed Low Back Pain Syndrome, *First Interdisciplinary World Congress on Low Back Pain and its Relation to the SI Joint* 1992.

Greenman P E. Clinical aspects of sacroiliac function in walking. *J Manual Med*. 5:25,1990.

Guan, Yu, Wng and Liu. The role of cholinergic nerves in electroacupuncture analgesia - influence of acetylcholine, eserine, neostigmine, and hemichonum on electroacupuncture analgesia. In: Zhang XT (ed) *Research on acupuncture, moxibustion, and acupuncture anesthesia*. Science Press, Beijing 1986.

Guizhou Institute for Drug Control. Proceedings of the first symposium of the *Chinese Parmaceutical Association*. 324,1962.Galletti R, Procacci P. The role of the sympathetic system in the control of pain and of some associated phenomena. *Aceta Neurovegetativa* 28:495,1966.

Gunn CC. Tennis elbow and the cervical spine. CMA J. 114:803, 1976.

Gunn CC. "Bursitis" Around the Hip. *Am. J. Acup*. 5:53, 1977.

Gunn CC. Shoulder Pain, Cervical Spondylosis and Acupuncture. *Am J Acup*. 5:121, 1977.

Gunn CC. Tennis Elbow and the Cervical Spine. *Can Med Assoc J*. 114:803, 1977.

Gunn CC. *Treating Myofascial Pain Intramuscular Stimulation for Myofascial Pain Syndromes of Neuropathic Origin*. University of Washington 1989.

Gunn CC. Neuropathic Pain: A New Theory for Chronic Pain of Intrinsic Origin. *Annals RCPSC*. 22. 327, 1989.


# H

Hachett G S, Hemwall, GA, Montgomery GA.: *Ligament and Tedon Relaxation treated by Prolotherapy*. Gustav A Hemwall, Publisher 1991.

Hackett GS. Ligament and tendon relaxation. Treated by prolotherapy. 3rd ed. Springfield: Charles C. Thomas Publisher, 1958.

Hachisu M et al. Analgesic effect of novel organogermanium compound. Ge-132. *J Pharmacobiodyn* 6:814,1983.

Haeckel E. *Report on the scientific results of the voyage of the H.M.S. Challenger*, Radiolaria Edinburg 18:XL, 1887.

Haker E, Lundeberg T. Acupuncture treatment in epicondlylagia: a comparative study of two acupuncture techniques. *The Clinical J of Pain* 6:221,1990.

Hamba XT, Toda K. Rat hypothalamic arcuate neuron response in electroacupuncture-induced analgesia. *Brain Res* 21:31, 1988.

Hambly MF, Mooney V. Effect of smoking and pulsed electromagnetic fields on intradiscal pH in rabbits. *Spine.* 17:S83, 1992.

Hamilton W. *Traumatic Disorders Of The Ankle.* Springer Verlag, NY, 1984.

Han JS, Tang J, Zhou Z. Augmentation of acupuncture analgesia by peptidase inhibitor D-phenylalanine in rabbits. *Acta Zoologica Sinica.* 2:133, 1991.

Han JS. *The Neurochemical Basis of Pain Relief by Acupuncture*: A collection of papers 1973-1987. Beijing Medical University. 1987.

Han JS. Neurochemical Basis of Acupuncture Analgesia. *Ann. Rev. Pharmocol Toxicol* 22:193, 1982.

Han JS, Zhou ZF, Xuan YT. Acupuncture has analgesic effect in rabbits. *Pain* 15:83, 1983.

Han JS. Physiology and neurochemical basis of acupuncture analgesia, in Cheng TO (ed). *The International Textbook of Cardiology.* Pergamon Press, NY 1986.

Han JS. Recent Advances in the Mechanisms of Acupuncture Analgesia. *The World United J for TCM and Acup* 1:2, 1998.

Hanck A, Weiser H. Analgesic and anti-inflammatory properties of vitamins. *Int J Vitam Nutr Res* (supp) 27:189,1985.

Hanck A, Wiser H. Analgesic and anti-inflammatory properties of vitamins. *Int J Vitam Nutr Res* (supp) 37:189,1985.

Hansen PE, Hansen JH. Acupuncture treatment of chronic tension headache: a controlled cross-over trial. *Cephalalgia* 5:137, 1985.

Hardin JG, Halla JT. Cervical spine and radicular pain syndromes, *Curr Opin Rheumatol* 2:136, 1995.

Harper P, Nuki G. Genetic factors in osteoarthrosis. In: The aetiopathogenesis of osteoarthrosis. Pitman Press 1980.

Hascall VC, Hascall GK. Proteoglycans. In Cell *Biology of Extracellular Matrix*, edited by Hay ED. Penum, New York, 1981.

Hayes MA. Roentgenographic evaluation of lumbar spine flexion-extension in asymptomatic individuals. *Spine* 14:327, 1989.

Heine H. Anatomische Struktur der Akupunkturpunkte. *Dtsch Ztschr Akup* 31:26, 1988.

Helbig T, Lee CK. The lumbar facet syndrome. *Spine* 13:61, 1988.

Helms JM. *Acupuncture Energetics. A Clinical Approach for Physicians.* Medical Acupuncture Publishers, 1995.

Heinz, G.J., and Zavala, D.C.: Slipping rib syndrome. Diagnosis using the "hooking maneuver" *JAMA*, 237:794,1977.

Hendriksson, K.D., et al.: Muscle biopsy findings of possible diagnostic importance in primary fibromyalgia (fibrositis, myofascial syndrome). *Lancet* 2:1395, 1982.

Henriet JP. [Veno-lymphatic insufficiency. 4,729 pts. undergoing hormonal and procymidol oligomer therapy]. *Phlebolojie* 46:313,1993.

Hide JA, Stokes MJ, Saide M, et al.: Evidence of lumbar multifidus muscles wasting ipsilateral to symptoms in patients with acute/subacute low back pain 1994.

Hieber H. Die Behandlung vertebragener schmerezen und sensibilitatsstorungen mit hochdosiertem hydroxocobalamin. *Med Monatsschr* 28:545,1974.

Hilsrome C et al. Effect of ginseng on the performance of nurses on night duty. *Comp Med East West* 6:277,1982.

Hinz, P. Sektionsbefunde nach Schleudertraunmen der Halswirbelsäule. *Dt. Z Med* 64:204, 1968.

Hippocrates. *The genuine works of Hippocrates.* Francis Adams, trans. Baltimore: Williams & Wilkins 212, 1946.

Hirschberg GG, Lynn P, Ramsey T. The Incidence and distribution of skinfold tenderness in subjects with cervical sprain. *The J Orthop Med* 16:52, 1994.

Hirschberg G.G., Williams K.A., Byrd J.G.: Diagnosis and Treatment of Iliocostal Friction Syndromes, *J Ortho Med* 14:35, 1992.

Hirsch, S.A., Hirsch, P.J., Hiramoto, H. et al. Whiplash Syndromes: Fact or Fiction? *Orthop Clin North Am* 3:19, 1988.

Hohl M. Soft tissue injuries of the neck. *Clin Orthop.* 109:42, 1975.

Holbrook, T.L., et al.: *The Frequency of Occurrence, Impact and Cost of Selected Musculoskeletal Conditions in the US.* Chicago, American Academy of Orthopedic Surgeons,1984.

Hollinshead WH. *Functional Anatomy of the*

*Limbs and Back*. 4th Ed. W.B. Saunders, Philadelphia, 1976.

Holm S, Nachemson A. Nutrition of the intervertebral disc: acute effects of cigarette smoking: an experimental animal study. *Uppsala J Med Sci*. 93:91, 1988.

Holm S et al. Nutrition of the intervertibral disc: Solute transport and metabolism. *Connect Tissue Tes*. 8:101, 1981.

Hopwood JJ, Robinson HC. The molecular-weight distribution of glycosaminoglycans. *Biochem J* 135:631, 1973.

Houghton PJ. The biological activity of Valerian and related plants. *J Ethnopharmacol* 22:121,1988.

Howard JMH. Magnesium deficiency in peripheral vascular disease. *J Nutr Med* 1:39,1990.

Hu CJ. *Acta Academiae Medicinae Wuhan* 1:125, 1957.

Hubbard D,R. and Berkoff G,M.: Myofascial Trigger Points Show Spontaneous Needle EMG Activity. *Spine*.18:1993, 1988.

Huberti HH, Hayes WC. Patelofemoral contact pressures. *J Bone Joint Surg* 66A:715, 1984.

Hunt TK et al. Effect of vitamin A on reversing the inhibitory effect of cortisone on healing in animals and man. *Ann Surg* 170:203,1969.

Hyde AS. Crash Injuries: How and Why They Happen. Key Biscayne, Fla: Hyde Assoc;1992.


## I

Inman VT, Saunders JB, deCM. Referred pain from skeletal structures. *J Nerv Ment Dis* 99:660,1944.

Illingworth C. Pulled elbow. BMJ 1:672, 1975.


## J

Jackson R. *The cervical syndrome*. Springfield, Charles Thomas, 1977.

Jackson R. *The cervical syndrome*. 4th ed, Charles C Thomas; Springfield, 1958.

Jacobsen S., Samsoe D.S., Lund B.; Consensus document on fibromyalgia: The Copenhagen Declaration. *J of Musculoskeletal Pain* 1:295, 1993.

Jameson S et al. Pain relief and selenium balance in patients with connective tissue disease and osteoarthritis: A double blind selenium tocopherol supplementation study. *Nutr Res Supp* 1:391, 1985.

Janda V.: Evaluation of Muscular Imbalance. In *Rehabilitation of the Spine* (eds) Liebenson C. Williams & Willkins 1996.

Janda V: *Muscle Function Testing*. Butterworths, london, 1983.

Janda V. Muscle spasm-a proposed procedure for differential diagnosis. *J Manual Med* 6:136, 1991.

Janda V. *Muscle strength in relation to muscle length*. NY Churchill Livingstone, 1993.

Jelnes R et al. Improvement of subcutaneous nutritional blood flow in the forefoot by hydroxyethylrutosides in patients arterial insufficiency: Case studies. *Angiology* 37:198,1986.

Jensel MC et al. Magnetic resonance imaging of the lumbar spine in people without back pain. *N Engl J Med* 2:331, 1994.

Jensen LB, et al. Effect of acupuncture on headache measured by reduction in number of attacks and use of drugs. *Scand J of Dent Res*. 87:373, 1985.

Jenzel JH. U. of Missouri School of Med.-reported in *Med Trib* 10/26/70.

Ji Y. 776 cases of pain treated with auriculoacupuncture therapy. *J Trad Chin Med* 12:275, 1992.

Ji XJ et al. *Acta Physiologica Sinica* 23:151, 1959.

Jiang MX et al. *Acta Physiologica Sinica* 22:294, 1958.

Jin Gz et al. *Acta Pharmaceutica Sinica* 5:39, 1957.

Johansson JA, Rubenowitz S. Risk indicators in the psychosocial and physical work environment for work-related neck, shoulder and low back symptoms: a study among blue- and white-collar workers in eight companies. *Scand J Rehabil Med* 3:131, 1994.

Jose A. Orcasita, assistant clinical Pharmacology, U. of Miami School of Medicine-reported in Walker M. Therapeutic effects of shark cartilage. *Townsend Letter for Doctors*, June, 1989Jackson, R. *The Cervical Syndrome*. 4th ed. Springfield: Charles C. Thomas, 1958.

Jónsson H Jr., et al. Hidden cervical spine injuries in traffic accident victims with skull fractures. *J Spinal Discord*. 3: 251, 1991.

Jungmann, M: *The Jungmann Concept and Technique of Antigravity Leverage*. 2ed ed. Rangeley, Institute for Gravitational Strain Pathology, Inc., 1992.

# k

Kaartinen JAE. Diagnostic value of stress radiography in lesions of the lateral ligaments of the ankle. *Acta Radio* 18:711; 1988.

Kamada T et al. Dietary sardine oil increases erythrocyte membrane fluidity in diabetic patients. *Diabetes* 35:604,1986.

Kapandji I.A. *The Physiology of the Joints Vol 3 The trunk and the Vertebral Column*. Churchill Livingstone Edinburgh London and New York, 1974.

Kapandji I.A. *The Physiology of the Joints Vol 2 Lower Limb*. Churchill Livingstone Edinburgh London and New York, 1987.

Kapandji I.A. *The Physiology of the Joints Vol 1 Upper Limb*. Churchill Livingstone Edinburgh London and New York, 1974.

Katoh Y, Chao EY, Morrey BF. Objective technique for evaluating painful heel syndrome and its treatment. Foot Ankle. 16:60, 1984.

Kaufman W. The use of vitamin therapy to reverse certain concomitants of aging. *J Am Geriatr Soc* 3:927,1955.

Kellgren JH.:Observation of referred pain arising from muscles. *Clin. Sci*.3:175, 1938.

Kellner G. Bau und Funktion der Haut. *Dtsch Ztschr Akup* 3:1, 1966.

Kelmes IS. Vitamin B12 in acute subdeltoid bursitis. *Indust Med Surg* 26:20,1957.

Kime CE. Bell's palsy: A new syndrome associated with treatment by nicotinic acid. *Arch Otolaryngol* 68:28,1958.

Kho HG, Arnold BJ. As chronische benigne Schmerzsyndrom: Moglichkeiten und Rolle der Akupunktur. *Deut Zeits Aku* 40:51, 1997.

Kho HG, Robertson EN. The Mechanisms of Acupuncture Analgesia: Review and Update. *Amer J of Acup* 25:261, 1997.

Kinzler E, Kromer J and Lehamann E. Effect of a special Kava extract in patients with anxiety, tension and excitation states of non-psychotic genesis. Double blind study with placebos over 4 weeks. *Arzneim Forsch* 41:584,1991.

Kirkalldy-Willis WH, Burton CV. *Managing Low Back Pain* (3ed)edi Churchill Livingstone NY 1992.

Kitade T et al. Studies on the enhanced effect of acupuncture analgesia and acupuncture anesthesia, by D-phenylalanine (first report): effects on threshold and inhibition by naloxone. *Acupunct Electrother Res* 13:87,1988.

Kleijnen J, Knipschild P. Ginkgo biloba. Lancet 340:1136,1992Knight K, Aquino J, Urban C. A re-examination of lewis's cold-induced vasodilation in the finger and ankle. *Athl Train*. 15: 248, 1980.

Klein RG, Eek BJ, DeLong B, Mooney V. A Randomized Double-Blind Trial of Dextrose-Glycerine-Phenol Injections for Chronic Low Back Pain. *Journal of Spinal Disorders*. 6:1 22, 1993.

Knight KL. Cryotherapy in sports medicine. In: Schriber K, Burke Ej, eds. *Relevant Topics in Athletic Training*. Ithaca, NY: Monument Publications; 1978.

Koltringer P et al. Ginkgo biloba extract and folic acid in the therapy of changes caused by autonomic neuropathy. *Aceta Med Austriaca* 16:35,1989.

Konovalov MN et al (trans. by Lin Y). *Chine Med J*. 49:402,1963Kamimura M. Anti-inflammatory effects of vitamin E. *J Vitaminol* 18:204, 1972.

Kopell HP, Thompson WAL. Peripheral entrapment neuropathies of the lower extremity. *New Eng J Med* 262:56, 1960.

Kopell HP, Thompson WA. *Peripheral Entrapment Neuropathies*. Krieger Publishing Co Malabar, Fl, 1976.

Korr IM et al. Cutaneous patterns of sympathetic activity in clinical abnormalities of the musculoskeletal system. *Acta Neuroveget Bd* XXXV, Heft 4:589, 1962.

Korr IM, Wright HM, Thomas PE. Effects of experimental myofascial insult on cutaneous patterns of sympathetic activity in man, *J. Neural Transm*. 23:330, 1962.

Korr IR, Edi, The Neurobiologic Mechanisms in Manipulative Therapy; *Sustained sympathicotonia as a factor of disease*. Plenum Publishing

Corp, NY, 1987.

Korr IM. The neural basis of the osteopathic lesion. *J Amer Osteo Ass*. 47:191, 1947.

Korr I.M.,Edi.: Sustained sympathicotonia as a factor in disease in. *The Neurobiologic Mechanisms in Manipulative Therapy*. Plenum Publishing Corp, New York,1978.

Korr IM et al. Cutaneous patterns of sympathetic activity in clinical abnormalities of the musculoskeletal system. *Acta Neuroveget Bd. XXXV*, Heft 4:589, 1962.

Koslow SH et al. *The Neuroscience of Mental health II*. NIH publication 1995.

Kraus, H. Diagnosis and treatment of low back pain. *Gen. Pract*. 5:55, 1988.

Kraft, G.L.and Levinthal, O.H.,. Facet synovial impingement. *Sug Gynol Obstet* 19:439, 1951.

Kraus, H.: *Diagnosis and Treatment of Muscle Pain*. Quintessence Publishing, Chicago, 1988.

Krismer M, Haid C, Rabl W. The Contribution of Annulus Fibres Torque Resistance. *Spin* 21:2551, 1996.

Kroening R, Oleson T. Rapid narcotic detoxification in chronic pain patients treated with auricular electroacupuncture and naloxon. *International J of Addiction*. 20:1347, 1985.

Kroto H. Space, stars, C60, and soot. *Science* 242:1145, 1988.

Kuchera W.A., Kuchera M.L. *Osteopathic Principles in Practice* 2ed edi KCOM Press Kirksville, Miss 1993.

Kuhn, Thomas S. *The Structure of Scientific Revolution*. The University of Chicago Press, 1962.

Kunnasmaa KTT, Thiel HW. Vertebral Artery Syndrome: A review of the literature. *J. Ortho Med* 16:17, 1994.

Kunnasmaa KTT. Literature review of the prevalence of normal imaging modalities of the vertebrobasilar system in reported cases of cerebrovascular accidents following manipulation of the cervical spine. *BSc Project* Anglo-*European College of Chiropractic*, Bournemouth, England 1993.

**L**

Langohr HD et al. Vitamin B-1, B-2. and B-6

deficiency in neurological disorders. *J Neurol* 225:95,1981LaCourse M, Moore K, Davis K, Fune M, Dorman T. A report on the asymmetry of iliac inclination: A study comparing normal, laterality and change in a patient population with painful sacro-iliac dysfunction treated with prolotherapy. *J Orthop Med*. 12:3, 1990.

Laitenen J. Treatment of cervical syndrome by acupuncture. *Scandinavian J of Rehab Med*. 7:114, 1975.

Lambert, G.A., Bogduk, N. et al, Cervical Cord Neurons Receiving Sensory Input from the Cranial Vasculature. *Cephalgia*. 11:75, 1991.

Lankhorst GJ, Van de Stadt RJ, Van der Korst JK. The natural history of idiopathic low back pain. *Scand J Rehabil Med* 17:1, 1985.

Laude D, Girard A, Consoli S, Mounier-Vehier C, Elghozi JL. Anger expression and cardiovascular reactivity to metal stress: a spectral analysis approach. *Clin Exp Hypertens* 19:901, 1997)

Lavignolle B, et al. An approach to the functional anatomy of the sacroiliac joints in vivo. *Anat Clin* 5:169, 1983.

Lavignolle B, Vital JM, Senegas J, Destandan J, Toson B, Bouyx P, Morlier P, Delorme G, Calabet A. A new understanding of the human pelvis. An approach to the functional anatomy of the sacroiliac joints in vivo. *Mat Clin* 5:169, 1983.

Lawson GE, Walden T. Nutrition and the traumatized patient. *J Council Nutrition*. 12:1 1989.

Lawrence RM. The periosteum: Neurophysiology and its role in treatment. *Annu of Sport Med*. 3:85, 1987.

Lawrence, Dana J. *Chiropractic Diagnosis and Management* Williams & Wilkins, 1991.

Laxorthes Y, Esquerré, Simon J, Guiraud G, Guiraud R. Acupuncture meridians and radiotracers. *Pain* 40:109, 1990.

Leduc et al. The effect of physical factors on the vasomotricity of blood and lymph vessels. In Leduc, Lievens (eds) *Lympho-kinetics*. Birkhauser Verlag, Basel, 1979.

Lee MHM, Ernst M. The sympatholytic effect of acupuncture as evidenced by thermography: A preliminary report. *Ortho Rev*. 12:67, 1983.

Lee CS, Tsai TL. The relation of the sciatic nerve to the piriformis muscle. *J Formosan Med Ass* 73:75, 1974.

Lee MHM, Ernst M. Clinical and research observation on acupuncture analgesia and thermography. Presented at Duesseldorfer Akupunktur Symposium. 1987.

Lee Th et al. Effect of dietary enrichment with eicosapentaenoic acid and docosahexaenoic acids on in vitro neutrophil and monocyte leukotriene generation and neutrophil function. *N Engl J Med* 312:1217,1985.

Lenot G. Note sur l'aneurine, anesthesique general. *Ann Anesthesiol Franc* 7:173, 1966.

Levine JD, Fields HL, Basbaum AL: Peptides and the primary afferent nociceptor. *J. Neurosci* 13:2273, 1993.

Levine J, Taiwo Y. Inflammatory pain. In: *Textbook of Pain* (3ed)(edi) Wall and Melzack. Churchill Livingstone 1994.

Levin SM. *The icosahedron as the three-dimensional finite element in biomechanical support.* Proceedings of the Society of General System Research Symposium on Mental Images, Values and Reality Philadelphia 1986.

Lewis T. *Pain.* MacMillan, NY 1942.

Lewit K. *Manipulative therapy in rehabilitation of the motor system.* 2ed Ed. London, Butterworths, 1991.

Lewit K. Chain reactions in disturbed function of the motor system. *Manuelle Med* 3:27, 1987.

Li Y, Jin R. Clinical study on the sequelae of cerebral vascular accident treated with temporal-point acupuncture. *Chen Tzu Yen Chiu* 19:4, 1994.

Li C, Peoples RW, Weight FF. Acid pH augments excitatory action of ATP on a dissociated mammalian sensory neuron. *Neuroreport* 7:2151, 1996.

Liao SJ, Liao MK. Acupuncture and tele-electronic infrared thermography. *Acupunct Electrother Res Int J* 10:41, 1985.

Liberman HR et al. Mood, performance and pain sensitivity: Changes induced by food constituents. *J Psychiatr Res* 17:135,1983.

Liebenson C. *Rehabilitation of the Spine.* Williams & Wilkins 1996.

Lietti A et al. Studies on vaccinium myrtillus anthocyanosides. I. Vasoprotective and anti-inflammatory activity. *Arzneim Forsch* 26:829,1976.

Lin Zj. *Chinese Medical J* 2:114,1954.

Lindenberg D, Pitule-Scodel H. Dl-kavain in comparison with oxazepam in anxiety disorders. A double-blind study of clinical effectiveness. *Fortschr Med* 108:49,1990.

Lindh, M.: Biomechanics Of The Lumbar Spine. In *Basic Biomechanics of the Skeletal System.* Lea & Febiger, Philadelphia 1980.

Lindstrand A. Diagnosis. *Acta Radiol* 18:529, 1977.

Linzer M, Van Atta A. Effects of acupuncture stimulation activity of single thalamic neurons in the cat. *Adv Neurol* 4:799, 1975.

Liu JE, Tahmoush AJ, Roos DB, Schwartzman RJ. Shoulder-arm pain from cervical bands and scalene muscle anomalies.*J Neurol Sci* 128:175, 1995.

Loh L. et al. Acupuncture versus medical treatment for migraine and muscle tension headaches. J of Neuro, Neurosurg, and Psychiatry 47:333, 1984.

Long T el al. *Acta Pharmaceutica Sinica.* 14:429,1979.

Lord, SM, Barnsley L, Wallis BJ, Bogduk N. Third Occipital Nerve Headache: a Prevalence Study. *J Neurol Neurosurg Psychiatry.* 57:1187, 1994.

Lunsford LD et al. Anterior Surgery For Cervical Disc Disease: Treatment Of Lateral Cervical Disc Herniation In 253 Cases. *J Neurosurg.* 53:1, 1980.

Lowman CL. The sitting position in relation to pelvic stress. *Physiother Rev* 21:3033, 1941.

Loy TT. Treatment of cervical spondylosis: electoacupuncture versus physiotherapy. *The Medi J of Australia* 2:32, 1983.

Lu FH et al. *Acta Physiologica Sinica* 5:113, 1957.

## M

Maciocia G. *The Foundations of Chinese Medicine.* New York: Churchill Livingstone, 1989.

Mackenzie J. *Symptoms and their interpretation.* Shaw, London 1989.

Mackenzie MA et al. The influence of glycyrrhetinec acid on plasma cortisol and cortisone in healthy young volunteers. *J Clin Endocrinol Metb* 70:1637,1990.

Macintosh JE, Pearcy MJ, Bogduk. The axial

torque of the lumbar back muscles: torsion strength of the back. *Aust N Z J Surg* 63:205, 1993.

Macintosh JE, Bogduk N, Pearcy MJ. The effects of flexion on the geometry and actions of the lumbar erector spinae. *Spine* 18:884, 1993.

MacNab I. *Backache*, Williams&Wilkins, 1977.

MacNab, I. Acceleration Injuries of the Cervical Spine. *J of Bone and Joint Surgery*. 46a:1655, 1964.

MacNab, I. Whiplash Syndrome, *J. Clinical Neurosurgery*. 20:232, 1973.

MacNab I. The "whiplash syndrome." *Orthop Clin North Am*. 2, 2:389, 1971.

Madan BR, Khanna NK. Anti-inflammatory activity of L-Tryptophan and DL-tryptophan. *Indian J Med Res* 68:708,1978.

Magora, A: Conservative treatment in spondylolisthesis. *Clin. Ortho*. 117:74, 1976.

Main CJ, Spanswick CC. Personality assessment and Minnesota multiphasic inventory. 50 years on: do we still need our security blanket? *Pain Forum* 4:60, 1995.

Malarky WB et al. Influence of academic stress and season on 24-hour mean concentrations of ACTH, cortisol and beta-endorphin. *Psychneuroendocrinology* 20:499; 1995.

Mann M Glasjeen-Wray M, Nyberg R: Therapist Agreement for Palpation and Observation of Iliac Crest Heights. *Phys Ther* 64:223, 1984.

Maquart FX et al. Simulation of collagen synthesis in fibroblast culture by a triterpene extracted from Centella asiatica. *Connect Tissue Res*. 24:107,1990.

Marcus A. *Acute Abdominal Syndromes. Their Diagnosis & Treatment According to Combined Chinese-Western Medicine*. Boulder: Blue Poppy Press, 1991.

Marcus A, Gracer R.: A Modern Approach to Shoulder Pain Using the Combined Methods of Acupuncture and Cyriax-Based "Orthopaedic Medicine". *American J of Acupuncture* 22:5, 1994.

Markelova VF et al. Changes in blood serotonin levels in patients with migraine headaches before and after a course of reflexotherapy. Zh Nervopatol Psikhiatr 84:1313, 1984.

Martin R M. *The gravity guiding system*. Essential Publishing Co. 2823 Cumberland Rd. San Marino, CA. 1975.

Matin P. Basic principles of nuclear medicine techniques for detection and evaluation of trauma and sports medicine. *Smin Nucl Med*:18:90, 1988.

Matin PJ. The appearance of bone scans following fracture, including immediate and long term studies. *J Nuc Med* 20:1227, 1979.

Matthews PM, et al. Enhancement of natural cytotoxicity by beta-endorphin. *J of Immunology* 132: 3046, 1984.

Matsuo K et al. Influence of alcohol intake, cigarette smoking and occupational status on isiopathic osteonecrosis of the femoral head. *Clin Orthop* 234:115, 1988.

Matsumoto K, Birch S. *Hara: Reflections on the Sea*. Brookline: Paradigm Press 1988.

Maver DJ, Price DD, Rafii A. Antagonism of acupuncture hyperalgesia in man by the narcotic antagonist naloxone. *Brain Res*. 121:368, 1977.

Mazzara JT. The effect of C1-C2 rotation on canal size. *Clin Ortho Relat Res* 237:15, 1989.

McConnell WE et al. Analysis of Human Test Subject Kinematic Responses to Low Velocity Rear End Impacts. paper 930094. Society of Automotive Engineers, 1993.

McCann P, Wootten M, Kadaba M Bigliani L. A kinematic and electromyographic study of shoulder rehabilitation exercises. Cil Orthop Rel Res. 288:179, 1993.

McCarthy, W.J., Yao, S.J., Schafer, M.F. et al. Upper Extremity Arterial Injury in Athletes. *J Vasc Surg* 9:317, 1989.

McGeer, T. Passive Dynamic Walking. *Int J Robotics Res* 9,2.1990.

McKenzie and Jacobes In: Liebenson C. *Rehabilitation of the Spine*. Williams & Wilkins 1996.

Mcleod Dw, Revell P, Robinson BV. Investigations of Hapagophytum procumbens (Devil's claw) in the treatment of experimental inflammation and arthritis in the rat. *Br J Pharmacol* 66:140,1979.

McLennan H Von, Gilfillan K, Heap Y. Some pharmacological observations on the analgesia induced by acupuncture in rabbits. *Pain* 15:83, 1977.

McNair JFS. Acute locking of the cervical spine. In: Gieve GP (eds). *Modern Manual Therapy of the Vertebral Column*. Churchill Livingstone, London 1986.

McNeil Alexander, R. *Elastic Mechanism in Animal Movement*. Cambridge University Press, New York, 1988.

Medelson, G. Not "cured by verdict." Effects of Legal Settlement on Compensation Claimants. *Medical Journal of Australia*. 1:132, 1982.

Meenen NM, Katzer A, Dihlmann SW, Held S, Fyfe I, Jungbluth KH. Whiplash injury of the cervical spine--on the role of pre-existing degenerative diseases. *Unfallchirurgie* 3:138, 1994.

Mehta AK, et al. Pharmacological effects of Withania somnifera rot extract on GABA receptor complex. *Ind J Med Res* 94(b):312,1991.

Mellin G. Chronic low back pain in men 54-63 years of age, correlations of physical measurements with the degree of trouble and progress after treatment. *Spine* 11:421, 1986.

Melzack R, Wall P.:Pain mechanisms. A new theory. Science 150:971, 1965.

Mendelson G. Follow-up studies of personal injury litigants. *Int J Law Psychiatry* 7:179, 1984.

Mense S: Physiology of Nociception in Muscles. *J Advances in Pain Research and Therapy* 17:67-85,1990.

Mennell, J. *The Science and Art of Joint Manipulation*. New York, Blakinston, 1952.

Mennell J. *Back Pain*. Little Brown. Boston 1960.

Mennell JM. *Joint Pain*. Little, Brown, Boston. 1964.

Mercer S, Bogduk N. Intra-articular inclusions of the cervical synovial joints. *Br J Rheumatol* 32:705, 1993.

Metchnikoff Eli (1848-1916). *Lectures on the comparative pathology of inflammation*. Dover publications, NY 1968. original 1893.

Middleeditch A The cervical spine-safe in our hands? *World confederation for physical therapy 11th international congress book III* The Barbican center, London UK,1991.

Miehlke K, Schulze G, Eger W: Klinische und experimentelle Untersuchungen Zum Fibrositis-syndrom. *Z Rheumaforsch* 19:310, 1950.

Miles KA et al. The incidence and prognostic significance of abnormal radiology in soft tissue injury of cervical spine. *Skeletal Radiology* 17:493, 1988.

Miller JAA, Schamtz BS, Scjultz AB. Lumbar disc degeneration: correlation with age, sex and spine level in 600 autopsy specimens. *Spine* 13:173, 1988.

Miller J AA, Schultz A B, Andersson G B 3. Load displacement behavior of sacroiliac joints. *J Orthop Research* 5:92,1987.

Miller EJ. Chemistry, structure and function of collagen, in L manaker, Ed. *Biologic Basis of wound Healing*. NY, Harper and Row 1975.

Millinger GS. Neutral amino acid therapy for the management of chronic pain. *Cranio* 4:156,1986.

Mitchell FL Jr. In *Rational Manual Therapies* edi Basmajian JV and Nyberg R. Williams & Wilkins 1993.

Mitchell F.L. The balanced pelvis and its relationship to reflexes. *Yearbook, Academy Applied Osteopathy* 48:146, 1948.

Mitra M, Nandi AK. Cyanocobalmin in chronic Bell's Palsy. *J Indian Med Assoc* 33:129,195

Moldofsky, H., et al.:Musculoskeletal symptoms and non-Rem sleep disturbances in patients with "fibrositic" syndromes and healthy subjects. *Psychosom. Med.* 37:341,1975.

Molsberger A, Jille E. The analgesic effect of acupuncture in chronic tennis elbow pain. *British J of Rheumatology* 33:1162, 1994.

Mooney V. Where is the Lumbar Pain Coming from?. *Ann Med.* 21:373, 1989.

Mooney V, and Robertson J. The facet syndrome. *Clin. Orthop.* 115:149, 1976.

Morscher E, Finger G.Measurement of leg length. *Prog Orthop Surg* 1:21, 1977.

Moses Ma, Subhalter J, Langer R. Identification of and inhibitor of neovascularisation from cartilage. *Science* 248:1408,1990.

Moussard C et al. A drug used in traditional medicine, harpagophytum procumbens: No evidence for NSAID-like effect on whole blood eicosanoid production in humans. *Prostaglan Leukotri Essent Fatty Acids* 46:283,1992.

Murad S et al. Regulation of collagen synthesis by ascorbic acid. *Proc Natl Acad Sci USA*, 78:2879,1981.

# N

Nachemson AL. Newest knowledge of low back pain, *Clin Orthop* 279:8, 1992.

Nachemson, A., Elfstrom, G.: *Intravertibral Dynamic Pressure Measurement in the Lumbar Spine in Lumbar Disks: A Study of Common Movements, Maneuvers and Exercises.* Stockholm, Alwuist & Wikstell, 1970

Naeser MA, Alexander MP, Stiassny-Eder D, Galler V, Hobbs J, Bachman D. Acupuncture in the treatment of paralysis in chronic and acute stroke patients--improvement correlated with specific CT scan lesion sites. Boston University School of Medicine, MA, USA. *Acupunct Electrother Res* 19:227, 1994.

Naeser MA, Hahn KK, Lieberman B. Real vs. Sham Laser Acupuncture and Microamps TENS to Treat Carpal Tunnel Syndrome and Worksite Wrist Pain: Pilot Study. *Lasers Surg and Med* suppl. 8:7, 1996.

Naeser MA, Hahn CK and Lieberman BE. Home Naeser Laser Treatment Program for the Hand, AAOM Publication, 1996.

Naliboff BD et al. Comprehensive assessment of chronic low back pain patients and controls: Physical abilities, level of activities, psychological adjustment and pain perception. *Pain* 23:121, 1985.

Nash CL, Moe JH. A study of vertebral rotation. *J Bone Joint Surg* 51A:223, 1969.

*National Medical Journal of China* 7:444, 1978.

Neuhuber WL, Bankoul S. Specifics of innervation of the cranio-cervical transition Orthopade 23:256, 1994.

Newman NM, Ling RSM. Acetabular bone destruction related to non-steroidal anti-inflammatory drugs. Lancet:11, 1985.

Nielsen S. Radiologic findings in lesions of the ligamentum bifurcation of the midfoot. *Skeletal Radiol* 16:114, 1987.

Nordhoff LS. *Motor Vehicle Collision Injuries:Mechanisms, Diagnosis and Management.* Maryland, An Aspen Publication, 1996.

Norris SH, Watt I. The prognosis of neck injuries resulting from rear-end vehicle collisions. *J Bone Joint Surg* [Br] 65: 608, 1983.

Noyes F, Torvik PM, et al. Biomechanics of liga- ment failure: an analysis of immobilization, exercise and reconditioning effects on primates. *J Bone Joint Surg.* 56A:1406, 1974.

# O

Obodencheva GV. Farmakologiia I Toksikologiia 29:496, 1966.

Ochoa J, Mair EGP The normal sural nerve in man. *J. Neuropathological Berlin* 13:197, 1969.

O'Connor J, Bensky D (eds). *Acupuncture, A Comprehensive Text.* Chicago, Eastland Press, 1981.

O'Dell B et al. Zinc status and peripheral nerve function in guinea pigs. *FASEBJ* 4:2919,1990.

Oleson TD, et al. An experimental evaluation of auricular diagnosis: the somatotropic mapping of musculoskeletal pain at ear acupuncture points. *Pain* 8:217, 1980.

Ohuchi K et al. Glycyrrhizine inhibits prostaglandin E2 formation by activated peritoneal macrophages from rats. *Prostagland Metab* 70:143,1981.

O'Hara J. A double-blind-controlled study of Hexopal in the treatment of intermittent claudication. *J Int Med Res.* 13:322-27,1985.

Okimasa E et al. Inhibition of Phosphatase A2 by Glycyrrhizine, an anti-inflammatory drug. *Acta Med Okayma* 37:385,1983.

Ombregt L, Bisschop P, ter Veer HJ, Van de Velde T. *A System of Orthoaedic Medicine.* Saunders, London UK 1995.

Omura Y. Pathophysiology of acupuncture effects, ACTH and morphine-like substances, pain, phantom sensation, brain mirocirculation and memory. *Acupunct Electrother Res Int J.* 2:1, 1976.

Ongley MJ, Klein RG, Dorman TA et al. A new approach to the treatment of chronic back pain. *Lancet* 143, 1987.

Orloff S, Krieg T and Muller P: (+) Cyanidanol-3 changes functional properties of collagen. *Biochem Pharmacol* 31:3581,1982.

Ornstein R, Thompson RF. The Amazing Brain. Houghton Mifflin Company. Boston1984.

Orsay Em at al. Prospective study of the effect of safety belts in motor vehicle crashes. *Ann Emeg Med.* 19:258, 1990.

Orthopade 4:287, 1994.

Ouigley, Carroll. Tragedy and Hope, *A History of the World in Our time*. Collier MacMillan, London, 1966.

Owens J, Malone T. Treatment parameters of high frequency electrical stimulation as established on the electro-stim 180. *J Orthopaed Sports Phys Ther*. 4:162, 1983.

Owoeye I, Spielholx NI, Fetto J, et al. Low intensity pulsed galvanic current and healing of tentomized rat achilles tendons: Preliminary report using load-to-breaking measurements. *Arch Phys Med Rehabil*. 68:415, 1987.


**P**

Padova C. S-adenosylmethionine in the treatment of osteoarthritis. Review of clinical studies. *Am J Med* 83:60,1987.

Paladin F, Russo Perez G. The haematic thiamine level in the course of alcoholic neuropathy. *Eur Neurol* 26:129,1987.

Palmoski MJ, Brandt KD. Effects of some nonsteroidal antiinflammatory drugs on proteoglycan metabolism and organization in canine articular cartilage. Arthit Reum 23:1010, 1980.

Paris, S.V. Differential Diagnosis of SI joint from lumbar spine dysfunction, *First interdisciplinary world congress on low back pain and its relation to the SI joint*; 1992.

Parker GB, Tupling H and Pryor DS. A controlled trial of cervical manipulation for migraine. *Aust NZ J Med* 8:589, 1978.

Parry GJ. Sensory neuropathy with low-dose pyridoxine. *Neurology* 35:1466,1985.

Passatore M., Filippi M., Grassi C. In: *The Muscle Spindle*, Boyd I. and Gaden M.,(eds.) Macmillan, London 1985.

Patacchini R, Maggi CA and Meli A. Capsaicin-like activity of some natural pungent substances on peripheral ending of visceral primary afferents. *Arch Pharmaco* 342:72,1990.

Patterson M. *Hooked? NET: the new approach to drug cure*. Faber and Gaber London 1986.

Pearce P. Structures in Nature as a Strategy for Design. MIT Press Cambridge 1978.

Pearson EJ. Combined manual medicine and acupuncture in neck injury. *Manual Med*. 5:19, 1990.

Pecina M. Contribution to the etiological explanation of the piriformis syndrome. *Aceta Anat* 105:181, 1979.

Pennarola R et al. The therapeutic action of the anthocyanosides in microcirculatory changes due to adhesive-induced polyneuritis. *Gazz Med Ital* 139:485,1980.

Peterson B. *The collected papers of Irvin M. Korr*. Amer Acad. Osteo Indianapolis, IN 1979.

Petrou P. Double-blind trail to evaluate the effects of acupuncture treatment on knee osteoarthritis pain: a placebo controlled study. American J of Chin Med 19:95 1991.

Petrie JP, Langley GB. Acupuncture in the treatment of chronic cervical pain: A pilot study. *Clinical and Experimental Rheumatology*. 1:333, 1983.

Pettersson K, Hildingsson C, Toolanen G, Fagerlund M, Bjornebrink J MRI and neurology in acute whiplash trauma. No correlation in prospective examination of 39 cases. *Acta Orthop Scand* 5:525, 1994.

Penimak T et al. Progressive strengthening and stretching exercises and ultrasound for chronic lateral epicondylitis. *Physiotherapy* 82:522, 1996.

Penning L. Normal movements of the cervical spine. *Amer J Radiol* 130:317, 1978.

Penning L, Wilmick JT. Rotation of the cervical spine—A CT study in normal subjects. *Spine* 12:732, 1987.

Penning L, Wilmick JT. Rotation of the cervical spine—A CT study in normal subjects. *Spine* 12:732, 1987.

Piesse JW. Vitamin E and peripheral vascular disease. *Int Clin Nutr Res*, 4:178,1984.

Pietri-Taleb F, Riihimaki H, Viikari-Juntura E, Lindstrom K. Longitudinal study on the role of personality characteristics and psychological distress in neck trouble among working men. *Pain* 2:261, 1994.

Pintar FA, et al. Kinematic and anatomical analysis of the human cervical spinal column under axial loading. In: Proceedings of 33rd Strapp Car Crash Conference, P-227, 892436. Washington, DC: Society of Automotive Engineers: 191, 1989.

Pomeranz B, Cheng R, Law P. Acupuncture reduces electrophysiological and behavioral responses to noxious stimuli: Pituitary is implicated. *Exp Neurol*. 54:172, 1977.

Pomeranz B, Paley D. Electroacupuncture hypalgesia is mediated by afferent nerve impulses: An electrophysiological study in mice. *Exp Neuro* 66:398, 1979.

Pomeranz B, Nguyen P. Inrathecal diazepam suppresses nociceptive reflexes and potentiates electroacupuncture effects in pentobarbitol rats. *Neurosci Lett* 77:316, 1987.

Potter N, Rothstein J: Inter-tester Reliability for Selected Tests of the Sacro Iliac Joint. *Phys Ther* 65:1671,1985.

Prino G.,Pharmacological profile of Ateroid, *Mod. Probl. Pharmacopsychiatry*, 23, 68,1989.

Prodigal genius: The Life of Nicola Tesla. John J O'Neill. Angriff Press. P.O.Box 2726, Hollywood CA 90078.

Prudden, Jf and Balassa LL, The biological activity of bovine cartilage preparations, *Sem Arth Ruem*., 17:35, 1987.

Prudden JF, Allen J. The clinical accelerating of healing with a cartilage preparation; a controlled study. *JAMA* 192:352,1965.


**Q**

Quirin H. Pain and vitamin B1 therapy. *Bibl Nutr Dieta* 38:708, 1986.


**R**

Radanov P, Sturzenegger M, Di Stefano G. Prediction of recovery from dislocation of the cervical vertebrae (whiplash injury of the cervical vertebrae) with initial assessment of psychosocial variables. *Orthopade* 23:282, 1994.

Raja SN. Role of the sympathetic nervous system in acute pain and inflammation. *Ann Med* 2:241, 1995.

Ramani, P.S., et al.: "Role of Ligamentum Flavum in the Symptomatology of Prolapse Lumbar Intervertebral Discs," *J. Neurol. Neurosurg*. 38:550,1975.

Reeves KD. Treatment of consecutive severe fibromyalgia patients with prolotherapy. *The J of Orthop Med*. 16:84,1994.

Reddy CK, Chandrakasan G, Dhar SC. Studies on the metabolism of glycosaminoglycans under the influence of new herbal anti-inflammatory agents. *Biovhemical Pharmacol* 20:3527,1989.

Reider B, Marshall J, Warren R. Clinical characteristics of patellar disorders in young athletes. *Am J Sports Med* 9:4, 1981.

Rejhole V. Long term studies of anti-osteoarthritic drugs: An assessment. Semin Arth Rheum 17:35,1987.

Ren MF, Tu ZP, Han JS. The effect of hemicholine, choline, atropine and eserine on electroacupuncture analgesia in rats, in Han JS (ed) *The Neurochemical Basis of Pain Relief by Acupuncture; A Collection Papers*. Med Sci Press Beijing 1987.

Reshentinkova AD. *Sovetskaia Meditisina* 2:23, 1954.

Richmond, FJ, Abrahams,VC: What are the proprioceptors of the neck? Progr. *Brain Res*. 50:245, 1979.

Rivett HM. Cervical Manipulation: Confronting the Spectre of the Vertebral Artery Syndrome. *J. Ortho Med* 16:12, 1994.

Rheumatoid Arthritis Coordinating Research Group, First Teaching Hospital. *Acta Academae Medicinae Wuhan* 6:51, 1977.

Roaf R. *Spinal Deformities*. Philadelphia: JB Lippincott Co; 1977.

Roland M, Morris R. A study of the natural history of low back pain. Part I. Development of a Reliable and sensitive measure of disability in low back pain. *Spine* 8: 141, 1983.

Rong M. Comparing observations of treatments of periarthritis of the shoulder by acupuncture and massage. *Chin Acupun & Moxib* 6:3, 1986.

Ronningen, Langeland N. Indomethacin treatment in osteoarthritis of the hip joint. *Acta Orthop Scand* 50:169, 1979.

Rosenberg ZS. Ankle tendons: Evaluation with CT. *Radiology* 166:221, 1988.

Rosted P. Literature Survey of Reported Adverse Effects Associated with Acupuncture Treatment. *Amer J Acupu* 24:1, 1996.

Rothman Rh et al.: A study of computer-assisted tomograpy. *Spine* 9:548,1984.

Ruch T.C., Patton H.D (eds). *Pathophysiology of pain,* Physiology and biophysics. Sanders, Philadelphia, 1965.

Rupani HD. Three phase radionuclide bone imaging in sports medicine. *Radiology* 156:187, 1985.

Ruskin AP. *Current Therapy in Physiatry*: Physical Medicine and Rehabilitation. Philadelphia: WB Saunders Co; 1984.

Ryan GB, Majno G. *Inflammation a Scope Publication*. Upjohn Kalamzoo, 1983.


# S

Saal JA, Saal JS.: Nonoperative treatment of herniated lumbar intervertebral disc with radiculopathy. *Spine* 14:431, 1989.

Sabolovic D, Michon C. Effect of acupuncture on human peripheral T and B lymphocytes. *Acupunct Electrother Res Int J*. 3: 97, 1978.

Sakai F, Ebihara S, Akiyama M, Horikawa M Pericranial muscle hardness in tension-type headache. A non-invasive measurement method and its clinical application. *Brain* 118:52, 1995.

Saldinger, P., Dvorák, B., Rahn, S., Perren, M. The Histology of Alar and Transverse Ligaments. *Spine* 15:257,1990.

Sanders RJ, Pearce WH. The treatment of thoracic outlet syndrome: a comparison of different operations. *J Vasc Surg*. 10: 626, 1989.

Santini M, Ibata Y.: *Brain Res*. 33: 289, 1971.

Sawynok J, Reid A. Peripheral adenosine 5'-triphosphate enhances nociception in the formalin test via activation of a purinergic p2X receptor. *Eur J Pharmacol* 330:115, 1997.

Sheild MJ. Anti-inflammatory drugs and their effects on cartilage synthesis and renal function. *European J Rhemalol Inflam* 13:7, 1993.

Schultz AB. *Biomechanics of the spine. In Low Back Pain and industrial and social disablement*. American Back Association, London 1983.

Schultz DG, Fox NH. Kenneth Snelson Buffalo, Albright-Knox Art Gallery. 1981.

Schwarzer AC, Aprill CN, Bogduk N.:The sacroiliac joint in chronic low back pain. *Spine* 20:31, 1995.

Schwarzer AC, Aprill CN, Derby R, Fortin J, Kine G, Bogduk N. The relative contributions of the disc and zygapophyseal joint in chronic low back pain. *Spine* 19:801, 1994.

Schwarzer AC, Aprill CN, Derby R, Fortin J, Kine G, Bogduk N. Clinical features of patients with pain stemming from the lumbar zygapophyseal joints. Is the lumbar facet syndrome a clinical entity?. *Spine* 19:1132, 1994.

Schweiger U, Deuschle M, Korner A, Lammers CH, Schmider J, Gotthardt U, Holsboer F, Heuser I. Low lumbar bone mineral density in patients with major depression. *Am J Psychiatry* 151:1691, 1994.

Seifter E et al. Supplemental arginine: Endocrine, autocrine, and paracrine effects on wound healing. *J Am Coll Nutr* 8:437,1989.

Seitfer E et al. Influence of vitamin A on wound healing in rats with femoral fracture. *Ann Surg* 181:836,1975.

Selzer M, Spencer W A. Convergence of visceral and cutaneous afferent pathways in the lumbar spinal cord. *Brain Res*. 14:331, 1969.

Shapiro D, Goldstein IB, Jamner LD. Effects of cynical hostility, anger out, anxiety, and defensiveness on ambulatory blood pressure in black and white collage students. *Psychosom Med* 58:354, 1996.

Shaw, T.E.In.: Mennell J. *The Musculoskeletal System*. Anaspen Publication, Gaithersburg, Maryland 1992.

Shekelle, PG, Adams, AH, Chassin, MR, Hurwitz, EL, Brook, RH. Spinal Manipulation for Low-Back Pain. *Annals of Internal Medicine* 17:590, 1992.

Shen E, Tsai TT, Lan C. Supraspinal participation in the inhibitory effect of acupuncture on viscero-somatic reflex discharges. *Chin Med J* 1:431, 1975.

Shi GD et al. *J of Guiyang College of TCM* 1:59, 1980.

Shigata M. *J of the Pharm Socie of Jap* (Tokyo) 97:911, 1977.

Shibata M. Metabolism and Disease *Wakan Yaku* Supplement 10:687, 1973.

Shriber WJ. *A Manual of Electrotherapy*, 4th ed. Philadelphia, Lea & Febiger, 1974.

Shudo D. *Introduction to Meridian Therapy*. Seattle: Eastland Press, 1990.

Siegman AW, Snow SC. The outward expression of anger, the inward experience of anger and CVR: the role of vocal expression. *J Behav Med*. 20:29, 1997.

Simon L. The importance of cyclo-oxygenase selectivity in the efficacy of NSAID therapy.

*Proceedings of American Back Society,* 1997.

Sin YM. Acupuncture and inflammation. *Int J Chin Med.* 1:15, 1984.

Sincair DC, Weddell G, Feindel WH, Referred pain and associated phenomena. *Brain* 71:184, 1948.

Singer R, Roy S. Osteochondrosis of the humeral capitulum. *Am J Sports Med.* 12:351, 1984.

Singh GB, Atal CK. Pharmacology of an extract of salai guggalex Boswellia serrata, a new nonsteroidal anti-inflammatory agent. *Agents Action* 18:4,1986.

Singh YN. Effects of kava on neuromuscular transmission and muscle contractility. *J Ethnopharmacol* 7:267; 1983.

Smillie IS. The current pattern of internal derangements of the knee joint relative to the menisci. *Clin Orthop.* 51:117, 1967.

Smock T, Fields HL. ACTH (1-24) blocks opiate induced analgesia in the rat. *Brain Research.* 212:202, 1980.

Snelson KD. Continuous tension, discontinuous compression structures. U.S. Patent 3,169, 611, Washington Patent Office 1965.

Snijders C J, Vleeming A, Stoeckart R. Transfer of lumbosacral load to iliac bones and legs. Part I Biomechanics of self-bracing of the sacroiliac joints and its significance for treatment and exercise. *In Low back pain and its relation to the sacroiliac joint. First interdisciplinary world congress.* San Diego, Nov 1992.

Snook, S.H.: The Costs of Back Pain in Industry. *State of the Art Review. Spine,* 2:1 1987.

Sola AE, Kuitert JH, Myofascial trigger point pain in the neck and shoulder girdle. *Northwest Med* 54:980, 1955.

Solonen KA. The sacroiliac joint in the light of anatomical, roentgenological and clinical studies. *Acta Orthp Scand Suppi* 27, 1957.

Song ZY et al. *Acta Pharmaceutica Sinica* 10:708, 1963

Song ZY et al. *Acta Physiologica sinica* 22: 201, 1958.

Sorenson JRJ. Copper complexes offer a physiological approach to treatment of chronic diseases. *Progress in Medical Chemistry* Vol. 26,1989.

Sorenson J. Copper aspirinate: a more potent anti-inflammatory and ulcer agent. *J Int Acad Prev Med* 1980.

Sopranzi N et al [Biological and electroencephalographic parameters in rats in relation to Passiflora incarnata L.] *Clin Ter* 13:329,1990.

Srivastava KC and Mustafa T. Ginger (Zingiber officinale) in rheumatism and musculoskeletal disorders. *Med Hypothesis* 39:342,1992.

Srivastava R Srimal RC. Modification of certain inflammation-induced biochemical changes of by curcumin. *Indian J Med Res* 81:447,1973.

Spengler, Oswald. *The Decline of the West.* Alfred A. Knopf, New York, 1932.

Stammers T et al. Fish oil in osteoarthritis. Letter. *Lancet* 2:503,1989.

Stanish WD, Valiant GA, Bonen A, et al. The effects of immobilization and electrical stimulation on muscle glycogen and myofibrillar ATPase. *Can J Appl Sport Sci.* 7:267, 1982.

Stefano G, Radanov BP. Course of attention and memory after common whiplash: a two-years prospective study with age, education and gender pair-matched patients. *Acta Neurol Scand* 91:346, 1995.

Stevens, A. Side bending in Axial Rotation of the Sacrum Inside the Pelvic Girdle. *First Interdisciplinary World Congress on Low Back Pain and its Relation to the Sacroiliac Joint.* San Diego 1992.

Stiles TC, Landro NI. Information processing in primary fibromyalgia, major depression and healthy controls. *J Rheumatol.* 22:137,1995.

Stone S. Pyridoxine and thiamine therapy in disorders of the nervous system. *Dis Nerv Sys* 11:131,1950.

Sturzenegger M. Headache and neck pain: the warning symptoms of vertebral artery dissection. *Headache* 34:187, 1994.

Su HC, Su RK. Treatment of whiplash injuries with acupuncture. *Clin J Pain.* 4:233, 1988.

Su XR et al. Scientific Research Compilation (*Shenyang Medical College*) 3:6,1959.

Subotnick SI. *Sports Medicine Of The Lower Extremity.* Churchill Livingstone, NY., 1975.

Suessmann Muntner. *Moshe ben Maimon Medical Works.* Mossad Harav Kook, Jerusalem, 1957.

Suga T. Metabolism and Disease (may supp); *The References of Traditional Chinese Medicine* 4:39, 1976.

Sullivan MX, Hess WC. Cystine content of finger nails in arthritis. *J None Joint Surg* 16:1985,1935.

Sun AY, Boney F, Lee DZ. Electroacupuncture alters cathecolamines in brain regions of rats. *Neurochem Res* 10:251, 1984.

Surtees SJ, Hughes RR. Treatment of trigeminal neuralgia: Conservative management with massive vitamin B12 therapy. *N Carolina Med J* 14:206,1953.


**T**

Tait RC, Chibnall JT, Margolis RB.: Pain extent: Relations with psychological state, pain severity, pain history and disability. *Pain* 41:295, 1990.

Taillard, Meyer and Garcia. *Int Orthop* 5:117, 1981.

Tanaka TH. Professor Nishijo's Research-Acupuncture and the Autonomic Nervous System. *North Amer J of Orien Med.* 3:8, 1996.

Taren DL et al. Increasing the breaking strength of wounds exposed to pre-operative irradiation using vitamin E supplementing. *Int J Vitam Nut Res*, 57:133,1987.

Tasker RR.: *Deafferentation pain syndromes*: pathophysiology and treatment. Raven Press, NY 1991.

Tatlow Brown BSt, Issingtone Tatlow WF. Radiographic studies of the vertebral arteries in cadavers. *Radiology* 81:80, 1963.

Taussig S, Batkin S. Bromelain, the enzyme complex of pineapple (ananas comosus) and its clinical application. An update. *J Ethnopharmacol.* 22:191,1988.

Taylor JR, Twomey LT. Structure and Function of Lumbar Zygapophyseal (Facet) Joints: Review. *J Ortho Med* 14-3: 71, 1992.

Thiel H, Wallace K, Donat J, Yong-Hing K. The effect of various head and neck positions on vertebral artery blood flow-a study using Doppoler ultrasound. *Clinical Biomechanics* [in press].

Thompson D. On growth and form. Cambridge University Press, Cambridge 1961.

Tixier IM, et al. Evidence by in vivo and in vitro studies that binding of pycnogenols to elastin affects its rate of degradation by elastase. *Biochem Pharmacol* 33:3933,1984.

Trabrer MG et al. Lock of tocopherol in peripheral nerves of vitamin E deficient patients with peripheral neuropathy. *N Engl J Med* 317:262,1987.

Travell JG, Simons DG. Myofascial Pain and Dysfunction. *The Trigger Point Manual.* Williams & Willkins Baltimore, 1983.

Travell JG, Simons DG., *Myofascial Pain and Dysfunction The Trigger Point Manual.* vol.II. Williams & Wilkins 1992.

Travell J, Rinzler SH. The myofascial genesis of pain. *Postgrad Med* 11: 425, 1952.

Travers RL, et al Boron and arthritis: the results of a double-blind pilot study. *J Nutri Med* 1:127,1990.

Tripterygium Wilfordii Coordinating Research Group of Hubei, Institute of Combined Western and Chinese Medicine et al. *Health J of Hubei* 1:72, 1979.

Troup JD et al. The perception of back pain and the role of psychophysical tests of lifting capacity. *Spine* 12:645, 1987.

Tsuchisashi M. et al. Road traffic accidents and the abbreviated injury scale (AIS) in Japan. *Accid Anal Prev.* 13:37,1981.

Turek S.L.: *Orthopaedics*: Principles and Their Application. 4th ed. Philadelphia, J.B. Lippincott, 1984.


**U**

Yang YR et al. *Acta Physiologica Sinica* 8:101, 1966.

Uhlig Y, Weber BR, Grob D, Muntener M. Fiber composition and fiber transformations in neck muscles of patients with dysfunction of the cervical spine. *Orthop Res* 13:240, 1995.

Unruh AM. Gender variations in clinical pain experience. *Pain* 65:123, 1996.

Upadhaya L et al. Role of an indigenous drug Geriforte on blood levels of biogenic amines and its significance in the treatment of anxiety neurosis. *Acta Nerv Super* 32:1,1990.

Yu YX, Bao H, Zhou ZF, Han JS. C-fibers afferents are necessary for diffuse noxious inhibitory control (DNIC) but not for electroacupuncture analgesia, in Han JS: *The Neurochemical Basis of Pain Relief by Acupuncture; A Collection of Papers*. Med Sci Press Beijing 1978.

Yu PL et al. *Hunan Yiyao Zazhi* (Hunan Medical J) 5:52, 1979.

Yu QX et al. *Chinese Pharmaceutical Bulletin* 7:567, 1959.


**V**

Vallo MD, Ransohoff J. Thoracic disc disease in: *The Spine*, 2ed ed. WB Saunders Philadelphia 1982.

Veldhuizen AG. Kinematics of the scoliotic spine as related to the normal spine. *Spine* 12:852, 1987.

Vernon HT, Mior S.: The neck disability index: A study of reliability and validity. *J Manip Phsiol Ther* 14:409, 1991.

Verrier RL, Mittleman MA. Life-threatening cardiovascular consequences of anger in patients with coronary heart disease. *Cardiol Clin* 14:289, 1996.

Vidal Y Plana RR et al. Articular cartilage pharmacology: In vitro studies on glucosamine and non-steroidal anti-inflammatory drugs. *Pharmacol Res Commun* 10:557,1978.

Videman at al.: Changes in 35S-sulphate uptake in different tissues in the knee and hip regions of rabbits during immobilization, remobilization and the development of osteoarthritis, *Acta Orthop Scand* 47: 290, 1979.

Vicenzino B, Collins D, Wright A. The initial effects of a cervical spine manipulative physiotherapy treatment on the pain and dysfunction of lateral epicondlylagia. *Pain* 68:69, 1996.

Vincent CA. A Controlled trial in the treatment of migraine by acupuncture. *The Clin J of Pain* 5:305, 1990.

Vitamin A supplementation may be beneficial in peripheral vascular disease (PVD) *Acta Vitaminol Enzymol* 4:15,1982.

Vleeming A. et al. Mobility in the SI-Joints in old people: A kinematic and radiologic study. *Clin Biomech* 7:170, 1992.

Vleeming A et al. Load application to the sacrotuberous ligament: Influences on sacro-iliac

joint mechanics. *Clin Biomech* 4:204, 1989.

Vleeming A. *AAOM annual meeting* 1994.

Vleeming A, Stoeckart R, Volkers AC, Snijders CJ. Relation between form and function in the sacroililac joint Part I: Clinical anatomical aspects. *Spine* 15:130, 1990.

Vleeming, Volkers AC, Snijders CJ, Stoeckart R. Relation between form and function in the sacroiliac joint Part II: Biomechanical aspects. *Spine* 15:133, 1990.

Vreden SG et al. Aseptic bone necrosis in patients on glucocorticoid replacement therapy. *Netherlands J Med*. 39:153, 1991.


Vyklicky L, Knotkova-Urbancova H. Can sensory neurons in culture serve as a model of nociception?. *Physiol Res* 45:1, 1996.


**W**

Waddell G.: A new clinical model for the treatment of low back pain. *Spine* 12:634,1987.

Wang N, Butler JP, Ingber DE. Microtransduction across the cell surface and through the cyroskeleton. *Science* 260:1124, 1993.

Wang K, Yao S, Xian Y, Hou Z. A study on the receptive field of acupoints and the relationship between characteristics of the needle sensation and groups of afferent fibers. *Sci China* 28:963, 1985.

Wall PD, Gutnick M. Ongoing activity in peripheral nerves: the physiology and pharmacology of impulses originating from a neuroma. *Exp Neurol* 43:580, 1074.

Waxman SG, deGroot J. *Correlative Neuroanatomy* 22ed (edi) Appleton & Lange Northwalk, Connecticut 1995.

Weisl H. The movement of the sacro-iliac joint *Acta Mat* 23, 1955.

Weber H.: Lumbar disc herniation: A controlled prospective study with ten years of observation. *Spine* 8:131, 1983.

Webster BS, Snook SH. The cost of 1989 workers' compensation low back pain claims. *Spine* 19:1111,1994.

Wei Hui Publishing. *Chinese Medicine Secret Recipe*. Shanghai, 1990.

Weiner DS, Macnab I. Superior migration of the humeral head. *J Bone Surg* 52B:524, 1970.

Weingart, J.R., Bischoff, H.P. Doppler-Sonographische untersuchungen der a. vertebralis unter berucksichtigung Chirotherapeutisch relevanter. *Kopfpositionen Manuelle Medizin* 30:62, 1992.

Weintraub MI, Khoury A. Critical neck position as an independent risk factor for posterior circulation stroke. A magnetic resonance angiographic analysis. *J Neuroimaging* 5:16, 1995.

Weiss DS, Kirsner R, Eaglastein WH. Electrical stimulation and wound healing. *Arch Dermato.* 126:222, 1990.

Weinstein JN: The role of neurogenic and non-neurogenic mediators as they relate to pain and the development of osteoarthritis. *Spine* 105: 356, 1992.

Wenneberg et al. Anger expression correlates with platelet aggregation. *Behav Med* 22:174 1997.

Werback MR. *Nutritional Influences on Illness* (second edition) Third Line Press, Trazana, CA).

Werback MR. *Botanical Influences on Illness*, Tarzana, CA, Third Line Press 1994.

White AA, Panjabi. M.M.The basic kinematics of the spine. *Spine* 3:13, 1978.

White AA, Panjabi MM. *Clinical biomechanics of the spine*. Lippincott, Philadelphia 1978.

White G. Vitamin E inhibition of platelet prostaglandin biosynthesis. *Fed Proc* 36:350, 1977.

Whittingham W, Ellis WB, Molyneux TP. The effect of manipulation, toggle recoil technique for headaches with upper cervical joint dysfunction: a pilot study. *J Manipulative Physiol Ther* 6:369, 1994.

Wildy P, Home RW. Structures of animal virus particles. *Progressive Medical Virology* 5:1, 1963.

Williams KW et al. The effect of topically applied zinc on healing of wounds in animals and man. *Ann Surg* 170:203,1969.

Willburger RE, Wittenberg RH. Prostaglandin release from lumbar disc and facet joint tissue. *Spine* 19:2068, 1994.

Willis GC et al. Serial artheriography in atherosclerosis. *Can Med Assoc J.* Dec, Willis GC et al. Serial artheriography in atherosclerosis. *Can Med Assoc J.* 562:68,1954.

Willis WD.: Mechanical allodynia: A role from nocireceptive tract cells with convergent input from mechanoreceptors and nociceptors? *APS Journal* 2:23, 1993.

Woelk H. Multicentric practice-study analyzing the functional capacity in depressive patients. *4th International Congress on Phytotherapy.* Munich, Germany, Sep 10-13, 1992, abstract SL54.

Woldenberg SC. The treatment of arthritis with colloidal sulphur. *J South Med Assoc* 28:875,1935.

Wolf SL, Basmajian JV.: Assessment of paraspinal electromyographic activity in normal subjects and in chronic low back pain patients using biofeedback device. In: Asmussen E, Jorgensoen K, eds. *Biomechanics VI-B*, Baltimore: University Park Press,1979.

Wolff, HD. Comments on the Evolution of the Sacroiliac Joint in Progress and Vertebral Column Research, *First International Symposium on the Sacroiliac Joint, Its Role in Posture and Locomotion*. EcL Vleeming, A. European Conference Orgairrers, Rotterdam, 1991.

Woltring HJ, Long K, Osterbauer PJ, Fuhr AW. Instantaneous helical axis estimation from 3-D video data in neck kinematics for whiplash diagnostics. *J Biomech* 27:1415, 1994.

Wong J et al. The therapeutic effect of 154 cases of scapulohumeral peri-arthritis treated with electroacupuncture. *Chin Acup & Moxib* 8:20, 1988.

Wybran J, et al., Suggestive Evidence for Receptors for Morphine and Methionine-enkephalins on Hormonal Human T Lymphocytes. *Journal of Immunology* 130:168, 1979.

Wyke B. The neurology of joints. A review of general principles. Clinics in Rheumatic Diseases 7:233, 1981.

Wyke BD. Neurology of the cervical spinal joints. *Physiotherapy* 65:72, 1979.

Wyke BD. Clinical significance of articular receptor system in the limbs and spine. *Proc. of the 5th Int. Congress of Manual Medicine* Copenhagen 1977.

Wynne-Davis, R.: Hypermobility. Proc. Roy. *Soc. Med* 64:689, 1971.

Wynne-Davis, R.: Hypermobility. Manipulation of the spine: In: Basmajian JV (ed). *Manipulation, traction and massage*. Paris RML., 1986.

## X

Xie CW, Tang J, Han JS. Central norepinephrine in acupuncture analgesia: Differential effects in brain and spinal cord, in Takagi H, Simon EJ, (eds). *Advances in Endogenous and Exogenous Opioids: Proceedings of the Int Narcotic Res Conference / INRC*, Kodansha Sci Books, Tokyo, 1981.

## Y

Yahia LH, Garzon S, Strykowski H, Rivard CH. Ultrastructure of the human interspinous ligament and ligamentum flavum: a preliminary study. *spine* 15:262, 1990.

Yaksh TL, Hammond DL. Peripheral and central substrates involved in the rostrad transmission of nociceptive information. *Pain* 13:1, 1982.

Yi ZZ. *Acta Pharmceutica Sinica* 15:321, 1980.

Yin QZ, Duanmu ZX, Guo SY, Yu XM. Role of hypothalamic arcuate nucleus in acupuncture analgesia: A review of behavior and electrophysiological studies. *J Trad Chin Med* 4:103, 1984.

Ying Y, et al. Effects of acupuncture on adrenocortical hormone production. *Amer J Chin Med*. 22:160, 1976.

Yrjama M Vanharanta H. Bony vibration stimulation: a new, non-invasive method for examining intradiscal pain. *Eur Spine J*. 3:233, 1994.

Yoganandan N et al. Epidemiology and injury biomechanics of motor vehicle related trauma to the human spine. In: Proceedings of the 33rd Stapp Car Crash Conference, P-227, 892438, Washington, DC, 1989, SAE.

Yunus, M et al.: Primary fibromyalgia (fibrositis): Clinical study of 50 patients with matched normal controls. Semin. *Arthr. Rheum*. 11:151,1981.

## Z

Zang QZ et al. Abstracts of the symposium of the Chinese society of Physiology *Pharmacology* 1964. p.106

Zhang DF et al. *Jiangsu Zhongyi* (Jiangsu J of TCM) 3:23, 1965.

Zhang YZ, Tong J, Han JS. Potentiation of electroacupuncture analgesia by D-phenylalanine or bacitracine in mice. *Kexue Tongbao*. 24:1523, 1981.

Zhang Xinshu. Wrist and Ankle Acupuncture Therapy. *J Chin Med* 37:5, 1991.

Zang XT. Interaction in thalamus of afferent impulses from acupuncture point and site of pain. *Chin Med J* 93:1, 1980.

Zao FY, Meng JZ, Yu SD, Ma AH, Dong XY, Han JS. Acupuncture analgesia in impacted last molar extraction: effect of clomipramine and pargyline, in Han JS (ed). *The Neurochemical Basis of Pain Relief by Acupuncture; A Collection of Papers*. Med Sci Press, Beijing 1981.

Zhejiang Medical College. Proceedings of the national symposium on Chinese traditional anesthesia 1970.

Zhu Zong-Xiang. Research advances in the electrical specificity of channels and acupuncture points. *Amer. J. Acup.* 9:203, 1981.

Zhu Y. *Pharmacology and applications of Chinese medicinal materials*. People's Medical Publishing House. 1958.

Ziboh Va, Fletcher MP. Dose-Response effects of dietary γ-linolenic acid-enriched oils on human polymorphonuclear-neutrophil biosynthesis of leukotriene B4. *Am J Clin Nutr* 55:39,1992.

Zukauskas G et al. Quantitative analysis of bioelectrical potentials for the diagnosis of internal organ pathology and theoretical speculations concerning electrical circulation in the organism. *Acup & Electro-ther. Res Int. J.* 13:119, 1988.

# Works Consulted

## A

Anon. *A Barefoot Doctor's Manual*. Washington, DC: U.S. Department of Health, Education and Welfare: Public Health Service, 1974.

Anon. *The Canon of Acupuncture: Huangti Nei Ching Ling Shu*. Sunu K, translator. Los Angeles: Yuin University Press, 1985.

## B

Becker RO, Selden G. *The Body Electric: Electromagnetism and the Foundation of Life*. New York: William Morrow and Company, 1985.

Beijing College of Traditional Chinese Medicine, Shanghai College of Traditional Chinese Medicine, et al. *Essentials of Chinese Acupuncture*. Beijing: Foreign Languages Press, 1980.

Beinfield J, Korngold E. *Between Heaven and Earth*. New York: Ballantine Books, 1991.

Bensky D, Barolet R. *Chinese Herbal Medicine Formulas & Strategies*. Seattle WA: Eastland Press, 1990.

Bensky D, Gamble A. *Chinese Herbal Medicine Materia Medica*. Seattle WA.: Eastland Press, 1986.

## C

Chen Y, Deng L. *Essentials of Contemporary Chinese Acupuncturists' Clinical Experiences*. Beijing, China: Foreign Languages Press, 1989.

Chen Z-L, Chen M-F. *The Essence and Scientific Background of Tongue Diagnosis*. Long Beach: OHAI, 1989.

Croizier RC. *Traditional Medicine in Modern China*. Cambridge: Harvard University Press, 1980.

## D

Dosch M. *Illustrated Atlas of the Techniques of Neural Therapy with Local Anesthetics*. HAUG, 1985.

## E

Eckmann P. *The Book of Changes in Traditional Oriental Medicine*. Columbia, MD: Traditional Acupuncture Institute, 1987.

Ellis A, Wiseman N, Boss K. *Grasping the Wind*. Brookline, MA: Paradigm Publications, 1989.

## F

Faber W, Walker M. *Pain Pain Go Away*. ISHI Press International, 1990.

Flaws B. *Migraines and Traditional Chinese Medicine: A Layperson's Guide*. Boulder, CO: Blue Poppy Press, 1990.

Flaws B. *Sticking to the Point*. Boulder CO: Blue Poppy Press, 1989.

Flaws B, Zhang Ting-liang, Chace C, Helme M, Wolfe HL, and The Dechen Yonten Dzo. *Blue Poppy Essays: Translations and Ruminations on Chinese Medicine*. Boulder, CO: Blue Poppy Press, 1988.

## G

Griffin JE, Karselis TC. *Physical Agents for Physical Therapists* (2nd ed). Springfield: Charles C Thomas, 1982.

Gunn CC. *Treating Myofascial Pain: Intramuscular Simulation (IMS) for Myofasical Pain Syndromes of Neuropathic Origin*. Seattle WA: University of Washington press, 1989.

## H

Helms JM. *Acupuncture Energetics. A Clinical Approach for Physicians*. Bekeley: Medical Acupuncture Publishers, 1995.

Hoc KH, Seifert GM. *Pulse Diagnosis Li Shi Zhen*. Brookline, Mass: Paradigm Publications 1985.

Hsü TC. *Forgotten Traditions of Ancient Chinese Medicine: A Chinese View from the Eighteenth Century*. Translated and annotated by Unschuld PU. Brookline, Mass: Paradigm Publications, 1990.

Huang BS. *Treatment of Pain by Traditional Chinese Medicine*. Harbin, China: Heilongjiang Education Press, 1993.

Hui JL, Xiang JZ. *Pointing Therapy*. Shandong China: Shandong Science and Technology Press, 1990.

**J**

Jenkner FL. *Electric Pain*-Controle. Vienna Austria.

Jirui, C. and Wang, N., editors. *Acupuncture Case Histories from China*. Seattle: Eastland Press, 1988.

**K**

Kaptchuk TJ. *The Web That Has No Weaver: Understanding Chinese Medicine*. New York: Congdon & Weed, 1983.

Kikutani T. *Combined Use of Western Therapies and Chinese Medicine*. Hsu H-Y, translator. Long Beach: HOAI, 1987.

**L**

Lade A. *Acupuncture Points: Images and Functions*. Seattle: Eastland Press, 1989.

Lee J, Cheung CS. *Current Acupuncture Therapy*. Hong Kong: Medical Book Publications, 1978.

Lee M. *Master Tong's Acupuncture*. Boulder: Blue Poppy Press, 1992.

Lee HM, Whincup G. *Chinese Massage Therapy*. Boulder: Shambhala Press, 1983.

Legge D. *Close To The Bone*. Australia: Sydney College Press, 1990.

Lennard TA. *Physiatric Procedures in Clinical Practice*. Philadelphia: Hanley & Belfus Inc. 1995.

Leonhardt H. *Fundamentals of Electroacupuncture According to Voll*. Uelzen: MLV, 1990.

Leslie C, editor. *Asian Medical Systems*. Berkeley: University of California, 1977.

Liu Yanchi. *The Essential Book of Traditional Chinese Medicine*, Volume 2: Clinical Practice. New York: Columbia University Press, 1988.

Low R. *The Secondary Vessels of Acupuncture*. New York: Thorsons Publishers, Inc., 1983.

**M**

Maciocia G. *The Foundations of Chinese Medicine*. New York: Churchill Livingstone, 1989.

Maciocia G. *Tongue Diagnosis in Chinese Medicine*. Seattle: Eastland Press, 1995.

Maciocia G. *The Practice of Chinese Medicine: The Treatment of Diseases with Acupuncture and Chinese Herbs*. Edinburgh: Churchill Livingstone, 1994.

Manaka Y, Birch S. Chasing the Dragon's Tail. Brookline: Paradigm Publications, 1995.

Mann F. *The Treatment of Disease by Acupuncture*, 2nd ed. London: William Heinemann Medical Books Ltd, 1967.

Matsumoto K, Birch S. *Extraordinary Vessels*. Brookline: Paradigm Publications, 1986.

Matsumoto K, Birch S. *Hara: Reflections on the Sea*. Brookline: Paradigm Press 1988.

Matsumoto K, Birch S. *Five Elements and Ten Stems*. Higganum: Paradigm Publications, 1985.

Mori H. *Modern Acupuncture and Moxibustion III - Locomotor*. Tokyo: Ido No Nippon Sha, 1982.

**N**

Naeser MA. *Outline Guide to Chinese Herbal Patent Medicines in Pill Form*. Boston: Boston Medical, 1990.

Nakatani Y. *A Guide for Application of Ryodoraku Autonomous Nerve Regulatory Therapy*. Tokyo: Japan Ryodoraku Autonomic Nervous System Society, 1972.

Nogier PMF. *From Auriculotherapy to Auriculomedicine*. Paris: Maisonneuve, 1983.

Nogier PMF. *Handbook to Auriculotherapy*. Paris: Maisonneuve, 1981.

**O**

O'Connor J, Bensky D, translators. Shanghai College of Traditional Medicine (Shanghai). *Acupuncture: A Comprehensive Text*. Chicago: Eastland Press, 1981.

Oleson TD. *Auriculotherapy Manual. Chinese and Western Systems of Ear Acupuncture*. Los Angeles CA: Health Care Alternatives, 1990.

Ombrengt L, Bisschop P, ter Veer HJ and Van de Velde T. *A System of Orthopaedic Medicine*. Saunders 1995.

Weinstein JN: The role of neurogenic and non-neurogenic mediators as they relate to pain and the development of osteoarthritis. *Spine* 105: 356, 1992.

Omura Y. *Acupuncture Medicine: Its Historical and Clinical Background*. Tokyo: Japan Publications, Inc., 1982.


**P**

Peigen K, Yuanping W. *Acupuncture Treatment of Neurological Disorders*. Beijing China: Traditional Chinese Medical Publishers of China, 1991.

Pomeranz B, Stux G. *Scientific Basis of Acupuncture*. Berlin: Springer-Verlag, 1989.

Porkert M. *The Theoretical Foundations of Chinese Medicine*. M.I.T. East Asian Science Series, Vol.3. Cambridge: M.I.T. Press, 1994.


**Q**

Quan SX. Yuan JY, Mao GY, Lin Y, translators;. *Applied Chinese Acupuncture for Clinical Practitioners*. Shangdong China: Shangdong Science and Technology Press, 1985.


**R**

Ross J. *Zang Fu: The Organ Systems of Traditional Chinese Medicine*, 2nd ed. Edinburgh: Churchill Livingstone, 1985.


**S**

Seem M. *A New American Acupuncture: Acupuncture Osteopathy*. Boulder: Blue Poppy Press, 1993.

Serizawa, K. *Clinical Acupuncture: A Practical Japanese Approach*. New York: Japan Publications, 1988.

Shou-Zhong Y. Dan-Xi, translator. *The Heart & Essence of Nan-Xi's Method of Treatment*. Boulder: Blue Poppy Press, 1993.

Shudo D. *Introduction to Meridian Therapy*.

Seattle: Eastland Press, 1990.

Shudo, D. *Japanese Classical Acupuncture: Introduction to Meridian Therapy*. Stephen Brown, translator. Seattle: Eastland Press, 1990.

So J Tin Yau. *The Book of Acupuncture Points*. Brookline: Paradigm Publications, 1985.

So J Tin Yau. *Treatment of Disease with Acupuncture*. Brookline: Paradigm Publications,1987.

Stux G, Pomeranz B. *Basics of Acupuncture*. Berlin: Springer-Verlag, 1991.


**T**

Tan R, Rush S. *Twelve and Twelve in Acupuncture*. San Diego CA, 1991.

Tan R, Rush S. *Twenty-Four More in Acupuncture*. San Diego CA, 1994.

Tanner J. *Beating Back Pain. A practical self-help guide to prevention and treatment*. Doris Kindersley 1987.


**U**

US Directory Service. *Acupuncture Anesthesia* (A translation of a Chinese Publication of the same title) U.S. Directory Service, 1975.

Unschuld PU. Nan-Ching The Classic of Difficult Issues. Berkeley: University of California Press. 1986.


**W**

Wallach, J 1978): Interpretation of *Diagnostic Tests, A Handbook Synopsis of Laboratory Medicine*. Little, Brown and Cope Boston USA 1978.

Wexu M. *A Modern Guide to Ear Acupuncture*. New York: ASI Publishers, Inc. 1975.

Wiseman N, Ellis A, Zmiewaski P. Fundamentals of Chinese Medicine. Brookline: Paradigm Publications, 1985.

Worsley JR. *Acupuncturists' Therapeutic* Pocket Book. Columbia, Maryland: The Centre for Traditional Acupuncture, 1975.

## X

Xianmin S, et al. *Practical Traditional Chinese Medicine & Pharmacology: Clinical Experiences.* Beijing China: New World Press, 1990.

Xing Z. *The English-Chinese Encyclopedia of Practical Traditional Chinese Medicine: Simple and Proved Recipes.* Beijing China: Higher Education Press, 1990.

Xu X, You K, Bao X. *The English-Chinese Encyclopedia of Practical Traditional Chinese Medicine: Orthopedics and Traumatology.* Beijing, China: Higher Education Press, 1990.

## Y

Yau PS, editor. Scalp-Needling Therapy. Revised Ed. Hong Kong: Medicine and Health Publishing Company, 1984.

Yeung H-C. *Handbook of Chinese Herbs and Formulas Vol. 1 and Vol. 2.* Los Angeles: 1983.

Yoo TW. *Lecture on KoRyo SooJi Chim: About the Korean Hand Acupuncture.* Korea: Eum Yang Maek Jin Publishing, 1983.

## Z

Zhang R-F, Wu X-F, and Wang N. *Illustrated Dictionary of Chinese Acupuncture.* Hong Kong: Sheep's Publications, 1986.

Zang XT, editor. *Research on Acupuncture, Moxibustion, and Acupuncture Anesthesia.* Beijing: Science Press; Berlin: Springer-Verlag, 1986.

# Glossary

**ACTINE**
The thinnest of the myofibrils filaments and is half the size of the thick filament myosin.

**ALPHA MOTOR NERVES**
Supply the regular contractile, extrafusal, muscle fibers (not the spindle).

**ARACHIDONIC ACID**
An essential fatty acid that is a component of lecithin and a basic material for the biosynthesis of some prostaglandins.

**AXON**
The process of a neuron by which impulses travel away from the cell body.

**BABINSKI SIGN**
A sign of upper-motor lesion, seen when the bottom of foot is stroked resulting in the big toe pointing upward.

**BALANCE-AND-HOLD**
**An osteopathic technique in which** motion of the joint is introduced in seven directions to identify;
- the point of maximal ease within each movement
- the point of maximal ease within the respiration cycle
After identifying these positions the patient is asked to hold them as long as possible.

**BODY INCH**
See cun.

**BRADYKININ**
A peptide of nonprotein origin containing nine amino acid residues. It is a potent vasodilator.

**CAPSULAR PATTERN**
A specific standard, (for each joint), of range of motion restrictions seen when the joint is inflamed.

**CARTILAGE**
A non-vascular tissue, is comprised of a variety of fibrous connective tissues in which the matrix (intracellular substance of a tissue) is abundant and firm.

**CELLULAR IMMUNITY**
Part of inflammatory response dominated by T cell lymphocytes. It is involved in resistance to infectious diseases, delayed hypersensitivity, resistance to cancer, autoimmune diseases, graft rejection and allergies.

| | |
|---|---|
| CHANNELS | Conduits for various types of matter and energies. Connect various tissues distributed from exterior to interior, also called meridians. |

- **Connecting channels**; link Main channels with surrounding tissues, part of the blood vessel system, provide a functional connection between the ventral-dorsal and Yin-Yang aspects, store energy and Blood and release them to the Main channels when needed, important in prevention of chronicity, emotional disorders, excess conditions.
- **Divergent channels**; reinforce Main channels, provide functional connection between Yin-Yang channels and Organs, balance between the right and left, Important in Yin (substance) anatomical pathological disorders.
- **Extra channels**; store extra Qi and Blood, release Qi and Blood when Main channels are vacuous, balance between the left right, superior-inferior, and diagonal aspects, important in chronic disorders.
- **Main channels**; connect Organs to rest of system, the main channel system.
- Sinew channels; tendon-muscular channels, location of Defense Qi circulation, connection between main channels and connective tissue and skin, with the muscles, provides body's protective layer important in acute disorders such as sprain/strain.

| | |
|---|---|
| CHANNEL THERAPY | A term used to describe a variety of ways of treating the body via the channel. |
| CHANNEL CIRCADIAN CIRCULATION | Channel energy circulation said to take 24 hours and is stronger for a period of two hours at each channel. |
| CNS | Central nervous system; brain and spinal cord. |
| CONNECTIVE TISSUE | Consist mostly of fibroblast cells; the rest are mast cells, macrophages, plasma cells, pigment cells, lymphocytes and leukocytes. |
| CORD GATE MECHANISM | See *gate mechanism*. |
| COUNTERTENSION POSITIONAL RELEASE (STRAINCOUNTERSTRAIN) | An osteopathic treatment system especially effective for muscle spasm with an accompanying exquisitely tender point. |
| CUN | Body inch. The width of the patient's thumb, or the distance between the ends of the patient's interphalangeal creases on the radial surface of the middle finger. The distance between the outer edge of the index finger and the outer edge of the little finger is said to be three inches. |
| DENDRITE | A tree-like, branched process of a neuron. Dendrites conduct impulses to the cell body from the axons of other neurons. |
| DERMATOME | Superficial sensation innervated by a spinal root. |
| DIENCEPHALON | The division of the brain between the cerebrum and mesencephalon. Consisting of the hypothalamus, thalamus, metathalamus and epithalamus. |
| DOLOMETER | A pressure meter used to quantify subjective pain threshold. |
| DRY NEEDLING | Needling tissues with acupuncture needles based on neuroanatomical principals. |
| EIGHT PARAMETERS | A diagnostic paradigm that describe disorders according to their nature and location. |
| END FEEL | The characteristic sensation the practitioner perceives at the end of the patient's passive ROM. |
| ENDOGENOUS FACTORS | Influences that originate from within. Consist of the seven affects: Joy, Anger, Sorrow, Anxiety, Preoccupation, Fear, Fright. |

| | |
|---|---|
| **ENDORPHINS** | Function as synaptic neurotransmitters, possibly modifying the movement of sodium and potassium across nerve membranes and affecting action potentials. Researchers have isolated several endorphins, such as alpha, beta and gamma endorphin.s |
| **ENERGIES** | See types of Qi. |
| **ENKEPHALINS** | Two closely related polypeptides found in the brain called met-enkephalin and leu-enkephalin. Frequently enkephalinergic interneurons are localized in the same areas as opiate receptors that produce pharmacological effects similar to morphine. The amino acid sequence of met-enkephalin has been found in alpha-endorphin and beta-endorphin. |
| **EOSINOPHIL** | A granulocytic, bilobed leukocyte (white blood cell), that increase in number in response to allergy and in some parasitic infections. |
| **EXOGENOUS FACTORS** | Environmental influences that can cause disease: Wind, Cold, Fire, Damp, Dryness and Summer Heat. Can invade Interior or Exterior. |
| **FIBROBLASTS** | An undifferentiated cell in the connective tissue that gives rise to various precursor cells, such as the chondroblast, collagenoblast, and osteoblast, that form the fibrous, binding, and supporting tissue of the body. |
| **FIBROMYALGIA** | A painful, non-articular condition predominantly involving muscles, and is the commonest cause of chronic widespread musculoskeletal pain. |
| **FIVE PHASES** | The phases, five elemental configurations that can be found in all material and natural order, are called Wood, Fire, Earth, Metal and Water. |
| **FORNIX** | Nerve fibers that lie beneath the corpus callosum and connect the two cerebrum hemispheres. |
| **FRYETTE LAWS** | Rules pertaining to the coupling of vertebral movements. |
| **GAMMA MOTOR (EFFERENT) NERVES** | Supply motor innervation to the muscle spindles, comprise the small motor neuron system whose cell bodies are located in the ventral horn (spinal cord). |
| **GATE** <br> **GATE CONTROL MECHANISM** <br> **GATE MECHANISM** | A theory of pain modulation. |
| **GOLGI TENDON ORGANS** | Receptors that lie in series with the muscle fibers, serve as inhibitors of muscle spindles as well as contractile forces in the muscle. |
| **GROUND SUBSTANCE** | See nonfibrous ground substance. |
| **GUA SHA** | See scraping. |
| **HIPPOCAMPUS** | An elevation of the floor of the lateral ventricle of the brain. It is an important component of the limbic system and its efferent projections form the fornix of the cerebrum. |
| **HUMORAL RESPONSE** | One of the two forms of immunity that respond to antigens such as bacteria and foreign tissue. It is mediated by B cell lymphocytes. |
| **INDEPENDENT FACTORS** | Related to lifestyle: Diet, sexual activity, excessive consumption of physical resources, trauma, parasitic infection. <br> Can lead to obstruction and tissue damage. |
| **ION CORDS** | A wire with a diod used in acupuncture. |
| **ISOMETRIC CONTRACTION** | Muscle contraction that does not involve muscle shortening (no movement). |

| | |
|---|---|
| **ISOTONIC DONTRACTION** | Muscle contraction that involves movement of an object, constant tension contraction. |
| **JOINT DYSFUNCTION** | Describes the loss of intrinsic motions, joint play or function in the joint complex without obvious pathology. |
| **JOINT PLAY** | A motion within a synovial joint, in which the motion is separate from, and cannot be initiated by, voluntary muscle contraction. Joint play consists of fine movement (less then 1/8-inch) in any plane the natural laxity of the joint capsule allows. |
| **LATENT PATHOGENIC FACTORS** | Incubation period of pathogenic factors. |
| **LESION, MEDICAL** | A pathology of a tissue such as tendinitis. |
| **LIMBIC SYSTEM** | A group of cellular structures, rather than a single brain region, located between the brain stem and the cortex and associated with emotions. |
| **LYMPHOCYTE** | A type of white blood cell that increase in number in response to infection. |
| **MACROPHAGE** | Any phagocytic cell of the reticuloedothelial system including histocyte in loose connective tissue. |
| **MANIPULATION** | A thrust technique commonly used in many traditional therapies around the world. |
| **MCGILL PAIN QUESTIONNAIRE (MPQ)** | A pain questionnaire that uses classes of words that have been determined to represent affective (mood), sensory and cognitive components of pain experience. |
| **MCKENZIE SYSTEM** | A treatment system for disc derangements and other spinal disorders based on the patient's response to load strategies that either increase or decrease the patient's pain. |
| **MERIDIANS** | Conduits for various types of matter and energies. Connect various tissues. Distributed from exterior to interior. Also called channels. |
| **MINNESOTA MULTIPHASIC PERSONALITY INVENTORY (MMPI)** | The most thoroughly researched of the personality inventories in both psychopathology and pain management. |
| **MISCELLANEOUS FACTORS** | Secondary factors that can lead to channel obstruction and disease: Phlegm, Static Blood. |
| **MOTOR UNIT** | A motor neuron and the muscle fibers it innervates. |
| **MOTOR END PLATE** | A region of the muscle membrane together with the terminal portion of the axon. |
| **MOXIBUSTION (MOXA)** | A preparation of artemisia vulgaris that is either placed directly over or on a point, or is attached to a needle. Used commonly to treat cold pain and deficient patients. |
| **MUSCLE ENERGY** | Osteopathic technique developed by Mitchell Sr. which uses postisometric relaxation, reciprocal inhibition and isotonic contraction to restore mobility to joints. Also the use of the above mechanisms to treat muscular dysfunctions. |
| **MUSCLE SPASM** | Involuntary sudden movement or muscular contraction that prevents lengthening of the muscle involved. |
| **MUSCLES SPINDLE** | Specialized mechanoreceptive contractile fiber units containing intrafusal fibers surrounded by connective tissue. |

| | |
|---|---|
| **M**YOFASCIAL PAIN **S**YNDROME | A painful condition felt by some to be due to myofascial trigger point activation, either by direct causes or as a reactive mechanism to other dysfunctions. |
| **M**YOFASCIAL **R**ELEASE | An osteopathic technique that is a relatively new addition to osteopathic treatments. However similar techniques have been used for a long time and by many traditions. |
| **M**YOFIBRIL | Two fine longitudinal fibrils, lying side by side, comprised of many regularly overlapped, ultramicroscopic, thick and thin myosin and actin myofilaments that may extend the entire length of the muscle. |
| **M**YOSIN | The thicker of the myofibril filaments and is twice the size of the thin filament Actin. |
| **M**YOSITIS OSSIFICANS | A benign condition which can result from trauma to muscle tissue or can be inherited. |
| **M**YOTOME | Muscles innervated by a spinal root. The area of reference of those muscles. |
| **N**EUROGENIC **I**NFLAMMATION | Inflammation resulting from release of neuropeptides that interact with fibroblasts, mast cells and immune cells in the surrounding connective tissues. |
| **N**EURON | The basic functional and structural component of the nervous system which receives information, processes it, and sends it to other neurons. A neuron is composed of a cell body and its processes, a single axon, and one or more dendrites. |
| **N**EUROMUSCULAR **J**UNCTION | The junction that includes the axon terminal and the motor end plate. |
| **N**EUROPATHIC PAIN | Less common than nociceptive pain, can be caused by trauma or disease evoked damage affecting the peripheral nerves, posterior roots, splnal cord or certain regions in the brain. |
| **N**EUROTRANSMITTERS | Chemicals that regulate the nervous system. Some examples are epinephrine, norepinephrine, serotonin, acetylcholine, histamine, dopamine, and even some amino acids such as Gamma-aminobutyric acid (GABA) and glycine. |
| **N**EUTRAL TYPE **I** **MECHANICS** | Bending to one side coupled with rotation to the opposite side. |
| **N**EUTROPHILS | Circulating white blood cells essential for phagocytosis and proteolysis by which bacteria, cellular debris, and solid particles are removed and destroyed. |
| **N**OCICEPTORS | Pain nerve fibers that are classified by their fiber diameters, conduction velocities and physiologic characteristics (A-delta and C-fibers). Sensitive to noxious or potentially-noxious mechanical and chemical stimuli. |
| **N**ONFIBROUS GROUND **SUBSTANCE** | Composed of proteoglycans, which are polysaccharide molecules bound to protein chains in covalent complexes. Found in the extracellular matrix of connective tissue. |
| **N**ONNEUTRAL TYPE **II** **MECHANICS** | Side bending coupled with rotation to same side. Results in less stability than neutral spine mechanics. |
| **N**UCLEAR BAG REGION | The middle portion or receptor portion of a muscle spindle, noncontractile. |
| **N**ULLINESS | Referral of a numb-like ache from ligamentous disorders. |
| **O**RGAN | OM organ |
| **O**RGAN | Biomedical organ |

**ORTHOPAEDIC MEDICINE**  An updated version of the Cyriax approach to orthopedic medicine.

**ORTHOPEDIC MEDICINE**  The western medical specialty concerned with the musculoskeletal system, extremities, spine, and associated structures.

**OPIOD PEPTIDES**  Any of the opiod like endogenous opiates that are composed of many amino acids (peptides) that are secreted by the pituitary gland and that act on the central and peripheral nervous systems.

**PAIN**  A symptom of unpleasant sensation caused by obstruction of Qi or Blood flow in OM.

**PAINFUL OBSTRUCTION SYNDROMES (BI)**  Used to describe the majority of muscular and bony disorders. Characteristically these Bi syndromes are manifested as pain, soreness, numbness, and impaired movement.

**PARESTHESIA**  "Pins and needles" caused hy nerve disorders.

**PATTERN**  Syndrome.

**PATTERNS OF CORRESPONDENCES**  Defined relationships and effects between natural forces.

**PATTERNS OF DISCRIMINATION**  Differential diagnosis or the principal OM symptoms and signs, known as the pattern discriminations.

**PHAGOCYTE**  A cell that is able to surround, engulf and digest microorganisms and cellular debris.

**PHASES**  Phase, the elemental quality of; channel; Organ; points.

**PHASIC MUSCLES**  White muscles which consist predominantly of fast twitch (type II) fibers, are used for short periods when extra strength or quick response is needed.

**PHOSPHOLIPASE A2 (PLA2)**  PLA2 is an enzyme that controls the liberation of arachidonic acid (important in the inflammatory cascade) from membranes. PLA2 in circulation is inflammatory itself.

**PLATELETS**  The smallest cells in the blood. They are essential for the coagulation of blood.

POINTS
- Access Points; activate the Divergent channels.
- Accumulating (Cleft/Xi) points; are areas in the channels where channel Qi and Blood concentrate and accumulate.
- Activating points; activate the channels.
- Alarm(Mu) point; connect directly to the Organs and to reflect Organic health.
- Ankle points; part of the ankle/wrist acupuncture system.
- Ashi points; touch sensitive points that are outside the channels and giving rise to symptoms.
- Back Shu (Transport) points; located on the Urinary Bladder channel through which the Qi of the Organs circulates.
- Coupled points; points coupled with Master point for Extra channels.
- Entry Point; where the channel Qi enters the Main channel.
- Exit point; where Qi exits the Main channel.
- Five Phases(Transporting) points; region of the channel with a characteristic quantity and quality of Qi.
- Group Connecting points; four points on the extremities where several channels intersect.
- Influential (Meeting) points; empirical points effective for treatment of the tissue/ energy they influence.
- Return Point; return of Divergent channel.
- Master points; activate Extra channels.
- Master auricular points; A group of ear points that influence general function.
- Source points; the place in which the Original Qi resides within the channel. Termination points; termination of Sinew channels.
- Windows of the Sky points; group of points located around the neck and have the character for heaven (tian) in their name.
- Wrist points; part of the wrist and ankle acupuncture system.

POINTS, MUSCLE MOTOR    Points that are densely packed with sensory end-organs, causing muscle to be easily excitable and most liable to tenderness.

POSAIN    The experience of increased pain when any position is held for a long period, such as sitting, standing in one position due to ligamentous disorder.

POSTURAL MUSCLES    Also called tonic, or *red* muscles have a significantly larger number of type I fibers than phasic muscles have. Type I fibers are more vascular and resistant to fatigue than type II fibers.

PROSTAGLANDINS    Eicosanoids formed by fatty acids which are part of the arachidonic acid inflammatory cascade.

Qı                         Vital energy; the life force within all living matter. In Medicine: the dynamic
                           function of the body.

                           • Ancestral Chest Qi; formulated from the interaction of food Qi and air, the force
                             and strength of respiration that circulates Qi and Blood by regulating the heart
                             function, the force that nourishes the Heart and Lungs, limb circulation and
                             movement depends largely on Ancestral Qi.
                           • De Qi (energy experienced as needle sensation).
                           • Defensive Qi; flows outside of vessels, coarse and slippery in nature, enters the
                             channels; however, enters the organs at night, warms and moistens the
                             muscles and skin, controls the skin pores, regulating sweat, main function:
                             defense against exogenous, pathological Qi.
                           • Nourishing Qi; moves with the Blood, helps the Blood in nourishing functions.
                           • Organ Qi; physiological activity of the organs.
                           • Original Qi; inherited vitality and constitution; closely related to essence,
                             precursor to all other Qi, not renewable, resides in the Kidney, as well as
                             nourishes Kidneys.
                           • True Qi; formed by Ancestral and Original Qi assumes two forms; Defensive
                             and Nourishing Qi.

RETICULAR SYSTEM           A diffusely-organized neural apparatus that extends through the central region of
                           the brainstem into the subthalamus and the intralaminar nuclei of the thalamus.

ROM                        Range of Motion.
                           Range of Movement.

SELECTIVE TENSION          A process by which the practitioner isolates and tests tissues for pathology.

SCLEROTOME                 Sensation arising from connective tissues and bone innervated by a spinal root.

SCRAPING (GUA SHA)         Vigorous scraping of the skin, a useful OM technique for reducing pain and
                           loosening tight muscles.

SIMS POSITION              An osteopathic way of positioning a patient.

SOMATIC DYSFUNCTION        An osteopathic term that describes impaired or altered function of related
                           components of the somatic system (skeletal, arthodial, and myofascial structures)
                           and related lymphatic, vascular and neural elements. Somatic dysfunction in the
                           past has been called "osteopathic lesion".

SUBLUXATION                A non-physiologic dysfunctions, movement greater than normal joint motions.

SUBSTANCE P                One of the first polypeptides to be discovered is a neurotransmitter messenger
                           formed by 11 amino acids found in the hypothalamus, substantia nigra, and dorsal
                           roots of the spinal nerves. It acts to stimulate vasodilation and contraction of
                           intestinal and other smooth muscles. Substance P also serves as a transmitter for
                           signals carried by alpha and delta nerve axons traveling to and from the periphery,
                           into the dorsal horn of the spinal cord.

SYMPATHETICALLY            Also known as reflex sympathetic dystrophy, or complex regional pain syndrome.
MAINTAINED PAIN

SYNAPSES                   Functional connections between nerve cells.

SYNAPTIC TRANSMISSION      Communication across the thin synaptic space between the two neurons via the
                           release of neurotransmitters.

SYNDROME                   Pattern of symptoms and signs.

| | |
|---|---|
| **Synovium** | Colorless, viscous fluid that lubricates and nourishes the joint, including the avascular articular cartilage. |
| **TCM** | Traditional Chinese Medicine (modern times). |
| **Tenosynovitis** | Inflamed tendon sheath. |
| **Tensegrity structures** | Trusses formed by icosahedron; tension-integrity. |
| **Thalamus** | A pair of oval shaped organs forming most of the lateral walls of the third ventricle of the brain and part of the diencephalon. |
| **Tonic muscles** | See postural muscles. |
| **Trigger points** | A biomedical ashi point, a small locus in the muscle that is strikingly different from its surroundings and is sensitive to mechanical stimulation. |
| **Universal pattern** | A common adaptation to gravity and dysfunction. |
| **Vessels** | Channels.<br>Blood vessels.<br>Lymph channels. |
| **Visual analog scale (VAS)** | A common method of pain measurement. |
| **Wasting syndrome (Wei atrophy)** | Syndromes characterized by decreased muscular mass and strength, are seen in diseases such as multiple sclerosis. |
| **West haven-yale multidimensional al pain inventory** | A multidimensional pain inventory intended to supplement behavioral and psychophysiological observations developed specifically for evaluation of chronic pain patients. |
| **Wrist and ankle acupuncture** | A modern technique developed by a Chinese physician. |

# Index

# A note about the author

Alon Marcus received his licensed acupuncturist degree from the American College of Traditional Chinese Medicine in San Francisco, California in 1984, and his Doctor of Oriental Medicine degree from SAMRA University of Oriental Medicine in Los Angeles, California in 1986. He also trained in Japan and China, where he served his internship at the Traditional Chinese Medicine Municipal Hospital in Guangzhou. He studied Orthopaedic and Osteopathic medicines with several physicians through the American Association of Orthopaedic Medicine. Dr. Marcus has published numerous articles in both Eastern and Western medical journals and the book *Acute Abdominal Syndromes Their Diagnosis & Treatment According to Combined Chinese-Western Medicine* (Blue Poppy press 1991). In 1995 he became a diplomate of the American Academy of Pain Management. He has lectured internationally and taught courses in complementary orthopedics for several years. In 1997 he was named Educator of the Year by the American Association of Oriental Medicine. Dr. Marcus is currently in private practice in Oakland, California.